Dr Ante Bilić
liječnik - stomatolog

Ante Bilić
08. 12. 80

Textbook of Practical Oral Surgery

Trifles make perfection and perfection is no trifle.

MICHELANGELO

Textbook
of
Practical
Oral
Surgery

SECOND EDITION

Edited by DANIEL E. WAITE, D.D.S., M.S.

Professor and Chairman, Division of Oral and Maxillofacial Surgery, School of Dentistry, University of Minnesota, Minneapolis, Minnesota

LEA & FEBIGER • 1978 • PHILADELPHIA

Library of Congress Cataloging in Publication Data

Waite, Daniel E.
    Textbook of practical oral surgery.

    Bibliography: p.
    Includes index.
    1. Mouth—Surgery. I. Title. [DNLM: 1. Surgery,
Oral. WU600 T355]
RK529.W34 1978   617'.522   77-23401
ISBN 0-8121-0615-6

Published in Great Britain by Henry Kimpton Publishers, London

PRINTED IN THE UNITED STATES OF AMERICA

Print Number 3 2 1

No one saves us but ourselves

No one can and No one may

We ourselves must Walk the Path

Teachers merely Show the way.

NANCY W. ROSS

Preface

This second edition of *Textbook of Practical Oral Surgery* is again directed primarily to dental students. I hope it will adequately serve them as a text through their training years and forever be a reference as they progress to the practice of dentistry. The basic concepts in the text remain the same as those in the first edition. However, with the much appreciated counsel from oral surgeons, students using the text, and our own staff at the University of Minnesota, I have made some changes, which will be easily noted. The new chapters by outstanding authors add greatly to the text by the material covered and their authorship. A reorganization of the chapters has been done to reflect more accurately the usual sequence of the development of the thought and practice in the management of oral surgery problems.

The student is introduced to the broad field of surgery, and some of the basic information a surgeon must possess is discussed. The importance of taking an adequate history, interviewing the patient, conducting an oral examination, and using laboratory aids in diagnosing a condition is stressed. Operating room procedures and aseptic technique, with which the dentist must be familiar if he is to use hospital facilities, are described in detail, and instruments for oral surgery are described and amply illustrated.

In order to adequately discharge his duties, the dentist must have a full knowledge of the processes of inflammation, repair, and infection, and how to provide supportive therapy for the patient both before and after surgery. He must understand the phenomenon of pain and the administration of anesthesia. He must also be prepared to cope with hemorrhage and shock, and be capable of performing an emergency tracheostomy. All these topics so vital to competent patient care are discussed at length, as are the many various disorders and problems that will confront the dentist routinely.

A stronger emphasis in the care of the hospitalized dental patient has been offered in order to prepare the student for his experience in the community hospital. Details relative to the admission and management of hospitalized patients are part of the chapter on Hospital Dental Practice and Operating Room Protocol. In a new chapter, Office Emergencies, the reader will find practical consideration to assess in the management of emergent problems in the dental office.

In the first edition the attempt was purposely made to use one column of the page for text and the other for related illustrations. The additional space also was intended for the student to make notes alongside the discussion as he attended the lectures, since it is my belief that the lectures should supplement reading assignments and largely arise out of clinical experience. In actual fact, students do not customarily bring their texts to lectures so this particular space has not been valuable for that purpose. Therefore, in this edition we have supplemented the chapters with additional illustrations which should prove helpful and supportive throughout the text.

Minneapolis, Minnesota   DANIEL E. WAITE

Acknowledgments

A book such as this is always the accumulated effort of many more persons than can be identified. One could never determine and compliment or thank all persons who have contributed to one's knowledge and experience at a given time in one's life. Those persons who have contributed to my personal and professional life are too numerous to mention. There is no question that an effort such as this textbook represents the skills of many persons including secretaries, residents, and colleagues, and to these I do give special commendation and sincere thanks.

Specifically, in the compilation of the second edition, I need give credit to the same important persons that currently appear in the acknowledgements of the first edition. In addition, Dr. Hak Joo Kwon has helped materially in proofreading, coordination, organization of chapters, and illustrations, and has offered me great assistance in this edition. The illustrations and photographs continue to be done by the Division of Photography and Illustration under the able direction of Mr. LeRoy Christensen. Some of the new line drawings in this edition are the artwork of Mr. John Molstad and Mrs. Joan Dacko. Dr. Mark Omlie has been of valuable assistance in his review of the writings and for his suggestions and, of course, for his own chapter. Mrs. Gloria Carlson continues to be the principal secretary involved in all communications and the final typing, with the assistance of her associates, Judy Cummings, Barbara Olson, and Shari Helmers. Finally, of course, were it not for the expertise of Lea & Febiger and the continual encouragement by staff, especially Martin C. Dallago, Executive Editor, the work could not have been completed. And, as in the first edition, the contributing authors and especially those who are new to this edition lend great support, knowledge, and credibility. My thanks to all of them.

D.E.W.

Contributors

MERLE L. HALE, D.D.S., M.S., F.A.C.D.

Professor of Oral Surgery, Chairman, Department of Dentistry, University Hospitals and Clinics, University of Iowa, Iowa City, Iowa

NORMAN O. HOLTE, D.D.S., M.S.

Professor, Division of Oral and Maxillofacial Surgery, School of Dentistry, and Department of Pharmacology, School of Medicine, University of Minnesota, Minneapolis, Minnesota

MARK T. JASPERS, D.D.S., M.S.

Assistant Professor, Division of Oral and Maxillofacial Surgery, School of Dentistry, University of Minnesota, Minneapolis, Minnesota

MYER S. LEONARD, B.D.S., M.R.C.S., L.R.C.P., F.D.S., R.C.S.

Associate Professor, Division of Oral and Maxillofacial Surgery, School of Dentistry, University of Minnesota, Minneapolis, Minnesota

DONALD R. MEHLISCH, D.D.S., M.D.

Oral and Maxillofacial Surgery Austin, Texas

RICHARD G. OGLE, D.D.S., M.D.

Private Practice, Oral and Maxillofacial Surgery, Lakeville, Minnesota

MARK R. OMLIE, D.D.S., M.D.

Division of Oral and Maxillofacial Surgery, School of Dentistry, University of Minnesota, Minneapolis, Minnesota

CEDRIC A. QUICK, M.D., F.R.C.S. ED., F.A.C.S.

Associate Professor, Department of Otolaryngology, School of Medicine, University Hospitals, Minneapolis, Minnesota

EMIL W. STEINHAUSER, D.D.S., M.D.

Department of Oral and Maxillofacial Surgery, University of Nuremberg-Erlangen, West Germany

DANIEL E. WAITE, D.D.S., M.S., F.A.C.S.

Professor and Chairman, Division of Oral and Maxillofacial Surgery, School of Dentistry, University of Minnesota, Minneapolis, Minnesota

VERNE C. WAITE, M.D., F.A.C.S.

Honolulu, Hawaii

Contents

Textbook of Practical Oral Surgery

1 Scope and Objectives

DANIEL E. WAITE

The term "oral surgery" refers to a specialty of practice within the broad confines of dentistry that deals with the diagnosis and the surgical and adjunctive treatment of the diseases, injuries, and defects of the human jaws and associated structures. Thus, its scope may range from the extraction of a tooth to the surgical repair of injuries involving the face and jaws. Since the use of the hospital is often required for treatment and care of his patient, the oral surgeon must be a member of a hospital staff. Most major hospitals have a dental department which includes an oral surgery service.

Although, in actual practice, the scope of oral surgery will vary with the skills and training of the individual practitioner and his continued experience in the locale of his practice, the need for a broad educational background and experience is obvious. Courses in oral diagnosis, oral pathology, oral medicine, radiology, anesthesiology, and pharmacology should be well planned and integrated. A good course in internal medicine that includes clinical experience on hospital wards and the review of case histories will do much to broaden the student's foundation in surgery. The oral surgery course should direct the student toward a precise understanding of the problems that would be encountered by the general practitioner of dentistry as well as provide instruction and practice in those procedures that would be handled routinely. It is impossible for all undergraduate students to receive exactly the same experience—undoubtedly, some surgical procedures will never be done by the student during these formative years. This does not imply that the student should never perform them. Hopefully, the student will consider these years as foundation years, preparing him with basic principles of surgery relating to anatomy, physiology, and pathology. As he adheres to these basic principles and accumulates experience, his confidence should increase along with his grasp of the variety and complexity of oral surgery procedures.

General Objectives

General objectives in the instruction of the student include the following:

1. To provide a foundation of professional knowledge associated with surgical skills to enable the student to diagnose and treat competently the various disorders related to his practice.
2. To stimulate the student to recall basic science information and to correlate it

3

with the disease processes occurring in and about the oral cavity, particularly those lending themselves to surgical care.

3. To teach the student to examine his case findings critically and intelligently and to diagnose with competence.

4. To guide the student in developing a sense of confidence in his own skills and clinical judgment and to encourage the desire for continued professional study and self-improvement.

5. To help the student become familiar with and evaluate critically the scientific publications in the field of oral surgery.

6. To train the student to select cases that lie within the limits of his surgical ability and to exclude or refer those that he is not fully competent to handle.

7. To provide the student with a basis for continuing graduate or postgraduate study or for a teaching career.[1,2]

Specific Objectives

Upon completion of his course in oral surgery, the student should be able to provide treatment for surgical patients accordingly:

1. To administer a local anesthetic effectively and safely.

2. To extract teeth in uncomplicated cases and recover root fragments effectively and efficiently.

3. To prepare the mouth for the reception of a prosthesis, which may entail bone and soft tissue surgery.

4. To care for infection of the oral cavity resulting from dental disease.

5. To perform root canal and apicoectomy procedures.

6. To recognize, treat, and prevent, whenever possible, syncope and shock that might result from surgery.

7. To treat and control hemorrhage from oral surgical procedures.

8. To perform a biopsy of suspected lesions or neoplasms and submit the properly prepared specimen to an oral pathologist.

9. To reduce and immobilize fractures of the teeth, alveolus, and uncomplicated fractures of the jaws.

10. To be familiar with the hospital operating room and capable of managing hospitalized dental patients.

11. To utilize sedatives, analgesics, and antibiotic medications, when necessary, with confidence.

12. To be aware of the relationship between oral and systemic disease pathophysiology, to request medical consultation when appropriate, and to refer for medical treatment when necessary.

13. To diagnose oral and facial deformities that may be amenable to oral surgical management.

The dentist assumes an ethical as well as a legal responsibility when he accepts a patient for oral surgery. He must be qualified to diagnose and operate on patients presenting with surgical conditions; otherwise, it is his professional responsibility to refer the patient where he can be treated adequately. The health and welfare of the patient must always be the prime concern of the dentist. Good ethics and good surgical judgment based on his own surgical training and experience should clearly indicate to the dentist his responsibility for each surgical problem.

Since every oral surgeon is also a dentist, his background will make him sensitive to his patients' needs from a dental standpoint, and his hospital, anesthesia, and surgical experience will make him more aware of medical needs and medical counsel. The general dentist should rely upon the oral surgeon for assistance and guidance whenever complications arise as a result of surgically related diagnosis and treatment. At the same time, the oral surgeon should be sympathetic, alert, and willing to aid the general dentist in such instances. Difficult impaction procedures, roots or foreign bodies lost in the maxillary sinus or tissue spaces, are obviously within the experience of the oral surgeon. Fractures of the facial bones, skin grafts to the oral cavity for complicated prosthodontic cases, bone grafts, and problems relating to the temporomandibular joint will also have been a part of his training. The complicated hospital management for the dental surgical treatment of patients may become the joint responsibility of the general dental practitioner, the oral surgeon, and the physician. For example, the salivary glands and their disease processes often come to the attention of the dentist first. A detailed history and examination, which may include sialography or other special evaluations, have to be done before a diagnosis can be made (Fig. 1-1). Only at that time can one decide upon the best course of management, which may include a referral.

The relationship of oral surgery to orthodontics is close. Jaw deformities and severe malocclusion may necessitate both surgical and orthodontic management. Prognathism, micrognathism, maxillary retrognathism, and unilateral condylar hyperplasia are only a few conditions that require the cooperation of these two specialties (Fig. 1-2). Moreover, the general dentist must be able to recognize these deformities, obtain the appropriate records and history, and refer patients ac-

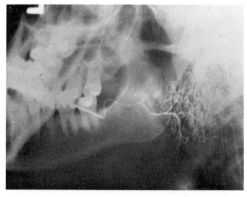

Fig. 1-1. Sialography. The use of a contrast medium placed within the salivary duct of the parotid gland. Normal filling of the duct and gland.

cordingly. Oral pathology is another dental specialty requiring close cooperation with oral surgery. The identification of tissue change through frozen section or conventional technique can only be done when adequate biopsy specimens and good case histories have been reviewed. Prosthodontics also requires close cooperation by the dentist in the surgical preparation of the denture base for a prosthesis. Alveolectomy, immediate denture surgery, frenectomy, tuberosity reduction, and alveoloplasty are a few situations in which this close cooperation must exist.

The relationship of oral surgery to the practice of medicine has become increasingly important. Even though preventive dentistry is making great advances, so is preventive medicine, and thus many patients outlive the life of their dentitions. Many surgical procedures will have to be carried out on patients receiving anticoagulant medication, antihypertensive drugs, tranquilizers, or immunosuppressive agents. Many patients are unaware of the significant relationship between a variety of medical conditions and even minor

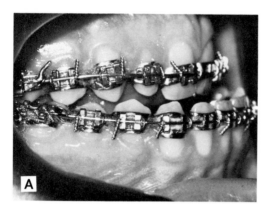

Fig. 1-2. Treatment of prognathism by the orthodontist and oral surgeon. (A) Before surgery. (B) After surgery and removal of orthodontic appliances.

surgical procedures (Figs. 1-3 and 1-4). This serves to emphasize the great need for the dentist to be knowledgeable about general medical problems. On occasion, patients will have to be hospitalized for medical reasons in order to perform otherwise routine office procedures. Laboratory procedures such as urinalysis, bacterial culture, and hematologic evaluation may have to be done on many surgical patients. This immediately draws the dentist into medical-dental discussion with physicians, nurses, and paramedical personnel. It may necessitate the writing of medication orders, pre- and postanesthetic care, and admission, progress, and discharge notes by the dentist when these patients are hospitalized. There is no substitute for experience and understanding when dental care is offered to the otherwise medically ill patient.

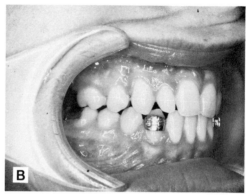

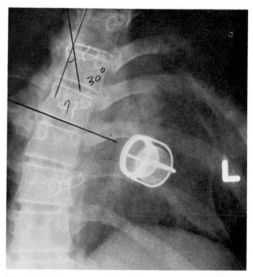

Fig. 1-3. Patient on dialysis machine for renal failure.

Fig. 1-4. Chest x-ray film of a patient with a prosthetic heart valve.

Finally, there is no substitute for the constant reading of up-to-date literature, discussion with dental and medical colleagues and, of course, just plain experience if the objectives of this text are to be realized. These pages are designed to be stimulating and to extend the invitation to learn more. An important concept is to do first things first. Thomas Henry Huxley has aptly said, "perhaps the most valuable result of all education is the ability to make yourself do the thing you have to do, when it ought to be done, whether you like it or not; it is the first lesson that ought to be learned; and however early a man's training begins, it is probably the last lesson that he learns thoroughly."

References

1. Reports of the Committees on the Teaching of Oral Surgery. University of Pittsburgh, 1952.
2. American Society of Oral Surgeons: Principles of undergraduate education in oral surgery. J. Dent. Educ., 30:403–428, 1966.

2 Principles of Surgery

VERNE C. WAITE

Scope and Philosophy

Perhaps the best way to approach the common denominator in all areas of surgical effort is to define the discipline called surgery. It is unfortunate that the term "surgery" is so often used synonymously with "operation," since illnesses cared for by the surgeon often do not require operation. Defining surgery, which encompasses the biologic sciences and art involved in the care of the sick, is difficult, but might be described as follows: *Surgery is a discipline which is devoted to the care of the sick and offers effective management for a large group of illnesses such as (1) congenital defects, (2) infections, (3) injuries, (4) neoplasms, (5) certain metabolic or functional derangements, (6) degenerative disease, and (7) organ replacement. Emphasis is placed on diagnosis, judicious selection of the patient for operation (if needed), preparation of the patient, timing of the procedure, tailoring of an operation to the person and his disease, and execution of the operative procedure with skill and expedience. But perhaps most important of all, the surgeon must provide attentive preoperative, immediate postoperative, and skillful long-term care with humanism, which includes all of the art, kindness, and compassion that the patient needs and deserves.*

The operative or transient technical phase, which takes place in the operative suite, though important, should be emphasized only occasionally, since it usually represents the lesser effort expended in the total care of these patients. This is perhaps fortuitous, since an operation constitutes *trauma*. A minor operation may be likened to a small injury, such as a localized laceration-contusion, whereas a major operation may be likened to a severe accident producing major musculoskeletal and internal injuries. Even though surgeons traumatize in the course of an operative procedure, such traumatization is justified in order to cure, palliate, or prevent disease. Obviously, the degree of injury must be minimal; therefore, the careful and gentle handling of tissues is a quality which the good surgeon must develop.

The Oral Surgeon

Surgery of the oral cavity and related structures, whether directly or indirectly related to dentition, has naturally become the province of the advanced trained dentist, and the oral surgeon has properly taken his place as a member of the head and neck team. Although in a relative sense a lot of dental surgery will be minor to the total body system, there are several

8

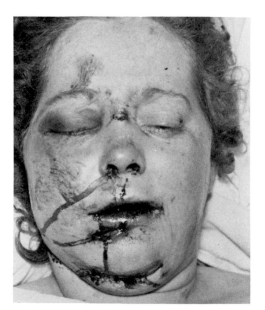

Fig. 2-1. Clinical photograph of patient with facial fractures and lacerations.

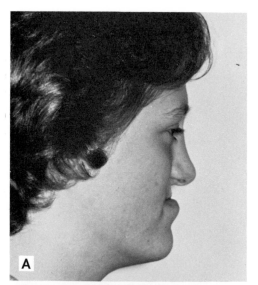

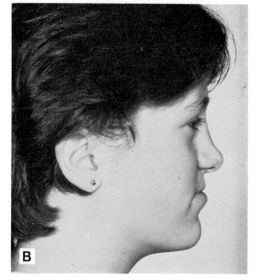

Fig. 2-2. (A) Maxillary hypoplasia and malocclusion. (B) Maxillary advancement by Le Fort I osteotomy.

major surgical procedures performed by the oral surgeon. In the treatment of trauma, deformity, tumors, and the like, however, the surgical principles involved in diagnosis, operation, and overall care of the patient until recovery are equally important in all surgery and require the same basic qualities common to all surgery; that is, a complete knowledge of the fundamentals of surgical care (Figs. 2-1, 2-2, and 2-3). But what are the basic requisite qualities of the good surgeon?

Basic Requirements of the Good Surgeon

Most modern surgeons, and particularly teachers, would agree that the qualities minimally required for the development of a good surgeon include the following:

1. *Personal insight.* "Know thyself and to thyself be true." The surgeon must be aware of his own limitations and able to work with others as a team, with complete professional honesty.
2. *Maturity of thinking,* which must be applied in making decisions, often

under stress, in caring for the patient in and out of the operating room. The good surgeon should be recognized for his "good surgical judgment." No two surgeons will achieve the same degree of

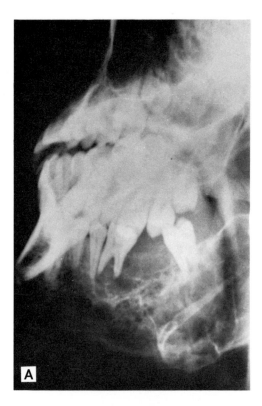

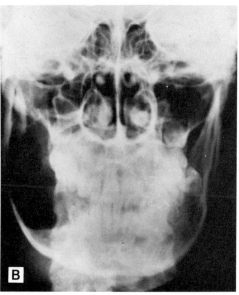

this quality—indeed, some may never achieve it at all. However, those who teach expect all their students to strive to reach their maximal potential.

3. *Profound respect and reverence for life,* sometimes expressed as "humanism." This is the possession of a warm human quality of being genuinely interested in one who is sick, not only in his disease but in him as a person, along with his family and immediate environment. Show the patient that you care.

4. *Respect for living tissue*—a profound, important quality. *Do no harm*—again, remember that the surgeon executes justifiable trauma during an operation, but he must be gentle in removing disease, handling tissue or correcting deformity, because the constitutional reaction of the patient postoperatively will be almost in direct proportion (Fig. 2-4).

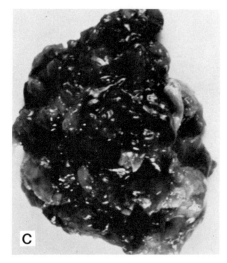

Fig. 2-3. Myxoma of the right mandible of 17-year-old girl. (A) Preoperative radiograph. Note splaying of teeth. (B) Postsurgical radiograph. Note continuity of inferior border. (C) Gross surgical specimen. There has been no recurrence in 15 years.

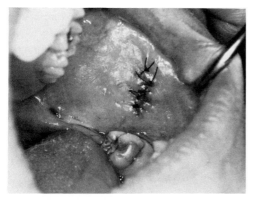

Fig. 2-4. Intraoral laceration of the buccal mucosa from a dental instrument, closed with interrupted black silk suture.

Therapeutic Factors Peculiar to Surgery

Wound Healing

Obviously, a complete knowledge of the physiology of wound healing is essential. Although the biochemical mechanism of healing is not completely understood, we know from research and clinical observation that optimal wound healing requires an optimal local and constitutional environment (Fig. 2-5).

In general, wound healing is categorized as (1) *primary*, which occurs when a clean

incised wound is promptly closed (Fig. 2-6); (2) *secondary*, which occurs when an open wound that is not bacteriologically clean is left open to permit granulation tissue to fill the defect, followed by the gradual peripheral growth of skin to cover

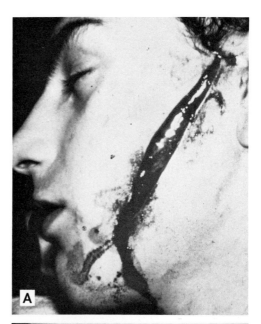

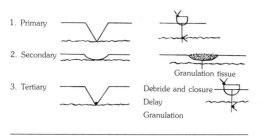

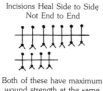

Fig. 2-5. Three modes of wound healing.

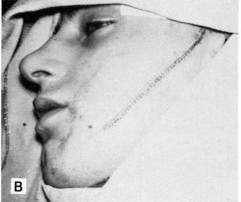

Fig. 2-6. (A) A superficial laceration of the left face with no severance of the facial nerve or parotid duct. (B) Primary closure of the facial laceration. (Courtesy of Dr. P. Morgan)

the defect (as in certain burns); and (3) *tertiary,* which is somewhat of a combined primary and secondary approach, and is used for war injuries and other highly contaminated wounds. In this approach, the wound is excised extensively to include all devitalized tissue and debris. A few days later, after the biochemical clean-up phase has been completed and the wound exhibits clean granulations, the skin and subcutaneous tissues can be closed.

Efficient wound healing depends upon the presence of normal circulating blood cells, clean healthy tissues, and humoral components that are associated with a series of biochemical events involving, at the least, protein, procollagen, mucopolysaccharides, sulfates, and ascorbic acid. Accordingly, total body health is important. Inadequate food intake, the presence of concurrent or debilitating disease (e.g., cancer, anemias, blood dyscrasias, prolonged infection) and endocrine and metabolic derangements may be present. *Local factors* involving tissues at the wound site may have equal importance. Foremost among these are local tissue immunity, blood supply, temperature (within limits), the presence of traumatized and devitalized tissue, and "dead space" with blood clots, foreign bodies, local edema, and the presence of microorganisms.

Technical factors affecting wound healing must be taken into consideration by the surgeon in performing the operation. These include placement of the incisions in a way that takes advantage of natural skin folds, reducing the tension and permitting ease in approximating the wound edges in areas where the blood supply is optimal (Fig. 2-7).

Suture and other supportive material

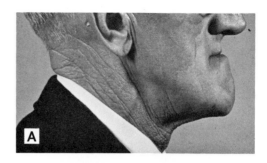

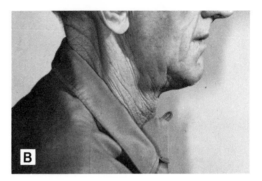

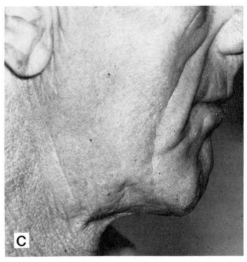

Fig. 2-7. (A) Prognathism. (B) Postoperative photograph. (C) A well-placed incision shows minimal scar along Langer's line of the face.

must be carefully selected and considerable care exercised in their use. Types of suture material that evoke the least local tissue rejection reaction are most desired, particularly if absorbable. Tissue reaction must be closely related to wound healing phases in order to exert maximal tensile strength until fibroplasia has produced secure tissue-holding power. In general, the finest local tissue reactive sutures should be used. It is most important regardless of the materials that sutures be accurately placed and approximate tissues only, they must not be tied tightly so that tissue pressure ischemia might be produced.

The preceding discussion briefly describes the general principles involved in the healing of all wounds; these principles also pertain to specialized tissues, such as bone, nerve, muscle, and tendons, although some variations occur in the healing process. Local tissue immunity exists where pathogenic bacterial flora are constantly present, as in the oral cavity and the inguinal and perianal areas. However, the surgeon does not rely upon such local immunity and does not forgo the basic principles of wound care when handling these areas.

Nutrition

The importance of oral intake of basic foods cannot be overemphasized. A complete knowledge on the part of the surgeon regarding the physiology of nutrition, nitrogen balance, fluid balance, and electrolyte content of tissues is of paramount importance. A firm understanding of organ function involved in food intake, absorption, assimilation, and distribution to the cell, as influenced by endocrine and enzyme systems, must be part of his working knowledge, since profound metabolic and endocrine disturbances may increase the operative risk, the incidence of complications, and affect the recovery of the surgical patient (Table 2-1).

Since many operative procedures immobilize the gastrointestinal tract or render the organ system incapable of receiving or assimilating a nutritious diet, in recent years the use of parenteral hyperalimentation has become a most helpful resort for the surgeon. This is accom-

Table 2-1. Recommended Daily Dietary Allowance (Normal activity and temperate climate)

	AGE (YR.)	CALORIES	PROTEIN (GM.)
Male			
70 kg., 175 cm.	18–35	2900	70
	35–55	2600	70
	55–75	2200	70
Female			
58 kg., 163 cm.	18–35	2100	58
	35–55	1900	58
	55–75	1600	58
		+ 200	+20
Pregnant		+1000	+40
Lactating		+1000	+40

plished by the insertion of a catheter within the venous system close to the junction of the caval systems in the patient's heart. Thus, high concentrates of glucose, amino acids, minerals, and other nutriments can be administered where the dilution factor quickly removes the danger of vessel damage. By this technique patients can receive adequate calories from glucose to prevent excess protein catabolism while receiving protein elements, and thus be kept in positive nitrogen balance. These techniques are particularly valuable in surgery of the head and neck, and thus to the oral surgeon.

The Bacteriology of Infections

The control and isolation of infections continue to require a major effort on the part of the surgeon. Burns, cellulitis, lymphangitis, bacteremia, suppuration, septicemia, and toxic shock are still problems in spite of the numerous "magic bullet" antibiotics now available.

Factors promoting favorable conditions in wounds for bacterial growth have already been mentioned. When infections occur in the upper digestive tract, the common contaminating organisms are streptococci, staphylococci, bacilli, and mycoses. In the lower intestinal tract, the agents most commonly encountered are *Escherichia coli, Pseudomonas,* and *Proteus.* Likewise, the skin and subcutaneous tissues that have low resistant fat and few regional lymphatics may be invaded by the entire spectrum of pathogenic bacteria. Here is the common site for the often lethal *Clostridium,* such as *tetani, welchii,* and *septicum,* and the mixed infections of microaerophilic streptococci of necrotizing fasciitis. In these instances, heroic incisional and excisional approaches in establishing drainage, along with hyperbaric compression, may be lifesaving (Fig. 2-8). Human bites deserve special mention due to the pathogenicity of human mouth organisms deposited in the subcutaneous tissues outside the oral cavity. Although local tissue immunity within the oral cavity is prominent, these organisms may spread to surrounding closed spaces, such as the retropharynx, sublingual, and fascial planes of the neck, to produce overwhelming infection.

The aforementioned types of infections and their recognition become of profound importance to the oral surgeon in particular, and to all surgical specialties in general. It should be unnecessary to point out the potentially lethal effects of these infections if therapy is inadequate. Cultures should be studied, and the most specific antibiotic agents selected. Moreover, a decision must be made regarding the most

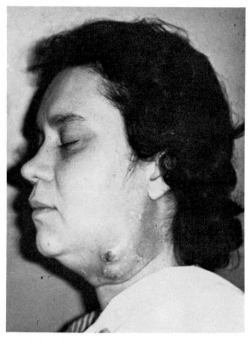

Fig. 2-8. Infection of the fascial space of the neck treated by incision, drainage, and removal of the offending teeth.

likely effective agent that can be used while the organism is being cultured for identification. All antibiotics must be given in therapeutic doses, but use of these drugs alone is rarely sufficient. The surgeon must also provide adequate drainage, nutrition, fluids and electrolytes, and immobilize the affected part. Such supportive management is regarded as basic, and has stood the test of time before and during the antibiotic era.

Body Fluids and Electrolytes

As our knowledge of body chemistry, physiology, and molecular biology has increased, no factor in homeostasis has become more important than that concerning body fluids and electrolytes. The physiology of water balance, urinary output, and compartmental shifting of fluids and electrolytes must be appreciated and controlled by the modern surgeon. Clinical observations combined with laboratory determinations permit the calculation of water or electrolyte imbalances, which must be fingertip knowledge if the surgeon is to create the best possible internal environment for the recovery of his patient. At the same time, he must evaluate concurrent metabolic, endocrine, cardiovascular, and excretory deficiencies. This can be a monumental task, but it is often considerably more important than the technical phase of operation.

BLOOD AND FLUID LOSS AND HYPOVOLEMIC SHOCK. Normal blood volume is essential to maintain normal tissue and organ perfusion, osmotic pressure, oxygen, carbon dioxide exchange, and cardiac output. Hypovolemic shock may occur following (1) acute blood loss from any site; (2) plasma, water, and electrolyte loss (e.g., in intestinal obstruction and burns); or (3) simple water and electrolyte depletion (Table 2-2). These three factors are usually present during a major operative procedure, and the surgeon should continuously be informed regarding such alterations and concurrently replace losses in kind and amount during the course of the operation. Blood replacement, with appropriate type and subfactor matching, is the most effective means of correcting hypovolemic de-

Table 2-2. Water Balance in 60 to 80 kg. Man

WATER GAIN ROUTES	AVERAGE DAILY VOLUME (ML.)
Sensible	
Oral fluids	800–1500
Solid foods	500–700
Insensible	
Water of oxidation	250
Water of solution	0
WATER LOSS ROUTES	
Sensible	
Urine	800–1500
Intestinal	0–250
Sweat	0

ficiency due to blood loss. Other substances, such as plasma and intravascular expanders (e.g., Dextran), and extracellular (interstitial) fluid replacement only partially meet the patient's needs when blood loss is acute.

The surgeon must be aware of fluid loss of any type, from any tissue source, into wounds, the gastrointestinal tract, or any expandable spaces. Derangements such as reduced cardiac output, inadequate pulmonary ventilation, reduced organ-tissue perfusion, capillary stagnation, or fluid loss to interstitial and intercellular compartments may precede, accompany, or in themselves produce a lethal series of events. Bacterial invasion, altered metabolism, acidosis, and electrochemical deterioration, followed by irreversibility of the process, may result in tissue and total body death. Therefore, the surgeon should know the following determinations for each patient while the patient is in a hydrated state: hematocrit, hemoglobin content, total blood volume, central venous pressure, efficiency of the cardiovascular and pulmonary systems, and the urinary output. Continued evaluation of these body functions is vital to patient recovery.

Until about 25 years ago, shock was considered more or less in terms of pure volume loss and replacement of kind and amount. We now know that there are many other factors producing shock, which may have several different predisposing causes, such as anemias, debilitating disease, toxicity due to bacterial endotoxins, adrenal cortical failure or medullary overactivity, and neurogenic factors.

This discussion is intended to emphasize a series of events that lead to tissue death, and several or all may occur concurrently. Therefore, it should be apparent that the doctor who manages surgical procedures must be knowledgeable in endocrinology, pathologic physiology, and biochemistry.

Patient Care Before Operation

All explanation of the reasons for operation, the nature of the procedure, the risks involved, anesthesia, and the expected results takes absolute priority in order to achieve the patient's confidence, and demonstrates complete professional honesty. It is important to establish sufficient rapport with the patient as a *person* in whom the surgeon is interested and cares about before discussing the need and nature of surgical treatment. The time required to establish this relationship is well spent and should precede any kind of patient management. A thorough, considerate explanation of the patient's problem—what the surgeon thinks should be done, how, and when—may be more important to both patient and surgeon than the technical phase. Certainly it will make the postoperative period easier for both.

Evaluation of the patient as a risk for "justifiable trauma" must accompany any decision for operative treatment. The nutritional and metabolic preparation of the patient is important in order to bring him to the operating area in the best possible biologic state. Occasions will arise in which, for the sake of expediency, a compromise must be made, requiring a determination of the "least of evils." These are times that "try a surgeon's soul" and require not only his reservoir of knowledge and experience, but sound surgical judgment, which often must be executed under duress.

Some specifics with which the surgeon must be concerned during the preoperative period are (1) tissue nutrition, state of hydration, and electrolyte balance; (2) blood volume and blood cellular content; (3) status of blood coagulation mechanisms; (4) cardiovascular status and reserve; (5) respiratory function; (6) kidney function; (7) association of concurrent disease (diabetes, tuberculosis, cancer, and other endocrine and metabolic deficiencies). All systems must be "go" or as close to such as is consistent with the risk involved. Again, the surgeon must ask himself: is an operation necessary? If so, is it emergent? urgent? or elective, and must defend not only his decision for operation, but also the type and the timing of the procedure.

Operative Care

The decision to operate should represent the most conservative approach to getting the patient well. *Operation is injury,* and to execute justifiable injury in order to cure disease constitutes the epitome of responsibility. An efficient, well-trained team of assistants, modern equipment, and expedient technical execution comprise the *sine qua non* for surgical success. The plan of operation may need to be altered in accord with the condition found—often unanticipated—or with changes in the patient's condition. Throughout the course of the operation, the operating team will be required to exercise keen and rapid judgment.

ANESTHESIA. All anesthetics are highly toxic agents, whether used for local infiltration, regional block (peripheral or subarachnoid), general inhalation, or intravenous administration. Regardless of the presence of a competent anesthetist or skillful anesthesiologist, the surgeon must have considerable general knowledge regarding the pharmacology of these potent drugs. This is of utmost importance to the oral surgeon, since most often anesthetic agents are administered by him or directly under his supervision (Fig. 2-9).

Patient Care Following Operation

It is so difficult, if not impossible, to single out one area of therapeutic surgical effort as being most important to the successful outcome of patient care. Nevertheless, most surgeons would agree that the understanding, compassionate installation of confidence, and genuine kindness so important in relations between the surgeon and his patient *before* surgical treatment are even *more* important during recovery. The "will to get well," if not manifested by the patient, must be instilled. Complete professional honesty with the patient and his kin is indispensable. Sympathy, understanding, gentleness, and reassurance will require time, but somehow must be made available in a manner that does not make the patient feel the surgeon is too busy to give him personal interest and attention. Patients usually need a personalized "hand-holding" chat, which should take place at the bedside, in the office, or at the chair. Points to be discussed include an explanation of things to expect, such as pain, change of dressings, drainage, ambulation, and elimination (Fig. 2-10).

Although personal management of the patient during recovery is important, such effort is not to be expended at the risk of

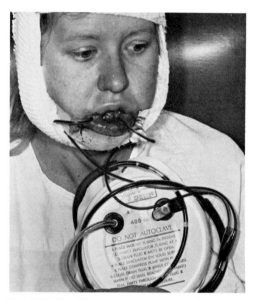

Fig. 2-10. The Hemovac is used to provide drainage during the first 24 hours after a bilateral sagittal split operation on the rami of the mandible for the treatment of prognathism.

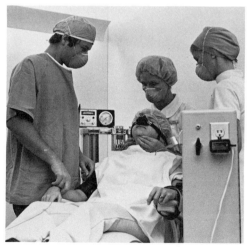

Fig. 2-9. Administration of general anesthesia to outpatients is an important part of the graduate training program in oral surgery and provides an excellent service to patients.

neglecting details of technical and clinical observation. The surgeon must anticipate possible complications and signs of retarded recovery *before* they "surprisingly" occur. Although regional operative approaches have special problems, many are common to all types of surgery, such as postoperative hemorrhage, atelectasis, delayed wound healing, ileus, infection, nutritional problems, depression, agitation, drug sensitivities, allergies, concurrent illnesses, heart failure, and pneumonia. The kind, compassionate surgeon-of-concern applying his professional and technical training is more often compensated by observing rapid patient recovery and rehabilitation. Relatively speaking, the joy in the practice of surgery comes from seeing a patient get well rapidly; thus, practice becomes a series of heartwarming and rewarding experiences.

3 History and Examination

DANIEL E. WAITE

Three important considerations in evaluating a patient are (1) taking the history; (2) conducting the examination; and (3) ordering a laboratory review, if indicated. Approaching each patient in this manner should become a habit if the doctor wishes to avoid mistakes and even tragedy.

The History

History-taking is an orderly, chronologic development of the patient's background to provide information that will permit the clinician to know more about his patient. Too frequently, this phase of dental practice is neglected. The careful, attentive listener will detect important diagnostic clues in the patient's narrative. Obviously, one cannot diagnose a condition unless he first knows of its existence, as Osler pointed out, so that an adequate history is not sufficient in itself. A knowledge of diseases that occur in the oral cavity is imperative, as is the etiology and treatment.

In general, history-taking and examination will involve three typical situations:

1. The patient who has been coming to the office for repeated treatment over the years. It is assumed that this patient originally had an excellent historical review, and all that is necessary now is

gaining additional information of pertinence since the last visit.
2. The patient who comes into the office for the first time for oral surgical procedures will need a careful examination and a review of the past medical history.
3. The patient who presents for dental care in the hospital will need the same careful workup by the dentist, to be documented in the patient's chart, in addition to a general physical examination by the physician.

The doctor must motivate the patient to communicate. It is his responsibility and opportunity to create an atmosphere in which the patient can focus on his problem with ease and without fear (Fig. 3-1). The doctor must make the patient comfortable with appropriate irrelevance and yet be professional. Rapport can be established by the usual "break the ice" questions, but the interview should be controlled by soon directing the patient to the problem at hand by effective questioning. The first few questions should be neutral in nature, becoming more direct. Neutral questions establish a topic ("What brings you to visit us today?"), whereas direct interrogation elicits either an affirmative or a negative response ("does heat aggravate the pain?"). The significance of the answers must be

18

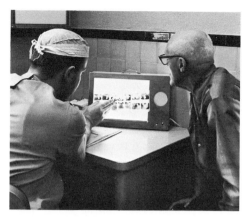

Fig. 3-1. Interview with patient in the office rather than in the dental chair provides a relaxed doctor-patient relationship.

evaluated accordingly and pursued dependent on their merit. On occasion the patient may have to be interrupted and brought back to the pertinent subject if he strays too far. If the doctor keeps the vo-

cabulary on the patient's level of understanding, coherent responses will be encouraged and the patient will feel that his background and experience are understood.

Valuable information regarding the patient's confidence toward the doctor, his temperament, outlook on life, and his problem can be gleaned from the interview if one will note the quality of the patient's handshake, his gait and coordination, the presence of tremors or roving eyes, and the general attitude of the responses (Fig. 3-2). For example, a patient with a weak handshake, a slow, shuffling gait, roving eyes, and a negative attitude might be quite

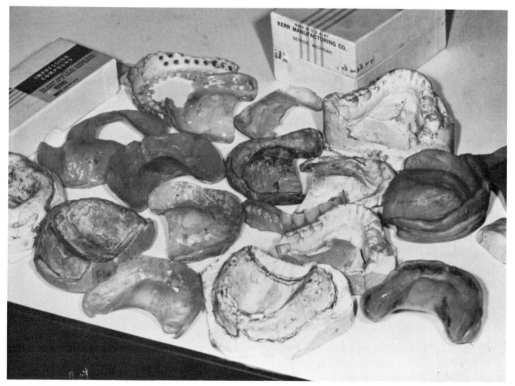

Fig. 3-2. These models, trays, and dentures were brought to the doctor's office by the patient, demonstrating involvement of the patient to such an extent that good doctor-patient relationships are questionable.

pessimistic about the prognosis of his problem and the doctor's ability to improve it.

Historical information should be taken down in the form of rough notes and then transferred to a more permanent record. The following outline is commonly employed to ensure an orderly and complete review of the patient's problem:

C.C.   Chief Complaint
H.P.I.   History of Present Illness
R.O.S.   Review of Systems
P.M.H.   Past Medical History
F.H.   Family History
S.H.   Social History

The history begins with the chief complaint, which should be in the patient's own words and uncoached. This is considered the keynote of the history, and is a statement of the main symptoms.

The history of the present illness is a chronologic account of the chief complaint and its related symptoms. This is probably the most important part of the history and the doctor should direct his effort accordingly. The time and mode of onset of the symptoms, as well as their duration and severity, must be noted. The relation of these to other activities, such as exercise, meals, medicines, and emotions, should be established. Occasionally, precipitating factors may be discovered by the latter line of questioning. If the patient has been treated previously for his chief complaint, the name of his doctor, hospital, medicines taken, and the course of the treatment can be invaluable information and should be thoroughly elicited.

The review of systems is a thorough exploration of the patient's systemic history and is most necessary for hospital admissions. The outline is readily available in any standard text of physical diagnosis[1-3] (see Chapter 18).

The past medical history is the delineation of the patient's medical problems of importance to the dentist. Examples include rheumatic fever, diabetes mellitus, allergies, heart diseases and/or murmurs, current medications, bleeding problems, hepatitis, and the like.[5]

The family history is of importance in tracing many syndromes and oral manifestations of systemic disease which have a genetic component. One should become familiar with the pedigree system of family tracing.

The social history allows the clinician to better understand his patients' habits and life styles. For example, a history of long smoking (40 to 50 packs/year) can alert the clinician to possible decreased pulmonary function and caution in the use of nitrous oxide analgesia, or the recommendation of general anesthesia.

A prepared questionnaire has often been suggested as an aid to history-taking, and we have included a sample in the text (Fig. 3-3).

Some years ago a group of workers in related disciplines working at Cornell University produced the Cornell Index. This was a health questionnaire of 195 questions designed to elicit from the patient appropriate knowledge of himself. There were two forms, one for men and the other for women. Technical terms were avoided and, where necessary, an explanation was given. In developing the questionnaire, more than 1,000 subjects showed that the items accurately collected data.[7] The questions in Figure 3-3 were modeled along similar lines and have proved effective in eliciting a good degree of broad information.

DENTAL HISTORY

Name of Former Dentist_____ Address_____

a. Are you having dental pain . . . . Yes No
b. Does food pack between your teeth. . . . . Yes No
c. Do your gums bleed when you brush your teeth . . . . Yes No
d. Do you grind your teeth during the night. . . . . Yes No
e. Do you have any pain in or near your ears. . . . . Yes No
f. Have you ever had periodontal (pyorrhea) treatment. . . . . Yes No
g. Have you ever been instructed on proper home care of your teeth . . . . Yes No
h. Do you have any sores or lumps in your mouth . . . . Yes No
i. Do you want to keep your teeth. . . . . Yes No
j. Approximate date of your last dental appointment_____

GENERAL HEALTH HISTORY

Name of Physician_____ Address_____
Approximate date of last appointment_____

a. Do you *now* have a sore throat or a cold . . . . Yes No
b. Have you ever had excessive bleeding from wounds or extractions . . . . Yes No
c. Has a physician ever told you that you have heart trouble. . . . . Yes No
d. Are your ankles often swollen . . . . Yes No
e. Do you get short of breath easily . . . . Yes No
f. Do you faint easily. . . . . Yes No
g. Do you frequently get overtired . . . . Yes No
h. Do you suffer from stomach trouble . . . . Yes No
i. Has a physician ever told you that you had kidney or bladder trouble. . . . . Yes No
j. Do you have to get up every night to urinate (pass water). . . . . Yes No
k. Do you frequently have loose bowel movements . . . . Yes No
l. As a child, were you confined to bed for a long time . . . . Yes No
m. Have you gained or lost much weight recently . . . . Yes No
n. Are you taking any medicine at the present time . . . . Yes No
   What_____For_____
o. Are you sensitive to any medicine. . . . . Yes No
   What_____
p. Have you had:

Asthma	Yes	No	High blood pressure .	Yes	No
Rheumatic fever.	Yes	No	Anemia.	Yes	No
Scarlet fever	Yes	No	Diabetes	Yes	No
Pneumonia	Yes	No	Kidney trouble.	Yes	No
Tuberculosis	Yes	No	Allergies	Yes	No
Heart trouble	Yes	No	Nervousness.	Yes	No

q. Have you taken:

Cortisone	Yes	No	Steroids	Yes	No

r. Injuries or operations:
   Treatment_____
   Hospital_____
s. Previous irradiation of head or neck . . . . Yes No
t. WOMEN: Are you pregnant. . . . . Yes No

Fig. 3-3. Health questionnaire.

The questionnaire, if used, should be done with the attitude that it is a guide to additional history to be taken during the interview and specific questions that should be asked. For example, if the question of shortness of breath is answered affirmatively (Fig. 3-3, General Health History, question e), the examiner would then seek to determine whether this relates to asthma or other pulmonary disease, coronary heart disease, congestive heart failure, metabolic disorder, or even a nervous disorder. If question j in the same section, concerning frequent urination, is answered positively, additional questioning would be appropriate relative to pregnancy (female), prostate gland (male), nervous disorder, diabetes, hypertension, chronic nephritis, cystitis, or excessive fluid intake at night. Each of these carefully selected questions has the potential of uncovering a host of additional information. The questionnaire should not be looked upon as an end in itself, but rather as a springboard from which many more questions could be launched and additional information gained.

Even such a minor item as the patient's signature on the questionnaire can be significant. Shaky, irregular penmanship could be indicative of a nervous disorder or senility (Fig. 3-4). The patient's name might suggest national or racial derivation which could contribute information to a diagnosis peculiar to race (e.g., sickle cell anemia—black) or geography. His occupation may have common hazards (e.g., miners—silicosis; x-ray technicians—radiation). Age may support a diagnosis of rampant decay, menopause, senility, or alveolar bone atrophy. Considerable additional information could well be available from a more detailed discussion of the patient's personal history.

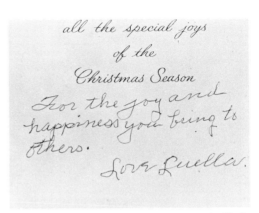

Fig. 3-4. Shaky handwriting of a normal elderly patient.

A prepared questionnaire, however, contains no magic and has some disadvantages. The most important is that the doctor might depend too heavily on the questions asked in the outline, which permit little deviation from a yes-or-no answer, thus decreasing the accuracy of the history. It is likely that such an outline more nearly applies to a hypothetical "average" patient. Certainly, the more complicated case or the vague historian will not give the pertinent data necessary for an accurate diagnosis. On the other hand, such a printed form has the advantage of giving patients time to think in the quiet of the waiting room as they ponder their past medical history. Under such circumstances, more accurate information can often be elicited than during pressured, rapid-fire direct questioning. If used properly, an outline can be a helpful, time-saving tool.

The Examination

The examination should proceed in the same orderly manner for every patient so that a good habit is established and nothing is overlooked. Inspection, palpation, percussion, and auscultation are performed when indicated, usually in that order. Bimanual and bilateral palpation should be used.

Careful utilization of the senses will

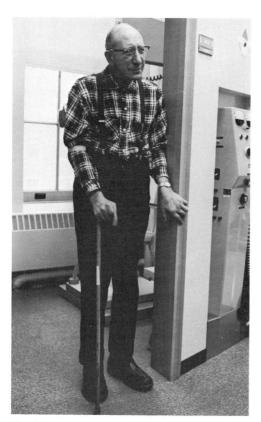

Fig. 3-5. First impressions of the patient may give valuable information relative to general health.

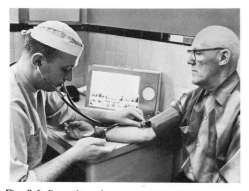

Fig. 3-6. Recording the preoperative blood pressure.

increase accuracy in the examination. Ashers excellent writing on sense emphasizes the need for a sense of perspective, a sense of reality, a sense of logic, plain sense, and even horse sense.[4]

When first viewing the patient, a general survey that includes posture, physique, nutrition, apparent age, severity and acuteness of illness, pallor, cyanosis, gait, voice and eye contact should be made (Fig. 3-5).

Vital signs should be established early to provide a baseline for the examination and subsequent treatment. These include temperature, pulse, respiratory rate, and blood pressure (Fig. 3-6) (see also Chap. 4).

A specific routine should also be followed for the oral examination. One can either begin examining from the anterior aspect and work posteriorly, or from the posterior aspect and work anteriorly; whichever, the same pattern should be followed for every patient. When examining any structure, keep in mind that you are looking for the "normal," rather than the "abnormal," so that when the latter is found it will be much more significant and easily noted.

The head and neck portion of the oral–facial examination should note facial growth patterns, symmetry or asymmetry, and include a general survey of the head, face, ears, eyes, nose, and neck. An important aspect is the examination of the lymph node system of the area. This is best done one side at a time; the submandibular nodes are palpated from in front of the patient and the cervical nodes from behind the patient.

The oral examination might well begin with the lips, taking note of symmetry, color (cyanosis or pigmentation), ulceration (Fig. 3-7), dryness, or the presence of keratosis. The evaluation of the parietes

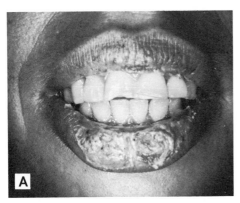 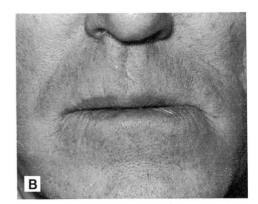

Fig. 3-7. (A) Severe, long-standing mucosal ulcerations of the lip in a 32-year-old woman. Diagnosed as cheilitis glandularis. (B) Normal lip contour.

and vestibular area includes a review of similar characteristics. The hard and soft palates should then be examined relative to clefts, tori, and deviation of the uvula (Fig. 3-8). The tongue should be reviewed in relation to all normal movements, color, papillae, and the lateral borders. Deep palpation should be done, including the posterior one third, and the floor of the mouth can be inspected (Fig. 3-9). The fauces and pharynx can be inspected with a mirror (Fig. 3-10).

The salivary glands, starting with one parotid and moving to the other, then to the submandibular glands, are bimanually palpated and evaluated relative to patency of ducts, quality and amount of saliva, and tenderness to palpation. A special examination for the salivary gland is provided in sialography. This is a technique of opacifying the duct system by injecting a radiopaque dye (Fig. 3-11). See Chapter 22 for details of this examination.

The gingivae are then carefully observed and palpated, and the pocket or crevicular depth is measured (Fig. 3-12). The teeth are the last part of the oral examination. The temporomandibular articulation is

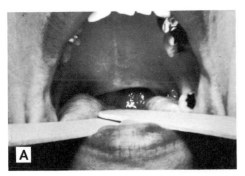 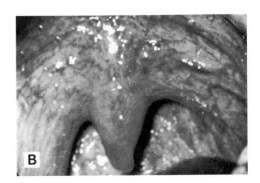

Fig. 3-8. (A) Absence of uvula. (B) Deviated uvula.

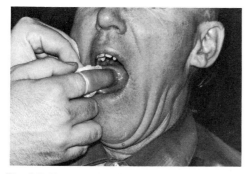

Fig. 3-9. Examination of the tongue.

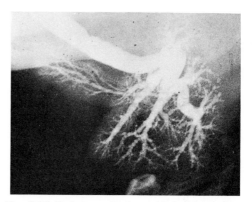

Fig. 3-11. Sialogram of submandibular gland showing dilation of ducts and stricture of the main duct.

examined when the history indicates that this structure is involved in the primary complaint. For details of this examination, see Chapter 23.

Any finding of the examination that indicates any degree of abnormality should be described in detail (e.g., size, duration, color, shape, and tenderness of a lesion). Following the oral examination, any indicated laboratory procedures are requested (see Chap. 4).

When all data have been assembled, the concluding part of the history and examination is then summarized and recorded on the Oral Surgery Examination Record (Fig. 3-13). First, the impressions of the doctor are listed; these are the possible diagnoses arranged in the order of their probability. Second, the recommendations are listed in the order that they are to be carried out. This may include additional

diagnostic studies as well as the exact treatment. Whenever possible, abbreviations should be used (see Chapter 18).

The Oral Surgery Examination Record is no different from any other record used to state clearly recommended treatments. There is no need to transfer the complete history from the history form to the examination sheet. Only facts and details relevant to the examination should be

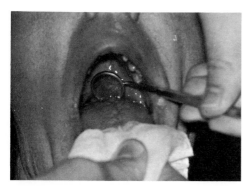

Fig. 3-10. Examination of the nasopharynx. Gauze is used to gently pull tongue forward.

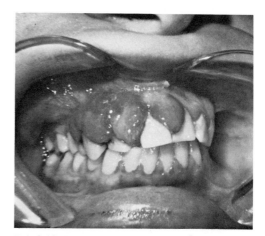

Fig. 3-12. Gingival hyperplasia in a patient who was receiving medication for the control of epilepsy.

ORAL SURGERY
EXAMINATION AND SURGERY RECORD

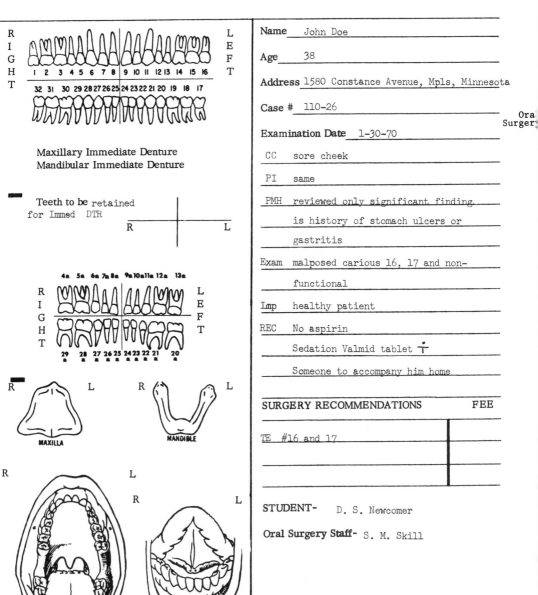

Maxillary Immediate Denture
Mandibular Immediate Denture

▬ Teeth to be retained
for Immed DTR

MAXILLA   MANDIBLE

Name   John Doe

Age   38

Address 1580 Constance Avenue, Mpls, Minnesota

Case # 110-26

Examination Date   1-30-70

CC   sore cheek

PI   same

PMH   reviewed only significant finding
      is history of stomach ulcers or
      gastritis

Exam malposed carious 16, 17 and non-
      functional

Imp   healthy patient

REC   No aspirin
      Sedation Valmid tablet $\dot{\top}$
      Someone to accompany him home

SURGERY RECOMMENDATIONS   FEE

TE #16 and 17

STUDENT- D. S. Newcomer

Oral Surgery Staff- S. M. Skill

Fig. 3-13. Surgical examination sheet.

included. If the history is complex, a note to the effect of "see additional history" might be helpful. Obviously, personal information for patient identification is required.

The assembly of the data gathered in the history and oral-facial examination is conveniently formulated using the SOAP format of the problem-oriented record.[6] In this system all historical data including past treatment are assembled under the "subjective," S, heading. The oral-facial examination and laboratory data are packaged under the "objective," O, category. Then the differential diagnosis is established under "assessment," A. Finally, under "plan," P, for procedures, either diagnostic or therapeutic measures are formulated to solve the problem.

Charting the mouth for both soft and hard tissues can be done on the appropriate dentulous or edentulous drawings. The hashmark ($/$) on a tooth indicates the tooth is to be extracted; it is placed at the time of the examination. The X is completed when the tooth has been removed. A horizontal line ⎯🦷⎯ through the tooth indicates that the tooth was missing at the time of the examination. Red ink can be used to mark in x-ray findings, such as cysts, roots, and granuloma. Soft tissue lesions can be drawn on the appropriate areas to indicate location and size, as can bony lesions on the edentulous jaw tracings. When immediate denture surgery has been planned, the teeth to be retained for the last surgical appointment are charted as

$$\underline{5\quad 6\quad 7\quad 8 \,\big|\, 9\quad 10\quad 11}\,.$$

The reverse side of the form is for the surgical write-up. This should be accomplished in a systematic manner, putting forth the facts relative to type and amount of anesthesia and the surgical procedure, noting specific teeth removed, the placement and number of sutures, and the purpose of the reappointment and its date. Any undue complications should be noted.

References

1. Brainerd, H., Krupp, M. A., Chatton, M. J., and Margen, S.: Current Diagnosis and Treatment. Los Altos, Calif., Lang Medical Publications, 1970.
2. DeGowin, E. L.: Bedside Diagnostic Examination. New York, Macmillan, 1976.
3. Morgan, W. L., and Engles, G. L.: The Clinical Approach to the Patient. Philadelphia, W. B. Saunders Co., 1969.
4. Jones, F. A., and Asher, R.: Talking Sense. Belmont, Calif., Pitman Publishing, 1973.
5. Freedman, G. L., and Hooley, J. R.: Medical contraindications to the extraction of teeth. Dent. Clin. North Am., 13:939–960, 1969.
6. Weed, L. L.: Medical Records, Medical Education and Patient Care: The Problem-oriented Record as a Basic Tool. Chicago, Year Book Medical Publishers, 1971.
7. Brodman, K., Erdman, A. J., Jr., Lorge, I., and Wolff, H. G.: The Cornell Medical Index: An adjunct to medical interview. J.A.M.A., 140:530–534, 1949.

4 Laboratory Aids

MARK R. OMLIE

This chapter deals with the various laboratory aids utilized by the clinician in establishing the diagnosis or in the presurgical preparation of the patient. It is beyond the scope of this text to provide a complete discussion of these tests; therefore, the objective will be to provide the student with an overview of some of the basic laboratory tests and their normal and abnormal values. The interested student is advised to consult the references for additional information.

The type of tests ordered will be determined by the historical data, physical examination, and the clinician's knowledge of physiology in normal and disease states. There will be differences in the type of tests ordered for an identical surgical procedure, one to be done in an office under local anesthesia and the other being performed in a hospital operating room (see Chap. 18). The types of laboratory tests that the clinician may find useful include:

1. Vital signs
2. Radiographs
3. Tissue examination
4. Bacteriologic culture and smears
5. Complete blood count
6. Coagulation studies
7. Urinalysis
8. Blood chemistry
9. Electrolytes
10. Electrocardiogram

Vital Signs

The recording of the patient's vital signs should be routine in all oral surgical procedures. Vital signs include the pulse, blood pressure, respiration, and temperature. All patients should have preoperative and postoperative blood pressure and pulse taken and recorded on their charts. The auscultation method of listening to the pressure is considered most accurate (refer to Fig. 3-6). The pulse is noted by its regularity or irregularity, rate, and strength. The student should be aware of the implication of the various blood pressure norms for different ages and sex.

Temperature is recorded routinely for hospital oral surgical patients, but is elective for outpatients except for those with suspected or proved infection. Remember that vital signs such as pulse rate and respiration can vary directly with temperature changes.

The respiratory rate can be elevated in the dental patient who is apprehensive and may manifest as the hyperventilation syndrome, with lightheadedness, perioral and extremity tingling, and occasionally chest pain, and can cause tetany and neuromuscular irritability.

Radiographs

The radiograph is employed in nearly every diagnostic evaluation and certainly in every surgical treatment of a patient. It is important for the clinician to understand the normal anatomy of extraoral, intraoral, and panoramic radiographs in order to properly diagnose and treat the wide spectrum of disease in the oral region. They include a panoramic film (Panorex) in diagnosis of a mandibular fracture (Fig. 4-1), a maxillary occlusal film demonstrating a maxillary cyst (Fig. 4-2), and a periapical film demonstrating a root fracture (Fig. 4-3). A chest radiograph is routine for all hospital admissions (Fig. 4-4). Surgical exodontia should always be preceded by a clear recent radi-

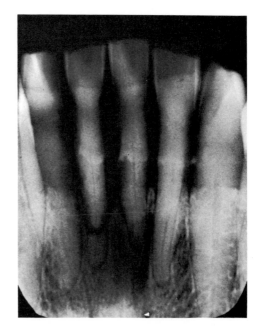

Fig. 4-3. Periapical film showing a fractured root, calculus, and alveolar bone resorption. (Courtesy of Dr. D. E. Waite)

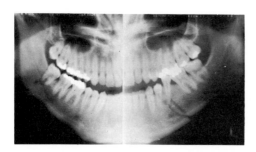

Fig. 4-1. Panoramic view of the jaws showing a fracture of the mandible bilaterally. A good screening film to show gross dental problems. (Courtesy of Dr. D. E. Waite)

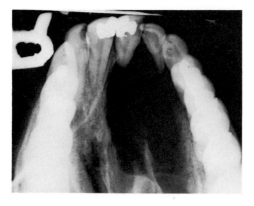

Fig. 4-2. Occlusal plane film demonstrating a globulomaxillary cyst. (Courtesy of Dr. D. E. Waite)

ographic survey with at least two views. The periapical radiograph is the most accurate and reveals the greatest detail of the dental and bony structures. One should not diagnose or attempt to treat on the basis of poor quality radiographs in which the area of interest is not centered on the film. Try not to focus on what initially seems to be the obvious pathologic lesion, but instead utilize a disciplined orderly assessment of the radiograph. When recording the radiographic findings in the record, be specific as to the lesion's size, location, radiolucency or opacity, relation to teeth, multilocularity or solitary, and ragged or well-defined outline.

The texts of Worth[4] and Stafne[5] are excellent sources for a review of normal

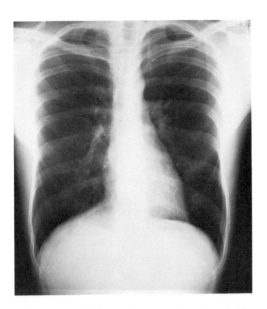

Fig. 4-4. Normal chest radiograph. Note lung fields, pulmonary vasculature, heart size, costophrenic angles, and bony structures.

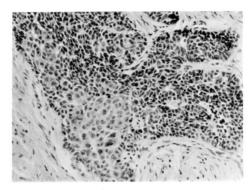

Fig. 4-5. Photomicrograph showing anaplastic cellular change. (Courtesy of R. Vickers)

radiographic anatomy[6] and examples of changes visible on x-ray films in various disease processes.

Tissue Examination

Tissue examination is frequently employed as an aid in establishing the final diagnosis in the wide spectrum of soft tissue and hard tissue pathologic lesions of the oral cavity.[2,3] Many times the differential diagnosis will include several entities which can be differentiated only on the basis of histologic examination. The ruling-out of malignancy will be one of the dentist's most important diagnostic responsibilities (Fig. 4-5). He must have a broad knowledge of oral pathology, know when to perform the surgical biopsy, and have good communication with the oral pathologist.

Bacteriologic Tests

Bacteriologic smears, cultures, and sensitivities are frequently used to aid in the diagnosis and treatment of infection. It is routine to culture specimens of all infections producing an exudate, abscess formations, or a fascial space involvement. Depending on the clinician's index of suspicion, he may order a smear to look for sulfur granules of *Actinomyces israelii*, a culture for coagulase-positive staphylococcus, or a culture and sensitivity test when a penicillin-resistant organism is suspected.

Principles for the collection of specimens for bacteriologic examination includes (1) do it before beginning antibiotic therapy; (2) if an anaerobic organism is suspected, utilize anaerobic culture containers; (3) rapid transmission to the laboratory; and (4) clear, concise explanation of the clinical situation on the laboratory slip, including suspected organisms. Blood cultures are often diagnostic in cases of bacteremia of septicemia. Specimens should be drawn from sites previously prepared in an aseptic manner.

Timing of collections is guided by the patients temperature spikes, because this is when the organisms will be present in the highest numbers (see Fig. 15-5).

Complete Blood Count

Complete blood count (CBC) includes the red cell indices, the white cell indices, and the platelet count.[7] This information is utilized preoperatively when attempting to assess systemic disease with oral manifestations, in cases of infection, or in assessing coagulopathies.

The red cell indices, of which hemoglobin determination is a part, give information regarding the oxygen-carrying capacity of the blood, the anemias, and impaired production.[7] Normal red cell values are given in Table 4-1. The white cell count is a valuable aid in evaluating the patient's defenses, infection, immunologic status, or blood dyscrasia.[7] Normal white cell values are given in Table 4-2. Platelets important in coagulation are

Table 4-1. Normal Values of Red Cell Series

	♂ MALE	♀ FEMALE
RBC count, MILLIONS/MM.[3]	4.5–5.5	4.2–5.2
Hemoglobin, MG%	14–17	12–16
Hematocrit, %	40–50	37–45
Mean corpuscular volume, μ^3	82–92	same
Mean corpuscular hemoglobin, $\mu\mu$g.	27–31	same
Reticulocyte count, %	0.5–1.5	

Table 4-2. Normal White Cell Indices

WBC count	5,000–10,000/MM.[3]
Differential count	(%)
Neutrophils	60–70
Lymphocytes	20–30
Monocytes	2–3
Eosinophils	1.6–3
Basophils	0.1–1

affected by a variety of diseases, physical agents, and drugs. Platelet defects may be qualitative (function), quantitative (number), or both.

The erythrocyte sedimentation rate (ESR) is a nonspecific reflection of a variety of diseases, such as infection, collagen diseases, rheumatic fever, rheumatoid arthritis, and some malignancies,[7] in which the ESR is increased. The test involves the settling of red blood cells in a glass tube over a given period of time.

Coagulation Studies

Coagulation studies may be useful in patients with a history of a bleeding problem.[7] The history is probably the most important tool in evaluating bleeding disorders. Hemorrhagic disorders are reviewed in Chapter 17. Tests commonly used include the prothrombin time (PT) for evaluation of the extrinsic coagulation system, the partial thromboplastin time (PTT) for the intrinsic system, the Ivy bleeding time for von Willebrand's disease and platelet function, and the tourniquet test for capillary fragility (Table 4-3).

Urinalysis

Urinalysis is routine for patients having surgery in the operating room under general anesthesia. This test can evaluate

Table 4-3. Coagulation Studies

Prothrombin time (PT), SEC.	11.0–12.5
Partial thromboplastin time (PTT), SEC. (varies with laboratory)	32–35
Bleeding time (IVY), MIN.	1–6

many aspects of renal disease and represents an important screening tool.[8,9] The first voided specimen is generally used for examination. The parameters of color, pH, specific gravity, protein, sugar, ketones, and blood breakdown products can be evaluated (Table 4-4). The microscopic examination of the urine detects red cells, white cells, casts, crystals, and bacteria.

Blood Chemistry

Blood chemistry evaluation includes a wide variety of enzymes, minerals, proteins, sugars, cations, anions, nitrogenous products, lipids, and blood breakdown products, to name a few.[8,9] The normal values and examples of disease entities in which they are elevated or decreased are shown in Table 4-5.

Serum glucose (fasting blood sugar) is normally 80 to 120 mg. per 100 ml. Glucose levels are increased in diabetes mellitus, acromegaly, adrenal tumors, anoxia, brain injuries, and hepatic dysfunction.

The levels are decreased in hypothyroidism. When the levels of the serum glucose are elevated, a glucose tolerance test and medical consultation may be indicated.

Normal serum calcium levels are 9 to 11.3 mg. per 100 ml. Elevations may occur when there is increased osteoclastic activity as in cases of hyperparathyroidism or hypervitaminosis D, or carcinoma metastatic to bone. Hypocalcemia is noted in renal failure and hypoparathyroidism. Tetany develops due to hypocalcemia.

Normal serum phosphorus levels range from 2.5 to 4.5 mg. per cent. The levels are increased in hypoparathyroidism and renal failure and decreased in hyperparathyroidism. Alkaline phosphatase is normally 4 to 17 King-Armstrong units. Increased levels are present in Paget's disease, rickets, and hyperparathyroidism.

Electrolytes

Electrolyte evaluation includes sodium, potassium, chloride, and bicarbonate.

Table 4-4. Normal Values of Urinalysis

	NORMAL	PATHOLOGIC	EXAMPLES
pH	4.5–8.0	Alkalosis ↑	Acidosis ↓
			Drugs ↓
Color	Straw	Red-hematuria	
RBC	0	Trauma	
		Glomerular damage	
WBC	<5 PER HPF	Infection	
Casts	Few	Tubular damage	
Bacteria	Sterile	Infection	
		Contamination	
Glucose	0	Diabetes	
Ketones	0	Ketosis	
Bilirubin	0	Liver disease	
Protein	2–8 MG./ML.	Nephrotic syndrome	

Table 4-5. Normal Blood Chemistry Profile

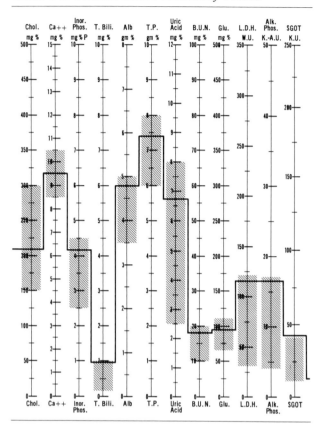

These values vary with the state of hydration, replacement and ongoing losses, endocrine problems, acid-base status, gastrointestinal losses, and water-salt balance.[8,9] Normal values with examples are given in Table 4-6.

Electrocardiogram

The electrocardiogram (EKG) measures the electrophysiologic forces of the heart during the phases of the cardiac cycle. It can assess rate, rhythm, old or new in-

Table 4-6. Normal Values and Examples of Major Electrolytes

ELECTROLYTES	NORMAL VALUES (mEq./L.)	↑	↓
Sodium	135–145	Dehydration	Aldosterone
Potassium	3.5–4.5	Renal disease	Diuretics aldosterone
Chloride	95–102	↑ ACTH	Ketosis diuretics
Bicarbonate	24–28	Alkalosis	Acidosis

farcts with their locations, the cardiac axis, ventricular hypertrophy, and patterns consistent with electrolytes or drugs.[10] An EKG would be ordered, for example, on a patient having surgery under general anesthesia or intravenous sedation in the operating room who is over 40 years of age or who has a history of cardiac disease.

Additional Tests

There are many other tests and procedures that are considered laboratory aids. The interested student is directed to the reference list. Procedures such as vital signs and radiographs are routine for nearly all patients. The others are ordered on the basis of the history, examination, differential diagnosis, and the clinician's understanding of the pathophysiology of not only oral-facial diseases but of systemic diseases.

The question of which tests are appropriate to order often arises. This can be partially answered by assessing whether the test in question will affect either the diagnosis, prognosis, or treatment. As alluded to before, some tests are ordered because they are part of standard admissions protocol for the hospital management of patients.

Test Results

When results are returned from the laboratory, what do the values mean? It must be noted that the range of normal values is determined from a curve including two standard deviations above and below the mean. This implies that normal includes 95 per cent of individuals tested and 5 per cent of normal individuals will fall outside of this normal range.

Any laboratory result must be scrutinized as to whether it is really abnormal, is it diagnostic, or is there another reason for the value.[11] Be sure to obtain a print-out of normal values for your laboratory because differences occur secondary to technique, controls, and/or procedures utilized.

The dentist and physician should be in close communication regarding many of these laboratory aids used in patient care. Much of the information gained will be used in discussion with the patient's physician. With the ever-expanding role of the dentist in the care of the patient's total health, it is critical that he or she have fundamental knowledge of disease pathophysiology. An integral part of this will be the ability to intelligently utilize laboratory aids.

References

1. Pickering, G.: Hypertension. London, Churchill-Livingstone, 1974.
2. Shafter, W. G., et al.: A Textbook of Oral Pathology, 3rd ed. Philadelphia, W. B. Saunders Co., 1974.
3. Gorlin, R. J. and Goldman, H. M.: Thoma's Oral Pathology, 6th ed. St. Louis, C. V. Mosby Co., 1970.
4. Worth, H. M.: Principles and Practice of Oral Radiologic Interpretation. Chicago, Year Book Medical, 1963.
5. Stafne, E. C.: Oral Roentgenographic Diagnosis, 4th ed. Philadelphia, W. B. Saunders Co., 1976.
6. Manson-Hing, L. R., et al.: Dental Radiology, 2nd ed. St. Louis, C. V. Mosby Co., 1969.
7. Wintrobe, M. M.: Clinical Hematology, 7th ed. Philadelphia, Lea & Febiger, 1974.
8. Bennington, J. L.: Laboratory Diagnosis. London, Macmillan, 1970.
9. Frankel, S.: Gradwohl's Clinical Laboratory Methods and Diagnosis. St. Louis, C. V. Mosby Co., 1970.
10. Dubin, D.: Rapid Interpretation of EKG's, 2nd ed. Tampa, Cover, 1973.
11. Zilva, J. F.: Clinical Chemistry in Diagnosis and Treatment. London, Lloyd-Luke, 1971.

5 The Armamentarium

DANIEL E. WAITE

The instruments for oral surgical procedures are varied and many. As a general rule, the fewer instruments needed to complete a task, the more efficient the operation becomes. Every time an instrument is picked up, the work for which it was intended should be completed. Wasted movements are an indication of disorganization and lack of self-confidence or knowledge of how to proceed. Before one can expect to use instruments correctly, he must have a fundamental knowledge of them and the indications for their use.

The Scalpel

For oral surgery, there are three blades in general use and two knife handles. The blades are Bard Parker nos. 11, 12, and 15, and the handles are nos. 7 and 3 (Fig. 5-1). The no. 11 blade is primarily used for incision and drainage when a puncture-type incision is preferred, and when blind cutting of deep tissue is necessary. The no. 12 blade is especially good for incision of the marginal gingivae and adapts well for following the cervical lines of the teeth (Fig. 5-2). The no. 15 blade is for general use and is used most frequently. It is excellent for most skin and mucosal incisions. Personal preference determines the choice of handles.

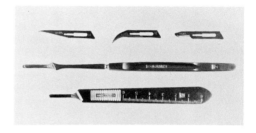

Fig. 5-1. Knife blades, nos. 11, 12, and 15; handles nos. 7 and 3.

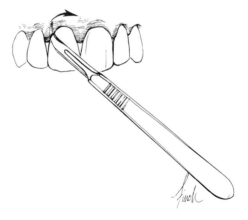

Fig. 5-2. Knife blade no. 12 being used to incise gingival attachment.

In using the scalpel, the pen grasp is utilized (Fig. 5-3). The fourth and fifth fingertips rest on a solid base. Tissue should be placed under tension while the curved portion of the blade is placed on

35

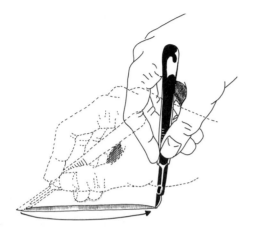

Fig. 5-3. No. 15 blade with no. 3 handle, showing pen grasp. (Clark, *Practical Oral Surgery*, Lea & Febiger, 1965)

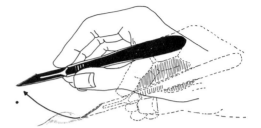

Fig. 5-4. Incising an abscess with no. 11 blade. (Clark, *Practical Oral Surgery*, Lea & Febiger, 1965)

the tissue surface. Firm pressure is then directed downward and the blade drawn with a steady stroke for the desired distance. Even pressure on the blade should be applied and when the stroke is completed, the handle is raised, finishing with the tip of the blade. When incising mucoperiosteum, the incision should be made direct to bone with one movement. Whenever possible, always make complete incisions. Stopping midway through an incision is unnecessary, even if bleeding is evident. Hemorrhage can be controlled as soon as the incision has been completed.

When incising an abscess, the no. 11 blade is most useful. Place the point of the blade at the dependent point of the swelling, usually near its lower edge, and direct it toward the center with the cutting edge up (Fig. 5-4). Again, one stroke is made, and the incision should extend well into the center of the abscess. If necessary, a curved hemostat can then be placed in the point of the incision to improve the drainage. Incision and drainage fre-

quently can be done without anesthesia because the pain is brief and may not be significant until after the incision has been made.

Periosteal Elevators

The no. 1 Woodson and the no. 9 periosteal elevators are excellent (Fig. 5-5). They are used primarily for the reflection of mucoperiosteum. The ease of flap reflection varies considerably. The mucoperiosteum of the anterior palate is attached tightly to bone and difficult to reflect throughout its entirety because of the heavy, thickened tissue and the roughness of the palatal bone. In contrast to this, the tissue overlying the palatal torus is extremely thin and tears easily. The mandibular lingual mucoperiosteum is also thin and must be raised with care, although it reflects rapidly and easily.

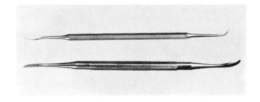

Fig. 5-5. No. 1 Woodson periosteal elevator (above) and no. 9 periosteal elevator (below).

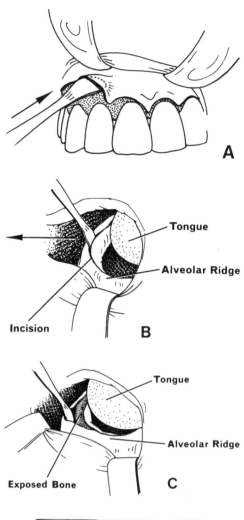

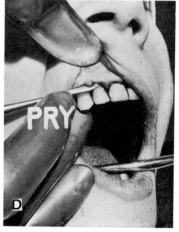

Fig. 5-6. Flap reflection with a periosteal elevator. (A) Push stroke. (B and C) Pull stroke. (D) Pry stroke.

When handling mucoperiosteal flaps, use the largest portion of the instrument that works well with its convexity toward the flap; less tearing and puncturing of the flap will occur. Three major strokes are used in the developing of a periosteal flap: the push stroke, the pry stroke, and the pull stroke. In each instance, the instrument is held at an approximate 45° angle to the surface. The convex portion of the elevator should be against the flap. Again, the pen grasp is best, with the fourth and fifth fingers resting on a solid base, usually the teeth. In initiating the pry stroke, the flap is developed first in the interdental papilla area with the small end of the instrument (Fig. 5-6). The point is inserted firmly under the papilla and the adjacent tooth is used as a fulcrum. It is wise not to reflect the mucoperiosteal flap beyond the area of tissue to be exposed, since a certain degree of bone resorption takes place whenever a flap is reflected. If the reflection of the flap extends too far into the sulcus, edema will accumulate in this area, thus retarding the healing process and shortening the overall depth of the mucobuccal fold.

The Retractor

A number of excellent retractors are available for oral surgical use. The University of Minnesota retractor and the Austin retractor are used most frequently. A ribbon retractor has several advantages, and is more commonly used for extraoral surgical procedures (Fig. 5-7). The tongue retractor is most serviceable when a gauze sponge is placed as a curtain in the pharynx and partially under the retractor.

The retractors are primarily used by the assistant, and should be used in the right

centrate on the surgical procedure so much that the retractor may gag the patient or otherwise be a hindrance to the operator. Remember that constant retraction of tissues minimizes the blood flow through them. Therefore, whenever possible and when retraction is not needed, one should relax the tissues to let the blood supply return. A heavy-handed assistant can greatly increase the trauma to the retracted tissues.

The Handpiece and Bur

The surgical bur is often used in the removal of bone and the sectioning of teeth. Carbide burs are much preferred over steel burs for cutting tooth structures and bone. The conventional handpiece and pulley system has the disadvantage of being dirty, slow, and inconvenient. When used in the hospital, nurses find this equipment difficult to set up and difficult to sterilize. Some of the newer, high-speed equipment do not have these disadvantages. Whenever possible, high-speed instrumentation is recommended. The burs most useful in general oral surgical procedures are the cross-cut fissure and round carbide burs. Water irrigation should be used while cutting, both to reduce the generation of heat and to keep the area clean, as well as to improve the efficiency of cutting.

The handpiece and burs should be available at all times. The time lost in setting up the equipment is considerable, and when it is needed, it is needed immediately, not 10 minutes later.

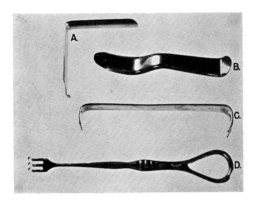

Fig. 5-7. Retractors useful in oral surgery. (A) Austin; (B) University of Minnesota type; (C) ribbon; (D) catspaw. (Clark, *Practical Oral Surgery*, Lea & Febiger, 1965)

hand to leave the left hand free for handling the suction, for malleting, and for cutting the sutures (Fig. 5-8). The assistant must be aware of what he is doing with the retractor. His main purpose is to retract the tissues gently but firmly and steadily in order that the surgeon has the area under direct vision. The assistant must be careful not to pinch the lip or other tissues; moreover, it is easy to con-

General Principles

Because mandibular bone is much more dense than maxillary bone, the bur can be used to much advantage here. The chisel is more often used in the removal of maxillary bone. Use a pen grasp with the straight handpiece, providing a steady, firm base with the fourth and fifth fingers

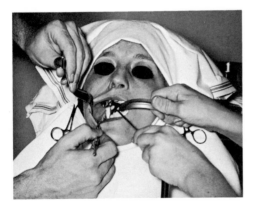

Fig. 5-8. Tongue retractor in place over gauze, depressing the tongue and also protecting the pharynx.

to assure secure handling. The assistant directs an intermittent stream of water at the area, and he regularly uses the suction tip to evacuate the waste water and debris. The periosteum must be carefully retracted away from the revolving bur, or it will be quickly mutilated if it becomes entangled in the instrument. Lingual reduction of bone with the handpiece should be done cautiously. Bony correction of lingual anomalies often can be best managed with chisels and smoothed with the bone file.

To recover a root with the bur, the overlying bone can best be removed by creating a necklace of holes above the area where the root tip is anticipated (Figs. 5-9 and 5-10). These holes are then connected

with a bur and the disc of bone is removed. This permits entry into the area of the root tip, making an easy removal. The bone overlying a third molar impaction can be similarly removed (Fig. 5-11).

When the bur is used for the sectioning of teeth, irrigation may be even more necessary (Fig. 5-12). The generation of heat can be considerable, and the tooth structure clogs the bur blades quickly. (The sectioning of teeth is discussed in detail in

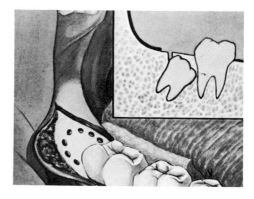

Fig. 5-11. Necklace of drill holes with surgical bur to gain access for surgical removal of impacted tooth. (Courtesy of M. L. Hale)

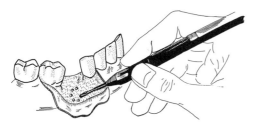

Fig. 5-9. Method of gaining entry to mandible for removal of root fragment. Circle of drill holes being made. (Clark, *Practical Oral Surgery*, Lea & Febiger, 1965)

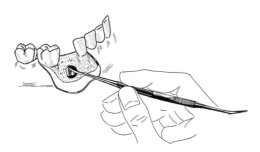

Fig. 5-10. Root revealed after circle of drill holes has been completed and disc of bone pried up. (Clark, *Practical Oral Surgery*, Lea & Febiger, 1965)

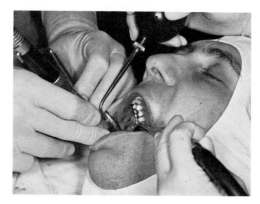

Fig. 5-12. Irrigation is necessary when bur is used for the sectioning of teeth.

Chaps. 10 and 11.) The bur can also be used to make a purchase point for elevation (Fig. 5-13).

Mallet and Chisel

The chisel is another fine instrument for the removal of bone. Maxillary bone, which is much more porous than mandibular bone, is reduced easily with the chisel using either hand pressure or the mallet (Fig. 5-14). The entire cranium acts as a countermass to receive the mallet blows, which causes much less irritation than when the mallet is used on the mandible. Of course, the use of the chisel guarantees greater sterility than the handpiece and bur, and it obviates the need for water as a coolant and irrigation.

The chisel is also used for splitting teeth, especially the bi-bevel chisel. The mono-angle chisel is preferable for bone reduction. The chisel must be razor sharp and should be honed after each use. When splitting teeth, give a single sharp bouncing blow with the mallet with no follow-through. When reducing bone with the chisel, the mallet should follow with a sequence of taps appropriate to the job being done. Additional information on tooth splitting can be found in Chapters 10 and 11.

The Elevator

One of the most valuable instruments to aid in the extraction of teeth is the elevator or exolever. Wherever possible, the

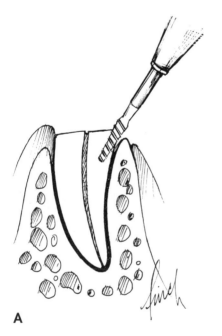

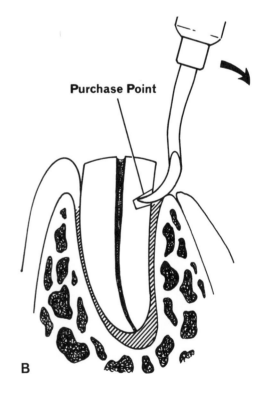

Purchase Point

Fig. 5-13. Purchase point. (A) The surgical bur is used to make a purchase point. (B) Elevator is used to lever the root out.

A

B

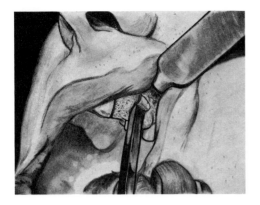

Fig. 5-14. Use of chisel to shave bone from root of upper tooth. (Clark, *Practical Oral Surgery*, Lea & Febiger, 1965)

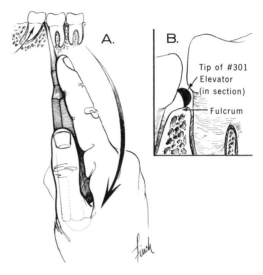

Fig. 5-15. The correct application of the elevator for the luxation of teeth.

elevator should be used to luxate all teeth before applying the forceps. This aids in the following ways: it facilitates the removal of the tooth; it minimizes the breakage of the tooth; it facilitates the removal of broken root tips if the tooth has been luxated prior to breakage; and it reduces the forcep pressure felt by the patient.

The elevator may be divided into three basic parts: the handle, the shank, and the blade. The blade of the straight elevator is concave and is used with the concave surface toward the tooth to be luxated. The occlusal edge of the blade engages the tooth while the gingival edge engages the interseptal bone, which is the fulcrum (Fig. 5-15). The determination of the occlusal edge and the gingival edge varies according to the arch quadrant. Some elevator designs vary from the straight elevator in that the blade is set at an angle to the shank and handle; this allows a better application of the elevator in certain areas of the mouth.

As used in the extraction of teeth, the elevator is a lever of the first class; that is, a lever with the fulcrum (which is the alveolar bone) between the resistance (which is the tooth) and the force (which is the hand of the operator) (Fig. 5-16). The function of a lever is to gain a me-

chanical advantage, which is calculated by dividing the input length by the output length. For example, 4 inches divided by 1 inch equals the mechanical advantage of 4 (Fig. 5-17). Thus, tremendous force is generated with this instrument.

Another type of lever application is that of the wedge. The force is supplied by the

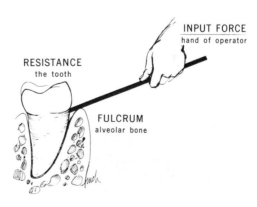

Fig. 5-16. Illustration of the lever principle.

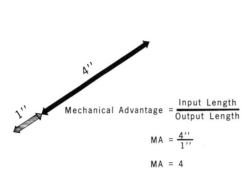

$$\text{Mechanical Advantage} = \frac{\text{Input Length}}{\text{Output Length}}$$

$$MA = \frac{4''}{1''}$$

$$MA = 4$$

Fig. 5-17. Formula demonstrating increased force using the lever principle.

hand of the operator and the resistance is supplied by the tooth or root tip. The size and shape of the wedge determine the force and the mechanical advantage. The mechanical advantage is the inclined length divided by the wedge height (Fig. 5-18). The wedge action of an elevator may be used to advantage in the delivery of fractured root tips.

Elevators may be grouped according to their primary usage. The 301, 46, and 34 elevators vary only in size and are used to luxate teeth and root tips (Fig. 5-19). The no. 41 elevator is designed to be used in the bifurcation of lower molars or on teeth with a prepared purchase point (Fig. 5-20). The root apex instruments 1, 2, and 3 are designed primarily for the recovery of upper molar root tips (Fig. 5-21).

For the luxation of the anterior teeth,

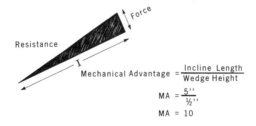

$$\text{Mechanical Advantage} = \frac{\text{Incline Length}}{\text{Wedge Height}}$$

$$MA = \frac{5''}{\frac{1}{2}''}$$

$$MA = 10$$

Fig. 5-18. Formula using the principle of the inclined plane as a wedge.

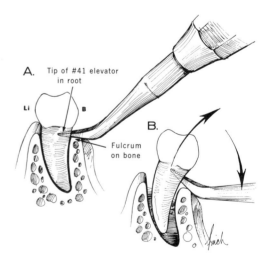

Fig. 5-19. The straight elevators are often used as a wedge for displacement of the root or tooth.

the 301 elevator is the instrument of choice. The blade of the elevator is inserted into the interproximal space with the concave surface toward the tooth to be extracted, and with the fulcrum edge of the blade well engaged on the alveolar process adjacent to the tooth. The blade is

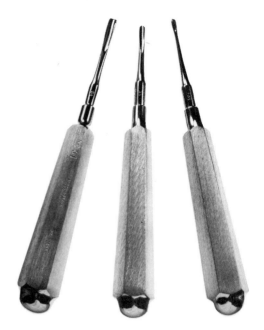

Fig. 5-20. Demonstration of the lever principle using the no. 41 elevator.

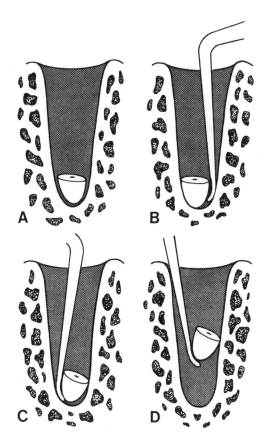

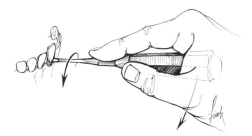

Fig. 5-22. The 301 elevator used to luxate an anterior tooth.

Fig. 5-21. The curved root pick is used to displace a retained root in the process of recovery.

then rotated toward the tooth and is engaged on its surface below the greatest point of convexity or at the cemento-enamel junction. The elevator is then rotated until engaged, and the handle is moved inferiorly so that the tooth is elevated vertically as well as slightly horizontally (Fig. 5-22). In the upper arch, the elevator handle would be moved superiorly after it has been rotated to engage the tooth. The 301 may also be used to advantage as a wedge-type lever for the recovery of root tips in some areas of the mouth,

such as the anterior maxillary area. The blade is inserted between the root tip and the alveolar bone, displacing the root tip by wedge action (Fig. 5-23). The 46 and 34 elevators vary from the 301 only in size. The increased size and strength of these elevators make their use more favorable for the posterior teeth.

The 3 and 4 elevators are specifically designed for the luxation of the upper third molars (Fig. 5-24). The blade of the elevator is placed between the alveolar

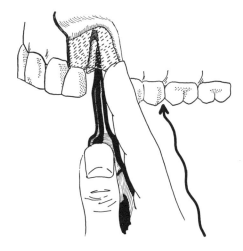

Fig. 5-23. Use of straight inclined plane elevator on upper cuspid root. (Clark, *Practical Oral Surgery*, Lea & Febiger, 1965)

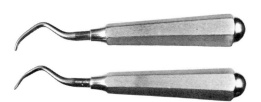

Fig. 5-24. No. 3 (top) and no. 4 (bottom) displacement elevators for removal of maxillary third molars.

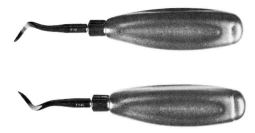

Fig. 5-26. No. 190 (bottom) and no. 191 (top) elevators.

crest and the mesial surface of the third molar. The gingival edge is engaged into the tooth. A slow, steady, upward distal and arc-like movement of the handle elevates the tooth in a distal and occlusal direction (Fig. 5-25).

The 190 and 191 elevators have an offset shank to facilitate access to the lower molar roots (Fig. 5-26). These elevators are designed primarily for the recovery of lower molar root tips that have been fractured during the extraction of the tooth. For example, if the crown and distal root of a lower right molar are delivered, and the mesial root remains in the socket, the blade of the 190 elevator is

inserted into the distal socket and rotated so that the point moves toward the apex of the mesial root and occlusally brings the root with it (Fig. 5-27).

The oral surgeon must adhere to certain basic precautions when using elevators. Proper application of elevator position, direction, and force is essential to prevent damage to the adjacent teeth, the alveolar process, and the mandible or maxilla. The danger of damage to adjacent tissues may be minimized by placing a finger along the shaft of the elevator and another on the lingual to act as stops in the event of a slip (Fig. 5-28).

The Rongeur Forceps

The rongeur is a forcep-like instrument used to remove bone by shearing or a planing action. There are basically two types: the side-cutting rongeur and the end-biting rongeur (Figs. 5-29 and 5-30).

The end-biting rongeur is good for en-

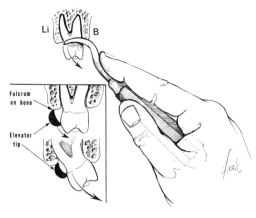

Fig. 5-25. The nos. 3 and 4 displacement elevators are used in an arc-like movement to elevate maxillary third molars.

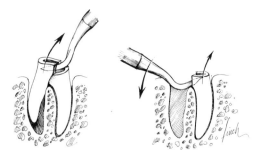

Fig. 5-27. Using the 190 and 191 elevators to remove the molar roots.

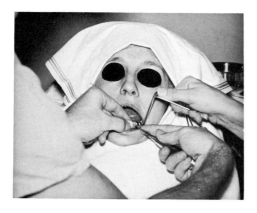

Fig. 5-28. The use of the straight elevator, showing finger protection on lingual and elevator grasp.

larging the bony wall of a cyst or the antrum, removing the peripheral bone by its biting action. It is also helpful in performing an alveolectomy. Occasionally it can be used to remove heavy fibrous tissue attachments, such as a pericoronal sac or scar tissue masses posterior to the third molar area. Finally, this instrument may be used on occasion for the extraction of a

portion of a tooth when the specific biting action of the rongeur is needed.

The side-cutting rongeur is ideal for alveolectomy procedures. It should be used in a horizontal position with one of the biting edges of the forceps locked high on the alveolus while the other blade is brought to it in a planing action. This provides a controlled reduction of the excessive bone and creates less fracture or the breakage of large amounts of bone. It is especially useful for approaching a root by inserting its spear-pointed blade into a socket to remove a portion of the socket wall.

Whenever the rongeur is used, a constant cleansing of the blades is necessary. The operator holds the instrument with open beaks toward the assistant after each

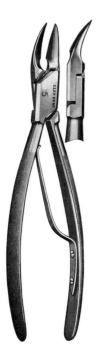

Fig. 5-29. The side-cutting rongeur. (Cleveland Dental Mfg. Co.)

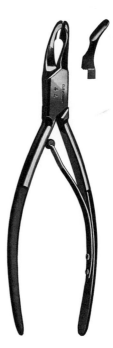

Fig. 5-30. The end-biting (blunt-nosed) rongeur. (Cleveland Dental Mfg. Co.)

rongeuring action, and the assistant wipes them clean with a gauze sponge. The rongeur is a radical instrument that reduces large amounts of bone rapidly. However, when carefully used with good judgment, it serves the surgeon well.

The Bone Rasp or File

The bone rasp or file is used for final trimming of the bony ridge after gross removal with the rongeur. Whenever a rongeur is used, it should be followed by filing. The file should be placed high on the interseptal crest and, using the pull stroke, drawn toward the crest. Cross filing should be avoided because it tends to fracture the small and unsupported interseptal bone (Fig. 5-31). Careful cleansing of the instrument is necessary; the assistant wipes the grooved ends with a sponge. Bone dust or chips may easily be left in the wound if careful cleansing is not done after each stroke or when filing is completed.

The Gilmore Probe

The Gilmore probe is a surgical explorer. A slender instrument, it can be broken easily. No leverage should be applied to it. Its purpose is for exploration and for teasing out small root tips near such structures as the inferior alveolar canal and the lining membrane of the antrum (Fig. 5-32). Remember that this is a sharp and dangerous instrument and can penetrate and injure these same structures.

The Double-Ended Curette

The double-ended curette comes in three basic sizes: small, medium, and large. Its function is to explore the apices of sockets and to enucleate granulomas, soft tissue tumors, cysts, and the like. The curette is a sensitive instrument designed to reveal to the surgeon the quality of the

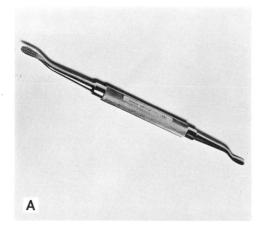

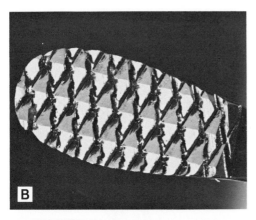

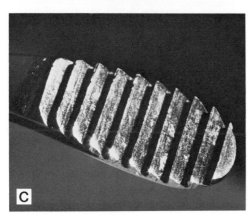

Fig. 5-31. Bone file or rasp.

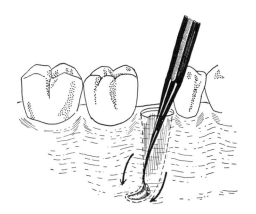

Fig. 5-32. Method of teasing out loosened root tip with Gilmore probe. (Clark, *Practical Oral Surgery*, Lea & Febiger, 1965)

structures with which it comes in contact. When one becomes skilled with this instrument, one can differentiate bone tissue from tooth structure and, of course, soft tissue.

When curetting the apices of a tooth socket, place the concave aspect of the curette near the superior edge of the socket wall and push the contents apically, following around the entire socket wall with this same movement. The total apical contents can then be drawn toward the surface in a scooping fashion until the socket is clean (Fig. 5-33).

The Scissors

A great variety of scissors are available to the surgeon. However, two main types are in general use, referred to as the suture scissors and the tissue scissors (Fig. 5-34). The curved Mayo 6-inch scissors with two sharp points works well for dissecting as well as for trimming wound margins. When trimming tissue margins, it is best to immobilize the tissue by means of the tissue forceps, which will permit accurate and careful trimming.

When dissecting or undermining with the scissors, the incised margins are again immobilized with the skin hook or forceps, and the scissors are inserted in the closed position and then forcibly spread apart (Fig. 5-35). The purpose of this technique is to bluntly dissect the tissues with minimal hemorrhage or risk of cutting significant anatomic structures. Undermining is often done to permit advancement of tissue to a new location, and to lessen tension as a flap is sutured into its new position.

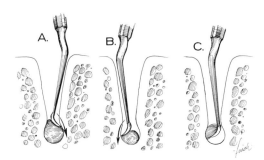

Fig. 5-33. Proper use of the curette.

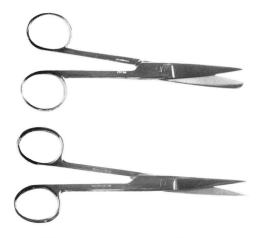

Fig. 5-34. Curved and straight 6-inch scissors.

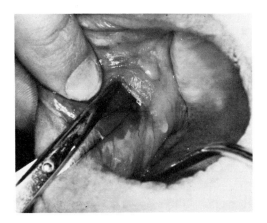

Fig. 5-35. After excisional biopsy of the left paries, the scissors is used to undermine the tissue flaps for closure.

Although tissue scissors can also be used for sutures in many instances, the specific suture scissors is a straight-bladed instrument with a Mayo 6-inch blunt surface and one sharp point which permits the assistant to slide the scissor blade down the suture strand until it stops on the knot, at which point the suture is cut. This is especially important for sutures that are to remain deep in the wound without a long tail.

The Tissue or Sponge Forceps

The forceps is a versatile instrument and the operator should establish the habit of having the thumb forceps in hand at all times during suturing. Tissue forceps are used to immobilize the tissue when the needle is passed through it. Several types are available; however, a good general tissue forceps for oral surgical use is the Rochester oral tissue forceps. In addition to this, there is a small O'Brien tissue forceps without teeth, the nasal dressing forceps, which is a bayonet-type instrument, the cotton pliers for the placement of dressings in sockets, and the tissue forceps with sharp teeth (Fig. 5-36).

Suture, Needle, and Needle Holder *

Specifications

SUTURE. For suturing oral mucosae use 3-0 black silk. This material is treated to be serum proof and braided to resist coiling and snarling. Nonabsorbable suture material has uniform tensile strength whether wet or dry, lending itself well to the time-saving technique of instrument tying of knots. Being black, the stitches are easily seen when the patient returns for their removal. One reason for using nonabsorbable material is to bring the patient back for the all-important postoperative "look." For tying bleeders or closing muscles or fascia, use Pycktanin catgut, plain type A, 000, or chromic or plain catgut, size 000.

NEEDLE. The needle should have a cutting edge for suturing oral mucosae; use Anchor Brand 1822–18 (large) or 1822–20 (small), or Hu-Friedy three-eighths circle, size 18 or 20. Use a round (noncutting) needle for stitch-tying or closing muscle or fascia: Anchor Brand 1833, number 2 or 3.

NEEDLE HOLDER. For all purposes, use Hegar-Mayo, 6 inches long.

HANDLING NEEDLE AND NEEDLE HOLDER. The needle is always grasped *just ahead* of the eye, to give maximal length of the needle for passing through tissue. Needles are readily broken when grasped *on* the eye (Fig. 5-37).

The needle holder is always grasped the same way, with just the tip of the thumb through one ring, one phalanx of the

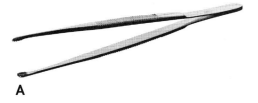

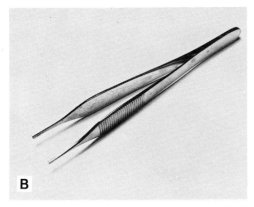

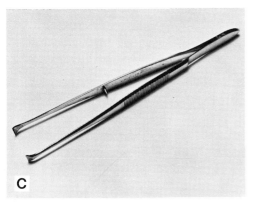

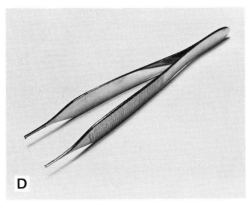

Fig. 5-36. (A) Rochester Russian tissue forceps, 6 inches. (B) Brown-Adson side-grasping forceps. (C) O'Brien fixation forceps. (D) Adson forceps with mouth tooth.

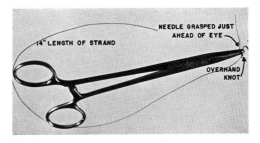

Fig. 5-37. Needle, suture, and needle holder. (Clark, *Practical Oral Surgery*, Lea & Febiger, 1965)

fourth finger through the other ring, and the index finger braced against the shaft, halfway down. The other fingers close on the instrument in a natural position, thus giving a secure grasp, but one that permits instant dropping of the instrument when all fingers are straightened (Fig. 5-38). (The same grasp is used for hemostatic forceps.)

Technique for Suturing Oral Mucosae

The tissue is immobilized with a tissue forceps and the needle thrust through at right angles to the surface, ¼ inch from the edge of the incised wound. The motion then becomes curved, since the needle is curved. The stitch should be so arranged that it crosses at right angles to the line of closure. When first learning to suture it is best to always go through each side of the wound with separate bites of tissue. When more experience has been gained, opportunities will be found to pass through both sides with one stroke.

After the first thrust of the needle the shaft should emerge to such an extent that the beaks of the needle holder can grasp it back of the point. The delicate tip of the needle is easily broken or bent by rough handling. The needle is drawn through

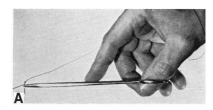

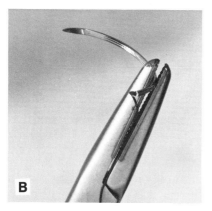

Fig. 5-38. (A) Proper grasp of needle holder. (Clark, *Practical Oral Surgery*, Lea & Febiger, 1965) (B) The needle is grasped with the needle holder at the junction of the middle posterior third of the needle.

the tissue with a curved motion. With the second side of the wound immobilized, this same procedure is repeated. The knot is then completed as a square knot or surgeon's tie (Fig. 5-39).

The Figure 8 Stitch to Control Bleeding (*Stitch Tie*)

Direct clamping of a bleeding vessel with a hemostat is preferred, but if this cannot be done due to inadequate facilities in an emergency, this method is acceptable and effective: The probable location of the bleeding vessel is estimated and the needle passed deeply through both edges of the wound slightly *ahead* of the bleeder. Another generous "bite" is taken

Fig. 5-39. Instrument tie of the surgeon's knot.

(A) Ready to tie the knot. Assistant retracts and holds back lip or cheek. Unlock needle holder, grasp needle between left thumb and forefinger (where it remains for the entire knot tie), pull forward until only 1 inch of suture remains.

(B) Place needle holder *on top* of the long strand of suture and pointed *up, toward the left shoulder.* Wrap needle holder around the long strand *two complete turns* (clockwise—to the right).

(C) With the left middle finger, stroke coils toward ring handles to keep suture away from box lock. Steady needle holder on left middle finger, carry open jaws of needle holder to the *very tip* of the short end.

(D) Grasp the *tip* of the short end and lock needle holder. (Grasping short strand in the middle will produce a bow knot.)

(E) Draw coils off of needle holder by pulling on the long strand. Keep short end 1 inch long. Direct short end toward the throat and pull long strand toward you, adjusting knot to desired tightness. Release suture from needle holder. From here on, if both strands are kept slack at all times, the double wrap will prevent knot from loosening.

(F) The second half of the tie is much like the first, but this time place the needle holder *under* the long strand, point it toward the left shoulder, wrap it around only *once* (counterclockwise—to the left).

(G) Repeat steps C and D as before.

(H) Draw coils off the needle holder by pulling on the long strand. Now you have a choice: (1) To form the surgeon's knot shown in the picture, draw the short end forward and the long end to the rear, or (2) *again* direct the short end toward the throat and draw the long end toward you. Opinions differ on the best technique for finishing the knot. Some prefer to draw the short end forward and the long end to the rear; this will produce the neat surgeon's knot shown in H. However I prefer to direct the short end to the rear both times. The great convenience of avoiding finger manipulation of suture material inside the mouth, especially in posterior areas, more than compensates for the altered appearance of the knot. In our experience knots made in the manner described fulfill the essential requirement of remaining tied for five to seven days.

In either event, now give one or two tugs on the strands, pulling in opposite directions, away from the knot, to set it firmly. Gather everything into the left palm—equal tension on both strands, then cut both $\frac{1}{4}$ inch from the knot.

Remove short piece from jaws of needle holder. Lock it on the needle just ahead of the eye in preparation for the next stitch. (Clark, *Practical Oral Surgery*, Lea & Febiger, 1965)

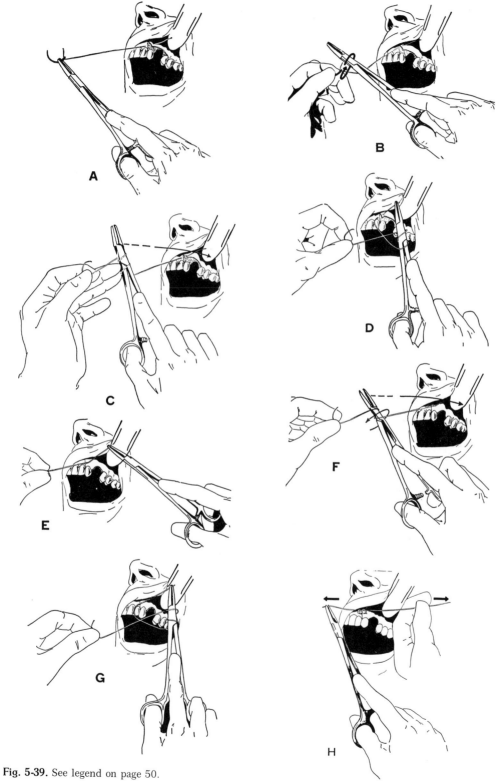

Fig. 5-39. See legend on page 50.

through both sides of the wound slightly *behind* the bleeder (Fig. 5-40). The suture is pulled up snugly and tied with a surgeon's knot, somewhat tighter than for an ordinary interrupted stitch.

The Mattress Stitch

There are two types of mattress stitch: the horizontal and the vertical (Fig. 5-41).

The mattress stitch is used to produce slight eversion of wound edges or to provide more absolute apposition of two raw surfaces, as in closure of an antra-oral fistula. The wound margins are considered as *near* and *far* edges. The needle is passed through the margins in the following sequence: *near, far, far, near* (Fig. 5-41A). The vertical mattress suture usually is used when more tension is needed (Fig. 5-41B). The suture is tied with a surgeon's knot.

The Traction Suture

Occasionally, when the steel retractor cannot be used, this atraumatic, nonslipping method of securing retraction can be used to good effect. The cutting edge needle is passed through the flap margin, 1/4 inch from the edge. The double strand of suture material is grasped with a hemostat attached (Fig. 5-42).

Use of Absorbable Suture Material

FOR TYING BLEEDERS. Refer to the section describing the hemostat. The catgut is held in the two hands and passed completely around the clamped vessel. The first half of the surgeon's knot is tied and tension maintained while the hemostat is

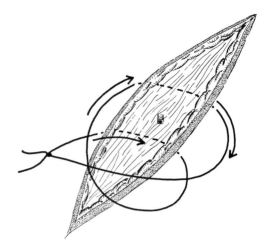

Fig. 5-40. The figure 8 stitch tie. (Clark, *Practical Oral Surgery*, Lea & Febiger, 1965)

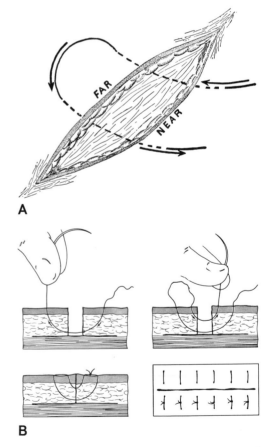

Fig. 5-41. (A) The mattress stitch. (Clark, *Practical Oral Surgery*, Lea & Febiger, 1965). (B) The vertical mattress stitch.

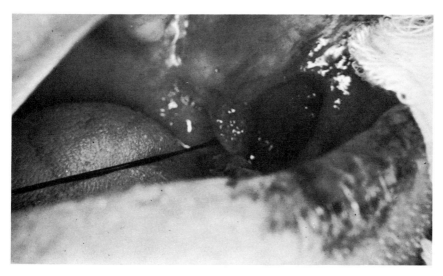

Fig. 5-42. Traction suture.

carefully opened and removed by the assistant. This step seats the knot on the stalk of the vessel where it has been crushed. With care not to jerk the strands and thus loosen the knot, the second half is tied tightly and the ends cut approximately ⅛ inch long.

The instrument tie may be used, but well-soaked catgut will often cut through when grasped with the needle holder or hemostat. If the bleeding vessel is difficult to clamp and tie, the figure 8 stitch tie, using a round (noncutting) needle, may be employed.

FOR CLOSING MUSCLE OR FASCIA. The catgut is threaded on a round (noncutting) needle, leaving one long and one somewhat shorter strand. Due to the greater friability of catgut, it is usually not practicable to secure it to the needle with an overhand knot. The fascial or muscle margin is immobilized with a traction hook or tissue forceps. Ample bites of tissue, at least ¼ inch from the wound margin, are taken. The catgut is tied by hand, with the surgeon's knot.

If the initial passage of the needle is made from beneath upward and the second passage from superficial to deep surface of the tissue, the resulting knot will come to rest in the depth of the wound so that there will be no projecting ends of suture material (Fig. 5-43).

Hemostat

Although there is a large variety of hemostats available for general operating room procedures in the hospital, the mosquito forceps and the Kelly forceps are generally used for intraoral use (Fig. 5-44). These come in both straight and curved designs. The Allis forceps is good for grasping tissue margins during dissection, and in some cases, retraction of the tissue segment that is to be removed.

When a hemostat is used to control bleeding, the area is first compressed with

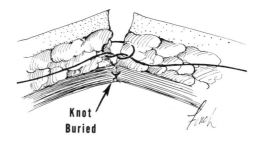

Knot
Buried

Fig. 5-43. Method of keeping the knot near the depth of the wound.

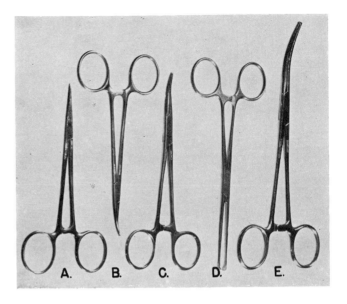

Fig. 5-44. Various types of hemostats. (A) Straight mosquito; (B) curved mosquito; (C) curved Kelly; (D) Allis; (E) Carmault. (Clark, *Practical Oral Surgery*, Lea & Febiger, 1965)

a gauze sponge and, as the assistant retracts the sponge from the previously bleeding site, the hemostat is quickly moved into position while the tissue is still blanched to grasp the bit of the tissue that appears to be bleeding. The bleeding vessel can then be tied beneath the hemostat or, in many instances, the hemostat can be left in position during the operative procedure and the hemorrhage controlled at the tissues as the tissues are sutured into position. The hemostat is also used to remove tooth fragments and root tips, and to grasp and hold tissues such as follicles or cyst membranes.

Aspirator

A necessary piece of equipment in oral surgery is the aspirator. The Frazier suction tip and the Hu-Friedy suction tip are excellent for oral surgical use. The aspirator is held in the assistant's left hand, freeing the right hand for retraction of

tongue or lip as necessary (Fig. 5-45). Effective suctioning means keeping several areas of the oral cavity free of blood, saliva, and debris at all times. Saliva quickly pools in the floor of the mouth and near the tongue and soft palate. Careful suctioning of this area must be done without gagging the patient. The operative field is

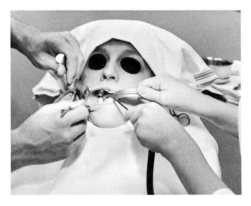

Fig. 5-45. The assistant uses his right hand to hold the retractor and his left hand to aspirate.

paramount and this too must be kept clean without interfering with the vision of the surgeon. Because the operator may occasionally see an immediate need for the suction which is not visible to the assistant, the assistant should be prepared to give up the aspirator to the surgeon quickly upon indication and be ready to accept it from him in the same manner.

The assistant should be much aware of the normal sound of the aspirator and able to detect when it is partially plugged or obstructed. Immediate freeing of the obstruction is necessary, which may necessitate the changing of the suction tip. These actions must be done quickly and efficiently. The effective use of the aspirator will greatly increase the efficiency of the surgeon and save considerable time that otherwise might be utilized by the patient attempting to use the cuspidor. Following surgery, good irrigation of the suction tip and its tubing is necessary to prevent blood clotting and general clogging of this instrument.

Tooth Extraction Forceps

Although there are many kinds of extraction forceps, they are all designed according to certain basic principles. In general, maxillary forceps are so designed that the beaks are in line with or parallel to the long axis of the handles, and mandibular forceps have the beaks at right angles to the handle. While extracting teeth, every effort is made to keep the beaks of the forceps in line with the long axis of the tooth in order to minimize root fracture. The forceps may be designed to correspond to the anatomy of particular teeth, or they may have a universal design.

The following are some examples of extraction forceps:

Clev-Dent (Stainless Steel) No. 150 (Fig. 5-46)—for maxillary incisors, cuspids, and biscuspids.

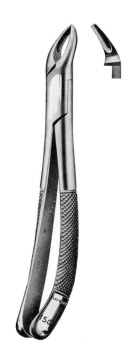

Fig. 5-46. No. 150 forceps. (Clev-Dent, Div. of Cavitron Corp.) MAX, INCIRORS.

Clev-Dent (Stainless Steel) No. 53R and 53L (Fig. 5-47)—anatomic forceps for maxillary molars.

Clev-Dent (Stainless Steel) No. 88R and 88L (Fig. 5-48)—nonanatomic forceps used when alveolar application is necessary in the presence of severely carious crowns or when the forceps beaks fit the bifurcation of the roots.

S. S. White (Tarno) No. 210 (Fig. 5-49)—for maxillary third molars.

Clev-Dent (Stainless Steel) No. 69 (Fig. 5-50)—universal root spicule forceps for grasping a tooth when the crown has fractured leaving a small portion of the root available.

S. S. White (Tarno) No. 151 (Fig. 5-51)—for mandibular incisors, cuspids, and bicuspids.

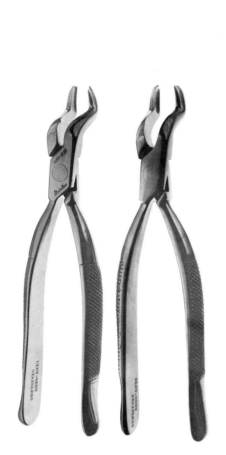

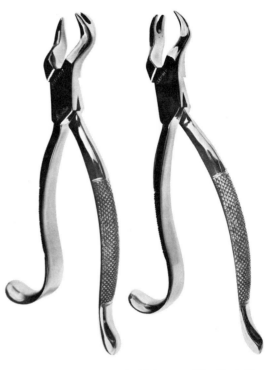

Fig. 5-48. No. 88R and 88L forceps. (Clev-Dent, Div. of Cavitron Corp.) *NEANATOMENA 20 MAXICCAR TIOLAR. LADA NCTA LRLNE- COWHORN*

Fig. 5-47. No. 53R and 53L forceps. (Clev-Dent, Div. of Cavitron Corp.) *MAXILLARY MOLARS*

Clev-Dent (Stainless Steel) No. 17 (Fig. 5-52)—anatomic forceps for mandibular molars.

Clev-Dent (Stainless Steel) No. 23 (Fig. 5-53)—nonanatomic forceps for broken mandibular molars. Often referred to as cowhorn forceps.

S. S. White (Tarno) No. 101 (Fig. 5-54)—universal forceps applicable for most deciduous extractions.

When using the extracting forceps, the removal of the tooth will be less difficult if some luxation by means of an elevator has preceded the extraction movement. The forceps is applied to the tooth by means of the "application grasp" (Fig. 5-55). Apply

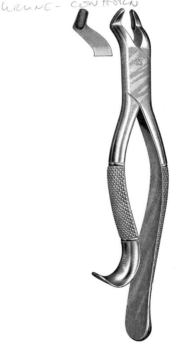

Fig. 5-49. No. 210 forceps. (S. S. White Div., Pennwalt Corp.) *MAXILLARY WISDOM TEETH*

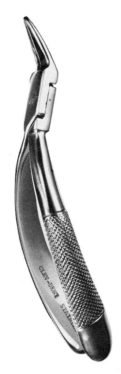

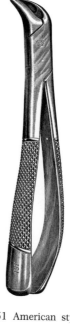

Fig. 5-51. No. 151 American style forceps (S. S. White Div., Pennwalt Corp.)

MAND. INCISORS.

Fig. 5-50. No. 69 forceps (Clev-Dent, Div. of Cavitron Corp.) ROOT FRAGMENTS.

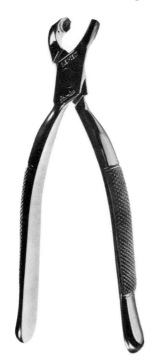

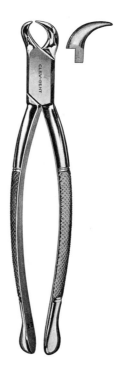

Fig. 5-52. No. 17 forceps. (Clev-Dent, Div. of Cavitron Corp.)

MAND. MOLARS.

Fig. 5-53. No. 23 forceps. (Clev-Dent, Div. of Cavitron Corp.) COW HORN LOWER MOLARS.

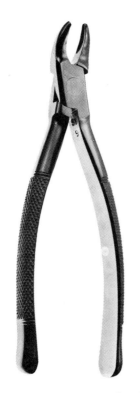

Fig. 5-54. No. 101 forceps (S. S. White Div., Pennwalt Corp.) DECIDOUS EX.

MOST OF

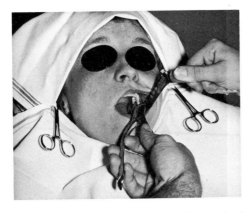

Fig. 5-55. Application grasp. Note lingual beak seated firmly in the ball of hand.

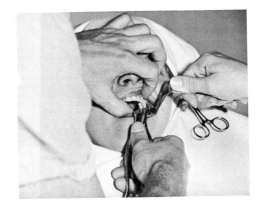

Fig. 5-56. Extraction grasp. Note position of left hand.

the forcep beak to the most difficult surface first, which is usually the lingual; the ball of the hand forces the beak well on to the surface of the tooth beneath the gingiva. The buccal or labial beak is then allowed to come into contact with the crown of the tooth, and the fingers encircle the handle to permit a firm grasp referred to as the "extraction grasp" (Fig. 5-56). A crushing force should be avoided, but apply firm and continuous pressure as the movements of the tooth extraction are developed.

Basic Forces Exerted During the Extraction of Teeth

A. Maxillary teeth
1. Central incisors: Labial pressure with mesial rotation.
2. Lateral incisors: Labial pressure with mesial rotation.
3. Cuspids: Labial pressure with mesial rotation.
4. First bicuspids: Buccal pressure, lingual pressure, remove to the buccal.

5. Second bicuspids: Buccal pressure, lingual pressure, remove to the lingual or buccal.
6. First molars: Buccal pressure, lingual pressure, remove to the buccal.
7. Second molars: Buccal pressure, lingual pressure, remove to the buccal.
8. Third molars: Buccal pressure, remove to the buccal.

B. Mandibular teeth
1. Central incisors: Labial pressure, lingual pressure, slight mesial and distal rotation.
2. Lateral incisors: Labial pressure, lingual pressure, slight mesial and distal rotation, remove to the labial.
3. Cuspids: Labial pressure, mesial rotation.
4. First bicuspids: Buccal pressure, slight mesial distal rotation.
5. Second bicuspids: Buccal pressure, slight mesial distal rotation.
6. First molars: Buccal pressure, lingual pressure, remove to the buccal.
7. Second molars: Buccal pressure, lingual pressure, remove to the buccal.
8. Third molars: Buccal pressure, remove to the buccal or lingual.

In all instances the final movement is traction.

The patient should be seated comfortably in the chair with the head and cervical spine in line with the back. The chair should be tipped back one to two notches from the center. In general, the chair will be low for extractions of mandibular teeth and somewhat higher for maxillary teeth. The elbow of the operator should be level with the surgical site. When the forceps has been appropriately applied, the left hand should grasp the alveolar process. Either the right front or right rear position can be used when appropriate (Figs. 5-57 and 5-58).

Before the first movement of the tooth is initiated, take a second look to be sure the

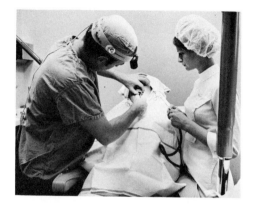

Fig. 5-57. Right front position for extraction.

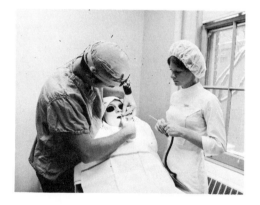

Fig. 5-58. Right rear position for extraction.

forceps is on the right tooth to be extracted. The extraction movements are then instituted depending on the anatomy of the tooth to be extracted. This coupled with slight traction as luxation increases should provide a smooth integrated extraction procedure (Figs. 5-59 to 5-63). The tooth is then carefully inspected to be sure it is intact, and the curette is used to gently explore the socket. Once satisfied of a clean wound, the thumb and forefinger are used to compress firmly the socket walls expanded during the extraction pro-

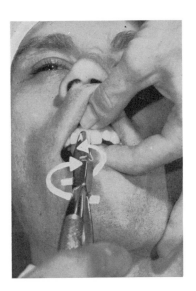

Fig. 5-59. Extraction of upper anterior tooth (rotation emphasized). (Clark, *Practical Oral Surgery*, Lea & Febiger, 1965)

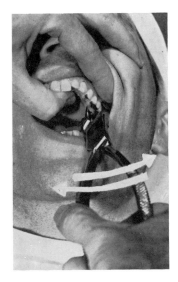

Fig. 5-61. Extraction of upper molar (buccolingual movement emphasized). (Clark, *Practical Oral Surgery*, Lea & Febiger, 1965)

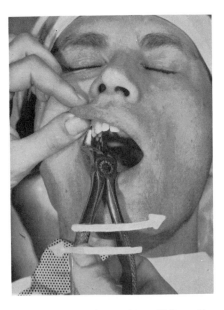

Fig. 5-60. Extraction of upper bicuspid (buccolingual movement emphasized). (Clark, *Practical Oral Surgery*, Lea & Febiger, 1965)

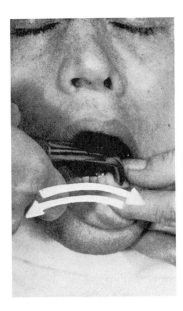

Fig. 5-62. Extraction of lower bicuspid (rotation emphasized). (Clark, *Practical Oral Surgery*, Lea & Febiger, 1965)

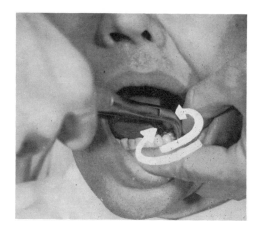

cedure. Suturing of an uncomplicated extraction site is unnecessary. The procedure is complete when a small moistened gauze is placed over the extraction site and the patient is requested to hold it in position for 20 minutes. Appropriate postoperative instructions are then given.

Fig. 5-63. Extraction of lower molar with cowhorn forceps (handles rotated to give buccolingual movement of tooth). (Clark, *Practical Oral Surgery,* Lea & Febiger, 1965)

6 Pain and Anesthesia

DANIEL E. WAITE

Diagnosis of Pain

One of the most serious and demanding clinical problems that confront the dentist is that of pain. There are many painful conditions related to the oral cavity that are not easily diagnosed. The great problem in diagnosis lies in detecting the cause of symptoms that range from specific acute dental pain to complicated facial pain of ill-defined origin. The problem may appear as a specifically organic one related to a carious lesion, a cracked tooth, or a broken jaw, or it may lie in the area of anxiety and apprehension that give rise to psychogenic pain. Through his knowledge and experience, the dentist must be able to initiate the proper and immediate treatment for the symptoms presented, or make appropriate referrals to dental or medical specialties in order to achieve the accurate diagnosis and treatment.

Again, the history is of prime importance. First, listen to the patient's subjective description, which later can be used to arrive at the diagnosis. Since only the effect of pain can be seen, it is a mistake to think solely in terms of organic disease; therefore, the patient should not immediately receive the usual dental examination. Rather, the patient should be seen in the private confines of a pleasant office background where he may express in detail the elements of his pain. Only under such circumstances can an appropriate history be taken. A good listener, surprisingly enough, may do much to relieve a patient's problems just by listening. Remember that patients react differently to pain depending upon their experience of it, and fear often greatly affects a given reaction to a stimulus. Once the history has been completed, it is then appropriate to perform a more complete physical and oral examination. This examination should be primarily directed to the sensory nerve patterns.

It is paramount that the dentist know regional anatomy expertly and have a thorough working knowledge of the neuroanatomic aspects relating to anesthesia and pain. He should be able to provide a good examination of all cranial nerves pertaining to the oral cavity. This is the area of his expertise, in which he is expected to be knowledgeable (Fig. 6-1).

It is important to consider most of the motor and sensory nerves when tracing pain problems. Although the effects of most motor nerve disturbances can be seen, those of sensory nerve disturbances cannot. For example, a disturbance of the seventh cranial nerve would produce paralysis of the face, and a disturbance of the twelfth cranial nerve would produce

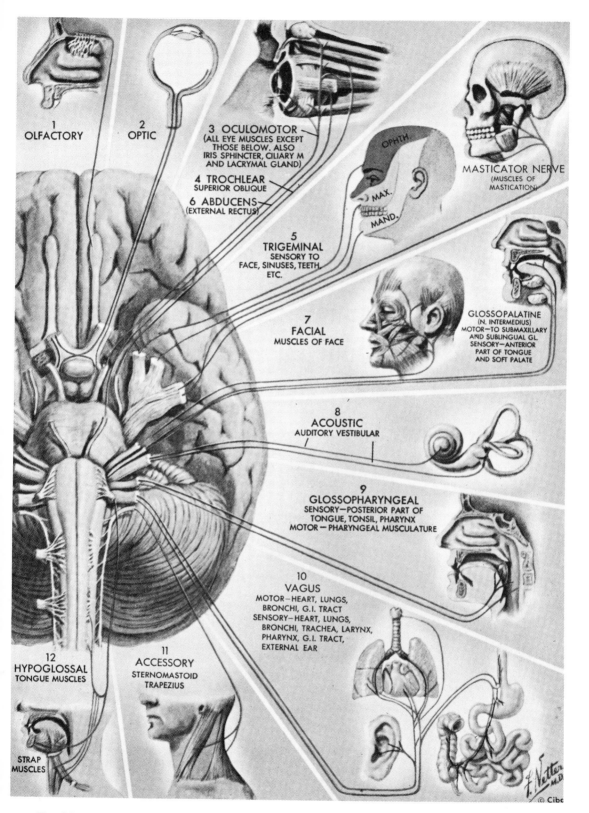

Fig. 6-1. Cranial nerve distribution. (Frank C. Netter, M.D., courtesy of CIBA Pharmaceutical Products, Inc., Summit, New Jersey)

deviation of the tongue; both are motor nerves. However, sensory nerve patterns have been accurately recorded, and some of the more important disturbances that concern the dentist are the following.

Neuralgia

Trigeminal neuralgia (tic douloureux) is a painful condition affecting branches of the trigeminal nerve: it is more commonly associated with the second and third divisions. Since these are the two main nerves innervating the dentition, many of these patients come first to the attention of the dentist. Dental causes must be ruled out; dental extraction for pain of unknown origin is inexcusable (Fig. 6-2A).

The classic symptoms are sharp, unilateral, lancinating pain of short duration. Some patients describe this condition as flashes of lightning, indicating the intensity and short duration of the pain, and in many instances a trigger zone will be described. Diagnostic nerve blocks are helpful in locating the trigger area and the specific nerve distribution area involved. The painful episodes occur most frequently during the fourth and fifth decades of life. They may be so severe a patient may refuse to talk, eat, shave, or permit examination for fear of the recurring pain. The patient may experience weight loss, severe apprehension, and depression, and even contemplate suicide (Fig. 6-2B).

Treatment for this condition has ranged from the administration of vitamin B, diphenylhydantoin (Dilantin), and carbamazepine (Tegretol), to nerve evulsion, alcohol injections, and rhizotomy. Alcohol injections used in peripheral areas may be expected to provide relief for 6 to 18 months. However, each injection may produce sufficient fibrosis that subsequent injections are of little avail. Sometimes a neuropathy occurs, in which continuous burning pain and odd sensations are experienced rather than good anesthesia.

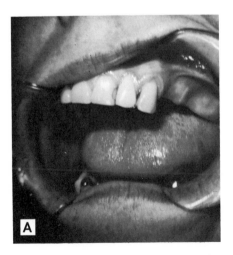 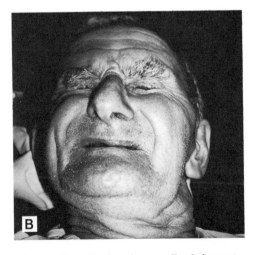

Fig. 6-2. (A) Loss of posterior maxillary dentition, one tooth at a time. No dental cause. Final diagnosis: trigeminal neuralgia. (B) Severe grimace of pain during episode of trigeminal neuralgia.

A new technique in treating trigeminal neuralgia has been introduced recently. The procedure involves percutaneous radiofrequency hyperthermia (70° C for a few seconds) of a specific area in the gasserian ganglion from which the involved branch of the fifth cranial nerve arises. The advantage of this method is that the patient remains conscious during the insertion of the insulated needle electrode through the foramen ovale. Surgical opening of the cranial vault is eliminated and transection of any branch of the nerve is unnecessary.

There are a number of other neuralgias that pertain to specific nerves, such as the ninth cranial nerve, known also as glossopharyngeal neuralgia and vidian neuralgia, and sphenopalatine neuralgia. However, these disturbances become difficult to diagnose and require a detailed neurologic evaluation, and they frequently are not dentally related.

Neuritis

The term "neuritis" refers to inflammation of a nerve. The condition is more irritating than painful, and is usually due to some infection of the area or injury to the nerve. Clinically, patients complain of paresthesia, which is a tingling or prickling sensation, or a degree of anesthesia.

Referred Pain

Referred pain is the transfer of painful stimuli over nerve pathways seemingly unrelated to the initial etiogenic condition. This is particularly true in the area of the temporomandibular joint (see Chap. 23).

Atypical Face Pain

Atypical face pain is somewhat of a basket term, but basically refers to those painful conditions of the face that cannot be evaluated in relation to the usual pat-

terns of specific neurologic problems. Many times these painful states are related to emotional stress or general psychogenic problems. Temporal arteritis, migraine, and histaminic cephalgia are similarly confusing to diagnose. Headache is also a symptom of brain tumor but may not always be the prime complaint. Figure 6-3 represents a case of salivary gland pain that had persisted for a period of three months when this lesion of the tongue was diagnosed as a grade 2 squamous cell carcinoma. Figure 23-32 (p. 445) is a patient who spent one and one-half years searching for the source of pain reflecting primarily in the temporomandibular joint with mandibular deviation and maxillary dental pain, finally resolved in the discovery of a nasopharyngeal tumor.

Other painful conditions that bear em-

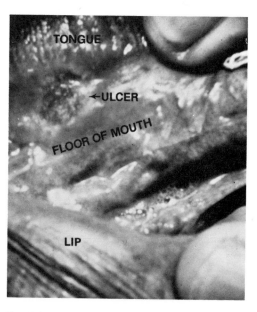

Fig. 6-3. Squamous cell carcinoma of tongue. Note 2 to 4 mm. ulcer on lateral border.

phasis are specific dental pain relating to pulpitis, dental injury, periodontal disease, and, of course, maxillary sinusitis. Each of these is discussed separately in its appropriate chapter.

Anesthesia

Intraoral Anesthesia

The proper administration of local anesthetic agents intraorally prior to routine dental or oral surgical procedures is undoubtedly the practitioner's most valuable asset for alleviating pain. Because intraoral local anesthesia is of such necessity and commonplace to the practicing dentist, it behooves the operator to become skillful and efficient in the use of these agents. Also, the dentist's ability to perform dental injections with relatively little patient discomfort can contribute significantly as a practice-building asset.

Technique

For many patients, the intraoral injection is the most anxious and trying moment of the dental procedure. The dentist should inform the patient that there will be momentary discomfort at the beginning of the injection and confidently reassure the patient during the injection procedure. The patient should be informed prior to the puncture that the injection will be made slowly and consequently with less discomfort. The tissue should be under slight tension when the insertion is made, and following the initial puncture, the needle is advanced slowly through the tissues to the point where the solution is to be delivered.

When the appropriate site has been reached, aspirate and deposit approximately 1.0 to 1.5 cc. of solution to provide proper anesthesia, and then withdraw the needle.

The anesthetic solution should be deposited slowly and the patient observed carefully for abnormal reactions.

The two basic injection techniques for attaining dental local anesthesia are the supraperiosteal (infiltration) and the nerve block injections. In the supraperiosteal injection, the anesthetic solution is deposited on the periosteum opposite the root apices of selected teeth. The solution diffuses through the periosteum and bony plate and penetrates the nerve fibers entering the apices of the roots and those supplying the periodontal membranes. Supraperiosteal injections will provide proper anesthesia for operative procedures on any of the maxillary teeth and often on the mandibular incisor teeth. It must be remembered that, for the extraction of a maxillary tooth, a palatal injection must be performed in conjunction with the supraperiosteal injection. The intraoral nerve block injections are described in the following sections.

There are several basic principles applicable to intraoral injections:

1. Sterile technique must be observed and applied.
2. The mucosa should be dried with a sterile gauze prior to the needle puncture.
3. Topical anesthetic solution and/or Metaphen may be used at the operator's discretion.
4. Prepackaged sterile, disposable needles and sterile, measured carpules of anesthetic solution should be used.

5. The needle should not be reused, but discarded after each injection.
6. The aspirating-type syringe should be utilized, especially for block injections.

Intraoral Nerve Block Injections

ZYGOMATIC INJECTION. This injection will anesthetize the posterior superior alveolar nerve before it enters the bony canals located in the zygomatic aspect of the maxilla above the third molar (Fig. 6-4). The maxillary third and second molar teeth, as well as the distobuccal and palatal roots of the first molar, are anesthetized. The puncture is made in the mucous membrane opposite the distobuccal root of the second molar, the needle being directed upward and inward to a depth of about 20 mm. Keeping the needle close to the periosteum will minimize the chances of entering the pterygoid venous plexus. To extract maxillary molar teeth, a posterior palatine injection is necessary as well as a supraperiosteal injection above the second bicuspid tooth to complete anesthesia of the first molar.

INFRAORBITAL INJECTION. This injection

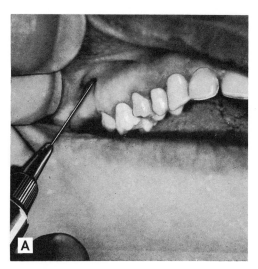

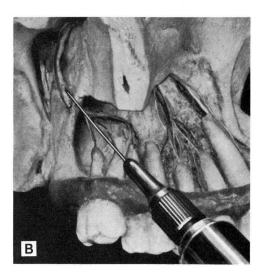

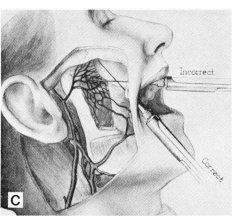

Fig. 6-4. (A) Point of insertion and direction of needle for zygomatic injection. (B) Direction of needle and distribution of posterior superior alveolar nerve. (*Manual of Local Anesthesia in General Dentistry.* Courtesy of Cook-Waite Laboratories) (C) Proper placement of needle for posterior superior alveolar injection avoids penetration of pterygoid plexus. (Archer, *A Manual of Dental Anesthesia.* Courtesy of W. B. Saunders Co.)

is indicated when infection contraindicates the use of a supraperiosteal injection, when a procedure on the maxillary antrum is contemplated, or when several teeth are to be extracted (Fig. 6-5). The anterior and middle superior alveolar nerves are anesthetized with subsequent anesthesia to the mesiobuccal root of the first molar, the second and first bicuspids, the cuspid, and the lateral and central incisors. The infraorbital foramen is palpated extraorally, and the cheek is retracted, keeping the palpating finger always over the foramen. The puncture is made opposite the second bicuspid tooth, about 5 mm. outward from the buccal surface. The needle is advanced superiorly until it is felt to enter the foramen beneath the palpating finger.

MANDIBULAR (INFERIOR ALVEOLAR) INJECTION. The inferior alveolar nerve and subsequently the mandibular teeth on the same side posteriorly from the central incisor will be anesthetized by the mandibular block injection (Figs. 6-6 and 6-7). The central and lateral incisors may receive innervation from overlapping nerve fibers from the opposite side and therefore require labial infiltration at this point. For mandibular injection, the patient is placed in such a position that when the mouth is opened wide, the occlusal plane of the mandible is parallel with the floor.[7] The anterior border of the ascending ramus is palpated with the index finger until the greatest depth of curvature is detected. With the barrel of the syringe lying between the bicuspids on the opposite side, the needle is directed parallel to the occlusal plane and toward the ramus. Insert the needle at the apex of the pterygomandibular triangle and guide it along the internal surface of the ramus until it

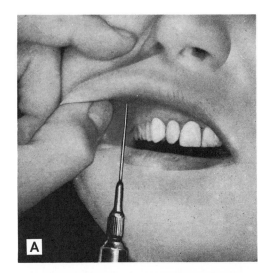

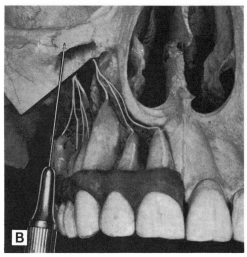

Fig. 6-5. (A) Point of insertion and direction of needle for infraorbital injection. (B) Direction of needle and distribution of infraorbital nerve. (*Manual of Local Anesthesia in General Dentistry.* Courtesy of Cook-Waite Laboratories)

reaches the posterior wall of the mandibular sulcus. The lingual nerve is usually anesthetized by injecting a small amount of solution halfway along this path of insertion. To complete anesthesia for the extraction of a lower molar tooth, the long buccal nerve must also be anesthetized. This can be accomplished by inserting a needle in the mucobuccal fold opposite the first molar and advancing it posteriorly parallel with the occlusal plane to a point opposite the second or third molar, where a small amount of solution is deposited on the mandible.

MENTAL INJECTION. As with the infraorbital injection, the mental injection can be performed either extra- or intraorally (Fig. 6-8). The intraoral approach provides the same anesthesia as does the extraoral. Palpate the area at the apices of

the lower bicuspid teeth to locate the mental foramen. Make the puncture in the mucous membrane above this point and advance the needle at a 45° angle to the

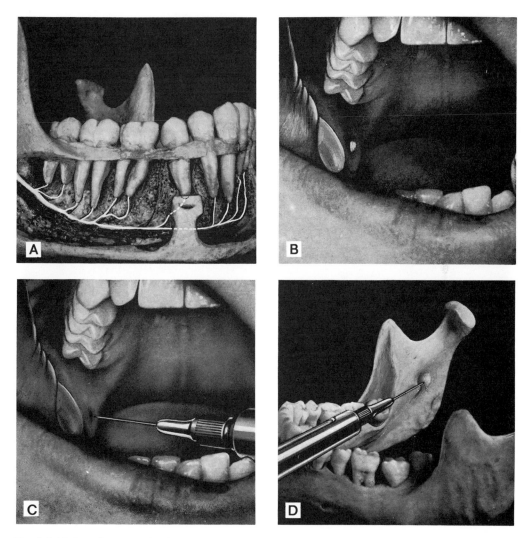

Fig. 6-6. (A) Bone dissection of right mandible showing inferior alveolar nerve and mental foramen. (B) Intraoral photograph showing finger in the retromolar fossa and pellet of cotton resting in the apex of the pterygomandibular triangle. (C) Needle entering apex of pterygomandibular triangle. (D) Position of syringe and needle for the mandibular injection. (*Manual of Local Anesthesia in General Dentistry.* Courtesy of Cook-Waite Laboratories)

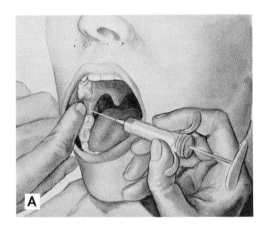

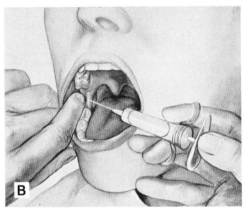

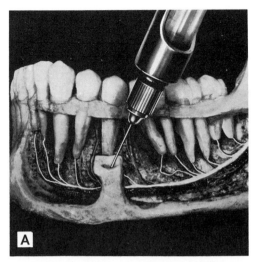

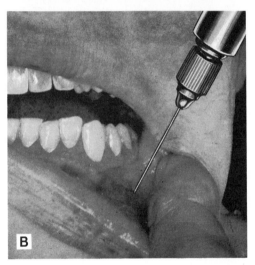

Fig. 6-7. (A) Inferior alveolar nerve injection utilizing the pen grasp. (B) Inferior alveolar nerve injection anesthetizing lingual nerve. (Archer, *A Manual of Dental Anesthesia.* Courtesy of W. B. Saunders Co.)

Fig. 6-8. (A) Bone dissection showing mental foramen and alveolar nerve. (B) Needle entering foramen for mental injection (*Manual of Local Anesthesia in General Dentistry.* Courtesy of Cook-Waite Laboratories)

buccal plate of the mandible. When the needle touches bone, deposit about 0.5 cc. of anesthetic solution, and explore the area with the needle until the foramen is located. Then deposit another 0.5 cc.

NASOPALATINE INJECTION. This injection anesthetizes the anterior third of the palate from cuspid to cuspid (Fig. 6-9). However, there is usually some overlapping from the anterior palatine nerve in the

cuspid region. The puncture for the nasopalatine injection is made alongside the incisive papilla. The needle is directed upward to the anterior palatine canal.

POSTERIOR PALATINE INJECTION. The anterior palatine nerve is blocked with this injection, resulting in anesthesia of the palatal mucoperiosteum from the tuberosity to the cuspid region and from the median line to the gingival crest on the side

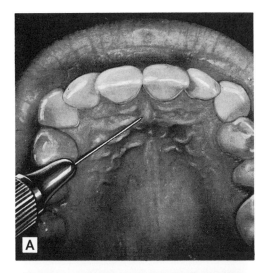

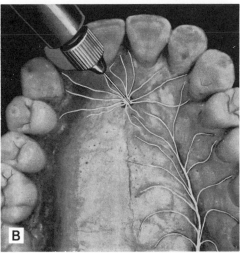

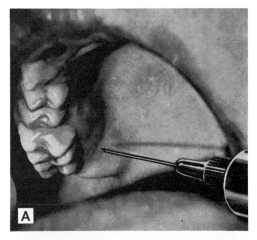

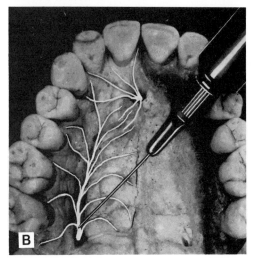

Fig. 6-9. (A) Point of insertion and direction of needle for nasopalatine injection. (B) Direction of needle and distribution of nerves in nasopalatine injection. (*Manual of Local Anesthesia in General Dentistry* Courtesy of Cook-Waite Laboratories

injected (Fig. 6-10). The puncture is made just mesial to the palatal root of the maxillary third molar with the syringe directed from the opposite side of the mouth.

Extraoral Nerve Blocks

Anesthesia of the trigeminal, or fifth cranial, nerve by the extraoral approach

Fig. 6-10. (A) Point of insertion and direction of needle for posterior palatine injection. (B) Direction of needle and distribution of nerves in posterior palatine injection. (*Manual of Local Anesthesia in General Dentistry*, Courtesy of Cook-Waite Laboratories)

was first described by Braun[2] in 1903. Although intraoral nerve block is a daily matter in dentistry, the extraoral approach has never been popular owing to the lack of acceptance by the patient, the technical skill involved, and the necessity for a strict aseptic technique. Anesthesia by means of the extraoral approach may at times be most important. A thorough understanding of regional anesthesia includes the ability to perform these procedures.[3,4]

Before employing this method of injection, the surgeon should consider the psychologic reaction of the patient. The patient should be told what is going to be done and assured that no disfiguring blemish will occur at the site of the injection. Premedication might be necessary. The needles should be sharp and of proper gauge. Postoperative instructions should be explicit and detailed.

Indications

1. When there is an infection or a tumor present at the site of an intended intraoral injection.
2. When trismus or false ankylosis makes the intraoral approach difficult or impossible.
3. When a large area is to be anesthetized using a minimal amount of anesthetic solution (e.g., when it is desirous to block all the subdivisions of the maxillary nerve using only one needle insertion).
4. For diagnostic and therapeutic purposes (e.g., in trigeminal neuralgia or temporomandibular joint problems).
5. When treatment under general anesthesia would be considered impossible or impractical (e.g., in the presence of systemic complications).
6. When attempts to give anesthesia by the intraoral approach have proved ineffective (e.g., when there is accessory innervation or anatomic deviations in the course of nerves).

7. When anesthesia of the entire distribution of the major nerve trunk is required for extensive surgery.
8. To relieve intractable pain in the jaws from any condition.

Contraindications

1. The presence of infection in the area of the needle insertion, or when aseptic conditions cannot be maintained.
2. When landmarks are difficult to locate.

All extraoral blocks should be done using aseptic technique. The operator should complete a surgical scrub and use sterile gloves. The area to be injected should be prepared and draped. The sterility of all armamentarium should be assured.

A thorough understanding of the anatomy of the head and neck—especially the nerve distribution—is essential to successful results. The anesthetist should review this area again for a complete understanding of the neuroanatomy, landmarks, and related structures involved in the technique of extraoral nerve blocks.

Neuroanatomy of the Trigeminal Nerve[5,6]

The trigeminal (cranial V) nerve takes its origin from the lateral surface of the pons (midbrain) and enlarges via the presence of many afferent nerve cell bodies into the gasserian, or semilunar, ganglion. It has three divisions: (1) the ophthalmic, (2) the maxillary, and (3) the mandibular (Fig. 6-11).

1. The first, or ophthalmic, division leaves the cranium through an opening of a fissure in the posterior wall of the orbit called the superior orbital fissure. Its branches supply structures within

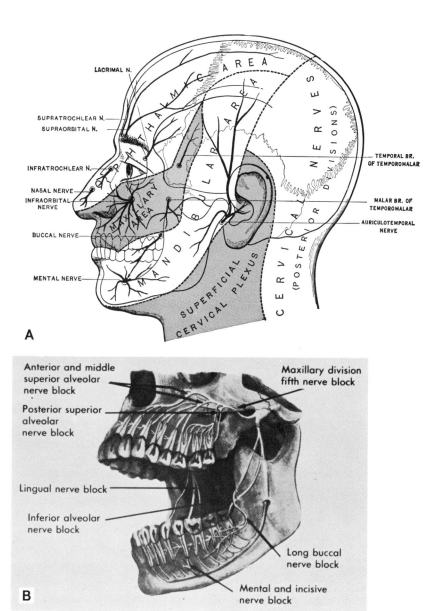

Fig. 6-11. (A and B) Fifth cranial nerve distribution. (A, from Goss, C. M. (Ed.): *Gray's Anatomy of the Human Body*, 28th ed. Philadelphia, Lea & Febiger, 1966. B, from Monheim, L. M.: *Local Anesthesia and Pain Control in Dental Practice*, 4th ed. St. Louis, C. V. Mosby Co., 1969.)

the orbit, the forehead, the scalp, the frontal sinuses, and the upper eyelids.

2. The maxillary division of the trigeminal nerve passes through the foramen rotundum into the pterygopalatine fossa, where it gives off branches to the sphenopalatine ganglion. Among them:

a. A pharyngeal branch, which passes

through a bony canal to the mucous membrane of the upper part of the nasopharynx.

b. The palatine nerves, which pass through the pterygopalatine canal and exit through the greater and lesser palatine foramina to supply the mucous membrane of the palate.

c. A sphenopalatine branch, which

enters the nasal cavity and sends a branch along the nasal septum to the palate through the incisive foramen.

The posterior superior alveolar nerves arise from the trunk of the maxillary division. They enter the maxilla and supply the molar teeth and related supporting tissues. The maxillary nerve continues as the infraorbital nerve, which gives off the middle and anterior superior alveolar nerves in the infraorbital canal. After reaching the face, a branch goes to the upper lip.

3. The mandibular nerve reaches the infratemporal fossa through the foramen ovale. It is the largest of the three divisions and consists of two portions, one motor and one sensory. The sensory is larger. Both arise from the lower anterior part of the semilunar ganglion. The mandibular division emerges from the skull as one trunk through the foramen ovale to separate under cover of the external pterygoid muscle into the anterior, or motor, division and the posterior, or sensory, division.

The posterior division passes downward under the external pterygoid muscle, and after giving off the auriculotemporal and lingual branches, passes between the ramus and the sphenomandibular ligament to enter the mandibular foramen as the inferior alveolar nerve, where it advances to supply the posterior teeth including the first bicuspid. The incisive branch continues forward in the body of the mandible to supply the canine and incisor teeth, and the mental branch emerges from the foramen to supply the skin of the chin and mucous membrane of the lower lip.

The lingual branch, after receiving the chorda tympani segment from the facial nerve, passes inward and downward under the mucous membrane of the floor of the mouth to supply general sensation to the anterior two thirds of the tongue, the floor of the mouth, and mucosae on the lingual aspect of the teeth.

The buccinator (long buccal) nerve, the only sensory branch of the anterior, or motor, division, joins with the buccal branch of the seventh, or facial, nerve to form a plexus around the facial vein; it also sends branches to supply the mucous membrane of the cheek as far forward as the angle of the mouth and the skin of the cheek.

The anterior division gives off branches to the muscles of mastication (masseter, temporalis, internal and external pterygoids), and to the anterior belly of the digastric, the mylohyoid, the tensor palati, and the tensor tympani muscles.

Infraorbital Nerve Block

The purpose of the infraorbital injection is to block the efferent nerve impulses of the maxillary anterior teeth and the labial supporting structures at a point within the infraorbital canal where the anterior and middle superior alveolar nerves are given off from the infraorbital nerve, which is the terminal division of the maxillary nerve. The injection can be used to obtain profound anesthesia of the anterior teeth for any operative or surgical procedure. It is of special value in cases of acute infection, or in cases of deep curettement following endodontic procedures when an intraoral technique is contraindicated or may prove inadequate.

Although entrance into the infraorbital

foramen presents some difficulties by the intraoral technique, it becomes a relatively simple matter when approached through the surface of the skin. There are certain definite landmarks that make locating the infraorbital foramen a routine matter. By placing a straight edge on a skull, it will be noted that the supraorbital foramen or notch, the infraorbital foramen, and the mental foramen all lie in a straight line (Fig. 6-12A). The pupil of the eye of a patient looking straight forward also falls in this line (Fig. 6-12B).

The infraorbital surface of the maxillary bone presents a marked concavity. There are two important muscles in this area. The caninus muscle (levator anguli oris) originates from the deepest surface of the infraorbital foramen, and inserts into the angle of the mouth; the head of the quadratus labii superioris (levator labii superioris) originates from the inferior border of the orbit and inserts into the muscular substance of the upper lip.

The infraorbital foramen exits into the infraorbital fossa below the levator labii superioris and above the caninus muscle. The foramen is in line with the aforementioned anatomic landmarks and lies 3 to 5 mm. beneath the lower margin of the orbit. Palpation with the index finger may give the patient a feeling of dull pain when deep pressure is applied exactly over the foramen.

The external maxillary artery follows a tortuous path from the corner of the mouth to the ala of the nose where it turns upward to terminate along the side of the nose as the angular artery. This vessel lies below and medial to the infraorbital foramen. The anterior facial vein crosses the inferior margin of the orbit lateral to the foramen in an oblique direction from the inner angle of the eye.

The maxillary nerve is referred to as the infraorbital nerve after it enters the orbital cavity. Both the middle and anterior superior alveolar nerves branch from the infraorbital nerve to descend within the

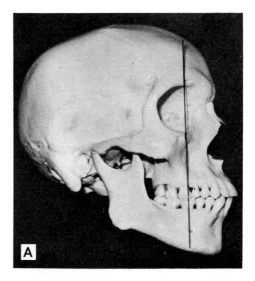

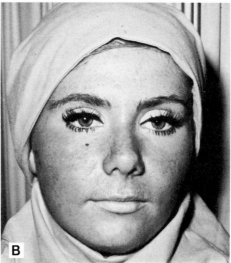

Fig. 6-12. (A) Skull showing relationship of foramina. (B) Facial view. Note relationship of pupil to dye mark over infraorbital foramen.

maxillary bone to supply the incisors, cuspid and bicuspid teeth, and their associated investing and supporting structures. The central incisor may demonstrate only partial anesthetization due to crossover fibers from the opposite side of the midline. Labial infiltration at the apex of this tooth will intercept these fibers, providing complete anesthesia.

Usually, a thin bony plate separates the orbital contents from the infraorbital canal. Since this is not always present, the needle should not penetrate more than 5 or 6 mm. into the canal. If some of the anesthetic solution enters the orbit, the unpleasant, though transient, symptoms of oculomotor paralysis and possible double vision will occur.

NERVES ANESTHETIZED
1. Infraorbital nerve.
2. Inferior palpebral, lateral nasal, and superior labial nerves.
3. Anterior and middle superior alveolar nerves.
4. Sometimes the posterior superior alveolar nerve.

AREAS ANESTHETIZED
1. The incisors and bicuspids together with the corresponding labial (buccal) alveolar plate and overlying soft tissues.
2. The upper lip, portions of the side of the nose, and the lower eyelid on the injection side.
3. At times, the maxillary molars and their buccal supporting structures.

ANATOMIC LANDMARKS
1. The pupil of the eye when the patient is looking straight forward.
2. The infraorbital ridge.
3. The infraorbital notch.
4. The infraorbital depression.
5. The supraorbital notch.

ARMAMENTARIUM
1. One $1\frac{5}{8}$-inch, 25-gauge needle.
2. One 5-cc. aspirating syringe.

3. Antiseptic solution for preparation of the skin.
4. Antiseptic dye for marking skin.
5. Sterile 4″ × 4″ sponges.
6. Local anesthetic, 2 cc.

PROCEDURE. Place the patient in the dental chair with his head, neck, and chest in a straight line. Tilt the chair back so that the maxillary occlusal plane is at a 45° angle to the floor and on a level with the operator's elbow.

Prepare the skin overlying the foramen with a suitable antiseptic agent. Then locate the infraorbital foramen by palpating the infraorbital ridge to the infraorbital notch. This should be directly below the pupil of the eye. Locate the infraorbital depression by moving the finger downward about 0.5 to 1 cm. The infraorbital foramen lies in this area, and its position on the face should be marked with skin-marking ink. Since the direction of the infraorbital canal is downward and medially, make another mark about $\frac{1}{4}$ inch below and $\frac{1}{4}$ inch medial to the foramen. Direct the needle upward and laterally so that its point contacts bone under the first mark, all the while keeping the needle under the palpating left index finger.

With a gentle probing motion, locate the foramen (Fig. 6-13). Advance the needle $\frac{1}{8}$ inch into the canal, and after aspirating, slowly inject 1 to 2 cc. of anesthetic solution. Then withdraw the syringe and apply pressure over the foramen. The upper lip should become numb as an indication of anesthesia.

While executing this block, the needle passes through the following structures:
1. Skin.
2. Subcutaneous tissue.
3. Levator labii superioris muscle.

Although there are many blood vessels in the immediate vicinity of the foramen, and the infraorbital artery and vein lie in the canal, the incidence of hematoma with subsequent ecchymosis is remarkably low.

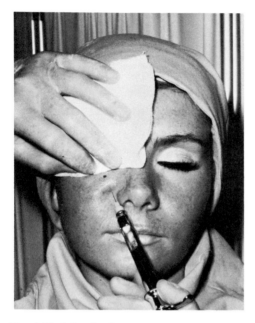

Fig. 6-13. Infraorbital nerve injection. Note gauze pad over eye and fingers held firmly against infraorbital rim.

Maxillary Nerve Block

The second, or maxillary, division of the fifth cranial nerve supplies the maxilla. The maxillary nerve leaves the skull through the foramen rotundum, crosses the upper part of the pterygopalatine fossa, and enters the orbit through the inferior orbital fissure. It follows the infraorbital groove in the superior surfaces of the maxilla to enter the infraorbital canal, terminating at the infraorbital foramen. The maxillary nerve trunk is therefore accessible and the pterygopalatine fossa can be approached by the extraoral method.

NERVES ANESTHETIZED
1. Two short sphenopalatine nerves to Meckel's, or the sphenopalatine, ganglion.

2. Pterygoid, pharyngeal, posterior palatine, middle palatine, anterior palatine, nasopalatine, and superior nasal nerves.
3. Posterior, middle, and anterior superior alveolar nerves.
4. Infraorbital nerve.

AREAS ANESTHETIZED
1. Anterior temporal and zygomatic regions.
2. Lower eyelid, side of nose, and upper lip.
3. Anterior cheek.
4. Maxillary teeth on side of injection.
5. Maxillary alveolar bone and investing structures.
6. Hard and soft palates.
7. Tonsils.
8. Part of pharynx.
9. Nasal septum and floor of nose.
10. Posterior lateral nasal mucosa and turbinate bones.
11. Maxillary sinus.

ANATOMIC LANDMARKS
1. The midpoint of the zygomatic arch (sigmoid notch).
2. The mandibular notch of the ramus of the mandible.
3. The lateral pterygoid plate.

ARMAMENTARIUM
1. One ¾-inch, 25-gauge needle for skin anesthesia.
2. One 8-cm., 22-gauge needle with stylette.
3. One 5-cc. aspirating syringe.
4. One metal centimeter rule.
5. Rubber or cork marker.
6. Other items same as for all extraoral procedures.

PROCEDURE. Strict aseptic technique should be followed for this procedure as

well as for all other extraoral block procedures.

Palpate the external bony landmark,
which is the sigmoid notch of the zygomatic arch (Fig. 6-14A). Have the patient
open and close his mouth as the operator
holds his finger in contact with the sigmoid notch—the operator should feel the
head of the condyle moving into the area.
Mark the depression below the inferior
surface of the zygomatic arch. Using a
25-gauge needle with accompanying syringe, make an insertion perpendicular to
the sagittal plane, which should pass
through the mandibular notch just inferior to the midpoint of the zygomatic arch.
A skin wheal is raised. Then place a
marker on an 8-cm. needle at the 4.5-cm.
position.

Using a pen grasp, insert the marked
needle through the skin wheal perpendicular to the median sagittal plane (skin
surface), and advance it slowly until it
contacts the lateral pterygoid plate. This
should occur before the marker reaches
the skin surface; never insert the needle
beyond the depth of the marker. Adjust
the marker so that it is 1 cm. from the
skin surface (Fig. 6-14B). Withdraw the
needle until only its point is in subcutaneous tissue. Redirect it anteriorly and superiorly so that it is pointed toward the apex
of the opposite orbit (Fig. 6-14C). The
point of the needle should now lie within
the pterygopalatine fossa. After aspiration, slowly inject 2 or 3 cc. of anesthetic
solution.

If bone is contacted prematurely, the
needle point is either still on the lateral
pterygoid plate or anterior to the pterygomaxillary fissure on the maxilla. Before
withdrawing the needle to redirect it, turn
the bevel toward each of these bones and

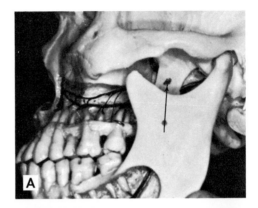

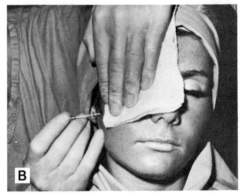

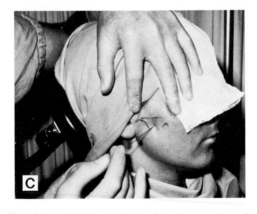

Fig. 6-14. (A) Skeletal relationship of ramus, lateral
pterygoid plate, and zygomatic arch. (B) Needle penetration to lateral pterygoid plate; marker adjusted to
1 cm. from skin surface. (C) Redirecting needle to
anesthetize the second division of the trigeminal
nerve.

exert slight pressure. If this is done, the needle may slide through the pterygomaxillary fissure and into the sphenopalatine fossa. Here, as always, aspiration should be carried out to ensure that a blood vessel has not been entered.

While executing the block, the needle passes through the following structures:

1. Skin.
2. Subcutaneous tissue.
3. Masseter muscle.
4. The mandibular notch.
5. The external pterygoid muscle.

While in contact with the lateral pterygoid plate, the needle approximates the following important structures:

1. Superiorly, the base of the skull.
2. The internal maxillary artery crosses inferiorly and curves up anteriorly to it, entering the lower part of the pterygomaxillary fissure.
3. Temporal vessels from the inferior maxillary artery may lie on either side of it.
4. Superficially, the transverse facial artery may lie above or below it.
5. Posteriorly, the foramen ovale, through which passes the mandibular nerve, and posterior to that, the foramen spinosum, through which passes the middle meningeal artery.
6. Anteriorly, the pterygomaxillary fissure, through which the needle may pass into the pterygopalatine fossa.

SYMPTOMS OF ANESTHESIA. The patient should feel tingling and numbness of the upper lip and side of the nose, and in some instances, anesthesia of the soft palate and pharynx. An accompanying gagging sensation may be experienced.

Both the maxillary nerve and the sphenopalatine ganglion are affected by this injection. Thus, there is complete anesthesia of the maxilla, including the palatal mucosa and the bone, as well as the walls and linings of the maxillary sinus on the side injected. This block,

therefore, is especially useful for operations involving the maxillary sinus or the bony structures of the palate.

Mandibular Block

The mandibular nerve leaves the skull through the foramen ovale, and after a course of 2 to 3 mm., divides into its various branches. It can therefore be anesthetized as it leaves the skull. The postcoronoid technique will be described.

NERVES ANESTHETIZED
1. Nerves of masseter, temporalis, internal and external pterygoids, anterior belly and digastric, mylohyoid, tensor palati, tensor tympani muscles.
2. Auriculotemporal nerve.
3. Lingual and long buccal nerves.
4. Inferior alveolar, mental, and incisive nerves.

AREAS ANESTHETIZED
1. Temporal region.
2. Auricle of the ear.
3. External auditory meatus.
4. Temporomandibular joint.
5. Salivary glands.
6. Anterior two thirds of the tongue.
7. Floor of the mouth.
8. Mandible.
9. Mandibular teeth and supporting structures to the midline.
10. Lower portion of the face (except at the angle of the jaw) and the lower lip.

ANATOMIC LANDMARKS. Identical to those for extraoral block of the maxillary nerve.

ARMAMENTARIUM. Same tray setup for maxillary nerve block.

PROCEDURE. The technique for blocking this nerve is identical to that for blocking the maxillary nerve up to the point where the needle contacts the lateral pterygoid plate. When this occurs, adjust the marker so that it is 1 cm. from the skin surface. Withdraw the needle until its point is in subcutaneous tissue only. Redirect it slightly posteriorly and superiorly and carefully insert it again until either the marker is flush with the skin (Fig. 6-15) or the point of the needle stimulates the mandibular nerve as evidenced by the patient's reaction. If bone is contacted prematurely, the needle is either still striking the lateral pterygoid plate or the base of the skull. If it does not slide into its proper position near the foramen ovale after exerting gentle pressure, check the needle position, withdraw, and repeat the procedure. When the needle is in place, carefully aspirate and then deposit the anesthetic solution.

The structures through which the needle passes and the structures adjacent to the needle when in contact with the lateral pterygoid plate are the same as those given in the maxillary nerve block.

Mental and Incisive Nerve Block

The mental and incisive block is the least called upon of the extraoral block approaches. However it may be useful when anesthesia of the mandibular teeth and the investing and supporting structures anterior to the mental foramen or lower lip is desired and a block of the inferior alveolar nerve is contraindicated.

NERVES ANESTHETIZED
1. Mental nerve.
2. Incisive nerve.

AREAS ANESTHETIZED
1. Skin of the chin.

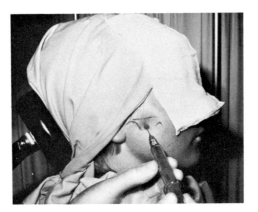

Fig. 6-15. Anesthetizing third division of the trigeminal nerve.

2. Skin and mucous membrane of the lower lip.
3. Canine and incisor teeth.

ANATOMIC LANDMARKS
1. Supraorbital notch.
2. Infraorbital notch.
3. Pupil of the eye when the patient is looking straight forward.
4. Lower border of the mandible.
5. Bicuspid teeth.

ARMAMENTARIUM. The same tray setup as for the infraorbital block.

PROCEDURE. To locate the mental foramen, the patient should first have his mouth closed and be looking straight forward. Draw an imaginary line through the supraorbital notch, the pupil of the eye, and the infraorbital notch. An extension of this line downward should pass through the mental foramen. Estimate a point on this line midway between the lower border of the mandible and the gingival margin and mark it with a dye. This point should lie over the mental foramen. If the lower teeth are present, the mental foramen should be located directly below the second bicuspid. Make a second point ¼ inch above and ¼ inch behind the first, since the mental foramen opens distally and superiorly. Make a skin wheal at this point using the 25-gauge needle. Then insert the needle with the syringe through

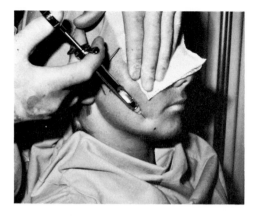

Fig. 6-16. Anesthetizing the mental nerve through the mental foramen.

the skin wheal and direct it downward, anteriorly, and medially until it contacts bone under the first mark. With a gentle probing motion, locate the foramen, enter, and after aspirating, deposit 1 to 2 cc. of anesthetic solution (Fig. 6-16).

While the block is carried out the needle passes through the following structures:

1. Skin.
2. Subcutaneous tissue.
3. Triangularis (depressor anguli oris muscle).

Complications of Extraoral Blocks

PARALYSIS OF BRANCHES OF FACIAL NERVE. This may be due to an excessive amount of anesthetic solution, or to some solution escaping the needle as it is being inserted or withdrawn. It is of no consequence and will resolve as the block dissipates.

NEEDLE POINT ENTERING THE ORBITAL CAVITY. This should not occur if the operator had used a marker as directed in the case of the maxillary nerve block, or if the needle did not enter the infraorbital foramen more than $\frac{1}{8}$ inch in the case of the infraorbital block. If the patient complains of pain in the eye, stop the injection and check the needle position. If some solution has entered the orbit of the eye,

as already mentioned, temporary loss of vision or diplopia may result but will be relieved as the anesthetic solution dissipates. Hemorrhage into the orbit, however, might be serious and the patient should be examined by an ophthalmologist.

SWELLING OF THE TISSUES AROUND THE ORBIT. If caused by the anesthetic solution, this may be prevented or reduced by exerting firm digital pressure on the infraorbital ridge during injection.

INTRADURAL INJECTION. This is extremely rare, and is managed as if a high spinal anesthetic had occurred. The treatment is supportive in nature; respiration and circulation may have to be artificially and pharmacologically maintained until the solution dissipates.

References

1. Manual of Local Anesthesia in General Dentistry. New York, Cook-Waite Laboratories, Inc., 1947.
2. Braun, H.: The influence of the vitality of the tissues on local and general toxic effects of anaesthetics and the importance of adrenal chloride for local anaesthesia. Brit. J. Dent. Sci., 46:681–685, 1903.
3. Thompson, R. D.: Extra-oral nerve blocks. Anes. Prog., 15:65–68, March, 1968.
4. Topazian, R. G., and Simon, G. T.: Extraoral mandibular and maxillary block techniques. Oral Surg., Oral Med., Oral Path., 15:296–299, 1963.
5. Shapiro, H. H.: Maxillofacial Anatomy. Philadelphia, J. B. Lippincott Co., 1954.
6. Monheim, L. M.: Local Anesthesia and Pain Control in Dental Practice, 4th ed. St. Louis, C. V. Mosby Co., 1969.
7. Archer, W. H.: A Manual of Dental Anesthesia, 2nd ed. Philadelphia, W. B. Saunders Co., 1958.

7 Office Emergencies

MYER S. LEONARD

Webster's Dictionary defines emergency as "an unforeseen combination of circumstances that calls for immediate action, sudden bodily alteration, such as is likely to require immediate medical attention." This chapter discusses those circumstances that may occur in the dental office and their management. Examination of the first part of the definition of emergency offered by Webster provides the clue as to what is probably the best way of minimizing the frequency of emergencies in the office—an adequate medical history. If a patient tells you that he is allergic to certain drugs, it is important to ask him about his previous experience with those drugs. Many patients confuse the word "allergy" with "side effects." This is perfectly understandable, as the former word is widely used by laymen, whereas it also has a specific or technical meaning for the clinician.

It is the commendable practice of many dentists to take a full medical history from their patients when the patients first visit their office, and it should be updated every six months. One must not forget that people grow older and may suffer illnesses with a bearing on their dental treatment which they did not have a year or more earlier.

Syncope

Syncope is a frequent and potentially hazardous emergency that occurs in dental practice. The normal blood pressure (BP) is 120/80 mm. Hg in healthy young people. The function of the heart is obviously to pump blood, and that it could adequately do at a much lower pressure. There are three principal reasons for the BP being 120/80 mm. Hg. The first reason is that a lower systolic pressure could not maintain an adequate filtration pressure to the kidney, resulting in renal shutdown—a most serious condition occurring at a systolic pressure of less than 60 mm. Hg. The second reason is to maintain a blood supply to the heart muscle itself. The coronary arteries have to force blood through cardiac muscle which is contracted during systolic contraction. The last reason is because without a hydrostatic pressure of at least 100 mm. Hg (at heart level) the upright posture cannot be maintained. This appears to be a failsafe mechanism, whereby a fall in pressure to the brain brings about collapse and the patient falls to the ground. In the horizontal position, flow is more easily achieved and cerebral ischemia avoided. The deleterious effects of cerebral ische-

82

mia are well known; epileptic-like seizures may be followed by coma and severe cerebral damage due to the hypoxia which occurs following cessation of flow.

Males suffer from syncope more frequently than females, and a recent paper showed that the incidence of fainting increased the longer the patient had been without nourishment.[1]

Typically, the patient tells the dentist that he is feeling faint. But the astute dentist looks at his patient frequently and does not allow himself to have "tunnel vision," just focusing on the cavity preparation and forgetting or becoming oblivious to everything or everyone about him. Whether it be the clinical order of the surgery, the thought or sight of the instruments, or the apprehension he suffers, the patient becomes pale, sweaty, yawns, complains of feeling sick, and then loses consciousness. The explanation for the condition is not known with certainty, but it is frequently described as a vasovagal attack. This means that the parasympathetic (vagal) nerves to the heart and the vasodilator nerves to the muscles have been stimulated, thus slowing the heart and dilating the skeletal vessels, which lowers the venous return and the cardiac output, and therefore the blood pressure. It is so common that treatment is instituted before confirmatory signs are elicited. The patient lies motionless and is quite pale, with low blood pressure, faint pulse, commonly a few clonic jerks of the limbs and shallow respiration.

Recovery is prompt if the correct steps are taken. First, tilt the chair back so that the patient is in a horizontal (Trendelenburg's) position, the head being level with the heart. The legs should be raised to a level slightly above that of the heart to improve the venous return. The loosening of tight clothing (collar, belt, and the like) will make the patient feel much better at once. The administration of odoriferous stimulants, for example ammonia, is often advocated, but I have often observed that

when the stimulant is removed, the patient frequently lapses back to "feeling faint." The administration of a cold pack to the forehead, face, and back of the neck—even allowing some cold water to run down the back—is remarkably stimulatory. If the patient has been without food for several hours, he will feel better after a drink of 50 g. of flavorless dextrose in water.

That adequate tissue perfusion is present in the supine syncopal patient can be shown by vigorously rubbing the patient's ear. If the ear becomes pink and flushed, it indicates that no hypoxia is present, and a rapid capillary refill with pink blood after a short compression indicates adequate tissue perfusion. One can assume that if the ear is being adequately perfused then the brain is. In dark-skinned people, this sign (in addition to that of pallor) is nondetectable, thus examination of the nail beds is advocated.

Angina Pectoris

Less common than syncope is an anginal attack. Angina pectoris is a clinical syndrome characterized by paroxysmal attacks of chest pain, usually substernal or precordial, exacerbated by physical or emotional stress and ameliorated by rest.

Seventy-five per cent of these patients are males in the fifth or sixth decade. Typically, the pain is described as a tightening or squeezing of the chest; it often radiates down the left arm and may radiate to the left jaw and simulate toothache. It lasts 5 to 10 minutes after the patient has rested. The cause of the pain is unknown, but is thought to be due to release of lactic acid, histamine, and related kinins by ischemic cardiac muscle. These substances are not removed rapidly enough and stimulate the pain endings in cardiac muscle, which are conducted by way of the sympathetic nervous system.

Treatment is to place a fresh 0.5 mg. tablet of glyceryl trinitrate under the patient's tongue. It is absorbed rapidly and brings relief from pain within 2 to 3 minutes. For many years, it was thought that this and similar drugs produced dilatation of the coronary arteries, but now the notion of these calcified and atherosclerotic vessels being capable of dilatation is rejected. The present theory is that the drug produces a generalized systemic arterial dilatation, thus lowering blood pressure, venous return, and cardiac output. This generalized arterial dilatation is responsible for the headaches, flushing, and occasional reflex tachycardia that follow their use.

Alternatively, an ampule of amyl nitrite is broken and the patient inhales the vapors. This produces more headaches than glyceryl trinitrate, and thus it is not so pleasant. The patient who becomes anxious and stressed is best placed in a semirecumbent position, oxygen should be administered, and the dental treatment is discontinued. Glyceryl trinitrate can be taken in anticipation of stress when a patient may imbibe it prior to dental treatment. Of course, mild sedation of the patient with 5 mg. diazepam prior to treatment is also of great benefit. There are no physical signs of angina pectoris and an electrocardiogram cannot rule out the diagnosis.

Myocardial Infarction

Myocardial infarction is the result of a sudden, severe arterial insufficiency to the heart. Classically this is an affliction of obese or heavily built individuals, almost always overweight, more commonly in men in the fourth and later decades of life than in women. For many years, the cause of this condition was held to be due to a thrombus or embolus forming from or in an atheromatous plaque in a coronary vessel subsequently blocking the vessel, which resulted in ischemia and necrosis of the muscle distal to the point of infarction. This view is no longer ubiquitously held, because thrombi were often *not* found at autopsies of patients who died rapidly after infarction but, as the interval between attack and death increased, so the incidence of coronary thrombosis found at autopsy increased.

Thus, the hypothesis has been presented that the myocardial necrosis occurs first followed by the thrombosis of the coronary vessels. The reason for the necrosis is not known, but those who agree with this hypothesis suggest that the underlying atherosclerosis of the vessels, the hypoxic state of the muscle, and the stagnating flow of the blood, all combine to cause a necrosis with subsequent thrombosis.

The patient who suffers a myocardial infarction in the office presents a challenge to the clinical abilities of the dentist and his assistants. The patient's first complaint is pain—severe, "squeezing, crushing, or heavy pain"—midsternal, occasionally radiating to the arm. The pain is not relieved by rest or nitrates and is often accompanied by belching with a feeling of acute indigestion. The patient looks pale, ashen gray, sweaty, and anxious, and feels nauseous. The patient's blood pressure falls, and he may die.

All dental treatment should cease. The patient is best placed in the semirecumbent position (45° position), since this is often the most comfortable. The oxygen mask is placed and oxygen is given at 4 to 5 liters per minute. If morphine is available, 10 mg. (combined with 25 mg. chlorpromazine as an anti-emetic) or 50 mg. meperidine (Demerol) are administered intramuscularly.* Some authorities advocate administration of 100 mg. hydrocortisone intramuscularly, and others advocate a vasopressor or 30 mg. (2 ml.) mephentermine intramuscularly as well. The patient must be transferred to a coronary care unit and the faster this is done, the better the prognosis.

Cardiac Arrest

When the heart ceases to pump blood, it has arrested. The failure to supply the brain with oxygen leads rapidly to death of the most oxygen-sensitive cells first and these are usually concerned with the "higher centers" (e.g., intellectual ability and memory). It is not surprising that some persons who have sustained periods of cerebral anoxia and been resuscitated are left vegetative. The lack of oxygen leads to incomplete metabolism of glucose by way of pyruvic acid in the citric acid cycle of Krebs. Accumulated pyruvic acid is thus metabolized to lactic acid and other ketone acids, which lower the pH of the blood (and cells) with subsequent necrosis (death) of the cells. Thus, one can see at once that the hallmark of successful treatment will be prompt diagnosis, followed by cardiac massage to prime the pump, artificial respiration to help deliver oxygen (the lungs rapidly cease to function after the heart has arrested), and alkaline solutions to counteract the acidosis. After five minutes or less of hypoxia brain damage occurs and after ten minutes, severe damage ensues. After the brain, the organs most susceptible to hypoxia are the adrenal glands, the liver, and the kidneys.

---

* All dosages are based on average-sized people. Recommended drugs and their dosages often change with the passage of time. Thus it is the responsibility of the clinician to be aware of these changes.

Cardiac arrest may follow a myocardial infarct or it may follow the most simple and benign maneuver (e.g., injection of local anesthetic). Sudden loss of consciousness, absence of radial and carotid pulses, dilating and nonreacting pupils, gasping respirations, and cessation of the blood flow, the blood becoming dark and tarry, are the signs of arrest.

The heart may be in asystole or in ventricular fibrillation; it is impossible to diagnose which without the aid of an electrocardiogram because there are no heart sounds or pulse with either condition. Many persons are of the opinion that the majority of arrests in patients in the dental office are due to ventricular fibrillation. The treatment of fibrillation is to defibrillate the heart, a maneuver which obviously cannot be done in the office. A maneuver that can be performed and is often efficacious (whether the arrest is due to ventricular fibrillation or arrest) is to give the midportion of the sternum a sharp, quick blow from 12 to 18 inches away, with the fleshy, or ulnar, part of the fist.

If there is no response after a couple of blows, then cardiopulmonary resuscitation is started. This procedure is described and illustrated in many texts, but personal practical illustrations using "Resusciann" or similar models are the only way one can discover such things as how much pressure is to be applied to the sternum and how effective one is at artificial respiration. There are not many steps but they should be done in the following order: (1) airway, (2) breathing, (3) circulation, and (4) drugs; thus the mnemonic ABCD.

Once cardiac arrest is suspected, a firm blow to the chest as described previously is thought to be a worthwhile procedure, then the patient must be laid on either the floor or a board. The usual dental chair is too soft to offer sufficient resistance to the chest when it is being compressed during cardiac massage, thus rendering the whole effort useless. Once the patient is on the floor, the mouth is swept clear of debris or dentures, a hand is placed beneath the neck in order to tilt back the head, the nose is pinched, and three deep expirations are made into the mouth (Fig. 7-1). There are special tubes which allow a more aesthetic approach to this situation, but time and efficiency must not be sacrificed (Fig. 7-2).

Effective cardiac compression requires sufficient pressure to depress the sternum 3 to 5 cm. This compresses the heart against the spine and thus squeezes blood out of the heart in a jet. Therefore, one can see the need for a firm surface beneath the spine. The pressure achieved is

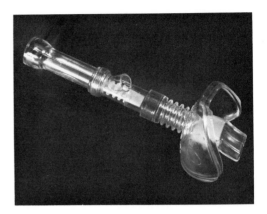

Fig. 7-2. Brook airway (Woodlets, Buffalo. N.Y.).

usually about 80 to 100 mm. Hg. One hand is placed cephalad to the xiphoid process, the other is placed with the heel (thenar eminence) on the back of the first hand, and then downward, short, firm compressions are made. The rate is 60 to 80 times a minute. If working alone, one stops every 15 compressions to inflate the lungs two or three times and then resumes the cardiac massage. If assistance is at hand, then ventilation is 15 times per minute without stopping the cardiac massage (Fig. 7-3).

If available, oxygen can be administered under pressure 15 to 20 times per minute. If the equipment is at hand, a nasoendotracheal tube can be passed, but unless the operator is expeditous and accomplished, he would be better advised to proceed with mouth-to-mouth respiration. Similarly, in the absence of oxygen, an AMBU bag is useful.

That one's efforts are successful is shown by (1) improved color of the face, (2) the presence of carotid or femoral pulse, (3) pupils responding to light, and (4) resumption of respiration.

In a hospital, there are numerous peo-

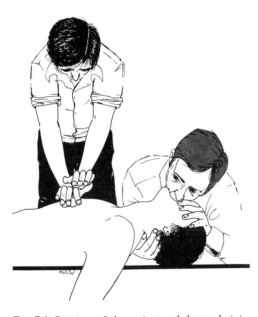

Fig. 7-1. Positions of the patient and those administering resuscitation.

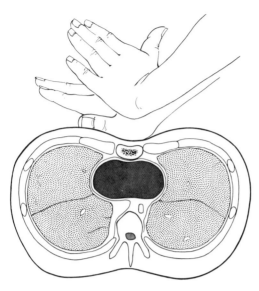

Fig. 7-3. Cardiac compression.

ple on hand, each able to carry out some act that will help resuscitate the patient. In the office, help is more limited, nevertheless, after one minute or less an intravenous injection of sodium bicarbonate is needed to counteract the acidosis which is almost inevitable. Most bottles of sodium bicarbonate carry 44 mEq./L. and two bottles (approximately 1 mEq./kg. body weight) at least should be injected. It is probably wise to defer further injections until blood gases have been measured on arrival at the hospital. Putting up an intravenous saline or dextrose solution drip is even better, because it maintains the vein open and affords ready access for intravenous drugs.

Resuscitory efforts should be maintained for at least 15 to 20 minutes or until a medical practitioner pronounces the patient dead.

Respiratory Obstruction

Modern dentistry is frequently performed on the supine patient. The only sure way not to risk any materials (e.g., root canal reamers, inlays, crowns, and the like) from falling into the pharynx and being inhaled or swallowed is to use the rubber dam or a gauze curtain (p. 128). If an object falls into the back of the pharynx, it is sometimes possible to remove it carefully by use of either suction or a toothed instrument.

If the object catches in the valleculae, a spasm of coughing and choking immediately occurs. This may dislodge the object into the mouth or it may be swallowed. The chair immediately should be placed upright and the patient bent forward and thumped vigorously on the back. This may assist in propelling the object out of the pharynx. The Heimlich maneuver can also be performed. The patient is held from behind with the operator's hands firmly clasped below the patient's xiphoid process, then two or three vigorous thrusts are made into the abdomen, which usually succeeds in dislodging the object (Fig. 7-4).

If an object is inhaled, it will usually slip into the right bronchus. Respiratory embarrassment, stridor, cyanosis, and indrawing of the chest wall are the obvious signs, and there will be pain in the chest. The violence of the respiratory efforts is not so great as in complete block, but immediate transfer to hospital for x-ray examination and possible bronchoscopy is strongly advised.

The object, however, may block at the cords; violent but ineffective respiratory efforts occur with increasing cyanosis. Unrelieved, this can proceed to coma and the patient chokes to death in 10 to 15 minutes. Few dentists would undertake tracheostomy in the office. However, a cricothyroidotomy is not so hazardous and can be performed with a wide (30-gauge) needle pushed between the thyroid and cricoid cartilages and kept in place. A

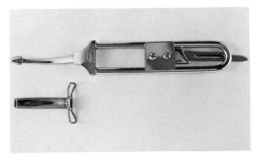

Fig. 7-5. Cawthorne knife (Down Brothers, Niagara Falls, N.Y.).

Hyperventilation

Some patients become acutely distressed in the dental chair and begin to hyperventilate. This means that they breathe rapidly and deeply and, therefore, exhale considerable volumes of carbon dioxide (CO_2). Normally, the pressure of carbon dioxide in solution in the blood is 40 mm. Hg. But if hyperventilation occurs, some of this CO_2 moves out of the blood and into the lungs and is exhaled, thus lowering the tension of CO_2 (or partial pressure of the gas in blood). Normally, the pH of the blood is finely balanced at about 7.4. The balance is between carbon dioxide levels on the one hand, and sodium bicarbonate levels on the other. The lowering of the CO_2 tension obviously swings the pH upward because now proportionately more bicarbonate is present. The plasma proteins (Pr) also contribute to maintenance of pH by buffering hydrogen (H) ions as HPr. In an alkaline medium, this acid dissociates to H^+ and Pr^+ ions in an attempt to prevent the pH rising too far. But calcium (Ca) ions have an affinity for protein ions in an alkaline medium, thus CaPr results which lowers the level of circulatory Ca ions. Calcium ions have an important, but as yet incompletely understood role in neuromuscular stability, and when the level of calcium ions drops, this stability is lost and the muscles contract, producing tetany.

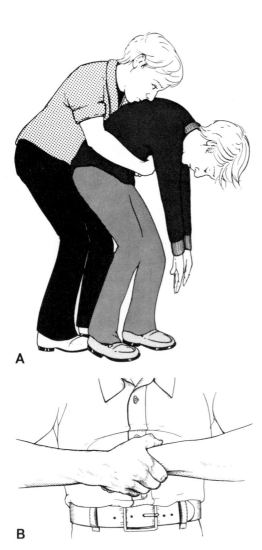

Fig. 7-4. Heimlich maneuver. (A) Positions of patient and person performing maneuver. (B) Position of hands on patient.

hissing sound will occur once the needle is correctly placed. Better than a needle is a Cawthorne knife (Fig. 7-5).

Obviously, after the patient is in a hospital, an elective tracheostomy must be performed.

It is obvious, therefore, that the treatment of the hyperventilating patient is to make him breathe into a paper bag or hold his breath for a minute or so, thus the inspired air will contain high levels of carbon dioxide and the normal pH will be maintained. If tetany occurs, 10 ml. calcium gluconate administered intravenously will rectify the problem.

Asthma

Asthma is a respiratory disease characterized by paroxysms of dyspnea and wheezing due to temporary narrowing of the bronchi by muscular spasm, mucosal swelling, or viscid secretion. Asthmatics have difficulty in expiring, not inspiring. Asthma may be due to allergies to dust, pollens, and the like, but in the dental office, it is usually psychogenic in origin. The patient usually has a history of the condition and it is more common in those who suffered from infantile eczema.

The patient feels an attack commencing, and it proceeds with astonishing rapidity to a distressful and alarming state. As the attack develops, the chair is tilted upright and the patient allowed to adopt the most comfortable position for him and permitted to take his own tablets or inhalant. If he does not have them or they have not helped, oxygen is administered and 0.5 ml. 1:1000 epinephrine (Adrenalin) is injected subcutaneously, which requires a couple of minutes to take effect. If there is no response, 10 ml. (250 mg.) aminophylline is injected intravenously over a 10-minute period. This will alleviate virtually all asthmatic attacks in the office. If these measures fail, the patient is in status asthmaticus and should be transferred to a hospital. Hydrocortisone hemisuccinate (100 mg.) is given intravenously prior to going, and oxygen (40 per cent) is administered on the way. Further management includes ventilatory assistance and steroids.

Hypoglycemia

The normal blood sugar level is 80 to 100 mg. in the fasting patient. Glucose is stored in the liver and also in the muscles as glycogen. (Glucose commonly is called sugar, but this is not correct. Glucose is dextrose; sugar is sucrose and before being available as glucose, must be metabolized in the liver.) Glycogen from the liver can be rapidly metabolized to glucose and released into the blood stream, thus raising the blood sugar level if the latter falls. Glucose is essentially the only source of energy that we have, and the cells are dependent on it in order to perform their functions as well as to maintain the life of the cell. The brain, which utilizes glucose at a considerable rate, has no way in which it can store glucose and thus lives a "hand-to-mouth" existence. A depletion of the level to 60 mg.% or less provokes symptoms of hypoglycemia—yawning, twitching of the limbs, profound hunger, faintness, nausea, and a feeling of weakness. As the level becomes lower (40 mg.%), confusion and disorientation with convulsions may occur. It is obvious, therefore, that the homeostatic mechanisms controlling blood glucose level are finely tuned and important. Insulin is the hormone that lowers the blood glucose; among those that tend to make the level rise are growth hormone, epinephrine, corticosteroids, and glucogon.

The diabetic patient is usually on a regimen which directs him to inject himself with insulin (or take an oral antidiabetic drug) each morning after breakfast. In this way, high postprandial blood glucose levels will be prevented and the patient will not exceed the capacity of his kidneys to retain all the glucose, meaning that he will not urinate it, as this, apart from other deleterious effects (e.g. polyuria), would simply be a waste of energy. Thus, if the patient takes the insulin but omits the meal, he can depress the glucose level precipitously. Again, the presence of infection (e.g., an abscessed tooth or extensive periodontal disease) can similarly provoke hypoglycemia, as may excessive exercise.

It is obvious, therefore, that if one has a full medical history of a patient, one is aware of this problem and can check on it before commencing treatment, which is best scheduled for mornings. The quickest and best treatment for hypoglycemia is 50 g. unsweetened dextrose in water. This is glucose and hence is available at once without prior metabolism in the liver. It should be unsweetened, because the sweetened form can be quite nauseous to some people.

An attack of hypoglycemia gives one warning so that an unconscious state occurring in the dental office should be an infrequent event. If it does occur, 20 to 40 ml. of 50% dextrose solution should be given intravenously. If this is not available, 0.5 ml. 1:1000 epinephrine administered subcutaneously will accelerate the metabolism of glycogen to glucose in the liver.

In patients who have failed to take their insulin, a hyperglycemic coma may occur. This is so different in onset and appearance from an attack of hypoglycemia, coupled with the fact that such a patient has been ill for several days, that confusion between these two conditions should not occur. The moist skin and tongue of a quietly breathing normotensive patient with hypoglycemia should not be confused with the dry-skinned, dry-tongued, hypotensive patient who is in hyperglycemic coma.

Anaphylaxis

The term "anaphylaxis" was first used in the early years of this century by two of the great immunologists, Richet and Portier. It means "against protection" (Gr. ana = against; phylaxis = protection), and was used by Richet and Portier to describe events that are the antithesis of immunity.

When one thinks of anaphylaxis in the context of the dental office, one thinks of the acute variety which presents with angioneurotic edema and respiratory collapse, and is a life-threatening event. Usually, it follows a penicillin injection or the administration of some other drug. Previous exposure to the drug is usually the cause but is not absolutely necessary.

Following the injection of the drug into a susceptible patient, there appears to be an interaction between the drug (antigen) and immunoglobulins (type E) on the surface of mast cells and basophils. This results in the release of chemical mediators which act on selected organs, primarily pulmonary and vascular in humans. Why these particular systems are selected is not known. The chemical mediators are (1) histamine, which provokes bronchial constriction, increased capillary permeability, and vasodilation; (2) SRS (slow-reacting substance of anaphylaxis), which is a powerful bronchoconstrictor and is not responsive to antihistamines; and (3) bradykinin, which provokes further vasodilation and increased capillary permeability.

The initial symptoms occur within seconds to minutes, and thus the patient must be observed for 20 minutes or so after he has received penicillin or other agents.

The reactions can be grouped as follows:

Eye: Lacrimation, ocular itching, conjunctivitis.
Nose: Sneezing, rhinorrhea, nasal congestion.
Respiratory: Laryngeal edema, dyspnea, stridor, wheezing (asthma).
Cardiovascular: Weak, thready, low-volume pulse; hypotension; cyanosis; syncope; cardiac arrest.
Gastrointestinal: Nausea, vomiting, diarrhea.

At one time, antihistamines were advocated as the first line of therapeutic attack, but contemporary expert advice is to administer 0.5 cc. 1:1000 epinephrine (Adrenalin), either squirted on the floor of the mouth or given intramuscularly (collapse of the peripheral circulation would impair the efficiency of subcutaneous administration). The patient is laid flat and his legs are elevated; antihistamine (50 mg. Benadryl, intravenously over a 2-minute period) is injected. If cardiac arrest has occurred, then the regimen described previously should be followed. Bronchospasm recalcitrant to epinephrine can be treated by 10 ml. (250 mg.) aminophylline administered intravenously over a 10-minute period.

The hypotensive state will almost always be rectified by the adoption of the supine position with legs elevated (Trendelenburg's position), and after 10 minutes epinephrine may be given and repeated at 10- to 20-minute intervals. Some authorities prefer to administer a vasopressor such as metaraminol bitartrate (Aramine),

2 to 10 mg. intramuscularly or 0.15 to 3 mg. intravenously.

It is interesting to note that steroids are no longer in the upper hierarchy of recommended drugs. This is because their effects are not seen for 30 to 90 minutes although they may be administered after the immediate crisis has been overcome (hydrocortisone hemisuccinate, 100 mg. intravenously).

Attention to the airway must also receive regard. Dentures must be removed and suction used to remove vomit. An airway is inserted and either artificial respiration given or an AMBU bag used. The nose must be pinched, otherwise the air will escape. If epinephrine has not ameliorated the pharyngeal edema, a cricothyroidotomy should be performed.

Most drug reactions, particularly those of drugs absorbed by digestion, are cutaneous in form and easily managed with an antihistamine cream or elixir. The reactions may occur several days after administration and the pathophysiology of their mechanism is different from other reactions.

Many patients report an allergy to lidocaine or other local anesthetics, but this is quite rare. Eyre and Nally described a simple technique of testing for local anesthetic sensitivity.[2] Five drops of the suspected allergen were placed on the nasal mucosa within one nostril. Although results of skin patch tests had been negative, in the event of an allergy, gross mucosal swelling and erythema occurred, resulting in unilateral nasal blocking. Epinephrine nasal drops rapidly reduced the swelling, leaving no tissue damage.

The one way to minimize the chance of an anaphylactic episode occurring in the office is to take a good history from the patient. Particular attention must be paid to a history of eczema, hayfever, or asthma, since drug reactions are more frequent in patients with these disorders.

Epilepsy

The fundamental pathophysiology of epilepsy is not known, but there is a recurrent disturbance of the central nervous system manifested by fits and loss of consciousness. There are several varieties, but the only one which presents as an emergency is grand mal, or "generalized seizures."

There is a stereotyped pattern to epilepsy and the patients recognize it but are unable to do much about it. The prodromal phase, marked by change of mood, lasts several hours. It is followed by the aura, a brief feeling that the fit is coming. In the tonic phase, in which consciousness is lost, the patient falls to the ground and may do himself severe injury. After 30 seconds, the tonic phase gives way to the clonic phase of sustained jerking movements of the face and body, and it is in this phase that the tongue may be bitten. This phase lasts a minute or so, and then a stage of relaxation ensues, a placid comatose state of sleep lasting a short period or several hours.

Once the attack has started, there is no way of abating it. The main aim of anyone present must be to prevent the patient from injuring himself, and so he must be moved away from electrical appliances and any dangerous objects. Protecting the tongue is difficult. If a wooden tongue blade or a rubber cup can be placed between the teeth to prevent this mishap, so much the better, but it must be done during or prior to the tonic phase.

If one fit follows another without the patient's regaining consciousness, then status epilepticus is diagnosed and this condition may be fatal. An intravenous injection of 10 to 20 mg. diazepam is given slowly until the fit stops.

Again, it is prudent to note that in patients with a history of epilepsy, dental treatment may provoke an attack, hence it is best to have a small mouth prop in place during treatment of these patients.

Adrenocortical Insufficiency (Addisonian Crisis)

The adrenal glands secrete cortisone and hydrocortisone as well as aldosterone and the sex hormones. The function of these hormones is to maintain electrolyte and water homeostasis, to sustain the blood pressure, to promote metabolism of carbohydrate, fat, and proteins, to make an important contribution to the homeostasis of blood sugar, and to play an important role in the body's ability to withstand stress. Some of the different stresses that increase cortical release are trauma, pain, apprehension, fear, intense heat or cold, surgery, and debilitating illnesses. The control of the level of secretion of the cortisol is by way of the hypothalamic-pituitary axis and is more subtle than was once thought. The normal amount of cortisol secreted per day is 12 to 20 mg. In a stressful situation, this amount increases 2- or 3-fold. Patients may be unable to secrete cortisol for one of three reasons.

1. Primary atrophy of the adrenal gland, at one time tuberculosis was the principal cause of this condition, but now an autoimmune mechanism is held to be the cause.
2. Secondary atrophy, defined as a failure of the pituitary gland, thus ACTH is not secreted.
3. Steroids (prednisone or prednisolone) are prescribed in many conditions because they suppress the inflammatory

component of the condition. Such diseases include ulcerative colitis and Crohn's disease, rheumatoid arthritis, systemic lupus erythematosus. Steroids are used in the treatment of leukemias and in conjunction with cytotoxic drugs in the treatment of malignant disease. The doses used exceed the 12 to 20 mg. normal daily output and lead to suppression of ACTH secretion and atrophy of the adrenal gland.

The consequence of these three causes of adrenal gland atrophy is that when a stressful situation occurs and supplemen-

tary cortisol would be secreted, the gland is unable to respond and an adrenocortical, or addisonian, crisis ensues.

A patient with adrenocortical insufficiency will, therefore, need supplementary steroids prior to his dental treatment, although they are usually only prescribed for exodontia or extensive periodontal surgery. Supplements are usually prescribed if the patient has been on a course of steroids of two months' duration within the previous two years. The usual regimen is to double the patient's daily dose the day before, the day of, and the day after the procedure, and then reduce it to 1.5

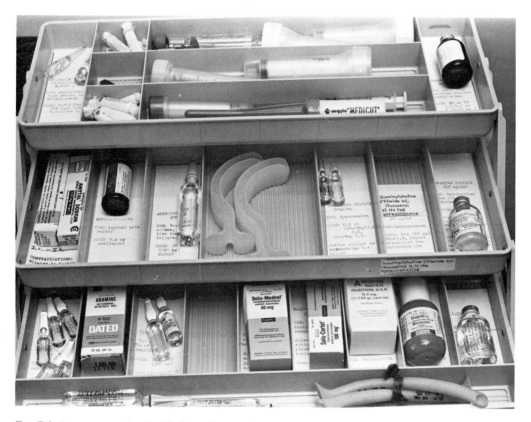

Fig. 7-6. An emergency kit should always be available in the dental office.

times the daily dose and then return to the normal dose.

An addisonian crisis can be circumvented by taking a good medical history. In the event that one does occur, the patient complains of headache, lassitude, nausea, and renal pains, and he has a low blood pressure and tachycardia. The treatment is to inject 100 mg. hydrocortisone succinate intravenously and transfer the patient to the hospital where the dosage may be repeated within several hours. Antibiotics are also usually prescribed.

This condition is not easy to diagnose and will only come to mind if the patient is known to suffer from adrenocortical insufficiency.

Summary

Despite what is often believed and espoused, most people have poor memories and are inept at that which they do rarely.

Only frequent rehearsals, about once a month, will ensure that not only the dentist but also his assistants are familiar with the office procedures in the event of an emergency. When designing a surgery, it is prudent to ask oneself, "If I collapse, can they get a stretcher in here and is there room and facilities for people to come to my aid?" If that question can be answered affirmatively, there is probably room enough to help someone else!

An emergency kit with medicaments and materials should always be available in the same place and updated once a month and after use (Fig. 7-6). Be sure your staff can carry out resuscitative maneuvers for cardiac arrest. "If you are the only person in the office who knows how to handle an emergency situation, and you are the victim, well it is your funeral"![3]

References

1. Muir, V. M. J., Leonard, M. S., and Haddaway, E.: Morbidity following dental extraction. Anaesthesia, 31:171, 1976.
2. Eyre, J. and Nally, F. F.: Nasal test for hypersensitivity. Lancet, 1:264, 1971.
3. Malamed, S.: Emergencies. Dental Management, August, 1976, p. 32.

8 Principles Involved in the Extraction of Teeth and the Flap Operation

DANIEL E. WAITE

General Considerations

Halstead stated: "the surgeon should use his head as well as his hands." Certainly this is especially true in operating in and around the oral cavity. The removal of teeth has a remarkable psychologic influence on the patient. Women, particularly, view the loss of teeth as a serious disfigurement. Teeth reflect personality and individuality. Their removal, regardless of the reason, often inflicts embarrassment and produces varying degrees of psychologic adjustment. The removal of teeth can be ominous to the patient.

The most important principle involved in the removal of teeth is to know the indications for extraction. One basic indication is specific disease of the teeth and periodontium, primarily caries and/or periodontal disease (Fig. 8-1). Because both conditions are controlled much better today, they are less frequently an indication for extraction than previously. Another indication for the extraction of teeth is to prepare tissues in which teeth are directly involved for irradiation to control a malignancy[1] (see also Chap. 21). While the evidence favoring extraction may be debatable in some cases, in others the teeth are sufficiently involved with the tumor and within the line of radiation that they must be removed (Fig. 8-2). In instances of trauma, the blood supply may be sufficiently embarrassed or the supporting structures sufficiently injured that extraction may be indicated (Fig. 8-3). Impacted teeth are another indication for removal, and may require special surgical techniques and manipulation (see Chap. 11).

It is assumed that the surgeon has taken a history of the patient and performed a preoperative evaluation before proceeding with extraction (review Chaps. 3 and 4). Moreover, he should carefully prepare a surgical plan beforehand that includes any difficulties that might occur. It is important to review the anatomy pertaining to the individual procedure. For example, knowing about the distal curvature of the maxillary lateral incisors would aid in their extraction, as would the knowledge that the central incisors have a conical root. The habit of sterile technique, and experience with infections both pre- and

95

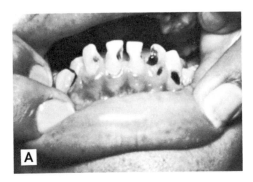

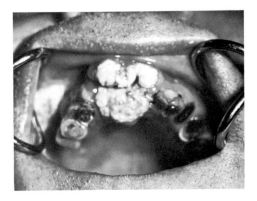

Fig. 8-2. Advanced squamous cell carcinoma of anterior maxillary ridge treated by radiation. Teeth in and near the tumor were extracted.

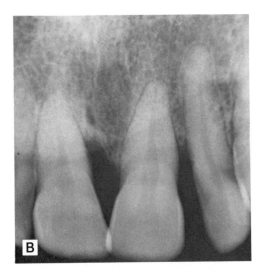

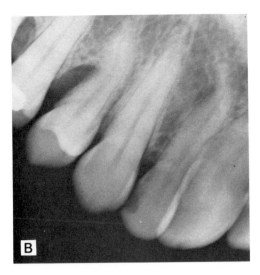

Fig. 8-1. (A) Several carious lower anterior teeth. (B) X-ray films show periodontal disease. Note the bony resorption between central incisor and premolar teeth.

postoperatively, will give the clinician confidence in the management of these surgical cases.

The selection of the appropriate anesthetic in terms of its beneficial vasoconstricting action and its duration, and the skill with which it is administered, will make the patient comfortable during the surgical procedure. Appropriate sedative and analgesic drugs will also increase the efficiency of the procedure and allow a smooth postoperative recovery period. All these matters must be considered before undertaking the actual procedure.

When teeth are indicated for removal, it is of the utmost importance that the clinician know how to proceed. Every patient presents different problems and requires specific management. Any patient who is to undergo a surgical procedure should have at least one presurgical visit; this permits careful arrangement and thoughtful consideration of all facts. Laboratory reports will be available and radiographs dried and mounted for proper study. The operator is then able to form a deliberate judgment that will represent his best preparation for his patient's needs.

After the diagnosis has been made, the treatment plan should be outlined. Some important questions to consider first are: "Does the patient need treatment?" "Is it

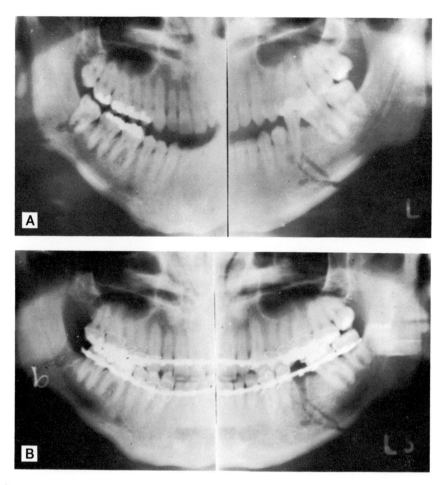

Fig. 8-3. (A and B) Bilateral fracture of mandible. Bicuspid and third molar teeth were removed at time of treatment of the fracture. Note intraosseous wire at mandibular angle for immobilization of the proximal segment.

within my scope of training?" "Am I capable of fulfilling this patient's needs?" If these questions can be answered affirmatively, then a decision to proceed should be made. The proposed treatment should be carefully gone over with the patient, or in the case of minors, with the parent. Such considerations as loss of work, postoperative pain, edema, and financial cost should all be mentioned. In this type of case presentation, several situations may become apparent:

1. An apprehensive patient.
2. Evidence of lack of confidence in the dentist.

3. A personality conflict or an attitude which may indicate lack of understanding of the operation or may prevent adequate communication during and after the procedure.
4. Medical-legal complications.
5. Consideration of hospitalization instead of outpatient care.
6. Need for general anesthesia instead of local anesthesia.

Any number of problems may come to light during the treatment planning appointment, and they must be appropriately answered before proceeding.

At this time also instruments must be

selected. From x-ray studies and the clinical examination, one can often ascertain whether the extraction can be made with or without a flap, bone removal, possible antral involvement, and so forth. A careful examination of the mouth may reveal mobile teeth, deep caries, areas of acute inflammation, or other situations that may dictate the order of the surgery. Depending on these findings, appropriate advice can be given to the assistant in regard to the selection of instruments, the time allotted for the surgery, whether someone should accompany the patient, and other details.

The Surgical Plan

In cases of a full mouth extraction, it is best to maintain the anterior teeth, if possible, until the last surgical appointment for aesthetic purposes (Fig. 8-4). One should maintain vertical dimension when possible by leaving a bicuspid tooth in occlusion until the last surgical procedure. It is usually best to do surgery in opposing quadrants. This allows a patient to maintain a good vertical relation and comfortable chewing on one side during a portion of the surgical and healing process (Fig. 8-5). The removal of two teeth is not

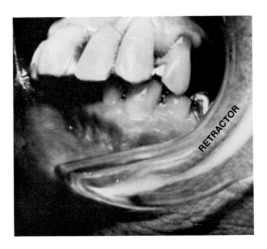

Fig. 8-5. Note retained maxillary bicuspid tooth serving as vertical stop to maintain the natural vertical dimension.

necessarily twice as much surgery as the removal of one. In fact, the removal of several teeth in one procedure is usually much less traumatic than their removal at individual surgical appointments.

When working in opposing quadrants, one must decide in which quadrant to start the surgery. One consideration is the duration of anesthesia. In the maxillary quadrant, where infiltration anesthesia is used, the anesthetic will dissipate early and therefore should be administered just prior to the commencing of the surgery. If the maxillary quadrant is done first, hemorrhage from it interferes with vision while working on the lower quadrant. If the lower quadrant is completed first, pieces of filling material or other foreign bodies may drop into the open mandibular sockets while doing the maxillary surgery. Since maxillary teeth are extracted by significant buccal and labial movement, the presence of mandibular teeth does not limit access. Because extraction forces of mandibular teeth are significantly more vertical, there is increased access for mandibular extraction when maxillary teeth have been removed first. In general, the decision regarding the first quadrant to be worked on must be made on an indi-

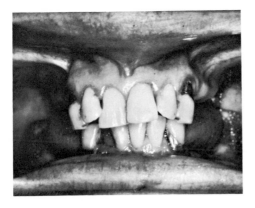

Fig. 8-4. A case for immediate maxillary denture. Posterior teeth have been removed, retaining anterior teeth for final surgical appointment.

vidual basis, keeping in mind these related problems.

Extraction begins with the most posterior tooth in the quadrant. When more than one or two teeth are removed, it is often necessary to consider a ridge trim or alveolectomy. When teeth from opposing quadrants are removed, attention must be directed toward providing adequate vertical dimension. To leave a pendulous or bulbous tuberosity after the molar complement has been removed only serves to create inadequate space or vertical dimension and buccal undercut (Fig. 8-6). If other conditions, such as periapical granulomas, cysts, tori, or enlarged tuberosities are also present, they may be considered for removal at the same time, depending on the skill of the operator, the time required, and the cooperation of the patient.

The removal of teeth need not be a totally frightful experience. Quiet, controlled, planned movements will assure the patient of a good extraction procedure. If a tooth resists the general exodontic movements, a flap should be reflected and appropriate bone reduced, and/or planned tooth sectioning instituted (Fig. 8-7). No detailed discussion should be made about the decision to proceed with the flap procedure. If the patient has been prepared

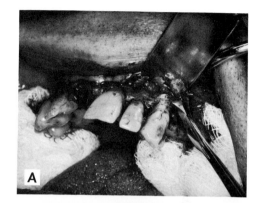

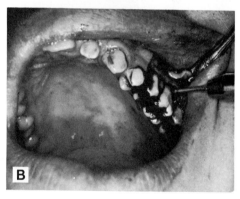

Fig. 8-7. (A) Cuspid tooth to be extracted showing collar of bone reduced with mono-angle chisel. (B) Difficult maxillary first molar extraction showing flap and tooth being sectioned with dental surgical bur.

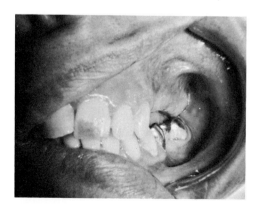

Fig. 8-6. Posterior quadrant of maxillary teeth previously removed without adequately gaining vertical dimension in tuberosity region.

properly and gives evidence of confidence in the dentist, this shift in the surgical plan should be a planned, integrated procedure.

The Flap Operation

Certain basic principles are to be followed in the planning, design, and manipulation of mucoperiosteal flaps. The indications for a flap operation are (1) to increase vision; (2) to gain surgical access;

(3) to remove bone; and (4) to avoid injury to soft tissue that might occur from the contemplated work. The surgical principles underlying the design of the flap are (1) that it has a broad base that will ensure a good blood supply; (2) that it is large enough to allow good access without stretching; (3) that the flap is full-thickness and includes the periosteum when it is reflected; and (4) that when the flap is returned to its original site, the flap margins rest on a good bone table to minimize shrinkage, scarring, and contraction.

The healing time for a short flap is comparable to that for a long one; therefore, the incision length is not critical, and the necessary length of the incision should not be compromised. Incision of the flap should begin in the interdental papillae; this allows easier repositing and suturing and provides a better blood supply at the termination of the incision.

Some have recommended a vertical incision at one end of the flap, and others, two vertical incisions (Fig. 8-8). If vertical incisions are used, they should be made in the interproximal area at least one tooth away from the margin of the bony wound, so that a plateau of bone will support the flap margin when it is sutured in position. The incision line should be so designed that the free corner of the flap does not have an acute angle (Fig. 8-9). This is important in order to avoid compromising the blood supply of the flap while obtaining adequate access without stretching or tearing. The envelope flap will often best serve these goals (Fig. 8-10).

An important consideration of flap design is to ensure appropriate reattachment. This is true whenever repositioning tissue to gain a good tissue base on the ridge for a prosthesis and to avoid perio-

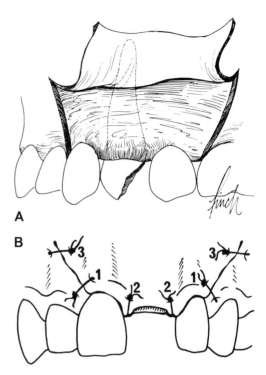

A

B

Fig. 8-8. (A) Broadly based flap. However, two vertical incisions are rarely necessary. (B) Placement of sutures to best reposition the flap. Note the order of the sutures.

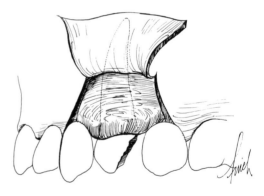

Fig. 8-9. Incorrect flap design showing narrow base limiting blood supply and narrow neck of tissue on tip of flap.

dontal pocket formation around teeth, particularly when third molars are being removed. Providing the appropriate bevel to the incision is helpful, because it basically decapitates the rolled epithelial-lined papillae and gingival crevice tissue,

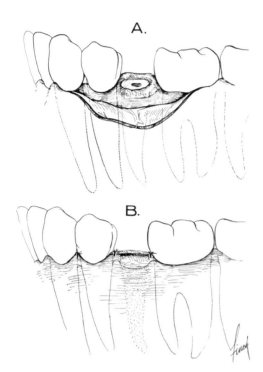

Fig. 8-10. The envelope flap is best for most surgical procedures. It provides the broadest base and fully covers the bone cavity.

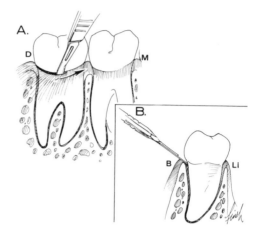

Fig. 8-11. The no. 15 blade is shown incising at a 45° angle, thinning the mucosa to create an internal bevel.

permitting new epithelialization and attachment[2] (Fig. 8-11).

All tissue must be handled gently. Sharp scissors and needles, fine suture, and tissue forceps without teeth are all part of the good surgeon's armamentarium.

Technique of Flap Operation

1. The "seven minimum essentials" as originally described by Clark (see p. 106) should be carefully reviewed.
2. Adequate anesthesia is necessary. In mucoperiosteal flaps, additional anesthesia by injection of saline solution under the flap allows dissection and reflection (e.g., when reflecting the flap from a torus). However, when a Z-plasty flap or a sliding soft tissue flap is planned, too much fluid injected near the surgical site could distort the soft tissue architecture, making flap design and planning difficult. For such cases, deposition of the anesthetic at appropriate innervation sites is better.
3. Prepare a flap tray (Fig. 8-12).
4. Make the incision with a sharp scalpel, keeping in mind the principles of flap design.
5. Reflect the flap with a periosteal elevator. Recommended instruments include the no. 7 wax spatula, the no. 1 Woodson, the no. 9 periosteal elevator, and the no. 4 molt curette (Fig. 8-13). To start the flap reflection, use the sharp portion of the elevator and immediately turn the instrument over so that the convexity of the elevator is against the flap (Fig. 8-14). Use the largest instrument appropriate to the situation and less tearing of the tissue

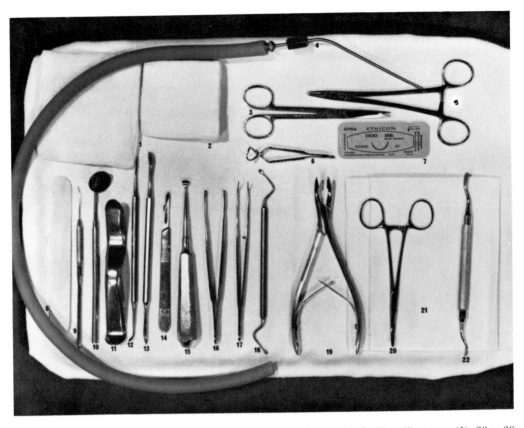

Fig. 8-12. The flap tray should always be readily available. It should include 4″ × 4″ sponges (1); 3″ × 3″ sponges (2); scissors (3); suction (4); needle holder (5); towel clip (6); 3-0 silk (7); tongue blade (8); Gilmore probe (9); mirror (10); retractor (11); no. 1 Woodson elevator (12); no. 9 periosteal elevator (13); no. 15 blade and Bard Parker handle (14); no. 4 molt elevator (15); pick-up forceps (16); cotton pliers (17); small double-ended curette (18); rongeur (19); Kelly hemostat (20); pads to adjust light (21); bone file (22); and appropriate forceps and elevators.

will occur. Avoid overreflection of the flap, as well as heavy-handed retraction. Periodic relaxation of the flap by letting up on the retractor permits a return of the blood flow and general nourishment of the tissues. This is especially necessary during a long procedure.

6. After completing the surgery, smooth the bony margins with rongeurs and files and perform a complete toilet of the wound. Curettement, debridement, and irrigation are performed just prior to flap closure. The flap is then returned over the solid bone table and adequately sutured into place. The edge of the flap (interdental margin) is trimmed to permit appropriate proximation of the tissues but not allowing an overlap of the tissue margins. Either the running continuous lock stitch or the interrupted suture technique may be used (Fig. 8-15). Deep portions of the flap should then be milked toward the incised surface to ensure good adaptation with the appropriate pressure packs placed.

On occasion, the operator may wish to place a drain of gauze wick or rubber in a wound under a flap. For such instances, use only one piece of a given material, so that when it is removed,

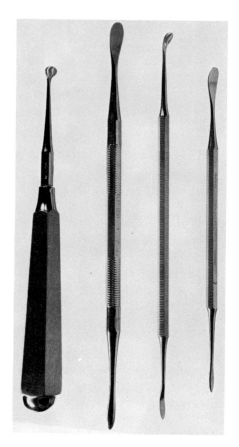

Fig. 8-13. The instruments recommended for initiating and carrying out flap reflection are the nos. 7, 1, and 9 periosteal elevators or the no. 4 molt curette.

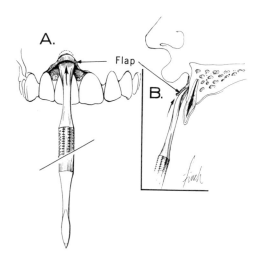

Fig. 8-14. Use of the no. 9 periosteal elevator during flap reflection. The curved portion of the instrument should be against the soft tissue.

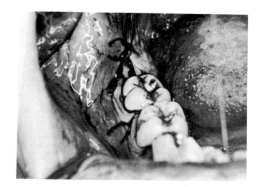

Fig. 8-15. Flap returned after third molar removal, showing three interrupted sutures.

one can be certain that nothing has been left behind as a foreign body and source of irritation.

7. The final responsibility after a flap procedure entails discussing with the patient the expected sequelae (e.g., pain, edema, ecchymosis), giving appropriate explanations, prescribing medication, and arranging the return appointment.

8. In general, sutures can be removed in three to five days, often coinciding with the next surgical appointment, if such is necessary. Patients often view the removal of sutures with undue apprehension. With good vision, light, suction, and assistance, the operator can make this procedure comparable to the examination.

Additional information on the flap operation appears in Chapter 9.

References

1. U.S. Dept. H. E. W.: Oral Care for Cancer Patients. June, 1968.
2. Friedman, N.: Mucogingival surgery: The apically repositioned flap. J. Periodontol., *33*:328–340, 1962.

9 Multiple Extractions, Alveolectomy, and Immediate Denture Surgery

DANIEL E. WAITE

Multiple Extractions

Regardless of the surgical procedure, the surgeon should have a definite routine for his evaluation and examination before beginning treatment. The record should be carefully reviewed and, as previously pointed out, a prior examination appointment is best. The x-ray studies are then evaluated. A review and an evaluation of the patient's history should be coordinated with specific reference to questioning the patient for any recent changes in his health status. Once the above have been satisfied, the patient should be seated comfortably in the chair. This usually means tipping back the chair one or two notches to give the patient the security of being seated well back into it (Fig. 9-1). When extracting teeth from the mandible, it is best to have the occlusal plane approximately parallel with the floor. For the extractions of the maxilla, the maxillary occlusal plane is best at a 45° angle with the floor. In any event, the patient should be comfortable, as should the operator.

The operator then systematically goes over the work to be accomplished. He makes a decision regarding the anesthesia to be used, and meticulously examines the tooth or teeth to be extracted clinically and roentgenologically. He must make a mental decision whether or not he can accomplish this procedure with or without a flap and whether bone removal will be necessary. His choice of elevators and forceps needs to be considered, as well as the general selection of instruments. It is well to form a mental picture as to how one thinks the case will go, both in terms of patient cooperation and of difficulties anticipated. Dr. H. B. Clark, Jr., in his text, *Practical Oral Surgery*, has given several guidelines in this area, from which the following has been adapted.

Operative Guidelines*

To achieve uniform success in the technical side of oral surgery, it is important to develop good working habits. A habit is a custom or aptitude acquired by repetition and marked by facility of perform-

*Adapted from Clark, H. B., Jr.: *Practical Oral Surgery*, ed. 2, pp. 151–159. Philadelphia, Lea & Febiger, 1965.

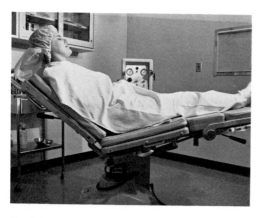

Fig. 9-1. The chair should be tipped back one to two notches from the center.

ance. Good working habits ensure good patient care.

As the prospective dentist contemplates his lifetime of operative work, he would do well to ponder the consequences of failing to operate systematically. Every act of the surgeon should advance the operation closer to its conclusion. An aimless, hit-and-miss approach to a surgical task becomes laborious, time consuming, and uncertain of result.

Some professional men feel it is undignified to standardize the method of caring for patients. To be sure, the total care of the patient cannot be carried through according to an ironclad plan, because individual differences in cases are always present. However, areas of treatment lend themselves well to standard disciplines, and the thoughtful operator is prepared to apply these separate, individual skills to his surgical problem in proper sequence. Serious mishaps are rather uncommon in oral surgery, and usually are avoidable. Wasted time, fatigue of the patient and operator, and substandard working conditions are far too common.

Increased efficiency takes effort, thought, planning, and some added cost, but it is a goal that is always worth working toward. As efficiency improves, it may be confidently anticipated that accidents,

operating time, and trauma will be reduced, and there will be a proportionate increase in the pleasure of operating and in the surgical result.

In order to achieve more efficiency in operating, the following possible measures come to mind:

1. MORE ASSISTANCE. Up to a certain point, more competent assistance helps. This limit is seldom reached in practice because of (1) the cost of salaries and (2) the labor of training assistants.
2. PAINSTAKING PREPARATION AND PLANNING OF OPERATION. (1) A complete diagnosis—history, examination, radiographs, medical opinion, and the like—is mandatory. (2) When indicated, a review of textbooks or periodical literature to determine the best procedure may be done.
3. AVOID UNNECESSARY MOTIONS. This takes discipline, a methodical temperament, and means working in steps.
4. WORKING BY DIRECT VISION. This is achieved by adequate opening of the wound, maintaining a bloodless field, and having brilliant illumination on the field all the time.

H. B. Clark, Jr., has compiled all of these measures into a basic set of operating conditions known as "The Seven Minimum Essentials." Although originally adopted for tooth removal operations, they have come to be regarded as a checklist or set of standards for all oral surgical work, whether performed under local or general anesthesia, and whether conducted in the dental clinic or the hospital operating room.

The Seven Minimum Essentials

R 1. *Radiograph:* a clear, recent radiograph of the tooth and some of the surrounding structures.

A 2. *Anesthetic:* a suitable anesthetic agent for the task at hand.

F 3. *Forceps and elevators:* appropriate for the teeth to be removed.

F 4. *Flap tray:* a tray of instruments for performing flap operations, sterile and ready.

L 5. *Light:* brilliant illumination on the site of operation 100 per cent of the time. This is best achieved with the headlight (Fig. 9-2).

E 6. *Efficient assistance* throughout the entire operation, on every operation.

S 7. *Suction aspiration.*

For ease in memorization, the initial letters have been arranged to form a key word: RAFFLES.

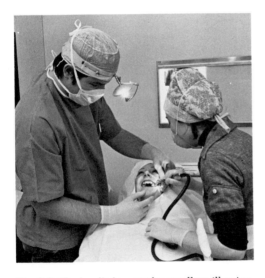

Fig. 9-2. The headlight provides excellent illumination to the oral cavity.

1. RADIOGRAPH. No tooth extraction operation should be attempted without a clear recent radiograph of the tooth and some of the surrounding area. Time taken to secure a good radiograph is not wasted; on the contrary, it is a good investment in safety and efficiency. The dentist must firmly believe in the principle of invariably working from radiographs if he is to convince his patients that it is essential. Some patients are astonished at the thought of "wasting" an x-ray picture on a tooth which is about to be sacrificed. The dentist should refuse to operate if an understanding cannot be reached on this point.

Operating with the constant advantage of good preoperative radiographs affords many benefits: they give a good view of the shape, size, and curvature of the root, the density of bone, the presence of pathologic processes such as cysts, tumors, or fractures that may not have been suspected, and they verify the clinical diagnosis of the condition of the tooth itself in matters of depth of caries, location of pockets, and so forth. Be certain that the object of the surgery appears near the center of the film; do not be forced to read accurately the periphery of any radiograph (Fig. 9-3).

2. ANESTHESIA. The anesthetic agent used for an operation must be suitable for the case at hand. The dentist must make this decision; the patient's whim or demands must not be the deciding factor. It is a good plan to ask the patient if he has a preference for any particular agent, and if the choice is suitable, use it. On the

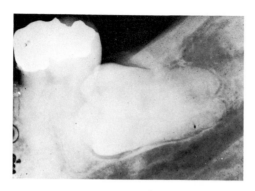

Fig. 9-3. A good x-ray study of proper density and with the surgical object in the center of the film. One should not be forced to read the periphery of a film.

other hand, if there is disagreement between the patient and the operator, the difference must be resolved. The following are indications for general anesthesia:

a. Children who are too young to adequately understand or who are extremely apprehensive.

b. Brief procedures, in the presence of acute infection, such as incision and drainage or the extraction of a single tooth.

c. Patients who are sensitive or allergic to some component of the local anesthetic solution.

d. Prolonged operations on patients whose physical or mental condition would be inadequate to give the surgeon ideal working conditions. These patients should be cared for by general anesthesia in the hospital operating room.

3. FORCEPS AND ELEVATORS. It is self-evident that, in the surgical removal of teeth, forceps and elevators must be available and ready for use. The choice of extraction instruments poses few problems when one has mastered the proper method of using each and has become familiar with those features of instrument design that afford greatest efficiency. Whenever possible, elevation of a tooth should be attempted, to make the extraction easier and less subject to root fracture.

4. FLAP TRAY. This is a standard rectangular surgical tray upon which are the desired instruments for reflecting a mucoperiosteal flap and performing the usual dentoalveolar surgery involved with the extraction of difficult teeth, recovering roots, alveolectomy, and other procedures. The flap tray may not be needed for every extraction and therefore is not a part of the regular instrument setup. However, it should be in readiness at all times and added to the basic tray setup when needed (see Fig. 8-12).

5. LIGHT. Brilliant illumination on the field of operation at all times is imperative. There are many rational arguments for the use of the headlight as the only instrument that can meet these criteria. It eliminates the possibility of shadows caused by the operator's head, and it permits variation of the direction of the beam when the patient's position changes or when a small cavity such as a tooth socket must be illuminated (see Fig. 9-2).

To adequately utilize the headlight, habit and practice are most important. From the standpoint of specialties such as oral surgery, otolarnygology, and ophthalmology, the headlight is superb and should be used. However, in the general practice of dentistry, it is not customary to use the headlight routinely. Much oral surgery, therefore, will be done under the "regular" light. Good overhead lights are available and ready for use in difficult situations.

6. EFFICIENT ASSISTANT. Attempting to do surgery alone is difficult and invites accidents, frustrations, and wasted energy. The use of an assistant is mandatory and he or she should be well trained in the specific functions and hand motions that will be required. The assistant is to:

a. Use the suction aspirator constantly to remove blood, saliva, and debris from the floor of the mouth, the dorsum of the tongue, the right and left retromolar areas, and the wound itself. If this duty is faithfully performed, the patient should never have to use the cuspidor, and the operation proceeds more efficiently and with cleanliness. If the aspirator tip becomes plugged, he must instantly clear the obstruction with the reaming wire.

b. Use the water syringe (in conjunction with the aspirator) to cool the bur or clear the film of blood from the surface bone. This should be done without a specific request from the operator.

c. Provide retraction.

d. Mallet with the left hand when possible, since the right hand will most often be used for retraction of the cheek.

e. Reassure the patient with a pleasant, affirmative manner.

f. Make appointments.

When scrubbed for an operation, the assistant must remain at the chairside until the completion of the procedure. An additional nonsterile attendant is highly desirable to answer the telephone, receive and discharge patients, and procure items that might be needed during the operation. This person is referred to as a circulator.

7. SUCTION ASPIRATOR. This is perhaps the greatest contribution to oral surgical technique in recent times. It provides an entirely new concept in operating. Formerly, many of the arm and hand motions of the operator or assistant were devoted to sponging with gauze or cotton. By the use of the aspirator, a bloodless field is maintained effectively throughout the entire operation.

These "Seven Minimal Essentials" must be used for every oral surgical procedure. In the various operations described in subsequent chapters, it may always be assumed that these facilities are present and functioning. They are equally essential in the dental clinic, office, or hospital operating room.

Instruments

Nurses and dental assistants should know the exact instruments needed for a given operation and the order they should be placed on the tray. During operative procedures the doctor should establish the habit of replacing an instrument on the tray to the same place from which he picked it up. A clean and orderly tray will always result from this habit.

1. The instruments that should be on every tray when *single extraction* is indicated and a flap procedure not contemplated are shown in Figure 9-4.

2. The instruments that should be included on the tray whenever *two or*

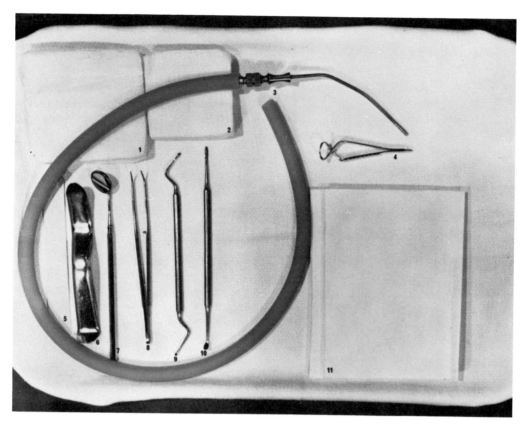

Fig. 9-4. A basic tray should include 4″ × 4″ sponges (1); 3″ × 3″ sponges (2); suction (3); towel clip (4); tongue blade (5); retractor (6); mouth mirror (7); cotton pliers (8); double-ended curette (9); no. 1 Woodson elevator (10); pads to adjust light (11); and forceps and elevators according to the case.

more extractions and a flap procedure are indicated are shown in Figure 8-12, (p. 102).

Alveolectomy

When difficulty with the extraction is anticipated, or two or more teeth are to be removed, an alveolectomy will probably be necessary, including the reflection of the flap (Figs. 9-5 and 9-6). The terms alveolectomy, alveoloplasty, and alveolotomy are often used synonymously. I choose to define alveolectomy as the appropriate reduction of the alveolus primarily for the reception of a prosthesis. An important consideration during the alveolectomy procedure is the conservative reduction of bone rather than the radical removal of it. Alveolotomy is defined as removal of specific portions of the alveolar bone to gain access, for example, to retained roots, residual areas of infections, or cysts. Alveoloplasty refers more to the specific surgical management of the soft tissues and improving soft tissue attachments to the alveolus.

One should mentally review the nerve and blood supply of the incision in order to provide the flap with the maximal blood supply. The incision should be kept on the crest of the ridge whenever possible, and angle cuts are rarely necessary. The flap should always have a wider base than its three margins, and it should be wider than the anticipated bone cavity (see Fig. 8-8). Once the surgical site has been exposed adequately, the alveolectomy should be done. If an alveolectomy is indicated to remove thick cortical bone to ease the removal of the teeth, the excessive bone is reduced prior to the extraction by either chisel or rongeur techniques (Fig. 9-7). If, however, the alveolectomy must be done to remove gross undercuts or sharpness to the alveolar ridge in order to enhance the reception of the prosthesis, the alveolectomy should be completed following the extraction of the teeth. Under good visualization, bone is reduced in a controlled manner. If rongeurs are used, one blade is placed high on the crest of the ridge with the other blade beneath the undercut; a shaving or planing technique

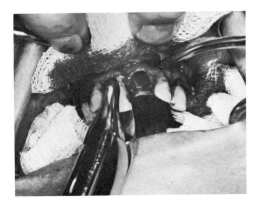

Fig. 9-6. More than one tooth is being removed, and in order to smooth the alveolar margins and compress the expanded sockets, an alveolectomy procedure should be anticipated.

is used, bringing the one blade to the other (Fig. 9-8). Smoothing is done with bone rasps or files, the area carefully debrided by irrigation, and the flap returned. The entire area is then manually palpated to be certain no sharpness or loose fragments of bone remain.

When reviewing the tooth or teeth to be extracted, one should pay attention to the degree of caries, severe abrasion, or long-standing attrition that may be evident. In such instances, the root structure and bony relationships may make the extraction more difficult. If large fillings are present, it is wise to counsel the patient that one may hear crumbling and there

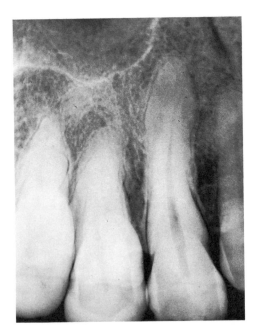

Fig. 9-5. Because of the bulbous curvature of the root of the cuspid, a difficult extraction is expected, therefore, a flap should be anticipated as well as possible root recovery and alveolectomy.

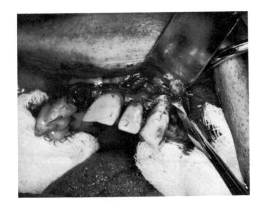

Fig. 9-7. Envelope flap has been reflected. A bony prominence is evident over the cuspid, and is being reduced by chisel technique.

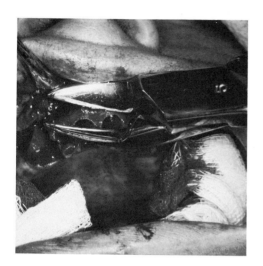

Fig. 9-8. Bone reduction using no. 5 rongeur: the superior blade is locked on alveolar bone and the inferior blade is brought to it in a planing manner.

may be slippage of the forceps. Should a large filling be adjacent to the tooth to be removed, fracture of it may be unavoidable (Fig. 9-9). In such anticipated instances, the patient should be advised of the possibility of a fracture of these restorations. It is important to review the size of the tooth and its roots, particularly if

they have been distorted on the radiograph. The formation and number of roots, the possibility of root fracture, and the type of bone in regard to its density are matters for consideration that would create fewer surgical problems if they are reviewed in advance. The relationship of the tooth to the maxillary sinus or the mandibular canal, and the presence of root canal fillings and large maxillary tuberosities may require a considerable change in the surgical approach (Fig. 9-10).

The examination should also include the supporting hard and soft tissues; low frenum attachments or complete loss of

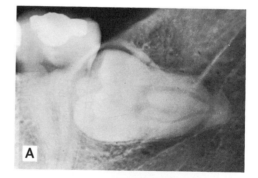

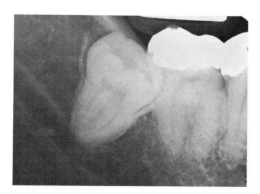

Fig. 9-9. There is a large filling in the second molar; the third molar is to be extracted.

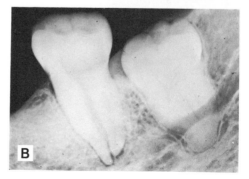

Fig. 9-10. (A and B) Teeth impinging on the inferior alveolar canal make surgical delivery more difficult and increase the postoperative sequelae.

alveolar bone with deep gingival pockets would be significant (Fig. 9-11). The thickness of the labial or buccal cortical plates will provide information on the need for bone reduction. Bone density may also be judged by the age and size of the patient. Teeth are often less brittle in younger patients than in older ones; the bone permits easier expansion of the sockets, and less root fracture occurs.

There is a technique for the reduction of buccal and labial undercuts by removing the V-shaped area of bone between the buccal and lingual cortical plates. Once this intermedullary bone has been excised, firm pressure is used to collapse the labial and buccal plate toward the lingual plate. This creates a greenstick fracture high in the buccal or labial sulcus; sutures are used to hold the overlying lingual and buccal tissues together (Fig. 9-12). No mucoperiosteal flap is reflected in this procedure. Although the technique does

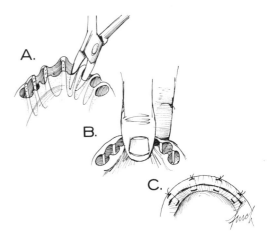

Fig. 9-12. Intermedullary alveolectomy. (A) Excision of interseptal bone. (B) Compression of cortical plates. (C) Mattress sutures in place.

accomplish the reduction of the undercuts and some bony irregularities while avoiding the reflection of the mucoperiosteal flap, it has some essential disadvantages:

1. A fracture is created in the alveolar bone, which we try to avoid as a basic principle.
2. Vital medullary bone, which contributes so much to the healing process, is sacrificed.
3. A sharp, knife-like edge on the ridge may result where the edges of the two cortical bone plates come together.
4. Because these plates are both comprised of cortical bone, they are subject to resorption.

While this procedure may be less time consuming and causes less hemorrhage than the other methods, it is not the procedure routinely recommended for acceptable alveolectomy.

The order of the extraction of teeth may be altered and dictated by individual cases, but basic guidelines can be stated.

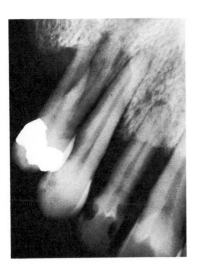

Fig. 9-11. Deep periodontal pocket formation changes the bony fulcrum, often making the extraction more susceptible to root fracture.

The surgery should be done in opposing quadrants when possible, maintaining the anterior teeth until the last surgical appointment. Extraction should begin with the most posterior tooth to be extracted, working toward the anterior. Complete each quadrant, including the alveolectomy and suturing, before proceeding to another arch.

Immediate Denture Surgery

The disciplines of prosthodontics and surgery become closely related in immediate denture cases. The complexities inherent in the construction of the prosthetic appliance make it mandatory that every possible avenue be pursued to present the individual patient with a prosthesis that is both aesthetic and functional. Therein lies one of the major advantages of the immediate denture insertion technique. With this procedure, the anterior teeth are still present in the arch and serve as a guide to the correct and natural positioning of the artificial teeth. The surrounding oral structures are also maintained close to their normal position and vertical dimension. There is less postsurgical discomfort because the prosthesis acts as a protecting splint. In addition, there is no period of edentulous adjustment, which is an important consideration for all patients, and especially those who by necessity are constantly before the public.

Some disadvantages of immediate denture surgery are:

1. Earlier relining of the denture will be necessary, and possibly a new prosthesis.
2. An increased number of office visits are necessary during the first few months.
3. Cost is increased with this type of management.

The most desirable plan is to utilize the maxillary immediate denture while maintaining the natural lower anterior teeth.

The maxillary posterior teeth are removed, except for one maxillary bicuspid that is maintained temporarily for vertical dimension (see Fig. 8-5). This is left as an occlusal rest to maintain the existing interarch distance during the healing period. Care should be taken to assure adequate surgical reduction of the tuberosity area in both vertical and lateral directions so that sufficient space exists for the base plate material and the posterior teeth (see Fig. 8-6).

Obviously, appropriate methods of obtaining good impressions, casts, and complete prosthodontic relation are indicated. As has already been mentioned, the preservation of the exact relation of the teeth in the arch is of great value and advantage in the immediate denture service. Part of this relation will be lost unless the plaster teeth are removed one at a time and replaced by porcelain teeth in the desired position. In this manner, the adjacent teeth serve as an accurate guide for vertical position, mesiodistal inclination, and rotational position (Fig. 9-13).

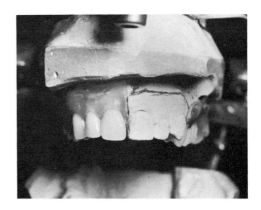

Fig. 9-13. By individually removing the plaster teeth, the prosthetic tooth placed in wax gives personal individuality to the prosthesis.

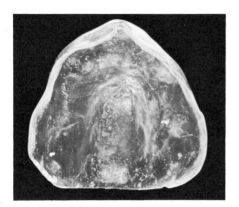

Fig. 9-14. The surgical splint is made of clear acrylic.

Prior to the surgical appointment the occlusion is corrected as much as possible before the processed dentures are removed from their casts. The labial flange of the denture must be well-rounded, shortened, and thinned. The inner surface of the denture should also be recessed in the region where the socket prominences protrude. A surgical splint is constructed with clear acrylic, using as a model the stone casts from which the anterior teeth have been cut away and bony trimming simulated by scraping the casts (Fig. 9-14). The splint should be a full palatal splint to record accuracy during the surgical reduction and trimming of bone. The operation then consists of fitting the alveolar process and tissues to the previously constructed splint.

Surgical Approach

If local anesthesia is used, both the lingual and labial tissue must be adequately anesthetized. Premedicating drugs may be used to the great advantage of the surgeon and the comfort of the patient.

If it is likely that a flap will have to be raised sometime during the operation, it should be done initially. This permits better vision and access, especially for bone contouring and smoothing, and generally expedites the procedure (Fig. 9-15). Excessive reflection of the surgical flap may lead to the formation of unnecessary scar tissue and immediate swelling accompanied by hematoma under the tissue at the denture periphery. This would obviously be detrimental to the stability and retention of the prosthesis. The object is to prepare the mouth so that the denture can rest firmly upon normal tissue.

The teeth are then removed by the usual careful techniques. The transparent surgical template is placed in the mouth after all the teeth have been removed, but before surgical trimming of the bone or soft tissue is done. The template must be seated perfectly or it will not reveal the proper areas to be trimmed. When the template has been securely seated against the palate and posterior maxillary ridge, the areas at the surgical site that are blanched from the pressure indicate the need for additional reduction (Fig. 9-16). The template is removed and soft tissue or bone is trimmed as indicated to relieve areas of excessive pressure. Insufficient trimming or excessive trimming will cause the denture to be positioned incorrectly. This results in improper occlusion and unnecessary pain and discomfort for the patient.

Following the alveolectomy, the flap may also have to be reduced in circumference with a pair of soft tissue scissors. The reduction of this excess tissue is easily accomplished by removing a small wedge at the extremity of the incision (Fig. 9-17). The interdental papillae are then trimmed and sutures placed over the interseptal

Fig. 9-15. Minimal envelope flap reflection for controlled reduction of bone if necessary prior to tooth removal.

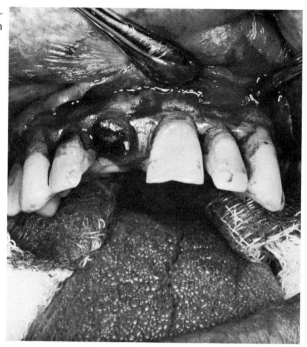

Fig. 9-16. The surgical template is repeatedly tried in place. Blanched areas indicate where additional reduction may be necessary.

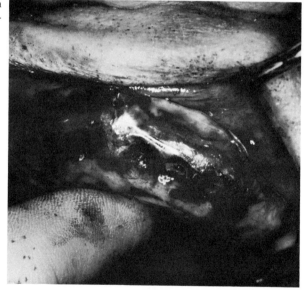

bone. If not adequately reduced and sutured firmly, the tissue is likely to become flabby, predisposing the area to subsequent denture injury.

Sutures may be interrupted or continuous, and 3-0 or 4-0 silk is excellent for this purpose. The denture should have been previously placed in a bichloride solution bath, after which it is rinsed in sterile saline solution and placed in the mouth. The occlusion is checked and, if satisfactory, the patient is instructed to keep the

Fig. 9-17. By reducing the bony circumference of the arch, there may be an excess of labial tissue. This can best be reduced by taking a small vertical triangular wedge of tissue from the extremity of the incision.

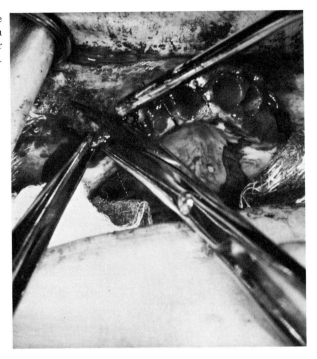

Fig. 9-18. Immediate denture, 24 hours postoperative.

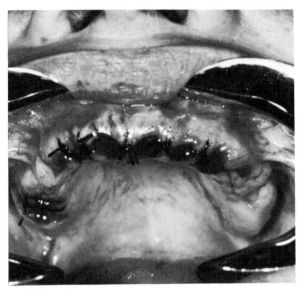

prosthesis in position for 24 hours, at which time the dentist performing the surgery will remove it for the first time (Fig. 9-18).

The postoperative instructions to the patient are extremely important, and should not be handled lightly by the dentist. The patient should be instructed to leave the prosthesis in place until his return to the office the next day. Premature removal may result in swelling that will make reinsertion of the denture impossible or at least extremely painful. It should be emphasized that the trauma of surgery will not be alleviated by the removal of the denture, and that adequate medication will be necessary.

To minimize swelling the patient is advised to apply ice packs to the face during the first 24 hours subsequent to surgery. Judicious use of the pack is recommended (i.e., 15 minutes out of each hour). Chewing is discouraged during the first 24 hours, and a liquid diet is prescribed. One should remember that the occlusion has not been finally adjusted, and thus mastication will be inefficient for a time. Stability of the denture will improve when the occlusion is perfected. If the loss of sleep is contemplated due to nervousness, stress, or discomfort, a sedative should be prescribed.

The prosthesis should be removed 24 to 48 hours subsequent to insertion and the mouth examined for border impingement and excessive pressure areas at the surgical site; the necessary adjustments are made. Sutures are removed in approximately five days postsurgery. Following adequate postsurgical management, the usual follow-up care for prosthesis management and adjustment is indicated (Fig. 9-19).

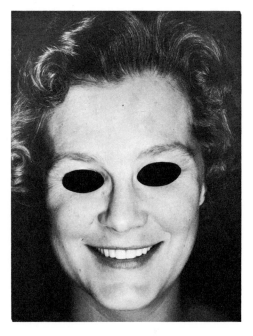

Fig. 9-19. Five days postsurgery: edema subsided, prosthesis in place, and patient happy.

10 Complications to Exodontia and Root Recovery Procedures

DANIEL E. WAITE

It is well known that the extraction of a maxillary or mandibular first molar can be as difficult as that of any impacted tooth. The assessment of the potential difficulty begins with correlating the radiograph of the tooth in question with the clinical impression at the time of evaluation. Evaluation of the patient regarding cooperativeness and general stability is also important. Specific clinical attention must be given to the quality of the tooth, the general soundness of the crown, caries, the amount of overlying bone, and the position in the arch.

When evaluating the x-ray picture, an important consideration is the quality of the roentgenogram. First, be certain that the tooth in question is in the center of the film; do not be forced to read the roentgenogram at its periphery. To be sure of the density and consistency of the x-ray study, look for some degree of soft tissue registration. The correct angulation of the roentgenogram can be assured if one looks for superimposition of cusps, open contact points, and normal pulp configuration (Fig. 10-1). Finally interpret the film from the standpoint of the normal, not the abnormal. For example, look for the intactness of the enamel cap, not caries, or for

the continuity of the periodontal membrane, not a periapical lesion. When the abnormal does exist, it is then more quickly recognized as a deviation from the known normal condition.

In the extraction of any tooth we have the option of performing the extraction by the closed technique, with no mucoperiosteal flap reflection, or by the open technique, with the reflection of the flap for access and some reduction of overlying bone. This can best be determined by the examination. As a basic principle, some form of elevation should always be attempted on the tooth to be extracted. Whenever some slight subluxation of a tooth has occurred, root fracture of that tooth is less likely and the extraction is that much easier. Moreover, if a root should fracture, the recovery of the root will generally be less difficult if the tooth has been slightly elevated. Once the gingival attachment has been severed by the no. 9 or no. 1 periosteal elevator, the appropriate tooth elevator is applied (see p. 40 on elevator technique).

If no movement is evident after elevation and reasonable extraction forces have been applied, it is probable that tooth sectioning and a flap procedure should be

A.

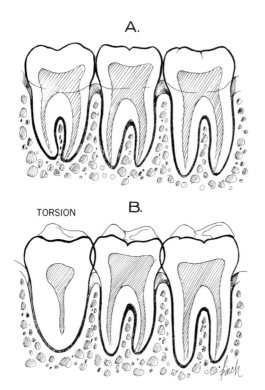

TORSION

B.

Fig. 10-1. Information regarding the position of the tooth and accuracy of the x-ray film can be determined from correctly reading the roentgenograms.

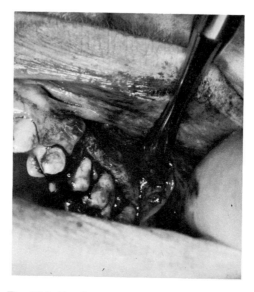

Fig. 10-3. For the removal of a difficult maxillary first molar, a vertical incision has also been used to provide more access.

done. Remember: "To do well what you see, you must see well what you do." Adequate exposure of the problem is necessary, which can usually be accomplished by the envelope flap technique (Fig. 10-2). However, if necessary, a vertical incision may be done for additional access (Fig. 10-3). To remove overlying buccal bone,

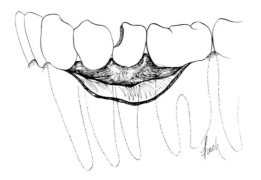

Fig. 10-2. The envelope flap exposing the surgical field. No vertical incision has been made.

one can use sharp mono-angle chisel or the rotary high-speed cutting instruments under irrigation. Controlled bone removal is always more conservative and less traumatic than permitting a fracture of the overlying bony plate to occur.

Tooth Division

Tooth division is necessary for erupted, multirooted teeth in certain standard situations: (1) divergent and curved roots; (2) fractured crown during extraction; (3) an extremely carious crown; (4) teeth in which no luxation occurs with either an elevator or a forceps. Controlled tooth division saves operating room time, requires fewer instruments than full-scale surgical removal, and often conserves bony tissue that otherwise would have to be sacrificed. Remember the philosophy:

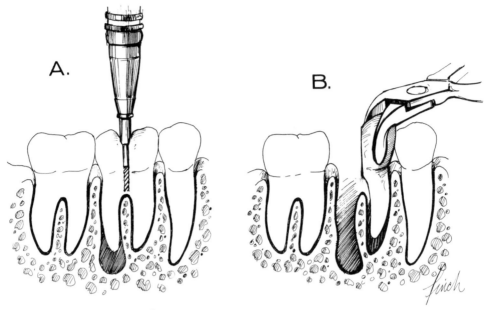

Fig. 10-4. Sectioning of lower molar.

"The tooth belongs to the surgeon, and the bone belongs to the patient."

The approach to sectioning multirooted teeth varies only slightly depending on the tooth. For lower molar teeth, the crowns may be sectioned buccolingually and the tooth extracted as two single teeth (Fig. 10-4). Other division techniques include (1) sectioning the tooth at the gingival crest and the remaining root structure mesiodistally, and recovering the roots separately (Fig. 10-5); or (2) sectioning one root through the bifurcation, removing the crown and the intact root, and recovering the remaining root separately (Fig. 10-6).

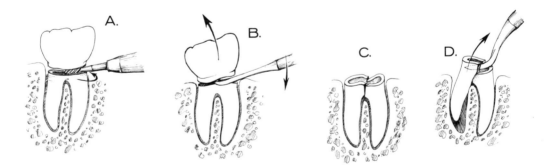

Fig. 10-5. Crown is severed at the gingival crest. The roots are then sectioned mesiodistally and elevated from their sockets individually.

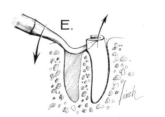

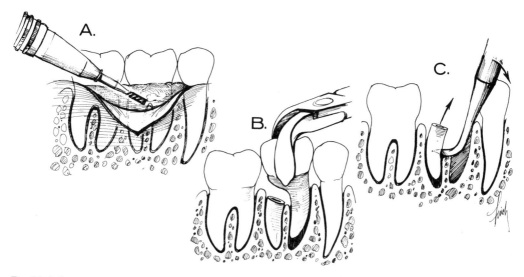

Fig. 10-6. Sectioning of molar for removal. (A) Envelope flap. (B) Tooth and one root being removed. (C) Root elevator being used.

Maxillary molar complications necessitating tooth division can be done by sectioning the crown at the junction of the mesiobuccal and distobuccal roots and removing the crown and the lingual root intact, and recovering the two buccal roots separately (Fig. 10-7). If this method is unsuccessful, the entire crown may be sectioned free and the roots all recovered separately (Fig. 10-8). Remember, however, that the maxillary antrum often dips low into the bifurcation of the lingual and buccal roots and therefore makes the approach to the lingual root from the buccal hazardous (Fig. 10-9).

When tooth division does not succeed in

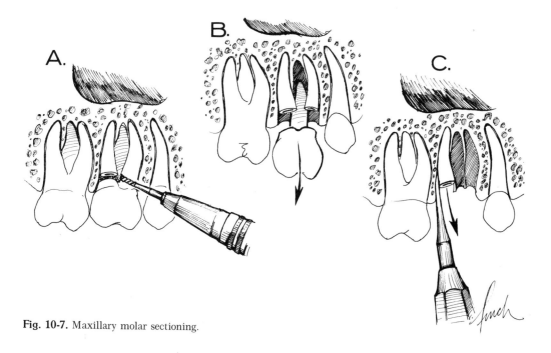

Fig. 10-7. Maxillary molar sectioning.

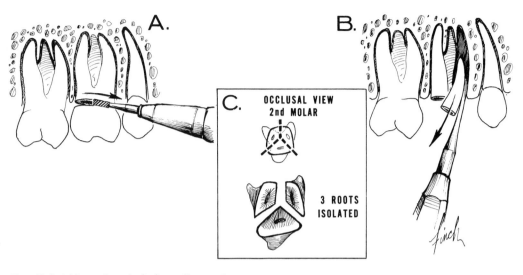

Fig. 10-8. Additional method of maxillary molar sectioning.

delivering the roots quickly, time should not be wasted; the operator should proceed immediately to full-scale flap operation and surgical removal.

Root Recovery

The fracture of a root should not necessarily be viewed as the result of negligence or an error, or faulty technique on the part of the operator. Many factors contribute to root fracture, including:

1. Ankylosis of tooth root to bone.
2. Hypercementosis.
3. Periodontal disease.
4. Dense or sclerotic bone.
5. Lack of alignment of forceps beaks with long axis of tooth.
6. Long, spiny, curved roots.

When root fracture occurs, the efficient surgeon will have in mind a treatment plan. As the particular problem presents itself, one should immediately move to the step in the root recovery outline that is appropriate to the problem. The use of forceps with a special design should be considered first. A variety of root spicule forceps are available: a standard root forceps is the no. 69. A long narrow beak for deep application may be all that is needed

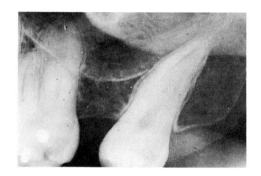

Fig. 10-9. Note maxillary antrum dipping low over the second molar and between the lingual and buccal roots.

(Fig. 10-10). If this is unsuccessful, proceed to the second step without delay. This entails utilizing the elevator as a displacement instrument. The no. 301 straight-blade elevator works well (Fig. 10-11). The instrument should be placed on the high side of the root, tipping the root to the lower side, then manipulating the elevator so as to displace the root, walking it down the socket wall. If a purchase point is indicated or a curved elevator more appropriate, the Hu-Friedy 190 and 191 elevators are excellent (see Fig. 10-5).

The third procedure for root recovery is to use the handpiece with a small round

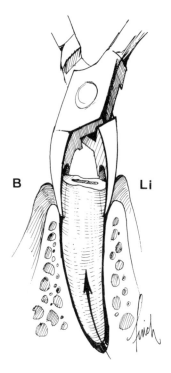

Fig. 10-10. Use of the root spicule forceps.

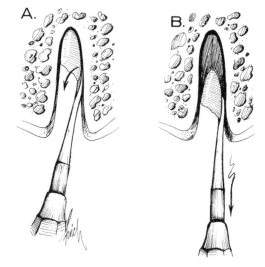

Fig. 10-11. Note the elevator inserted on high side of root.

bur as a retraction instrument. The size of the bur can be determined by the size of the root to be recovered. Thrust the rotary bur into the center of the root fragment, penetrating down the canal and binding

the bur in the tooth fragment at a slight angle to further increase the lock. Then stop the motor and withdraw the handpiece (Fig. 10-12).

The fourth step is the window tech-

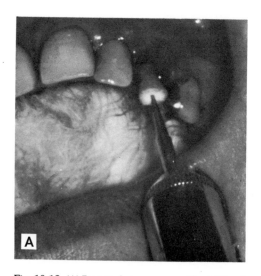

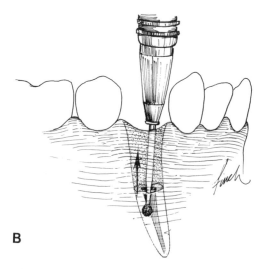

Fig. 10-12. (A) Root tip being recovered by drilling bur into the root content, killing the engine, and withdrawing the handpiece. (B) Illustration of the bur technique for root recovery.

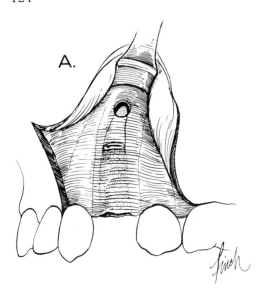

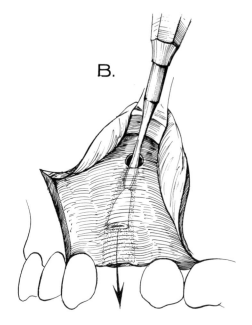

Fig. 10-13. Window technique for root recovery.

nique. On occasion, the decision to utilize this procedure may be made immediately, bypassing the others. A flap will be necessary. Once the flap has been reflected, a window is made with the bur or chisel near the apex of the root to be recovered. An instrument appropriate to the size of the window is then inserted and used to poke the root out of the socket. A primary goal here is to conserve alveolar bone (Fig. 10-13).

The final step is more radical and resorted to only when the others have failed or are not indicated. It involves a full flap and the removal of bone for access to the root (Fig. 10-14). A vertical flap incision should always be made at least one tooth away from the root to be recovered to assure the return of the flap over a solid bone table.

In review, the steps for root recovery are outlined as follows:

1. Root spicule forceps.
2. Appropriate elevator.
3. Bur technique.
4. Window technique.
5. Flap and removal of bone.

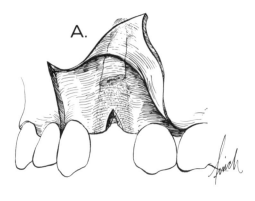

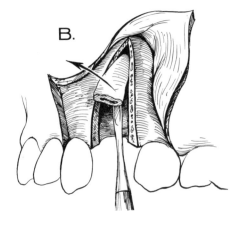

Fig. 10-14. Root recovery after removal of bone.

Vision is probably the most important adjunct to root recovery techniques. Excellent suction and a good light become important. Remember to avoid apical pressure on the root, especially in areas proximal to the antrum, the mandibular canal, or soft tissues.

If a root fragment is forced into the maxillary antrum, do not make the socket entry into the antrum any larger through attempted recovery. A moment could well be spent with good suction to see if recovery is possible through the socket, but no extensive surgical procedure is contemplated in this area. Occasionally the root may lie between the alveolar bone and the sinus membrane, making vision and recovery difficult. If a separate approach to the antrum is considered, make it above the bicuspids, leaving adequate gingival tissue with a good blood supply, and return the flap over a good bone table (Fig. 10-15). Special irrigation and suction may be used to float the root tip to the surface for removal. Antrum curettes are also helpful to recover these tips (Fig. 10-16); good radiographic coverage to locate the tips is important.

In most maxillary antrum complications, patient coverage with antibiotics should be considered. Vasoconstrictive nose drops may also help to assure normal flow of fluids and drainage from the sinus. Attention should also be directed to adequately closing the socket area, which can be done with one or two interrupted sutures. If necessary, a little alveolar bone may be sacrificed to allow closure, or use a relaxing incision. Additional information and description of maxillary antrum problems and surgical procedures appear in Chapter 16.

Root tips forced into the inferior alveo-

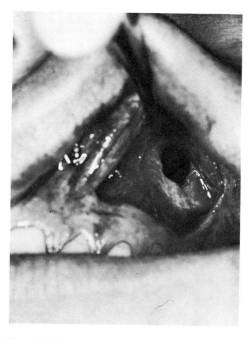

Fig. 10-15. Surgical entry into the maxillary antrum over apices of bicuspid teeth.

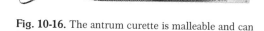

Fig. 10-16. The antrum curette is malleable and can be bent to contact the antral floor.

lar canal are difficult to recover. Vision and location are most difficult (Fig. 10-17). Complications in recovery include hemorrhage and nerve damage, resulting in possible anesthesia or at least paresthesia. The successful recovery is meticulous and should only be attempted by the experienced surgeon.

The loss of a root tip on the lingual to the third molar in the mandible places the tip in a difficult area for recovery (Fig. 10-18). It will be below the mylohyoid muscle and requires special positioning of the head of the patient. Place a finger

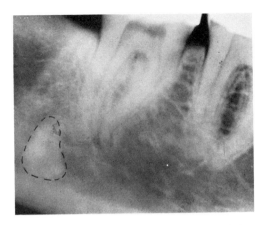

Fig. 10-18. Third molar root tip forced through lingual plate into the submaxillary space.

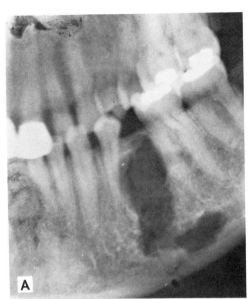

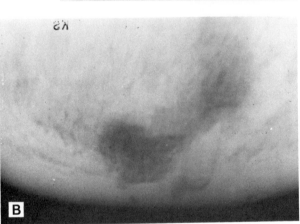

Fig. 10-17. Root tip dislodged into the inferior alveolar canal.

lingual plate, and as a result of swallowing by the patient and gravity, the tip tends to dissect its way inferiorly, making its location and recovery difficult.

Another area in which recovery of a lost tip or tooth is difficult is the infratemporal space posterior and superior to the maxillary tuberosity. Important neurovascular structures and the pterygoid plexus of veins occur within these tissues. Care must be taken to avoid working blindly in this area and to maintain contact always

extraorally to bring pressure on the submaxillary tissue to create a counterforce during exploration. A lengthy flap reflecting to the lingual is necessary for exposure (Fig. 10-19). The root tips of third molars are easily lost through the thin

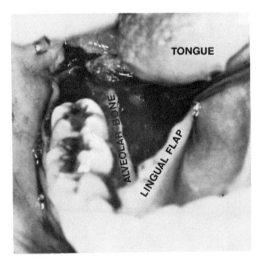

Fig. 10-19. Flap design for the recovery of root tip from the submaxillary space.

with the tooth or root by good vision and feel. Recovery from this area requires careful dissection or severe bleeding and nerve damage may result.

The loss of a root during the extraction procedure can be frustrating and discouraging. However, a well thought-out plan that includes various recovery procedures and a knowledge of the potential hazards will do much to alleviate this anxiety.

Other Complications

Additional complications occurring during the extraction of teeth include: injuries to adjacent teeth; fracturing alveolar bone, the tuberosity, or even the mandible; swallowing or aspirating a tooth or foreign body; and hemorrhage.

When a portion of the alveolus of the maxillary tuberosity has been fractured, the principle of conservation holds true. If the portion of bone fractured is of a reasonably good size and is still attached to periosteum, it should be left in place and immobilized with a suture or a splint. It will practically always heal and, of course, is valuable to the integrity of the alveolus. If, however, the segment is small and free from the periosteum, it will have lost its blood supply and, if permitted to remain, may sequestrate and contribute to infection. The large piece of bone removed with the maxillary third molar shown in Figure 10-20 was not replaced. Such a fracture and loss of bone might have been prevented had elevation techniques been used with a flap procedure and controlled bone reduction. In cases in which a piece of bone has been fractured and removed, a flap should be reflected and the sharp bony margins smoothed

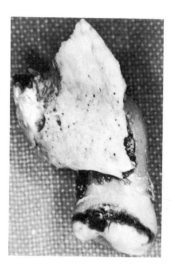

Fig. 10-20. Tuberosity removed with the extraction of maxillary third molar.

with files and rongeurs and the flap repositioned.

A much more serious problem exists in the event of a fractured mandible. Such an occurrence does not necessarily imply negligence; it is a potential complication of many difficult extractions. For management of these problems, see Chapter 19.

Breakage or injury to adjacent restorations and/or teeth and even the extraction of the wrong tooth can occur. Immediate repair (e.g., placement of a temporary filling or crown) must be done if appropriate. On occasion, a tooth may be displaced or completely dislodged. If the tooth is not fully developed, it can often be immediately repositioned and splinted and will probably survive. Such may not be the case with the accidental removal of a mature tooth. In such instances, prevention is better than treatment.

The swallowing or aspiration of a tooth

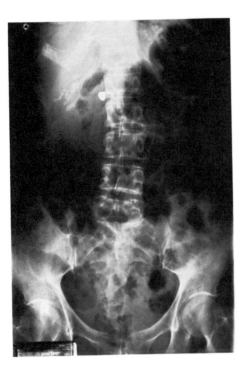

Fig. 10-21. Abdominal radiograph demonstrating a gold cast crown inadvertently swallowed by the patient.

or foreign body is an acute emergency (Figs. 10-21 and 10-22). The prevention of such an occurrence is most important; placing a pharyngeal curtain (gauze pack) across the throat helps in this regard. The contrast of the white gauze to the mucosa improves vision and the protection is worthwhile. If such an emergency does occur, the operator must immediately obtain chest films or flat plates of the abdomen to locate the tooth or foreign body. If it has dropped into the trachea, severe coughing will probably occur (Fig. 10-23). This, then, becomes a medical management case for recovery by bronchoscopy or esophagoscopy. Sometimes, when the gastrointestinal tract is involved, the specimen may pass without complications (Fig. 10-24).

Hemorrhage during surgery or postop-

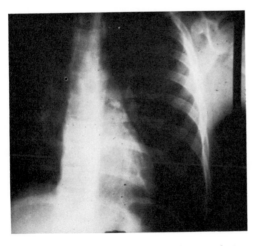

Fig. 10-22. A tooth lost into the pharynx during extraction and then aspirated into the lung.

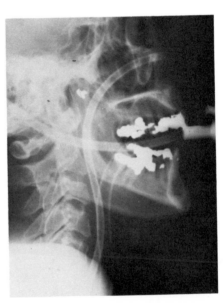

Fig. 10-23. A gold inlay, dislodged during an unrelated surgical procedure in a patient in the prone position, was recovered from the nasopharynx.

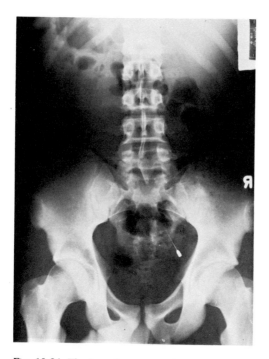

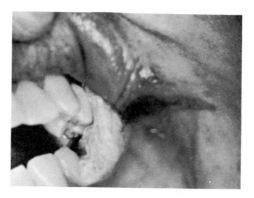

Fig. 10-25. Lip burn at angle of the mouth as a result of dental bur friction.

Fig. 10-24. The loss of a root canal reamer into the pharynx—now shown in bowel. (Courtesy of N. O. Holte)

eratively is one of the complications and will be discussed in Chapter 17.

The dental drill, while most useful for its intended purpose, can also be the cause of tissue irritation. This instrument can actually overheat when not working properly and burn anesthetized mucosa before the calloused hand of the operator detects how much heat is being generated. The rotary bur can unnecessarily cause a friction burn of the lip (Fig. 10-25). Puncture wounds can also occur if the unprotected bur slips under pressure and penetrates the soft tissue. The instrument may also be bumped inadvertently from its hanger by the doctor or assistant. Since patients are in the supine position for much of their dental work, all instruments should be kept carefully away from the head in case any instrument should be bumped and falls on the patient (Fig. 10-26).

The dental handpiece with its rotary attachment can inflict considerable in-jury, especially to tongue and lips. When the tongue is anesthetized, a patient is unaware of how mobile and in the way it is. Constant and careful attention to the work at hand is necessary to avoid a serious laceration (Fig. 10-27).

Another complication that may be stressful to both patient and doctor is immediate intraoral swelling upon making a posterior superior alveolar nerve injection. This probably results from lacerations of the pterygoid plexus of veins, causing an immediate release of blood that pools toward the mucosal surface. It occurs rapidly, at the time the needle is directed through the area or during its removal (Fig. 10-28). Pressure directed over the area will stop it with no serious sequelae. If a large hematoma occurs and a surgical procedure of the associated area has been contemplated, it would be well to postpone it. However, there would be no reason not to proceed with planned restorative work.

Too many persons in the operatory can create a variety of complications. Usually, no one does his best work with a large audience. Should an emergency develop,

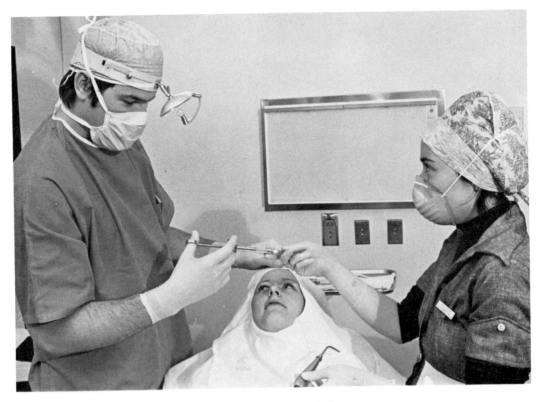

Fig. 10-26. No instrument should ever be passed over a patient's face.

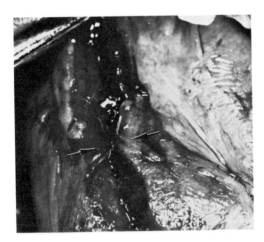

Fig. 10-27. Deep laceration of the tongue occurred with a dental disc. Top of photograph shows tip of tongue with proximating suture in center to control bleeding.

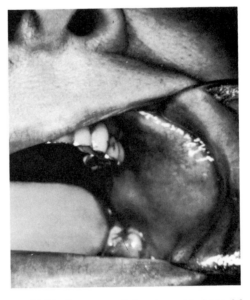

Fig. 10-28. Hematoma of the pterygoid plexus following injection of local anesthetic.

efficient measures cannot easily be carried out if there is a room full of people.

In spite of careful planning, diagnosis, and treatment, emergencies will occur. It is well to have a plan prepared for handling all anticipated emergencies, as well as a list of the person(s) with whom you intend to consult and/or refer such problems to. Good communication with the patient is most important and should be handled in a confident, sympathetic, but nonapologetic manner.

References

1. Thoma, K. H., and Goldman, H. M.: Oral Pathology, 5th ed., pp. 1241–1247. St. Louis, C. V. Mosby, 1960
2. Fader, M., Kline, S. N., Spatz, S. S., and Zubrow, H. J.: Gardner's syndrome (intestinal polyposis, osteomas, sebaceous cysts) and a new dental discovery. Oral Surg., Oral Med., Oral Path., 15:153, 1962.
3. Shafer, W. G., Hine, M. K., and Levy, B. M.: A Textbook of Oral Pathology. Philadelphia, W. B. Saunders Co., 1963.

11 Impacted Teeth

DANIEL E. WAITE

When teeth do not assume their normal position for function in the dental arch, they are considered impacted, or embedded, and with rare exceptions, should be removed (Fig. 11-1). Some exceptions would include (1) patients whose general health is so poor that such a surgical procedure is inadvisable;[1] (2) patients whose age is such that, in the presence of a totally asymptomatic tooth, such a surgical procedure is unnecessary and unwise. If a very young person requires total extraction for advanced caries or periodontal disease and unerupted third molars are present, it might be advisable to leave such impacted teeth until a later time for removal. This is done to ensure the protection of the valuable retromolar pad area and the maxillary tuberosity for prosthetic support during the long denture-wearing period. These teeth would be removed when eruption was such that it interfered with the prosthesis. Otherwise, it is my opinion that all teeth are intended to erupt and gain entrance into the oral cavity, and impacted teeth should be removed except in those instances when it is inadvisable or not possible.

Impacted teeth create a variety of complications, such as follicular cystic development (Fig. 11-2A), migration of the teeth, plus the erosion of adjacent normal teeth (Figs. 11-2B and 11-3). Degeneration of the follicular sac into ameloblastoma (Fig. 11-2C and D) and frank carcinoma (Fig. 11-2E) with its serious sequelae have been reported.

Common problems relating to third molars are infection and pain. The removal of third molars can contribute to a high incidence of periodontal pocket formation involving the distal aspects of second molars.[2] This is less likely to occur if they are removed early in their development, and close attention is given to flap design.

Secondary only to periodontitis is pericoronitis, which may be either transitory and mild or develop into a serious throat infection involving the fascial spaces, causing considerable debilitation. It occurs in the soft tissue of the partially erupted third molar, providing a fertile bed for bacterial growth and infection. Treatment may vary from local irrigation and debridement of the pericoronal flap to removal of the tooth. In instances in which the maxillary third molar traumatizes the mandibular third molar pericoronal tissue, it may be advisable to remove the maxillary tooth first and later extract the lower molar when inflammation, pain, and infection have subsided (Fig. 11-2F).

Impacted teeth have been defined as

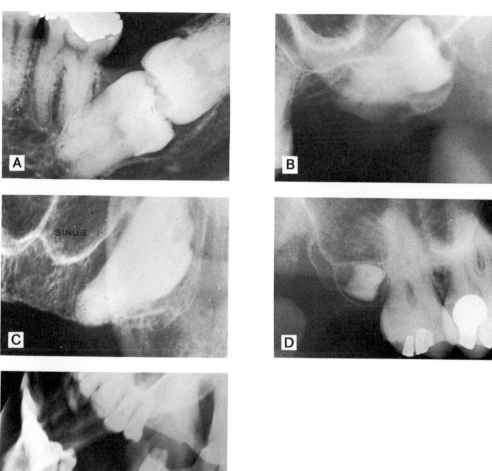

Fig. 11-1. (A) Impacted mandibular second and third molars. (B) Maxillary impacted third molar inverted. (C) Maxillary third molar inverted proximal to maxillary sinus. (D) Maxillary supernumerary impaction in third molar position. (E) Mandibular third molar migrating to sigmoid notch.

those whose eruption is partially or wholly obstructed by bone or other teeth (Figs. 11-4 and 11-5). Practically any tooth may become impacted, but the mandibular third molar is most frequently involved (Fig. 11-6). This frequency can be explained by the fact that the third molar is the last tooth to erupt normally, and any condition tending to lessen the space provided for it will naturally leave it without sufficient room. The canine, or cuspid, tooth is the last of the anterior

teeth to erupt, and it suffers similarly from lack of space when this part of the jaw is affected (Figs. 11-7 and 11-8).

Etiology

The cause of impactions is more theoretical than factual, and according to one author, should be discussed under three separate theories.[3] First and foremost is the *orthodontic theory.* Inasmuch as the normal growth of the jaw and the move-

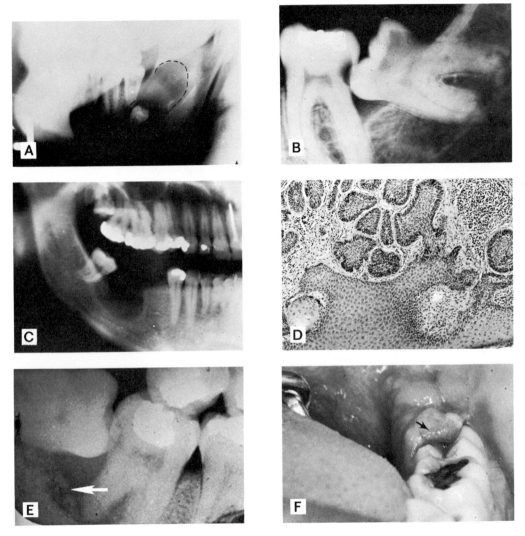

Fig. 11-2. (A) Dentigerous cyst forcing third molar inferiorly. (B) Mesioangular impaction demonstrates caries within the impacted tooth and erosion at the point of contact of the second molar. (C) Ameloblastoma of mandible. (Courtesy of Dr. Frantzich) (D) Microscopic section of ameloblastoma. (E) Bite-wing x-ray film partially showing impacted tooth and follicle that was positive for squamous cell carcinoma. Patient expired within five years. (F) Pericoronitis and operculum of mandibular third molar caused by constant traumatic irritation of maxillary third molar.

ment of the teeth are in a forward direction, anything interfering with such development will cause an impaction of teeth. Dense bone usually results in a retardation of such forward movement, and many pathologic conditions bring about a condensation of osseous tissue. For example, acute infections, fevers, severe trauma and malocclusion, and local inflammation of the periodontal membrane can cause increased bone density. Constant mouth breathing usually leads to contracted arches, and consequently, those teeth erupting last have no room. Occasionally, an early loss of deciduous teeth may cause arrested development of

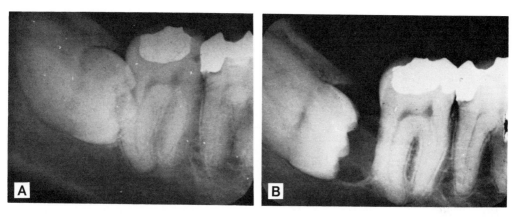

Fig. 11-3. (A) Impacted mandibular third molar. (B) Movement of third molar over a four-year period.

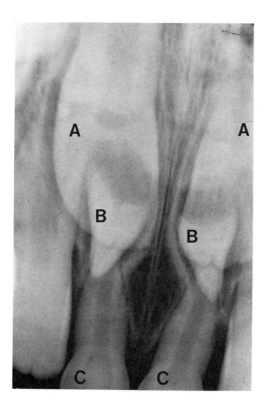

Fig. 11-4. Periapical x-ray film showing supernumerary teeth preventing eruption of permanent central incisors. Permanent incisors (A); supernumerary teeth (B); deciduous central incisors (C).

the jaw and/or malposition of the permanent teeth, resulting in impactions.

The second theory of interest is the *phylogenic theory*. Nature tries to eliminate that which is not used, and our civilization with its changing nutritional habits has practically eliminated the human need for large powerful jaws. As a result of this altered function, the size of the maxilla and mandible has decreased. In many instances, the third molar occupies an abnormal position, is malformed, and may be considered a vestigial organ without purpose or function. Moreover, it is frequently congenitally missing.

Mendelian Theory. It seems probable that heredity—such as transmission of small jaws from one parent and large teeth from the other—may be an important etiologic factor in impactions. Certainly, irregularities in some animals can be produced artificially by genetic manipulation—why should not the same thing occur accidentally in the human population?

Unfortunately, impactions follow no pattern; they have various shapes and

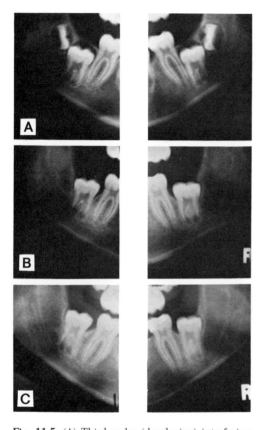

Fig. 11-5. (A) Third molar (developing) interfering with second molar eruption. (B) Third molar removed and second molar erupting (three months after surgery). (C) Second molar erupting into position (six months after surgery).

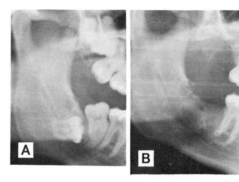

Fig. 11-6. Panogram views of third molar impaction, maxillary and mandibular. (A) Third molar impaction, with second molar overerupted. Impacted third molar in maxilla. (B) Third molar and second molar removed.

Diagnosis

The diagnosis is established at least partially by the clinical examination. It is imperative to have the area covered in detail by radiographs, followed by accurate interpretation. The dentist must know the true relationship of one tooth to the other;[4] this information is difficult to obtain if the teeth cannot be observed clinically, so it must then come from x-ray examination.

To form an overall, accurate interpretation of the radiograph, constant comparison of the visible teeth with the x-ray image is necessary. For example, if the clinical examination reveals teeth in their normal position but the radiograph records an overlap, it may be assumed that the angulation of the x-ray study was incorrect and should be repeated. If the clinical examination reveals lapping of the third molar over the second molar, it could theoretically be a buccal deflection, since lingual deflection seldom occurs.

sizes, and any tooth may be involved. They also vary widely in degree of impaction; some are partially erupted, whereas others are completely encased in bone. The literature presents many cases in which impacted teeth lie dormant in the jaw until long after the loss of the adjacent teeth, and then suddenly start to erupt, causing inflammation and pain.

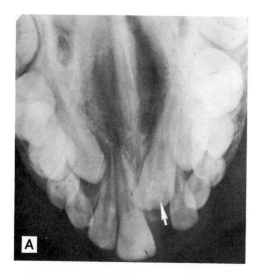

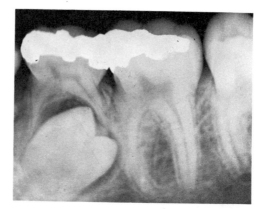

Fig. 11-8. Impacted mandibular second bicuspid and retained deciduous molar.

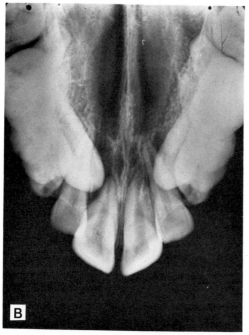

Fig. 11-7. (A) Bilateral maxillary impacted cuspids. Note odontoma (at arrow) overlying the impacted maxillary central incisor. (B) Occlusal x-ray film of bilateral maxillary impacted cuspids.

When teeth are in a normal, unrotated position, the enamel can be recorded on the radiograph as an "enamel cap," and if the rest of the teeth on the film are in normal alignment, their caps will be simi-

lar in appearance. However, if one of the teeth has a deflection, part of its occlusal surface will show and its cap will be distorted (see Fig. 10-1, p. 119). The outline of the pulp chamber on the x-ray film may also indicate torsion or rotation of the tooth in question. Other guides in reading the average radiograph are that (1) the area of concern should appear in the center of the film, and two views should be obtained; (2) the contact points should appear open, indicating the central ray has passed at a right angle to the area of exposure; (3) there should be some superimposition of the cusps of the posterior teeth; (4) some soft tissue registration should be seen; and (5) all roentgenologic interpretation should support clinical findings. Radiographic coverage of the third molar may include occlusal and lateral jaw films as well as regular intraoral films.

After a satisfactory radiograph has been secured, the operator should study it to interpret correctly every diagnostic point that may be present. First to be studied is the third molar, followed by the second and first molars.

Impacted Mandibular Third Molars

The diagnostic points of the impacted lower third molar are studied in the order of crown, roots, supporting bone, and mandibular canal.

The *crown* is observed in relation to the enamel cap, pulp, occlusal surface, and the buccal deflection. The crown may appear in various positions; this is discussed under the classification of third molar impactions (p. 140). When viewing the radiograph, an imaginary line should be drawn across the occlusal surface of the second molar in order to determine the vertical alignment of this surface with that of the impacted tooth.

If torsional deflection is present, it can be interpreted by studying the crown and root formation of the third molar and comparing the enamel cap, pulp chamber, and root formation of this tooth with those of another molar known to be in normal position. The pulp chamber may be small or obliterated, and the enamel cap will lose its sharp outline. Preoperative recognition of torsion is important because it will help in planning the operative procedure and lessen trauma. Caries are another important consideration; they often complicate removal since the strength of the crown is important to the plan of the operative procedure (Fig. 11-9).

After the crown has been thoroughly examined, the next consideration is the *roots*. They will vary in size from short to exceedingly long, in shape, from fused conical roots to two or more divergent roots, and may extend in any direction. If

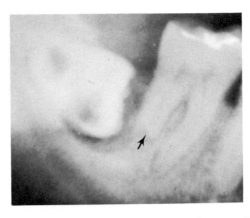

Fig. 11-9. Caries or internal resorption of impacted tooth. Note destruction of bone around the crown of the third molar and the distal roots of second molar.

the tooth is inclined lingually or buccally, the radiograph will not outline the entire tooth sharply. The sharpest images will always be those structures closest to the film.

The *surrounding bone* should be examined to determine whether it will interfere with the removal of the tooth. The density of the bone and/or the presence of bone destruction by infection may alter the surgical approach. The amount of bone to be removed is estimated by evaluating the crown and roots in relation to the bone and the line of removal.

The proximity of the *mandibular canal* must be accurately known in order to avoid injury to the nerve and vessels (Fig. 11-10). Where there is definite impinge-

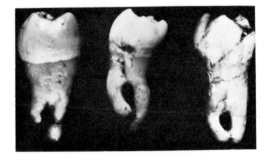

Fig. 11-10. Three different cases in which the third molar roots formed around the inferior alveolar nerve and vessels.

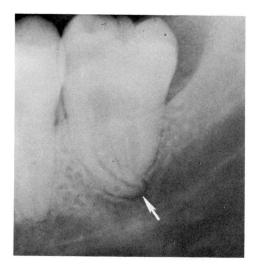

Fig. 11-11. Root apices close to mandibular canal. Note radiolucency of apex—not the result of bone destruction, but of proximity to the canal.

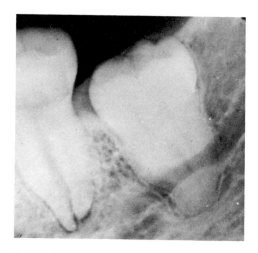

Fig. 11-13. Note proximity of canal to both second and third molar teeth and the constriction of the canal overlying the third molar.

ment, the root of the tooth appears to fade away, or the root of the tooth is darker at the point where it touches the canal. Sometimes, this fading away is so great that it is impossible to completely outline the root. When there is no impingement, the density of the roots is the same throughout the roentgenogram (Figs. 11-11 and 11-12). It is also well to note the lateral walls of the canal, and if impingement is present the canal will appear constricted (Fig. 11-13).

The nearness of the impacted tooth to the inferior border of the mandible is important from a pre- and postoperative viewpoint. The amount of bone inferior to the roots of the tooth should always be noted (Fig. 11-14).

A good classification of third molar impactions is given by Pell and Gregory.[5]

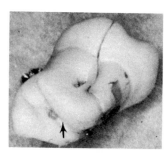

Fig. 11-12. Third molar removed. Note groove in apex of tooth created by mandibular canal.

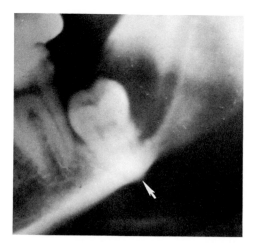

Fig. 11-14. Impacted tooth forced inferiorly by pressure within the follicular cyst. Apex of tooth palpable extraorally at inferior border of mandible.

This classification is based on an evaluation of the relationship of the second molar to the ascending ramus of the mandible, the relative depth of the third molar in the bone, and the position of the third molar in relation to the long axis of the second molar. It is explained in detail as follows:

1. Relation of the tooth to the ramus of the mandible:

    Class I. Sufficient space exists between the ascending ramus and distal of the second molar for the accommodation of the entire mesiodistal diameter of the crown of the third molar.

Class II. The space between the ascending ramus and the distal of the second molar is less than the mesiodistal diameter of the crown of the third molar.

Class III. All or most of the third molar is within the ramus.

2. Relative depth of the third molar in bone:

    Position A. The highest portion of the impacted tooth is on a level with or above the occlusal surface of the second molar.

    Position B. The highest portion of the tooth is below the occlusal line, but above the cervical line of the second molar.

    Position C. The highest portion of the tooth is on a level with or below the cervical line of the second molar.

3. The position of the tooth in relation to the long axis of the second molar:

    a. Vertical (Fig. 11-15).

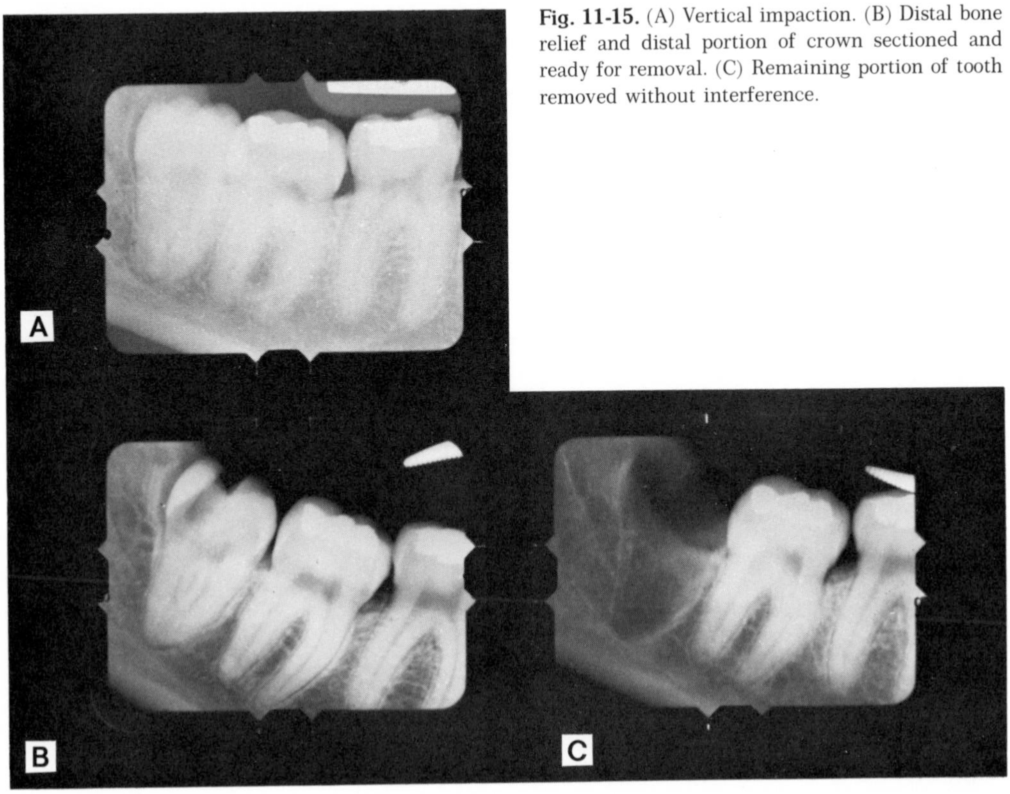

Fig. 11-15. (A) Vertical impaction. (B) Distal bone relief and distal portion of crown sectioned and ready for removal. (C) Remaining portion of tooth removed without interference.

b. Horizontal.
c. Inverted.
d. Mesioangular (Fig. 11-16).
e. Distoangular (Fig. 11-17).

The purpose of this classification system is to create an orderly approach to the diagnostic evaluation and surgical approach to third molar surgery. If the surgeon adheres to the classification procedure, he can make a quick decision regarding the types of impaction he wishes to personally handle and those he would choose to refer. It also provides valuable information for the well-qualified assistant, who will know the correct

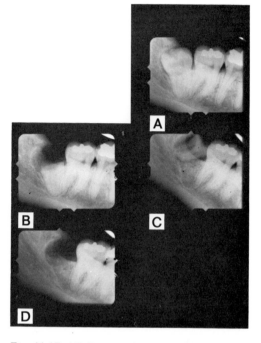

Fig. 11-17. (A) Distoangular impaction. (B) Distal and buccal bone relief and crown sectioned horizontally and removed. (C) Root portion of tooth raised into the superior space. (D) Total tooth removed with minimal trauma to surrounding bone and teeth.

instrument setup and the amount of time that should be reserved for the surgical appointment. The use of this orderly approach to impaction problems can do nothing but contribute to the success of the procedure and add harmony to what might otherwise be a discouraging experience for all concerned (Fig. 11-18).

Surgical Technique

After the patient has been evaluated, the history reviewed, the instruments selected, and the anesthesia established, attention can be directed to the details of the surgery. The patient should be prepared

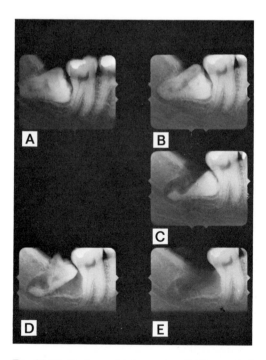

Fig. 11-16. Mesioangular impaction. (A) Bone relief on distal and buccal. (B) Tooth sectioned with high-speed drill. (C) Superior portion of tooth removed. (D) Inferior part of tooth raised into superior space. (E) Tooth removed with minimal trauma.

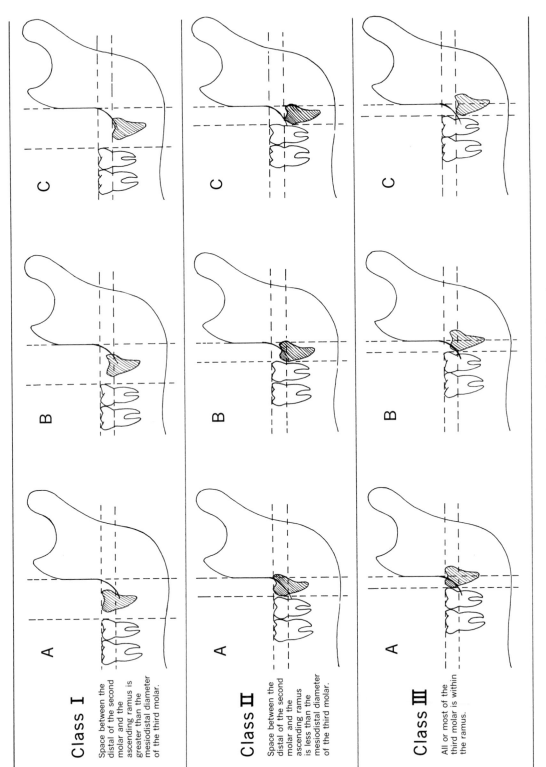

Class I

Space between the distal of the second molar and the ascending ramus is greater than the mesiodistal diameter of the third molar.

Class II

Space between the distal of the second molar and the ascending ramus is less than the mesiodistal diameter of the third molar.

Class III

All or most of the third molar is within the ramus.

Fig. 11-18. Classification of third molar impactions.

and draped in a manner acceptable for all basic oral surgical procedures. A mouth grossly poor in hygiene may require scaling, prophylaxis, or hydrogen peroxide rinses prior to surgery. Draping should include a sterile towel across the chest connected to a sterile head towel. The purpose of draping in oral surgery procedures is to drape out contaminated areas such as hair and whiskers, rather than to drape in a sterile area as would be done in the preparation of a skin surface. Reference is made again to the "seven minimum essentials," which is a standardized approach that will always stand the operator in good stead. After mentally checking each step, the procedure is begun.

For the average third molar impaction, the incision is made using the reverse bevel technique around the neck of the second molar;[6] it is kept on the ridge as much as possible (see Fig. 8-11, p. 101). The envelope-type flap is recommended. If access is inadequate, the incision can be extended in either direction. A common failure in impaction removal is inadequate exposure and therefore poor vision. Tissue does not necessarily heal end to end, but in all directions. Therefore a 1-inch flap takes just as long to heal as a 2-inch flap. In this sense, conservation is not always the best policy.

The no. 15 Bard Parker blade is used, making certain that the incision extends to bone, and the entire length of the incision is completed at one time. The no. 1 Woodson periosteal elevator is used to pull the interdental tissue free and the reflection of the flap is started. These first moments are tedious and may take a little extra time, but this will be time well spent. The push stroke for further reflection is used as soon as practical and the

total flap reflection is then complete. The flap is held back by means of a retractor, which should be placed lightly against the bone without constantly bearing against the flap. This technique will greatly minimize flap tearing, edema, and postsurgical pain (Fig. 11-19).

One should have a mental picture of where the embedded tooth lies in relation to the overlying bone (Fig. 11-20A), and this bone is carefully trephined with the surgical high-speed drill under irrigation (Fig. 11-20B). This area should be as large as necessary without endangering the second molar tooth and the distal bridge of bone. The bur holes are then connected and the bed of bone lifted off (Fig. 11-20C). At this point working space and displacement space must be created. Working space is that space created for the placement of the elevator or the bur for direct work on the tooth. Displacement space is created if the tooth is to be split or elevated to provide room for portions of the tooth during removal.

At this point one must decide whether

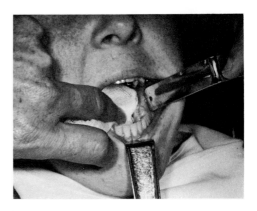

Fig. 11-19. Appropriate exposure of third molar site for surgery. Gauze positioned by surgeon's finger while assistant retracts cheek.

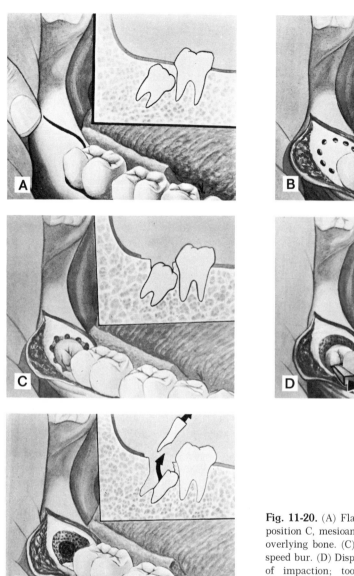

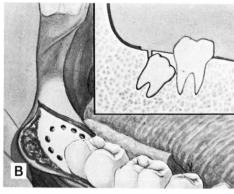

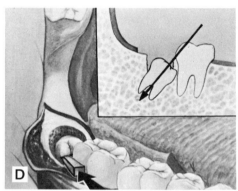

Fig. 11-20. (A) Flap design for removal of Class I, position C, mesioangular impaction. (B) Removal of overlying bone. (C) Exposure of crown using high-speed bur. (D) Displacement space evident on distal of impaction; tooth split with bi-bevel chisel. (E) Distal one half of tooth removed. (Courtesy of M. L. Hale)

to split the tooth with a chisel (Fig. 11-20D and E), or to section it with the bur and remove it in pieces; either technique works well. Elevators are used to remove the sectioned parts (Fig. 11-21). Additional sectioning methods may be utilized according to the type of impaction (Fig. 11-22).

Once the tooth has been removed, the toilet of the cavity must be carefully done.

The curette should first be used as an explorer to be sure the socket is clean. Irrigation can be used to remove bone dust and chips. A file may be needed to smooth interseptal areas or other bone margins. Bleeding is controlled and the flap returned and sutured (Fig. 11-21G). Before the pressure pack is applied the base of the flap should be milked upward to ensure no accumulation or pooling of blood

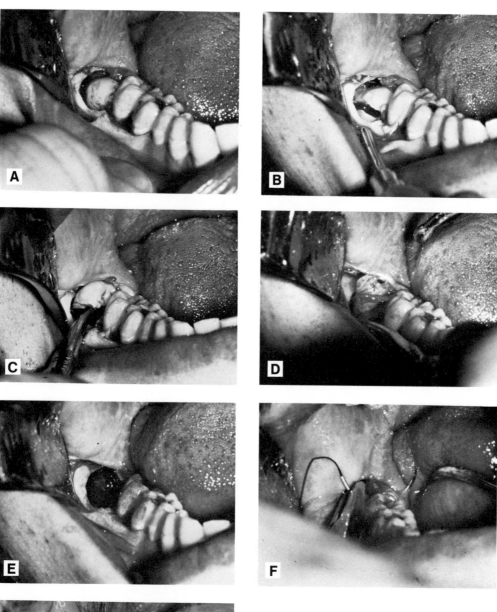

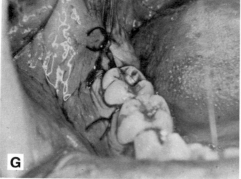

Fig. 11-21. (A) Envelope flap has been reflected and overlying bone removed with high-speed drill. (B) Impacted tooth is sectioned with bur in line with long axis of tooth. (C) Elevator is in place and superior portion of tooth is moved forward and out. (D) Inferior portion of tooth is elevated into the superior space and removed. (E) Socket is cleansed and free of debris, ready for closure. (F) Flap is returned and sutured with black silk suture. Suture distal to second molar is placed first. (G) Three sutures adequately position the mucoperiosteal flap.

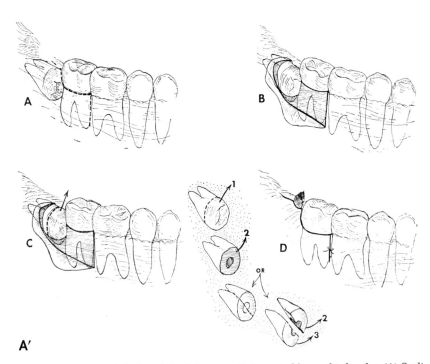

Fig. 11-22A'. Plan for removal of the less difficult horizontally impacted lower third molar. (A) Outline of flap. (B) Flap reflected, crown exposed. (C) Site of sectioning and path of exit of crown indicated; inserts show two methods of completing removal of tooth. (D) Wound sutured. (Clark, *Practical Oral Surgery*, Lea & Febiger, 1965)

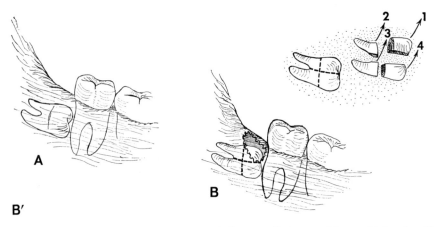

Fig. 11-22B'. Plan of removal of deeper, more difficult horizontally impacted lower third molar. Numerals indicate order of removal of sections for greatest ease and for greatest safety to second molar. (Clark, *Practical Oral Surgery*, Lea & Febiger, 1965)

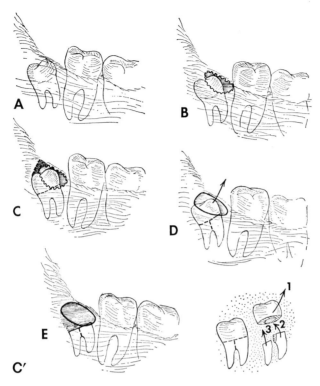

Fig. 11-22C'. Plan for removal of distoangular impacted lower third molar. (A) Preoperative situation. (B) Disc of bone removed for access. (C) Impinging bone above crown removed. (D) Sites for sectioning with bur to remove crown and divide roots indicated by dotted lines; path of exit for crown shown by arrow. (E) Crown removed and individual paths of exit for each root suggested by arrows. (Clark, *Practical Oral Surgery*, Lea & Febiger, 1965)

or saliva under the flap. A postoperative radiograph should be taken and postoperative instruction given. Appropriate medication for average third molar surgery should include analgesics and sedation. An appointment to return within three to five days should be arranged.

In the past few years, the literature has reflected an interest in the split bone technique for the removal of impacted mandibular third molars.[7] It is referred to as the lingual approach in contrast to the buccal, and is purported to be a shorter surgical procedure with fewer postoperative complications. The method requires removal of bone distolingually with final delivery of the tooth to the lingual. However, this method is not the best surgical technique for the novice or infrequent operator. Manipulation of lingual soft tissue, the proximity of the lingual nerve, and the severity of postoperative infection occurring in this area are deterrents to the procedure. Lingual soft tissue edema, lateral pharyngeal abscess formation, and trismus frequently accompany surgical procedures involving these tissues.

A careful review of the expected postoperative problems should be discussed. An estimation of the degree of discomfort, edema, and ecchymosis should be made (Fig. 11-23). Postoperative edema is difficult to predict due to patient individuality and propensity for swelling. The degree of trauma also dictates the postoperative course; the intermittent use of ice for the first 12-hour postoperative period, followed by heat applications, is helpful (see

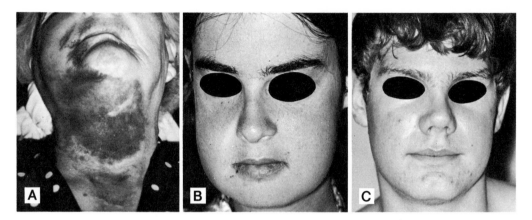

Fig. 11-23. Postoperative problems following removal of third molar impactions. All three cases similar in degree of surgical difficulty. (A) Ecchymosis. (B) Marked edema. (C) Minimal edema.

Chapter 15) (Fig. 11-24). The postoperative phase of third molar surgery can be devastating or it can be tolerated as expected, but, at best, it is not comfortable (Fig. 11-25).

Antibiotics may regularly be indicated in deep, difficult impactions and, when used, they should be prescribed in adequate dosage for a minimum of five to seven days. Good supportive therapy also includes adequate medication for pain and sedatives for two nights following surgery. An emergency contact should be provided. It is helpful to give the patient a written form that lists detailed instructions or at least the essential points of concern (Figs. 11-26 and 11-27).

Impacted Maxillary Third Molars

The indications for the removal of impacted maxillary third molars are similar to those that dictate mandibular third molar removal. These include such possible developments as pericoronitis, periodontitis, caries, pathologic resorption,

cysts, neoplasms, and idiopathic pain. However, the incidence of such sequelae is less than with impacted lower third molars. Maxillary third molars, like mandibular third molars, may also be found in the edentulous mouth, particularly if multiple extractions have occurred in the patient's younger years. In such cases, the developing third molar in either arch may have been purposely left in place in order to minimize the injury to the tuberosity or retromolar pad area, so necessary to prosthesis stability and retention.

As with impacted mandibular third molars, it is improbable that impacted maxillary teeth induce crowding of the dentition. No evidence exists that proves that impacted teeth cause orthodontic relapse.

Most impacted teeth will ultimately cause some difficulty. Since the operative and postoperative complications are significantly reduced when the impacted third molar is not pathologically involved, it is recommended that such teeth be removed as soon as it is obvious that there is

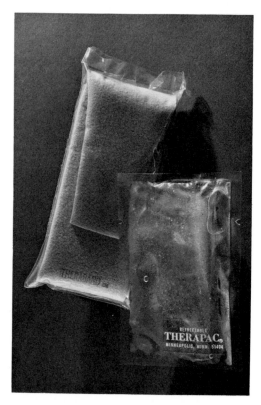

Fig. 11-24. Several types of proprietary cold pack preparations are available. The Therapac is a refreezable product that adapts well to the face or other areas where a cold pack may be useful. (Therapac Inc., Minneapolis, Minn.)

insufficient space or that they are not in a position for normal eruption. This decision can usually be made by the time the patient is 16 to 17 years of age.

Maxillary third molars are removed with less surgical difficulty than mandibular third molars because the bone of the area is less dense, which permits movement of the tooth by elevator technique. The flap design is usually the envelope type, but when necessary, a vertical arm may be added to the flap for increased exposure of a high impaction. Vision is difficult and the operator must become accustomed to the "feel" of these teeth as they are drawn out by the use of appropriate elevators (Fig. 11-28). The movement of the mandible into lateral excursion is helpful because it provides increased space between the ramus and the tuberosity.

Complications that may result include herniation of the buccal fat pad into the wound, affecting the vision of the operator, and the loss of the tooth into the buccal space, the pterygomaxillary space, or the throat. Osteitis or dry socket is not a common complication. Penetration of the maxillary sinus is a potential complication; this is discussed in Chapter 16.

Impacted Cuspids[8-11]

After the third molars, the cuspids are the teeth that are most frequently impacted. Several authors found that impacted maxillary cuspids occurred in both sexes but more often in girls.[8,9] A palatal impaction of these teeth was three times more frequent than a buccal one.[8] In a 1961 study, there was found a definite tendency for unilateral impactions rather than for bilateral.[9]

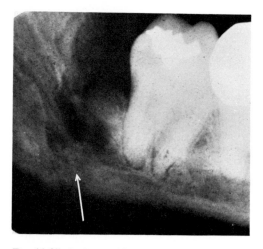

Fig. 11-25. At four weeks postoperatively, a pathologic fracture has occurred.

POSTOPERATIVE INSTRUCTIONS

Postoperative care is important after oral surgery and recovery may be delayed if this is neglected. Some swelling, stiffness and discomfort is to be expected. If this is excessive, please call or return for care.

THE DAY OF OPERATION

Bleeding
a. Keep gauze pack in place 30 minutes with constant, firm pressure.
b. Keep head elevated and rest quietly.
c. Do not suck or spit excessively. If bleeding persists, repeat the above.
d. Some oozing and discoloration of saliva is normal.

Swelling
Apply ice pack to region of surgery for 10 minutes per ½ hour for the first 6–8 hours.

Pain
Take prescribed tablets and rest.

Diet
Liquids, soft, or regular (as desired). Do not skip meals.

The Second Day
Brush teeth. Use hot water rinse (½ tsp. salt in glass of hot water [coffee temp.]) 3–5 times per day. Continue tablets for pain if necessary.

M_____

has an appointment with

_____

Day   **Date**   **Time**

Mon. _____

Tues. _____

Wed. _____

Thurs. _____

Fri. _____

The above time is reserved for you. If you are unable to keep your appointment, please notify the Clinic 24 hours in advance.

If care is necessary after clinic hours, please call:

000-0000

Fig. 11-26. Outline of instructions for postoperative care and postoperative appointment card.

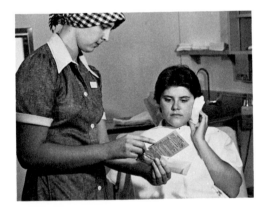

Fig. 11-27. The instructions for postoperative care should be explained when they are given to the patient.

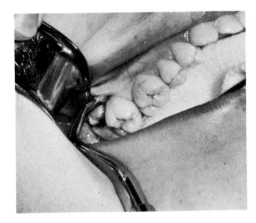

Fig. 11-28. Flap reflected and third molar exposed for elevation.

Several causes of impacted cuspids have been proposed, such as lack of space due to early loss of deciduous molars.[11] Odontoma, supernumerary teeth, cysts, and retained deciduous cuspids have also been reported as contributing to the impaction of maxillary cuspids (Fig. 11-29).

Roentgenologic localization and interpretation are important when evaluating impacted cuspids. The occlusal film, the

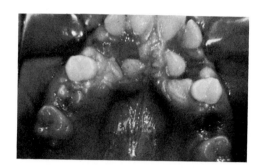

Fig. 11-29. Impacted maxillary cuspids uncovered by surgery; rapid eruption will often follow.

profile film, and the periapical film all become important. Since the great majority are palatally positioned, this is the usual surgical approach. The heavy palatal tissue is lowered and the bone relieved over the crown of the impaction. The crown can then be sectioned near its cervical line and removed, and the root drawn into the space thus created (Fig. 11-30). The flap is then returned and sutured.

References

1. Laskin, D. M.: Indications and contraindications for removal of impacted third molars. Dent. Clin. North Am., *13*:919–928, 1969.

2. Ash, M. M., Jr., Costich, E. R., and Hayward, J. R.: Study of periodontal hazards of third molars. J. Periodontol., *33*:209–219, 1962.

3. Durbeck, W.: *The Impacted Mandibular Third Molar.* London, H. Kempton, 1945.

4. Morris, H.: Anatomic considerations pertinent to the general practice of oral surgery. Dent. Clin. North Am., July, 1964, pp. 383–393.

5. Pell, G. J., and Gregory, B. T.: Impacted mandibular third molars; classification and modified technique for removal. Dental Digest, *39*:330–338, 1933.

6. Friedman, N.: Mucogingival surgery; the apically repositioned flap. J. Periodontol., *33*:328–340, 1962.

7. Rud, J.: The split-bone technic for removal of impacted mandibular third molars. J. Oral Surg., *28*:416–421, 1970.

8. Rohrer, A.: Displaced and impacted canines. Ortho and Oral Int. J., *15*:1002–1020, 1929.

9. Dachi, S. F., and Howell, F. V.: A study of impacted teeth. Oral Surg., *14*:1165–1169, 1961.

10. Thilander, G., and Jakobsson, S. O.: Local factors in impactions of maxillary canines. Acta Odontol. Scand., *26*:145–168, 1968.

11. Hitchen, A. D.: Impacted maxillary canine. Br. Dent. J., *100*:1–2 Disc. 12–14, 1956.

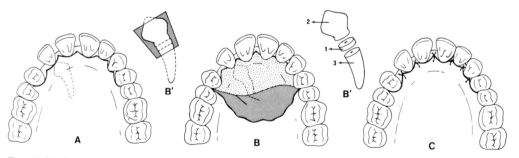

Fig. 11-30. Sectioning method for removing impacted cuspids. (A) Flap outline. (B) Flap reflected. (C) Flap returned and sutured.

12 Root Resection, Replant, Implant, and Transplant

DANIEL E. WAITE

Root Resection

There was a time when teeth were condemned and sacrificed if a root-end cyst or granuloma was evident. Now the conservative surgical approach of root canal filling with apicoectomy, or root resection, or the nonsurgical approach of endodontics has provided an excellent opportunity for maintaining these involved teeth.

In most instances, routine endodontic management of a tooth with a periapical lesion (abscess) will be adequate treatment, and surgical apicoectomy is not necessary (Fig. 12-1). The pulp contents are removed, and the canal reamed, cleaned, dried, and filled with silver points or gutta-percha and paste. Once this has been done, the apical injury should recover and heal normally. On this premise, the procedure of apicoectomy has been performed less frequently and good results have followed. To be confident of success, the clinician must be certain that he is dealing with a root-end granuloma and not a root-end cyst. This distinction is difficult, because the old criteria of a white line on the x-ray picture and the escape of cystic fluid upon opening the canal are not reliable for the accu-

rate diagnosis of a cyst. Statistically, about 45 per cent of the so-called root-end abscesses are granulomas, and about 55 per cent or less are cysts[1] (Fig. 12-2).

If the abscess is a cyst, enlargement is slow and no harm will be done if follow-up observation is provided. Follow-up evaluation and continued dental treat-

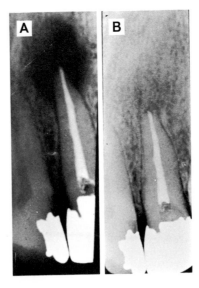

Fig. 12-1. (A) Root canal filling completed. (B) Apical lesion filled in with bone, six months later. (Courtesy of J. Jensen)

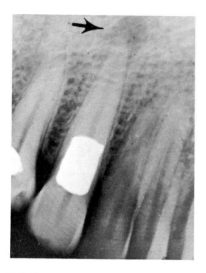

Fig. 12-2. X-ray picture of root-end lesion; periapical cyst confirmed by biopsy. (Courtesy of J. Jensen)

ment for all patients, however, are difficult because of the mobility of the population. Therefore, an apicoectomy may be indicated when follow-up is not possible, or when the work must be done in one appointment. Surgery is also indicated when it is impossible to fill the canal completely to the apex of the tooth, or when the canal is overfilled. In some cases a chronic infection may remain at the periapical site; in these instances, root resection or curettage should be done.

Surgical Technique

After an adequate radiograph has been taken and the decision made to proceed with the apicoectomy, the root canal may be filled prior to the surgical approach or after access to the root end has been obtained. The pulp is opened and the contents are removed. The surgical approach is then made, and with direct vision of the apical end, the canal can be reamed, filed, cleaned, dried, and filled. Finally, a good apical seal is made. Positive suction at the surgical site should be employed during the procedure to avoid contamination of the canal with blood. The alternative is to

complete the endodontic procedure and then proceed with the apicoectomy; either method is acceptable. A slightly curved incision is made over the apex of the tooth with the scalpel (Fig. 12-3). Adequate tissue with a good blood supply should be evident between the attached gingivae and the incised margin. An incision that extends around the cervical neck of the tooth and has one vertical arm may be used when greater exposure is needed or when a large amount of bone destruction exists. As with all alveolar surgery, the basic principles of flap design and reflection are followed.

After the flap has been reflected, a careful comparison of the surgical site with the x-ray film should be made. A surgical bur or chisel is used to perforate into the bony defect and locate the root end (Fig. 12-4). If the canal has already been filled, any excess paste or other filling material is removed. The bur is then used to reduce a small portion of the root, which is preferably beveled toward the labial side. This provides easy access to the apical canal for observation of the completeness of the canal filling or retrograde filling.

Following the control of hemorrhage

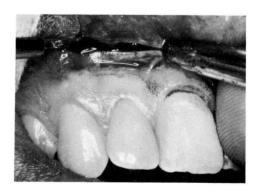

Fig. 12-3. Incision for apicoectomy.

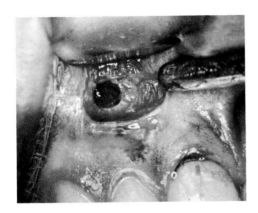

Fig. 12-4. Bone removed and root end exposed.

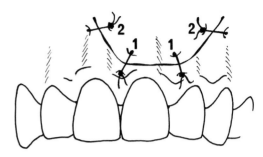

Fig. 12-5. Proper placement of sutures to reposition the flap correctly.

and debridement of the apical wound, the flap is returned and closed with interrupted silk sutures (Fig. 12-5). An immediate postoperative x-ray picture is taken, and a cotton roll or gauze is placed and pressure applied to the lip for 20 minutes. Sutures can be removed in four to six days and follow-up x-ray studies are taken at one-, three-, and six-month intervals or until the void has been completely filled with new bone.

Replantation, Implantation, and Transplantation

The history of replantation and transplantation of teeth dates back to the eighteenth and nineteenth centuries. John Hunter referred to "the practice of wrenching from the jaw of the indigent and helpless a tooth for a fine lady was done, all for the price of a meal."[2] Stack, in 1883, made the comment that transplants, replants, and repositioning should be done for the poor, who "cannot obtain the aid of artificial dentures."[3] On the battlefield of yesteryear, soldiers had to give up their teeth to officers who had lost theirs in battle.[4] Ambroise Paré indicated that "a certain princess had a tooth taken out and it was immediately replaced, being supplied by one of her ladies."[5]

Terminology becomes important when discussing the general area of transplantation and replantation. The following terms may help clarify the present status of this changing field:

A. Root resection—excision of the apical portion of a root.
B. Replantation—reinsertion of a tooth into the socket from which it was removed.
C. Implantation—insertion of a subperiosteal framework in the intact tissues of the recipient.
D. Transplantation:
   1. Autoplastic transplant (autotransplant, autogenous)—transplant between different parts of the same person.
   2. Heteroplastic transplant (heterologous)—transplant between different species.
   3. Heterotopic transplant—transplant of tissue typical of one area to a different recipient area.

4. Homotopic transplant—transplant of tissue typical of both the donor and recipient areas.

5. Isoplastic transplant (homoplastic, homologous)—transplant between members of same species.

6. Syngenesioplastic transplant—transplant between related members of the same species (e.g., mother to child, brother to sister).

7. Xenoplastic transplant—transplant of tissues between members of different species.

8. Anatomic relationship of origin and destination:

   a. Orthotopic transplant—transferred to an anatomically similar environment.

   b. Isotopic transplant—transferred to a topographic region which corresponds exactly.

   c. Heterotopic transplant—transferred to an atypical position, e.g., skin to mucosa.

9. Methods of transplantation:

   a. Free transplant—transferred completely free or separated from original environment.

   b. Pedicled transplant—connected to parent tissue and transplanted. Usually guarantees nutrition.

10. Vital or nonvital transplants:

   a. Homovital transplant—transferred vital and remains so.

   b. Homostatic transplant—successively loses vitality.

Replantation

The teeth most often involved in replantation are the anterior teeth of children following a variety of home accidents. The tooth can often be immediately replaced and reattachment and repair expected to occur when the apex of the tooth is still open, the tooth is only partially avulsed, and a minimal time (less than 90 minutes) has elapsed between the time of

the injury and treatment by the dentist.[4] When a tooth is repositioned and/or replanted, the tooth apices must be open in order for revascularization and reattachment to occur. The tooth should be immobilized by means of a splint, such as an Essig wire, criss-cross wire, or an acrylic overlay splint (Fig. 12-6). Of course, orthodontic banding would be ideal. If apical involvement develops at a later date, root resection and/or endodontic treatment may be done. However, if the tooth is completely out of the oral cavity and contaminated (e.g., by being on the ground), and more than 90 minutes have elapsed between the time of injury and

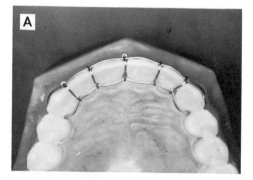

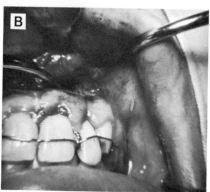

Fig. 12-6. (A and B) Essig wire stabilization.

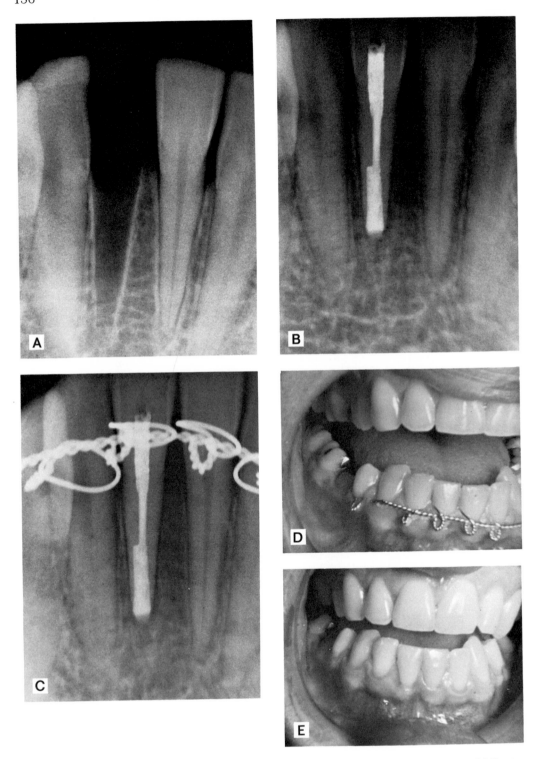

Fig. 12-7. Replantation. (A) Lower central incisor avulsed in athletic injury. (B) Tooth repositioned following retrograde endodontics. (C) Seven weeks after injury. Note Risdon wire used for fixation. (D) Clinical picture, the tooth firm and functioning seven weeks after injury. (E) Clinical appearance three months after injury. (Courtesy of Dr. N. O. Holte)

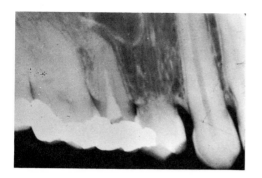

Fig. 12-8. Fifteen years after replantation of first bicuspid.

treatment, it is better to do immediate root canal therapy before reinserting the tooth and splinting it in place (Fig. 12-7). In such instances, resorption over a period of time will probably occur. Nevertheless, during this period the tooth will have served a functional purpose and maintained space in the arch; it may well remain in position for several years (Fig. 12-8). In such cases, antibiotics on a prophylactic basis should be administered for a period of seven to ten days; prophylactic protection for tetanus should be given.

It has been stated that healing in replantation occurs through resorption and replacement or ankylosis. With the loss of the periodontal membrane, progressive resorption of the root occurs, and it is replaced with bone. In other instances, healing may be entirely normal, with reestablishment of the periodontal membrane and total revascularization and vitalization of the tooth. Moreover, simple resorption may continue over a long period of time with no ankylosis.

Implantation

Implantation primarily refers to the placement of a subperiosteal framework or an osseous pin[6] to which a tooth or teeth can be attached. The implant denture has not been accepted by most prosthodontists as a regularly successful approach to the difficult edentulous patient (Fig. 12-9). The subperiosteal placement

of magnetic implants with the attracting magnet placed in the prosthesis has also been attempted, but resorption and migration of the implant magnet have made the technique difficult (Fig. 12-10).

The *mandibular staple* also has been used for stabilization of the denture. The staple is inserted extraorally under precise conditions and is indicated in patients with mandibular atrophy (Fig. 12-11).

Vitreous carbon was developed in 1963 and became commercially available in 1967. Prior to this time, carbon was known to be biocompatible;[7-9] however, not until the development of this new

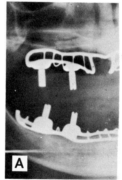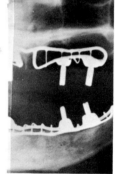

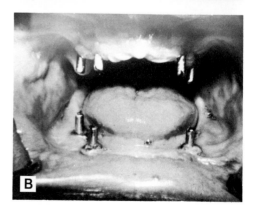

Fig. 12-9. Implant denture framework placed subperiosteally. (A) X-ray appearance. (B) Clinical appearance.

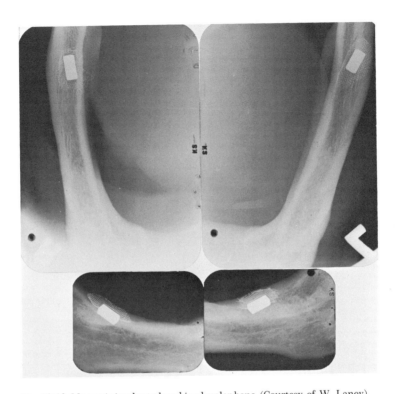

Fig. 12-10. Magnetic implant placed in alveolar bone. (Courtesy of W. Laney)

form of carbon was the pure material of sufficient strength to be used as a prosthetic device.[10] Research work began on establishing its biocompatibility and searching for medical applications.[11, 12]

Animal research was started in May, 1970,[13] and in 1971 a series of human dental implantations began. The animal studies showed minimal adverse tissue response, and a long-term (30 months) systemic study confirmed that vitreous carbon had no carcinogenic or toxic properties.[14] After establishing the safety of using the carbon implant in humans, several areas in the country carried out projects utilizing vitreous carbon as an endosseous dental implant. The University of Minnesota was one such center.

Vitreous carbon implants have been used in a variety of applications. They have been used as a single tooth replacement, a bridge abutment, and an aid in maintaining alveolar bone. They may be placed in fresh extraction sites or in healed sites. They have been used in individuals from 10 to 80 years old. The most important requirement is adequate bone to house the implant. A rolled, broad ridge of good quality cortical and cancellous bone free of any pathologic condition is an absolute requirement.

The surgical procedure is uncomplicated and within the scope of the general dentist. First, the proper position of the implant relative to the patient's occlusion must be determined. A mucoperiosteal

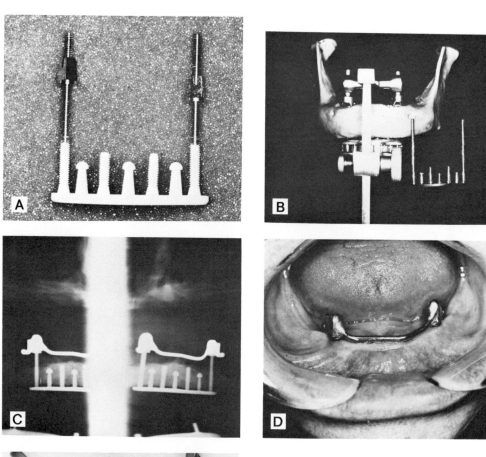

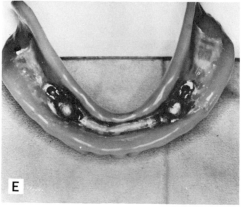

Fig. 12-11. Mandibular staple. (A) Seven pin mandibular staple. (B) Drill guide in place on specimen mandible. The drill guide provides parallel holes, so that the mandibular staples can be inserted into inferior border of the mandible. (C) Seven pin mandibular staple which has been functioning well for eight years. (D) Mandibular staple with superstructure and attachments, functioning well eight years after operation. (E) Undersurface of denture showing the female portion of the attachments. The denture is borne mostly by tissue and is stabilized by the mandibular staple. (Courtesy of Dr. I. Small)

flap is raised to gain adequate exposure of the surgical area. The socket is created using surgical bone burs and socket gauge to establish the correct depth and size for the cavity. The implant is tapped into place using a mallet and orangewood stick. Stabilization of the implant is necessary. It can be accomplished by splinting the implanted tooth to an adjacent tooth or by suturing the flap over the implant and allowing the mucosa to maintain the implant in position. The implant should be maintained in a stable position during the healing phase, much as an

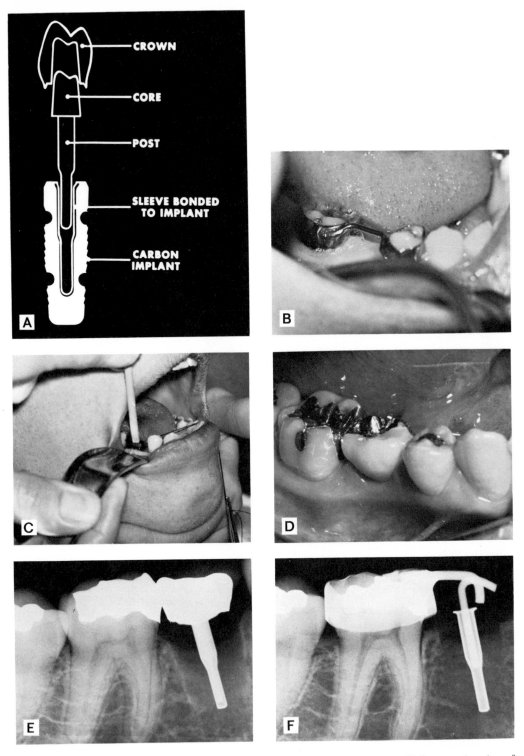

Fig. 12-12. Vitreous carbon implant. (A) Vitreous carbon implant and socket gauge. (B) Preoperative view of edentulous space and space maintainer. (C) Carbon implant being tapped into place with orangewood stick. Implant in this patient has been in place 34 months without any postoperative complications. (D) Final restoration with full-crown restoration on implant and splinted to an inlay in adjacent molar tooth. (E) Periapical radiograph immediately after operation. (F) Periapical radiograph six months postoperatively. Note cortical bone starting to outline the implant. (Courtesy of Dr. W. Frantzich)

160

avulsed tooth would be stabilized. The duration of the stabilization period may vary from six weeks to six months; however, this period may be shortened if the permanent restoration is splinted to an adjacent tooth (Fig. 12-12).

Experience at the University of Minnesota has shown the splinted implant to have a much higher degree of success than the free-standing or nonsplinted implant. The area of greatest success appears to be in the bicuspid region. Perhaps this is because of the more consistent good quality bone and ease of splinting to adjacent teeth.

Different techniques for implantation for a single tooth have been suggested. In such instances, a *Vitallium screw* has been placed through the apical portion of the tooth and inserted into the socket; postoperative healing and fibrosis are intended to anchor the implant screw. In other instances, a *Vitallium post* has been inserted into the bone, and the crown of the tooth fabricated upon it. The most difficult problem is the lack of an epithelial attachment to the foreign body, thereby maintaining a continual egress of tissue fluids along the implant material that permits contamination.

Transplantation

Much time, research, and investigation have gone into the study of tooth transplants. Homologous tooth transplantation has not been successful, primarily because of the rejection response and transplantation immunity. However, autogenous tooth transplants have had a fair measure of success. Autogenous tooth transplantation is taking a tooth from one portion of the oral cavity and placing it in a new

surgical site within the same mouth. This is not to be confused with surgical repositioning, which is the uprighting of a tipped or slightly embedded tooth by direct surgical technique (Fig. 12-13).

Developing teeth are utilized in autogenous transplants. The ideal method is to move a developing third molar forward to a first or second molar site when these teeth have been lost prematurely by caries or other causes. Under a careful surgical technique, such teeth can be expected to serve a useful purpose for many years. The tooth to be transplanted should at least have begun root formation with evidence of the bifurcation. The operator uncovers the third molar in the usual manner, being certain to direct no apical pressure on the developing root ends (Fig. 12-14).

The reduction of occlusal and overlying bone will be necessary to permit lifting the tooth from its donor site without injury. The tooth is not removed from the donor site until the recipient site has been prepared completely. For example, suppose a permanent first molar must be removed because of caries. Attention would be given to this tooth, making certain that the mesiodistal diameter of the host site will accommodate the donor tooth. If not, slight reduction of the third molar is permitted with a disc under irrigation. Following the extraction of the first molar, the socket is enlarged sufficiently to receive the tooth and hold it in an adequate position for acceptable alignment in the oral cavity and still have the root surfaces well impregnated in the new socket. Stabilization is accomplished by means of a fine wire or an acrylic splint, which is left in place until the tooth has stabilized (Fig. 12-15).

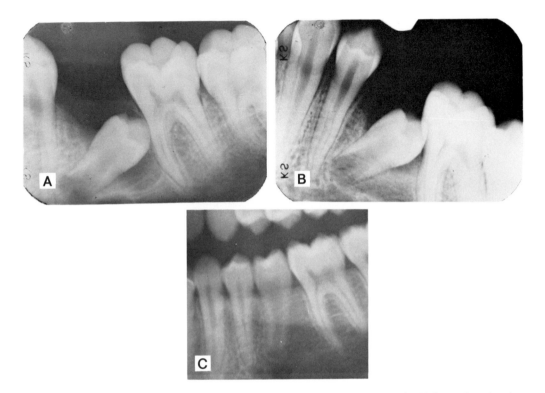

Fig. 12-13. A fourteen-year-old patient with embedded second mandibular bicuspid. (A) Surgical exploration with removal of overlying bone and minimal elevation of the tooth was performed. (B) Within three months the tooth is erupting and the root formation continues. (C) One year later, the tooth has completely erupted into the arch.

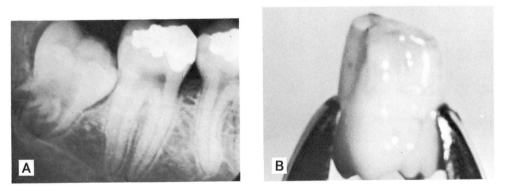

Fig. 12-14. (A and B) Appropriate development for transplant of third molar.

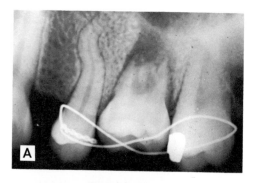

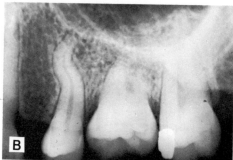

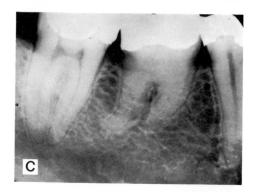

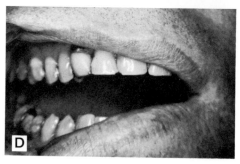

Fig. 12-15. (A) Case 1. Transplanted mandibular third molar placed in maxillary first molar site and stabilized by wiring. (B) Transplant five years postoperatively. (C) Case 2. Transplanted mandibular third molar to mandibular first molar site, 15 years postoperatively. (D) Clinical photograph of Case 2.

Another technique provides for the complete embedding of the entire transplant tooth into the new socket area and covering it with the gingival flap. Continued formation of the tooth and, finally, eruption are expected. A variety of successes have been reported.

References

1. Stafne, E. C.: Oral Roentgenographic Diagnosis. Philadelphia, W. B. Saunders Co., 1969.
2. Hunter, J.: Natural History of Human Teeth. London, J. Johnson, 1771.
3. Stack, T. R.: Replantation and transplantation of teeth. Trans. Acad. Med. Ireland, 1:314, 1883.
4. Andreasen, J. O., and Hjorting-Hansen, E.: Replantation of teeth. I. A radiographic and clinical study of 110 human teeth replanted after accidental loss. Acta Odontol. Scand., 24:263, 1966.
5. Emmertsen, E., and Andreasen, J. O.: Replantation of extracted molars; a radiographic and histological study. Acta Odontol. Scand., 24:327, 1966.
6. Branemark, P. I.: Intra-osseous anchorage of dental prosthesis. Scand. J. Plast. Reconstr. Surg., 3:81–100, 1969.
7. McCutcheon, M.: Chemotaxis in leukocytes. Physiol. Rev., 26:319, 1946.
8. Gott, V. L., Keopke, D. E., Daggett, R. L., Zarnstoff, W., and Young, W. P.: The coating of intravascular plastic prostheses with colloidal graphite. Surgery, 50:382, 1961.
9. Gott, V. L., Whiffen, J. D., and Dutton, R. C.: Heparin bonding on colloidal graphite surfaces. Science, 142:1297, 1963.
10. Cowlard, F. C., and Lewis, J. C.: Vitreous carbon—a new form of carbon. J. Materials Science, 2:507, 1967.
11. NASA: Carbon offers advantages as implant material in human body. NASA

Tech. Brief 69–10087. Technology Utilization Officer, Marshall Space Flight Center, Huntsville, Alabama 35812, April 1969.

12. Benson, J.: Pre-survey on biomedical applications of carbons. NASA Report, Contract NAS 8-5604, Report R-7855 Rocketdyne, North American Rockwell, 6633 Canoga Avenue, Canoga Park, California 91304, May 1969.

13. Grenoble, D. E., Melrose, R. J., and Markle, D. H.: Histological evaluation of a vitreous carbon endosteal implant in dogs. School of Dentistry. University of Southern California, 925 West Thirty-fourth Street, Los Angeles, California 90007, 1 July 1971.

14. Petten, L. E., v.: Report on chronic safety evaluation of Vitredent's Vc 1800 Vitreous carbon dental implants into the alveoli of dogs, vol. III. Huntington Research Center, Brooklandville, Maryland. (Private communication of Vitredent Corp.) December, 1973.

13 Preprosthetic Surgery

DANIEL E. WAITE

Soft Tissue Surgery

The oral surgeon will have to perform soft tissue surgery to correct and adjust such conditions as a limiting frenulum attachment, gingival hyperplasia and hypertrophy, and fibromatoses, as well as to manipulate soft tissue structures in order to create an acceptable ridge for a prosthesis. The manipulation of soft tissue attachments should only be considered in relation to the anatomy and physiology of the particular soft tissue and the underlying osseous structure. The maxillary sinus, the inferior alveolar canal, the mental foramen, muscle insertions and origins, and the salivary ducts are all important to consider when planning the surgical procedure.

Anatomy[1]

The dentist should clearly understand the basic anatomy of the desired edentulous ridge contour. The bulbous type of ridge, the U-shaped and the knife-edge ridges are encountered regularly and dealt with accordingly. However, in those cases in which no vestibular depth exists because of alveolar bone atrophy, trauma, or other causes, surgical intervention may become necessary for prosthodontic purposes. An awareness of the attachment of the muscles of facial expression to the surface of the mandible and maxilla is essential to understand the need for and the execution of these surgical procedures (Fig. 13-1). The mucobuccal and labial folds of the upper vestibule are determined by the bony origins of certain facial muscles.

Buccinator Muscle

The buccinator muscle of the cheeks derives its name from Latin, in which it means trumpeter. Its origin is from the outer alveolar process of the maxilla, the external oblique line of the mandible, and the pterygomandibular raphe. The terminal fibers blend into the orbicularis oris muscle. The function of the buccinator is to limit and control food within the dental arches and to aid the tongue in shifting the food and keeping it on the occlusal table until sufficiently masticated and prepared for swallowing. In the majority of vestibuloplasty procedures, portions of this muscle will be altered.

Levator Anguli Oris Muscle

The levator anguli oris muscle originates from the canine fossa of the maxilla and inserts into the soft tissue near the

165

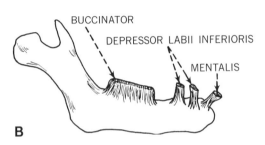

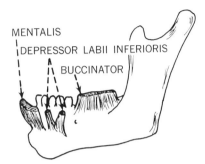

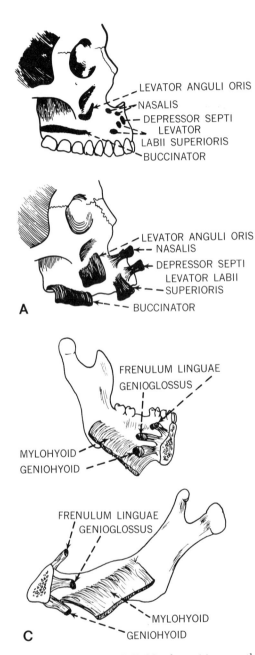

Fig. 13-1. (A, B, and C) Muscle positions on the lateral, labial, and lingual surfaces of the maxilla and the mandible in the dentulous as compared to the edentulous mouth.

angle of the mouth. When it contracts, together with the quadratus labii superioris, the nasolabial sulcus is accentuated. The lower portion of this muscle lies beneath the angular artery; therefore, surgical procedures affecting the two muscular origins may result in brisk arterial hemorrhage. However, blunt dissection of the tissues rather than sharp will often avoid severing of the vessel.

Levator Labii Superioris Muscle

The levator labii superioris muscle is a small muscle band that arises from the outer alveolar process of the maxilla. It has two points of origin just above the lateral and cuspid teeth, and inserts into the fibers of the orbicularis oris muscle. Its function is of little concern and probably serves only to tense the lip.

Nasalis and Depressor Septi Muscles

The nasalis and depressor septi muscles have a fairly low point of origin on the maxilla and frequently are severed in alveoloplasty procedures. However, their function is restricted almost completely to the action of the alae of the nose (Fig. 13-2).

Mentalis Muscle

The mentalis is an elevator of the chin and arises from the incisive area on the outer surface of the mandible. Its function is valuable in tensing and raising the lower lip in facial expression. During surgical procedures in this area, particularly vestibuloplasty, which is a supraperiosteal procedure, the entire muscle origin should not be sacrificed. In the surgical approach to this portion of the mandible for bone work, the degloving technique is subperiosteal and therefore permits reattachment without interfering with muscle function.

Depressor Labii Inferioris Muscle

The depressor labii inferioris muscle originates from the incisive fossa and inserts into the deep fibers of the lower lip. This muscle is located closer to the inner mucosae than the skin surface and often is involved in flaps designed to deepen the sulcus.

Mylohyoid Muscle

The origin of the mylohyoid muscular basket for support of the tongue is from the mylohyoid ridge, which is the same as the internal oblique ridge. A median fibrous raphe between this paired muscle serves as the insertion for the muscle fibers, which pass medially and posteriorly from their bony origin. The action of the mylohyoid raises the hyoid bone and also the floor of the mouth, thus enabling the tongue to exert pressure against the palate, aiding in deglutition. This muscle plays a minor role in depressing the mandible. It appears that most of this muscle can be sacrificed in surgical procedures without complication. During the procedure of lowering the floor of the mouth, the mylohyoid is carefully approached and sectioned close to its point of origin. This is a supraperiosteal technique, and

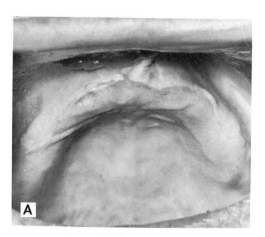

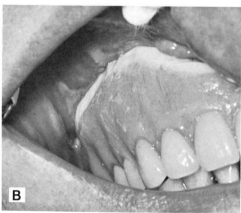

Fig. 13-2. (A) Vestibular extension into the lateral nasal area for denture stability is done with a skin graft. (B) A treatment denture with a soft tissue liner is worn for two months postsurgery, when the new denture is made.

after careful repositioning of the overlying mucosa, portions of the muscle probably reattach. Special care must be exercised when transecting the posterior portion of the muscle, since the lingual nerve is in close relation in this area.

Genioglossus Muscle

The genioglossus is a powerful extrinsic muscle of the tongue. This paired muscle arises from the superior genial tubercles, with its upper anterior fibers radiating toward the tip of the tongue and its remaining fibers passing back to the dorsum of the tongue and down to the upper border of the hyoid bone. When the upper fibers contract, the tip of the tongue is lowered and brought forward. The inferior fibers exert a pull on the hyoid bone,

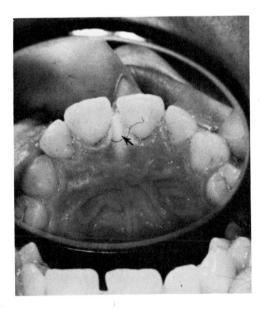

Fig. 13-3. Technique to determine lingual attachment of the frenulum. Note tissue blanching on the lingual.

raising it and drawing it forward. Because this is an important muscle for proper manipulation of the tongue, the entire attachment should not be sacrificed in surgical procedures, although the superior portions of it may be sectioned without causing apparent limitation of the tongue.

Geniohyoid Muscle

Originating from the lower genial tubercle and inserting into the anterior surface of the body of the hyoid bone, the geniohyoid muscle functions when the hyoid bone is fixed. It then acts as a depressor of the mandible. Its motor innervation is supplied by the loop of the cervical plexus between the first two cervical nerves by way of the sheath of the hypoglossal nerve.

Frenula

Frenula are rarely muscular in nature. They usually consist of mucosal folds in the labial, buccal, and occasionally the lingual surface of the alveolar ridge (Fig. 13-3). They act as flexible checkreins, limiting the movement of the lips, cheeks, and sometimes the tongue. A diastema between the maxillary incisors may appear due to the frenulum; however, when the lateral and cuspid teeth erupt this space almost always closes. If not, frenectomy is indicated. As the alveolar bone resorbs, the frenum attachments become more limiting and may need to be lengthened or excised (Fig. 13-4).

Surgical Correction of Soft Tissue Abnormalities

Frenectomy

Several techniques are available for labial frenectomy. Vertical or elliptical excision from the base of the frenulum attachment is a good method; the lip portion is closed by undermining the lateral

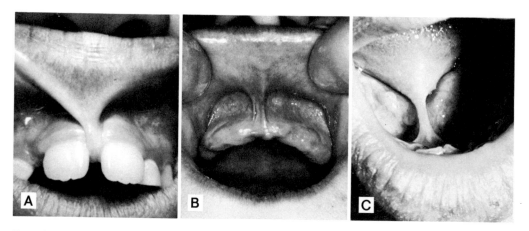

Fig. 13-4. (A and B) Maxillary frenulum attachments. (C) Lingual frenulum attachment to tongue.

borders and suturing together. A horizontal incision in the depth of the sulcus will provide more mobility of the tissue for closing (Fig. 13-5). The electrocautery unit may also be used to sever the attachment, and has the advantage of minimizing bleeding (Fig. 13-5).

Z-plasty is used to correct wide fibrous bands and muscle. A vertical incision is made along the length of the frenulum and undermined on both sides. Two lateral incisions are made, one on each side at opposite ends of the vertical incision—the three incisions resembling the letter "Z." The flaps are then transposed and sutured, obliterating the fibrous band and lengthening it (Fig. 13-6).

The hemostat technique is a good method for removing the labial frenulum. One clamp is applied to the lip portion of the frenulum and one to the ridge portion, with the tips of clamps both meeting in the depth of the fold. A scalpel is then passed beneath the clamps, removing the frenulum. The lip portion is sutured and the ridge portion is not. A surgical pack dressing or oral bandage may be placed in the alveolar void for a few days, if desired (Fig. 13-7).

To determine the need for excision of the lingual attachments of a labial frenulum when a diastema continues to exist

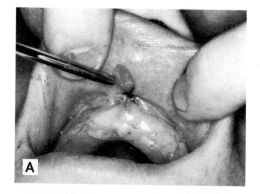

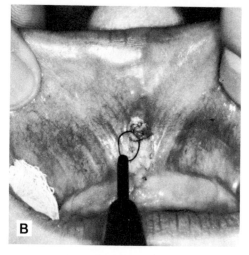

Fig. 13-5. (A) Elliptical excision technique for removal of frenulum; horizontal suture in place following the excision. (B) Frenectomy by electrocautery.

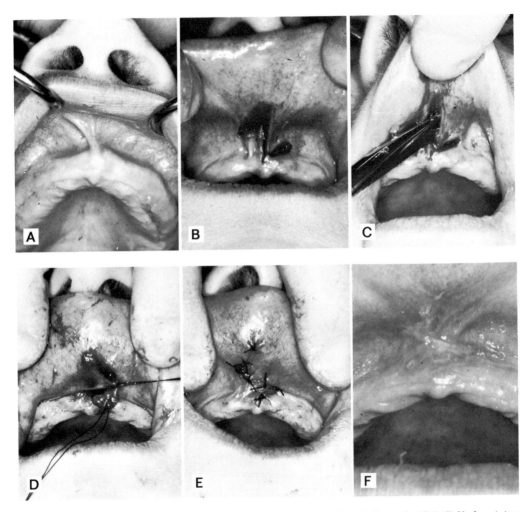

Fig. 13-6. (A) Frenulum to be corrected by Z-plasty. (B) Incision outlined in the form of a "Z." (C) Undermining of flaps. (D) Transposition of flaps. (E) Flaps sutured into new position. Note lengthening. (F) After suture removal.

after lateral and cuspid tooth eruption, place traction on the lip and observe whether blanching occurs on the lingual aspect (see Fig. 13-3). If so, excision of the lingual attachment is also indicated. In some instances the bony septa between the maxillary incisors may also have to be removed; this can be accomplished by carefully passing a tapered fissure bur a short distance between the teeth.

In cases of small muscle attachment on the buccal, an inverted semilunar incision supraperiosteally can be made at the base of the attachment (Fig. 13-8). With mini-

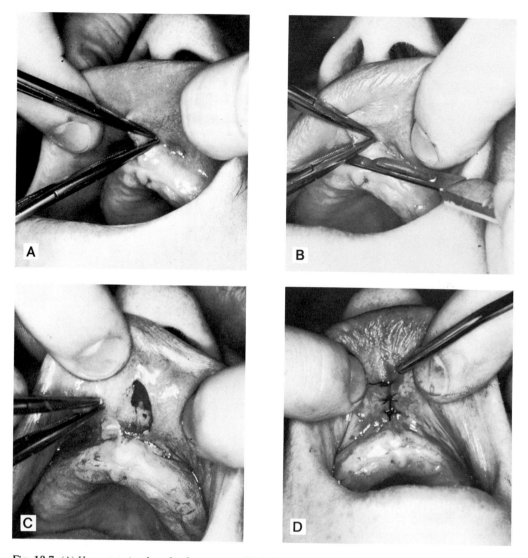

Fig. 13-7. (A) Hemostats in place for frenectomy. (B) Ridge incision of frenulum is made first. (C) Frenulum excised. Note elliptical shape of wound. (D) Sutures in place (lip portion only).

mal undermining, the attachment is raised and sutured to the periosteum (Fig. 13-9).

Lingual frenulum attachments on the tongue cause various degrees of ankyloglossia, which may interfere with speech and certainly limit the tongue in its cleansing ability. In such instances, the elliptical excision technique, the Z-plasty, or the V-Y advancement may all be acceptable procedures (Fig. 13-10).

Tuberosity Reduction

The surgical correction of the bulbous tuberosity is performed primarily to provide stability of the prosthesis and to increase posterior vertical dimension (Fig. 13-11A). The tuberosity can best be reduced by an elliptical incision with minimal undermining and the removal of two inverted triangles of tissue. The V-shaped incision is made first through the center of

osity. If bone removal is necessary, it is accomplished at the same time (Fig. 13-11C, D, and E).

Another technique for tuberosity reduction is to decapitate that portion of the soft tissue tuberosity that is pendulous or hanging down (Fig. 13-12A). If the tuberosity is entirely composed of soft tissue, this horizontal excision can be accomplished with slight contouring and minimal hemorrhage. In such instances the primary goal is to increase vertical dimension and still maintain a good solid base for the prosthesis (Fig. 13-12B).

Flabby Tissue

Flabby tissue beneath a poorly fitting prosthesis may constitute a difficult surgical problem (Fig. 13-13). If the denture can be removed for seven to ten days prior to surgery, the edema and inflammation will subside sufficiently to make the procedure considerably less difficult and necessitate less surgical correction. A variety of corrective procedures are available, such as excision (Fig. 13-13), removal by electrocautery, or special flap design plus undermining and repositioning with the excision of the excess tissue. The latter is referred to as the draping procedure. Since the hypertrophied or hyperplastic folds of tissue have a continuous epithelial covering, an incision can be made on the crest of the ridge and the soft tissue

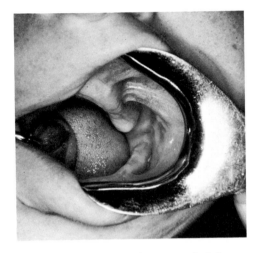

Fig. 13-8. Low muscle attachments on the left maxilla.

the tuberosity to a depth where contact is made with the crest of the ridge. After this wedge is removed, estimate the inverted V or triangle necessary to be removed on both the buccal and lingual aspects of the tuberosity (Fig. 13-11B). Following this minimal undermining, it will be necessary to adequately approximate the tissue flaps. This technique provides both a lateral and a vertical reduction of the tuber-

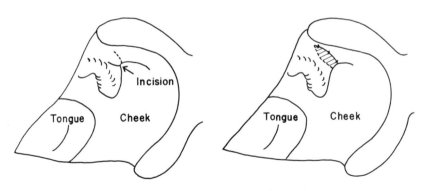

Fig. 13-9. Incision for raising the muscle attachment.

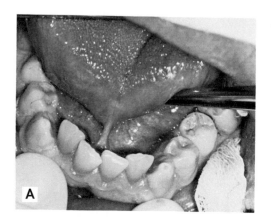

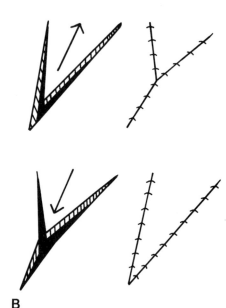

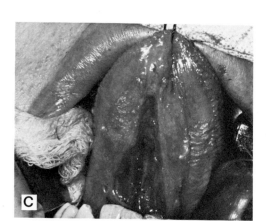

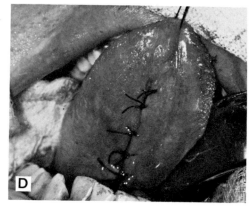

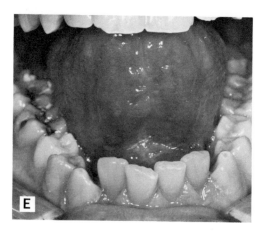

Fig. 13-10. Ankyloglossia. (A) Clinical appearance in a 21-year-old man. (B) The V-Y advancement flap. (C) Surgical correction by V-Y incision. (D) Sutures in place. (E) Three-month postoperative result. Note freedom of tongue movement.

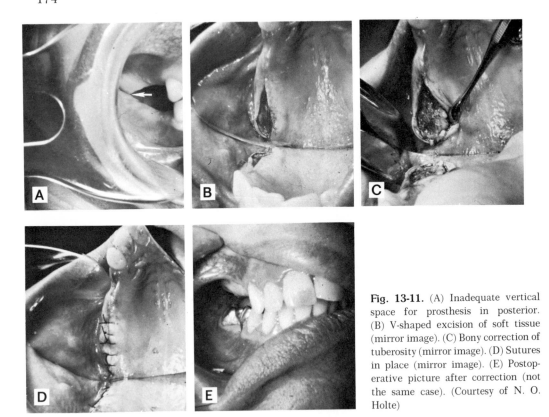

Fig. 13-11. (A) Inadequate vertical space for prosthesis in posterior. (B) V-shaped excision of soft tissue (mirror image). (C) Bony correction of tuberosity (mirror image). (D) Sutures in place (mirror image). (E) Postoperative picture after correction (not the same case). (Courtesy of N. O. Holte)

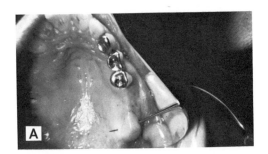
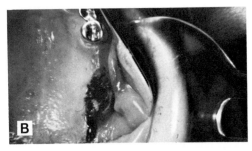

Fig. 13-12. (A) Probe in place shows that the tuberosity is composed entirely of soft tissue. (B) Complete excision of the tuberosity by decapitation. Note raw bleeding surface.

flap reflected. Undermining is continuous until all folds and wrinkles are free. The entire flap is then pulled out as a drape and the excess tissue excised (Fig. 13-14). The new flap margin is then sutured (Fig. 13-14B), and the denture reinserted as a splint.

Inflammatory Papillary Hyperplasia

Inflammatory papillary hyperplasia has specific characteristics. It appears on the palate and apparently is due to denture injury. In most instances there is an anterior-posterior shift to the denture. Its

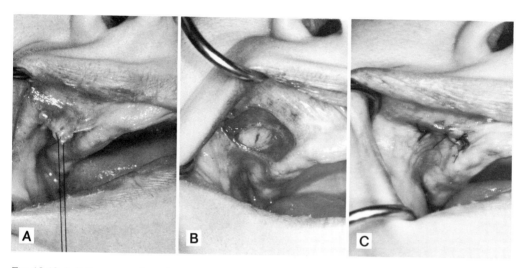

Fig. 13-13. Soft tissue mass from denture injury removed by total excision. (A) Preoperative view of soft tissue mass. (B) Lesion excised. (C) Postoperative view.

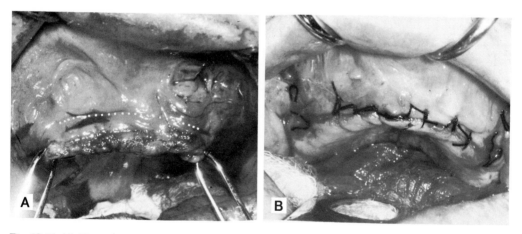

Fig. 13-14. (A) Many tissue folds due to ill-fitting denture; draping procedure following undermining. (B) Excision of excess tissues sutured in new position.

cause may have some relationship to the relief provided in the vault during denture construction, which affects the pressure on the palate. The lesion worsens with time and appears reddened, sore, and raspberry-like (Fig. 13-15A). One can play a stream of air on the lesions and note the small pedunculated stalks of tissue (Fig. 13-15B). Food and tissue fluid become embedded in the base and crevices of the lesion, adding to the injury and irritation. The lesion may be stripped supraperi-

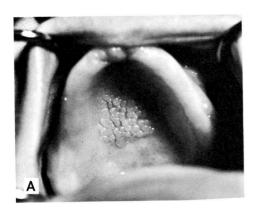
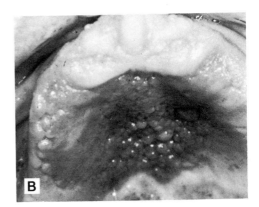

Fig. 13-15. (A and B) Inflammatory papillary hyperplasia. Note the numerous small papillary-like structures.

osteally, abraded with the high-speed drill using a large vulcanite surgical bur, or excised (Fig. 13-16). The electrocautery unit might also be used. The denture can be immediately inserted as a protective splint (Fig. 13-17).

Soft Tissue Tumors

A variety of soft tissue tumors occur within the oral cavity, and surgical management follows the same principles for the handling of all soft tissue.

Papillomas may be found on the tongue, cheek, or palate and are usually small pedunculated growths removed by excision (Fig. 13-18).

Hemangiomas appear as dark red or purplish compressible tumor masses located on lips, cheeks, or tongue (Fig. 13-19). Treatment is by excision or the injection of a sclerosing solution, and sometimes both. Incisional biopsy should not be done because of profuse bleeding that is difficult to control; aspiration of a suspected hemangiomatous lesion is the safer diagnostic method.

Lipomas may occur in the oral cavity

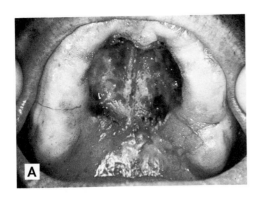
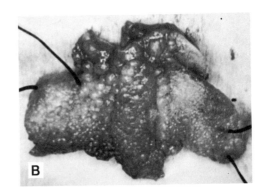

Fig. 13-16. (A) Excision of the palatal lesion including the periosteum. (B) Surgical specimen.

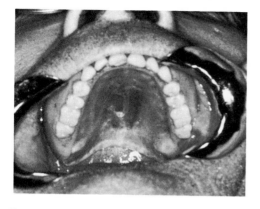

Fig. 13-17. Denture is reinserted and used as a protective covering; clear acrylic vault permits good visualization.

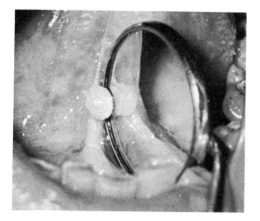

Fig. 13-18. Papilloma, (Courtesy of R. Gorlin)

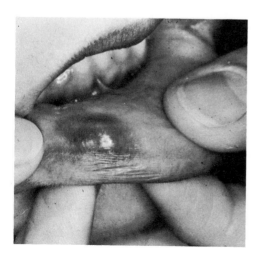

Fig. 13-19. Small hemangioma of the lip.

but are quite rare. A lipoma occurs so slowly and painlessly that it can attain a fairly large size before the patient may be aware of it. They are usually found in the cheek or the floor of the mouth, and are composed of fatty tissue, having a soft, doughy consistency (Fig. 13-20).

Occasionally, *pigmented lesions* may be found in the oral cavity. If a change in pigmentation has occurred, these lesions should be removed only by wide excision and considered potentially malignant until proved otherwise (Fig. 13-21).

The *mucocele* usually results from salivary secretion retention, and appears most commonly on the lower lip. It is best removed by elliptical excision, which is less likely to rupture the lesion and makes its dissection less complicated. This is followed by slight undermining and closure with interrupted sutures (Fig. 13-22).

Large *lesions of the tongue* can be removed by excision, and with extensive undermining, primary closure can be accomplished (Fig. 13-23). White lesions continue to cause controversy regarding diagnosis and treatment, and the terms describing these lesions vary among clinicians in both the medical and dental fields. However, most agree that red and white keratotic lesions should be evaluated by biopsy and histopathologic examination. The great majority will be found to be benign, but a significant number always turn up as precancerous or frankly cancerous, making such vigilance worthwhile.

The *ranula* is a soft tissue swelling of the floor of the mouth related to obstruction of one or more minor salivary glands (Fig. 13-24). The term "ranula" comes from the resemblance of this swelling to the color and consistency of the undersur-

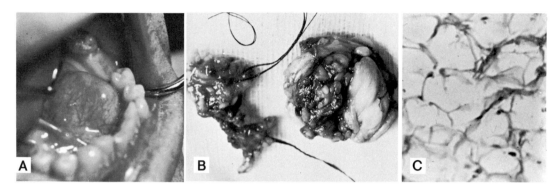

Fig. 13-20. (A) Lipoma on the floor of the mouth. (B) Surgical specimen. (C) Histologic section.

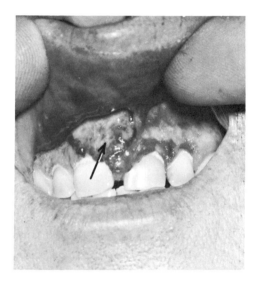

Fig. 13-21. Malignant melanoma. (From Catlin, D.: Mucosal melanomas of the head and neck. Am. J. Roentgen., *99*, 1967. Charles C Thomas, Pub.)

face of a frog. Treatment consists of establishing adequate drainage of the obstruction by creation of an epithelialized tract, marsupialization, or extirpation of the salivary gland.

Vestibuloplasty

Preprosthetic surgery includes the minor surgical corrections previously discussed, such as frenectomies and muscle attachments to the tuberosity, and the surgical correction of bony abnormalities of the jaws to provide an improved denture base. In addition to this, there may come a time in the life of the denture-wearing patient when he needs increased sulcus depth which is accomplished by vestibuloplasty. In 1965, there were over

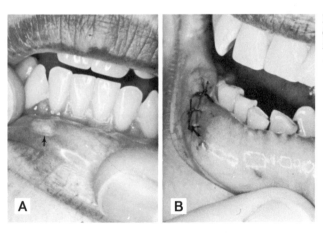

Fig. 13-22. (A) Mucocele of the lip. (B) Undermined enclosure with sutures in place following excision.

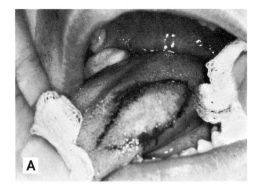

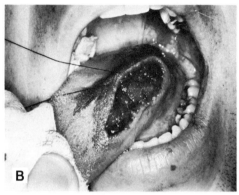

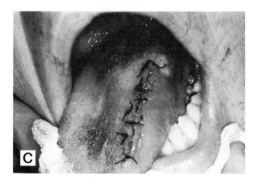

Fig. 13-23. (A) White lesion of tongue with incision lines marked. (B) Lesion excised. (C) Adequate closure by undermining and use of mattress sutures.

and the control of many diseases. A comparable advancement is in the knowledge of surgical procedures and the safety under which they can be performed.

Vestibuloplasty is necessary when no sulcus depth is available for prosthetic retention and support, as when alveolar resorption has been extensive, or when muscle, frenula, and mucosal attachments occur on or near the crest of the ridge (Fig. 13-26). A number of techniques can be utilized to improve the alveolar ridges for denture bearing and to increase the sulcus depth in relation to the alveolar process and muscle attachments. These include repositioning of the mucosa, as in Kazanjian and Clark's technique, and the procedures relying on immediate epithelial transfer of either mucosa or skin. Finally, ridge rebuilding by bone in extreme cases of alveolar bone atrophy may also be required.

The submucous procedure for vestibuloplasty as advocated by Obwegeser is best for increasing sulcus depth of the anterior maxilla.[2] A vertical incision is made in

nineteen million people in the United States who were 65 years and older. In 1967 thirty-three million people were edentulous. This gives some indication of the number of persons probably wearing a partial or a full prosthesis and perhaps most inadequately (Fig. 13-25).

The longevity of life has been extended as a direct result of medical knowledge

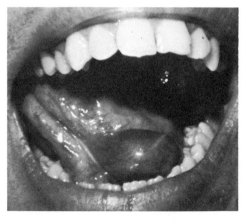

Fig. 13-24. Ranula. Note the dark color and nature of fluctuance.

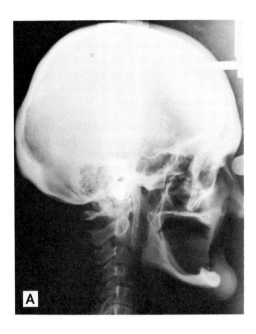

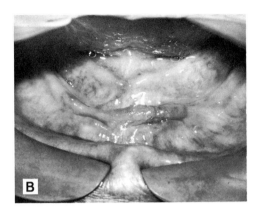

Fig. 13-25. (A) Lateral cephalogram showing severe alveolar bone loss. Note prominent genial tubercles remaining. (B) Photograph of inadequate ridge.

the midline just through the mucosa, permitting a blind supraperiosteal dissection with scissors. After all attachments have been released, the tissue is tacked high in the vestibular depth and a denture or surgical template is pressed against the new ridge and held in place by a perialveolar wire (Fig. 13-27).

The secondary epithelialization method involves the reflection of a supraperiosteal flap from the labial aspect of the ridge or the preparation of a mucosal flap on the inner surface of the lower lip, permitting the exposed surface to heal by secondary intention. A rubber catheter is then inserted in the depth of the newly created

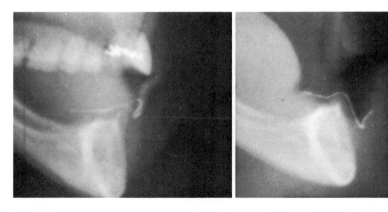

Fig. 13-26. Barium tracing of anterior sulcus depth before and after vestibuloplasty.

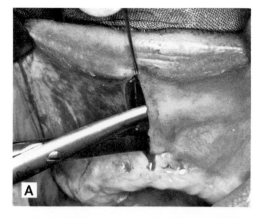

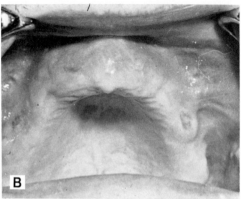

Fig. 13-27. (A and B) Submucous procedure for vestibuloplasty of anterior maxilla. See text for description. (Courtesy of E. Steinhauser)

sulcus and held in place by through-and-through sutures to the skin held in place by buttons. After seven to ten days, the sutures and catheter are removed, and within four to six weeks a new prosthesis can be made (Fig. 13-28). Experience has shown, however, that at least 50 per cent of the gained surgical depth is slowly lost. A similar procedure is accomplished by carefully dissecting the mucosal flap free from the periosteum and suturing at the new level, creating as much sulcus as possible (Fig. 13-29).

A more accurate method involves the utilization of a previously constructed splint. This is accomplished by taking a compound impression of the existing ridge and carving on the model the degree of extension that is potentially possible surgically, and then constructing a splint to fit the model. The surgery is accomplished as planned and the splint inserted and held in place by bone screws or circumzygomatic or mandibular wiring (Fig. 13-30.

The immediate extension technique has many of the same advantages as the immediate denture. The incision is made directly over the crest of the ridge through periosteum and gently curves into the mucobuccal fold distal to the areas where the extension is desired. The mucoperiosteal flap and muscle attachments are carried superiorly and buccally to the desired, or limit of, extension. This leaves a raw bony surface, which will be covered by the splint. This area becomes filled with a blood clot that will form granulation tissue and finally epithelialize over the exposed bone. It is important that the periphery of the overextended denture be thick and well rounded to prevent fissuring and undue irritation. In the maxilla, a single retention screw in the midline of the palate is often sufficient to stabilize the splint (Fig. 13-31). In the lower arch, at least two screws are necessary; however, three are advantageous, one in each of the retromolar pad areas and the other in the midline.

The swinging of buccal mucosal flaps with a pedicle base has also been a successful method of vestibuloplasty (Fig. 13-32). In such instances, the flap design is marked out on the cheek surface, keeping a broad base near the crest of the ridge in the retromolar area (Fig. 13-33). The flap (designated by a solid black dot in Fig. 13-34) is incised and freed to its base and then transferred into the new surgical site (designated by an open white dot), ex-

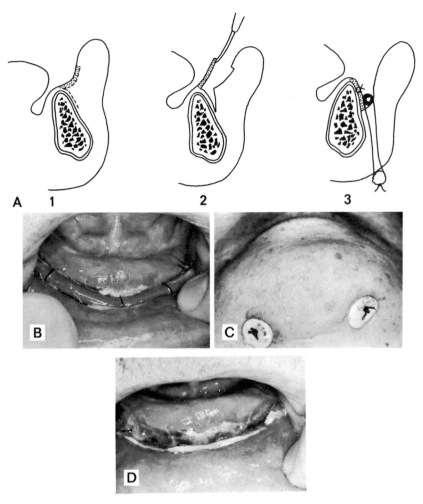

Fig. 13-28. (A) Secondary epithelialization technique. (B) Mucosa from lip attached to rubber tubing. (C) Tied to buttons on skin surface. (D) Seven days postoperative, tubing is removed. Note increased vestibule.

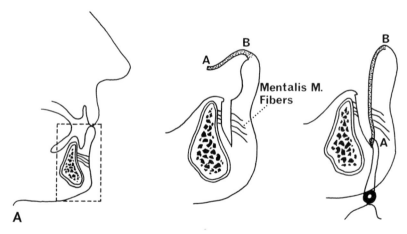

Fig. 13-29. (A) Secondary epithelialization technique, taking supraperiosteal flap from alveolar ridge of mandible. (*Continued on facing page.*)

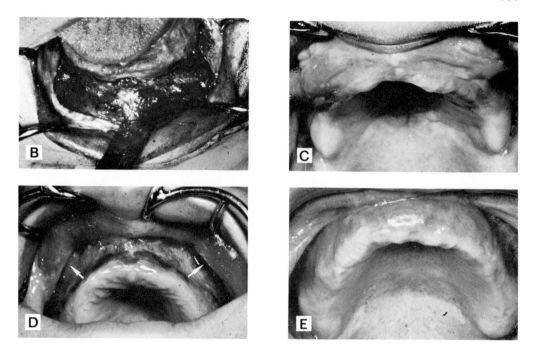

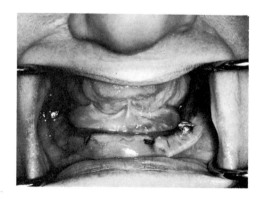

Fig. 13-29 (continued). (B) Secondary epithelialization technique for mandibular ridge. (C) For maxillary ridge. (D and E) Pre- and postoperative views. (Courtesy of E. Steinhauser)

tending the sulcus. The donor site is then undermined and closed by sutures (Fig. 13-35). Again, an overlying splint will have to be inserted and held in place by circummandibular sutures or screws (Fig. 13-36).

Skin Grafting

Although all techniques have varying degrees of success, the vestibular extension methods described previously frequently result in the eventual loss of much of the extension gained. This is caused by a gradually increasing fibrosis of exposed granulation tissue and resultant progressive contraction. However, this loss seems to be minimized when a split-thickness skin graft is used in conjunction with the vestibuloplasty. In such instances, the successful skin graft depends on rapid revascularization, which in turn depends on the vascularity of the host bed and adequate fixation of the grafted skin. The actual procedure of using skin in

the oral cavity to prevent infection or scar formation, or to cover defects from tumor surgery or trauma, dates back to the late nineteenth century. The Thiersch graft for defects of the buccal mucosa were among the first used.[3] Skin grafting was later described by Moskowicz and Esser in the early twentieth century.[4,5] Pichler, in 1931, presented probably the best series of

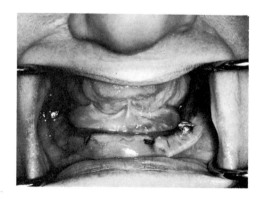

Fig. 13-30. Preconstructed acrylic splint with overextension.

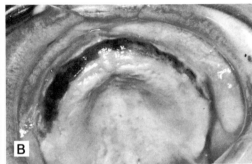

Fig. 13-31. (A) Immediate extension technique using retention screws. (B) Splint removed. Granulating tissue marks degree of vestibular extension.

covering intraoral defects with skin to prevent scarring and shrinkage of the soft tissue.[6] Obwegeser improved the "buccal inlay technique" originally described by Gillies.[7] This was the beginning of extensive skin grafting in the oral cavity for ridge extension procedures. In recent years, vestibuloplasty utilizing the split-thickness skin graft has gained considerable success.

TECHNIQUE. Prior to surgery, the operator takes impressions of the alveolar ridge

and constructs a duplicate plaster or stone model. A lateral cephalogram is also taken to provide accurate information on bony contours and outline. The duplicated cast is contoured to permit construction of the tray, allowing adequate relief in the area

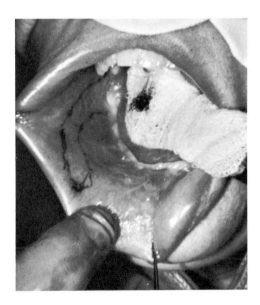

Fig. 13-33. Unilateral vestibular inadequacy due to trauma. Depth of vestibule was increased by pedicle graft.

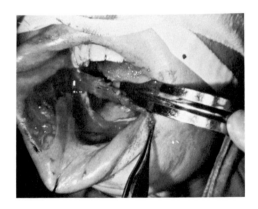

Fig. 13-32. Pedicled mucosal grafts from the parietes.

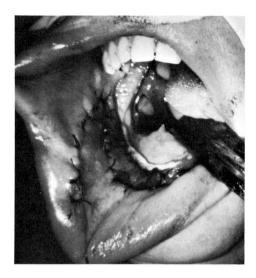

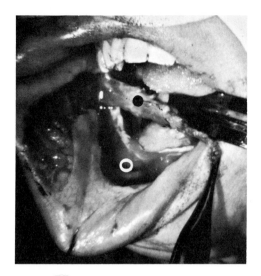

Fig. 13-34. Pedicle graft taken from right cheek; host site also prepared.

Fig. 13-35. Pedicle sutured into new position and donor site closed.

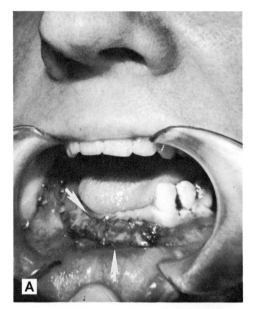

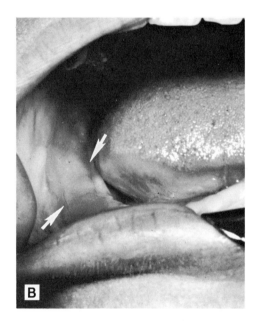

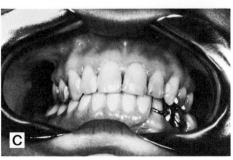

Fig. 13-36. (A) Seven-day postoperative view of pedicle graft. (B) Two-month postoperative view of pedicle graft. (C) Prosthesis in place.

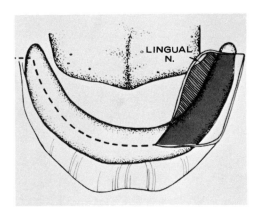

Fig. 13-38. Schematic drawing showing incision for vestibuloplasty with skin graft. Note extension of incision at 90° angle into vestibule; also note location of lingual nerve.

of the mental nerves. The buccal and labial aspects are extended along entire length of the periphery.

The dermatome is used to take skin from the outer aspect of the thigh or buttocks. A split-thickness graft best measures approximately 0.015 to 0.018 inch in thickness (Fig. 13-37). The graft is wrapped in a saline-solution-soaked gauze and the donor site covered with an appropriate dressing.

The recipient site is prepared in the following manner. The buccal, labial, and lingual tissues are injected with a local anesthetic solution containing a vasoconstrictor and an incision is made on the crest of the ridge throughout the arch (Fig. 13-38). It is carried through the mucosae only, without cutting into the periosteum, and the labiobuccal supraperiosteal flap is reflected by careful dissection (Fig. 13-39A and B). The incision for lowering the floor of the mouth is made in a sweeping manner at the junction of the lingual attached and unattached gingivae, extending from the retromolar area to the midline. The lingual nerve is near the posterior limit of this incision (Fig. 13-

39C). The mylohyoid muscle is cut free from its attachment, and the remaining lingual depth can be established by using the finger to strip away attachments of the submandibular gland and other visceral tissues in this area (Fig. 13-39D). The superior and lateral parts of the genioglossus muscle are also incised, but the entire muscle is not sacrificed. Sutures are then placed, using awls to draw the mucosal margins of both the lingual and labial buccal surfaces together near the lower, or inferior, portion of the body of the mandible, upon which the skin graft will be applied (Fig. 13-39E, F, and G). The previously constructed splint is lined with compound and carried to the mouth and an impression taken (Fig. 13-39H). This is immediately cooled and examined for reasonable accuracy. It can be further improved by the use of gutta-form (Obwegeser) for the final impression (Fig. 13-39I). A skin adhesive is applied to the newly formed impression and the skin graft transferred to it (Fig. 13-39J). The splint and graft are then carried to the mouth and a circumferential suture is placed on each side for immobilization (Fig. 13-39K). The splint is removed in six to eight days, when a "take" should be evident. A new prosthesis can be con-

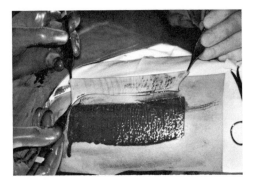

Fig. 13-37. Split-thickness skin graft taken from the thigh.

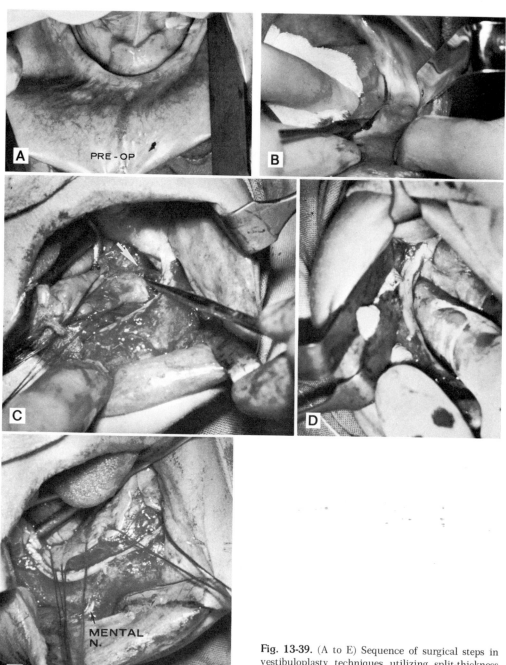

Fig. 13-39. (A to E) Sequence of surgical steps in vestibuloplasty techniques utilizing split-thickness skin graft. See text for details. (Continued on following page.)

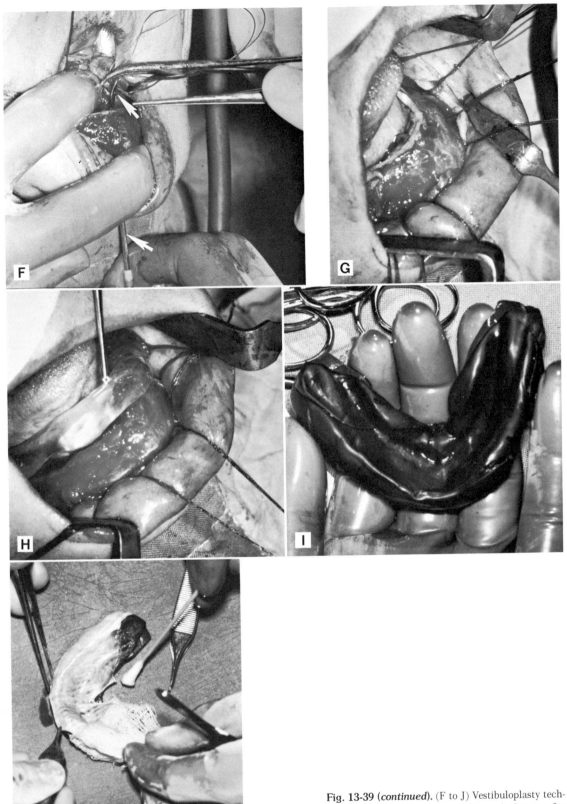

Fig. 13-39 (*continued*). (F to J) Vestibuloplasty technique utilizing split-thickness skin graft. See text for details. (Continued on facing page.)

188

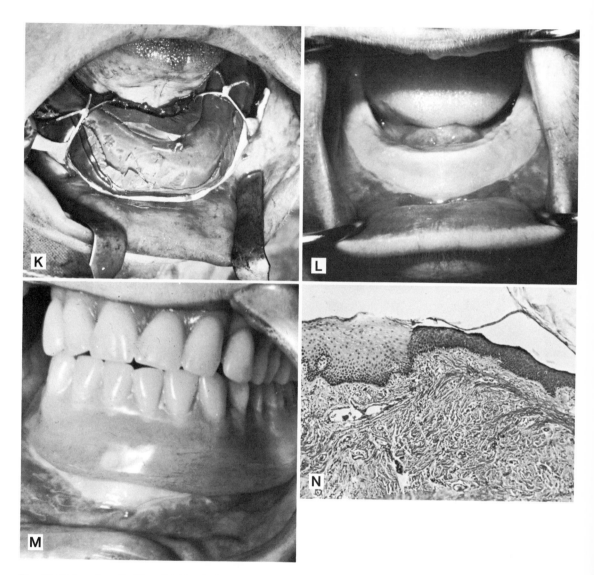

Fig. 13-39 (continued). (K to M) Vestibuloplasty technique utilizing split-thickness skin graft. See text for details. (N) Histologic section of mucosa and skin. Note thickness of skin compared to that of mucosa for denture-bearing surface.

structed in six to eight weeks (Fig. 13-39L, M, and N).

Mucosal grafts are also successful and more nearly reproduce the normal ridge tissue (Fig. 13-40). If the required vestib-

uloplasty is extensive, however, adequate mucosa may not be available. The mucosal strip graft is acquired from cheek, lips, and palate. Steinhauser recommends the mucosal grafting mainly in the atrophic maxilla, because adhesion and retention of the denture are more favorable with mucosal than with the skin grafting.[8]

Bone Rebuilding

In more severe cases of mandibular ridge atrophy when it is not possible to increase the vestibular space by any of the aforementioned procedures, bone rebuilding may be necessary. This may be accomplished by the use of rib, cartilage, or iliac crest bone with varying degrees of success. Boyne has reported limited use and success of rebuilding the ridge with a Vitallium casting lined with millipore filter filled with bone chips from the iliac crest.[9] A second stage procedure is required to

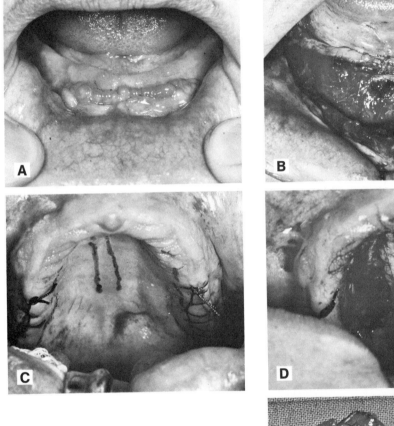

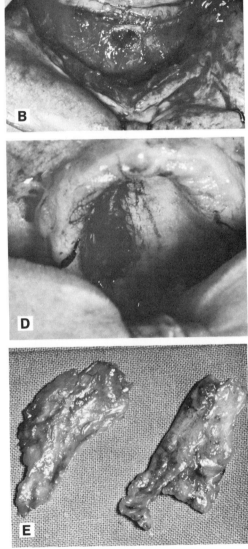

Fig. 13-40. (A) Tissue injury from denture. (B) Tissue excised and small root tip removed from anterior region. (C) Preoperative markings for mucosal graft from hard palate. Note tuberosity reductions done at the same time. (D) Mucosal graft donor site from the hard palate. (E) Two halves of the mucosal graft from the hard palate. (F) Mucosal graft sutured to mandibular anterior region. (G) Inflammation and edema 10 days after surgery. (H) Donor site three months postsurgery. (I) Palatal mucosal graft three years postoperatively. (J) Donor site in palate three years postoperatively. (K) Postoperative radiograph of palatal midline screw to maintain the splint.

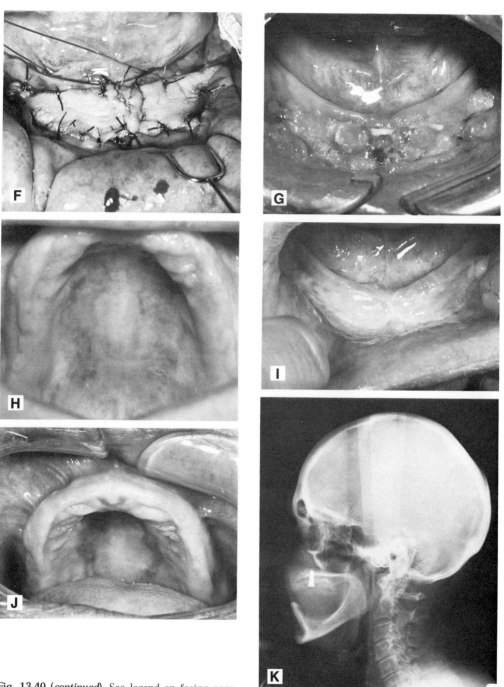

Fig. 13-40 (*continued*). See legend on facing page.

remove the Vitallium mold. We have been using cortical iliac crest bone and chips to rebuild the ridge with a secondary procedure of vestibuloplasty with skin graft with good success (Fig. 13-41).

Significant bone resorption has occurred (89% in some cases) within four years after surgery. However, most patients have indicated acceptable results. While some of the ridge height has been lost, a broad bony base seems to replace the previous knife-like, painful ridge, thus permitting the wearer of the prosthesis more comfort (Fig. 13-42).

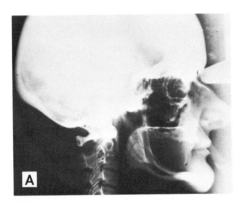

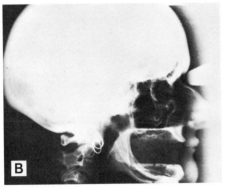

Fig. 13-41. (A) Preoperative cephalogram of patient, 38 years old. (B) Cephalogram following ridge augmentation with iliac bone crest.

Autogenous rib has also been used and perhaps with even increased success. However, this particular problem remains a difficult one to manage surgically and there is no ideal replacement for the normal alveolar ridge (Fig. 13-43).

Postoperative Problems

The postoperative problems are extremely variable. Why one patient will have so much difficulty and another does not has always been difficult to evaluate.

In regard to surgical procedures of the maxilla, the anatomic location of the tissues involved and their venous drainage are significant. The "facial system" comprises the facial vein which communicates with the superior ophthalmic vein, which empties directly into the cavernous sinus. The extension of infection by this route can result in encephalitis, brain abscess, meningitis, and cavernous sinus thrombosis.

Antibiotic coverage is most important in these cases, as well as the appropriate use of heat and cold. Careful attention to oral hygiene, general hydration, and nutrition is most important. Cortisone administered intravenously during the procedure and for two days postoperatively aids in the control of edema. Carefully planning the procedure, using sharp incisions, and giving meticulous attention to proper suturing materially aid in the success of these procedures.

Surgical Correction of Bony Anomalies

The surgical procedure for handling bony lesions or other hard tissues of the oral cavity is not particularly different

FOLLOW-UP STUDY ON RIDGE AUGMENTATION PROCEDURE

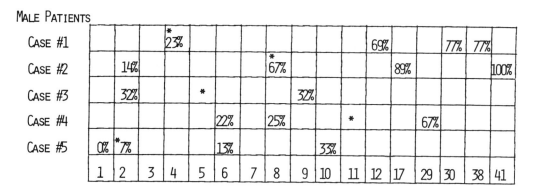

MALE PATIENTS

Case	1	2	3	4	5	6	7	8	9	10	11	12	17	29	30	38	41
CASE #1			*23%								69%			77%	77%		
CASE #2		14%				*67%						89%					100%
CASE #3		32%		*				32%									
CASE #4					22%	25%				*		67%					
CASE #5	0%	*7%			13%			33%									

% OF RESORPTION - (IN MONTHS) ILIAC CREST

A

* INDICATES THE DATE THE SKIN GRAFT PROCEDURE WAS DONE

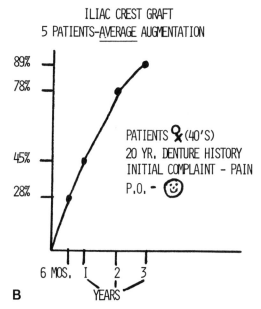

ILIAC CREST GRAFT
5 PATIENTS–AVERAGE AUGMENTATION

89%
78%
45%
28%

PATIENTS ♀ (40'S)
20 YR. DENTURE HISTORY
INITIAL COMPLAINT - PAIN
P.O. - ☺

6 MOS. 1 2 3
YEARS

B

Fig. 13-42. Documented studies of bone resorption of patients receiving a bone graft for ridge augmentation. (Courtesy of Wang and Waite)

from any other surgical procedure: the same careful and meticulous technique is indicated for all surgery. However, the removal of such conditions as the odontoma (Fig. 13-44), ossifying fibroma (Fig. 13-45), and tori (Fig. 13-46) or general-ized exostoses is among the more difficult bony surgical procedures to execute and can produce prolonged postoperative problems.

The operative approach to these calcified structures is by means of the flap, exposing them for excision by either the chisel or the bur. Some can be removed in toto, and others require a sectioning technique. In the case of an exostosis or torus, the intent may not always be complete removal, but simply trimming or smoothing the bulky mass to accommodate a prosthesis.

The most common enlargement of the palate is that of the torus palatinus. This condition has never been reported as a malignant growth; it is removed primarily to prevent irritation to the overlying mucosae and to permit the reception of a prosthesis. Its presence has been reported as high as 20 and 25 per cent.[10] The palatal tori are more prevalent than the mandibular tori, with no sex or race difference.[11] These bony masses have been known to increase in size during the first three decades of life, but stabilize after that period with no considerable change.

This growth of the palate often creates great anxiety in the patient when discovered for the first time. A cancerphobia may exist, and considerable reassurance and sometimes surgical removal may be necessary to satisfy such a patient. A frequent complaint may be that of trauma (Fig. 13-47). The bony growth, which occurs in the midline, takes considerable abuse from the mastication of food against the roof of the mouth by the tongue as well as from food passing through the oral cavity. Since the torus may extend posteriorly as far as the postdam area and occur lobulated and in a variety of shapes, it may also interfere with a prosthesis, preventing peripheral seal of the denture (Fig. 13-48). The surgical management for the reduction of the torus can be done under local or general anesthesia.

The double Y midline incision probably provides the best surgical access. This flap design preserves the nerve and blood supply to the flap entering from the nasopalatine and the bilateral greater palatine foramina. The mucoperiosteal flap is ex-

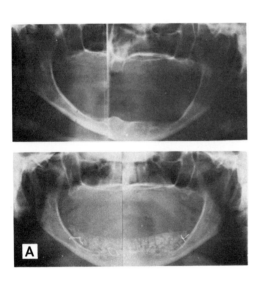

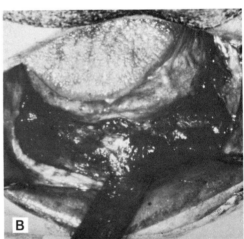

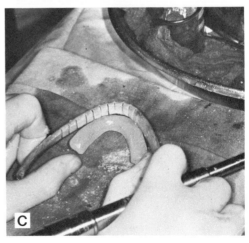

Fig. 13-43. (A) Preoperative and one-year postoperative radiographs of 40-year-old patient who had rib graft to mandible for pain of lower jaw and inadequate sulcus and ridge. (B) Surgical preparation of the mandibular ridge to receive the rib graft. (C) The patient's rib (autogenous graft) is contoured to fit a prepared model for placement to the atrophied mandibular bone.

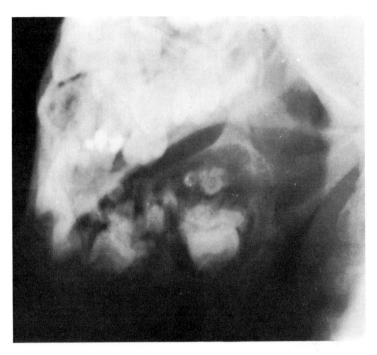

Fig. 13-44. Odontoma involving the body and ramus of the mandible in a ten-year-old boy.

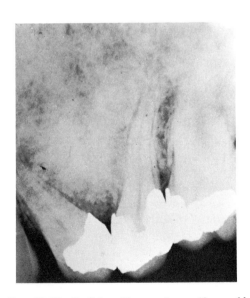

Fig. 13-45. Ossifying fibroma in a 48-year-old woman. Note divergence of roots of teeth.

tremely thin and tears easily, so it must be handled gently. A traction suture may be helpful (Fig. 13-49).

The injection of a local anesthetic near the base of the bony protuberance will control hemorrhage into the area and at the same time balloon the tissues sufficiently to make the dissection easier. The tumor mass is then sectioned into segments by means of the high-speed drill, with each segment removed separately (Fig. 13-50). The chisel may also be used to remove the individual segments. The torus is not removed in one large piece because of the possibility of fracturing the nasal floor. The high-speed drill may also be used to reduce the entire mass, utilizing copious irrigation. Smoothing of the raw bony surface is accomplished by

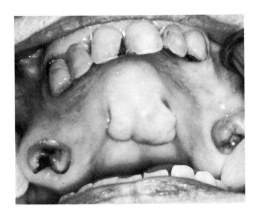

Fig. 13-46. Torus palatinus.

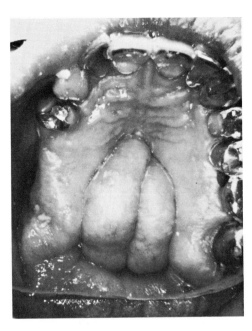

Fig. 13-48. Maxillary torus showing lobulations, undercuts, and posterior extension.

rongeurs and files or rotary bone wheels, and debridement is done by irrigation (Fig. 13-51A and B). The tissues are closed with mattress sutures (Fig. 13-51C).

A surgical splint is used to protect the flap during the first few postoperative days (Fig. 13-52). The splint not only physically protects the tissues from injury

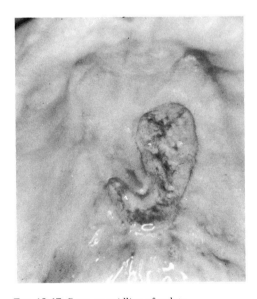

Fig. 13-47. Burn on midline of palate.

and food debris, but prevents dependent hematoma formation beneath the flap, which would retard the healing process. In the preparation of the splint, the surgeon should trim the cast himself to note the appropriate bony reduction necessary during the surgical procedure. If the relief provided is inadequate, pressure will be exerted against the wound. If a splint has not been prepared, an oral bandage will often suffice (Fig. 13-53). One can also insert a ball of gauze soaked in tincture of benzoin, which is held in place with a number of sutures criss-crossed from one side of the arch to the other like a basket. If teeth are present, they are used to anchor the criss-crossing sutures.

Mandibular tori are similar to the palatal tori except for location. They occur less frequently, develop above the mylohyoid muscle attachment, and occur bilaterally in most instances (Fig. 13-54). Their removal is similar to that for palatal tori, except when they occur with a narrow base, as on a pedicle. In this case, the chisel is best utilized for removal. Other-

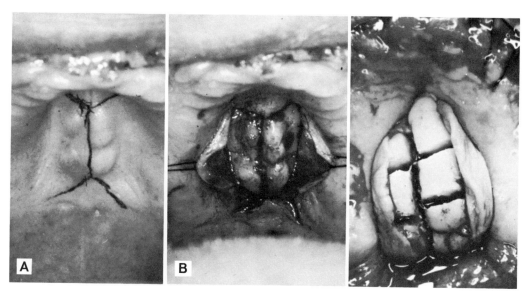

Fig. 13-49. (A) Torus showing outline of incision for the surgical approach. (B) Flap reflected and traction sutures used to hold the flap.

Fig. 13-50. Torus showing the bony mass sectioned by the high-speed drill.

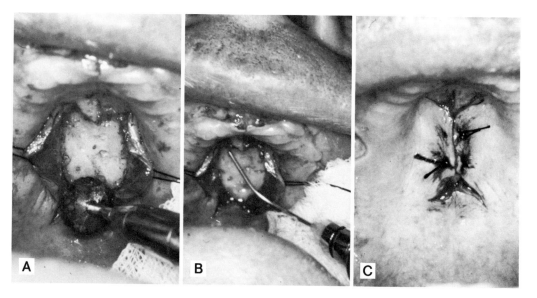

Fig. 13-51. (A) Smoothing of the bony surgical site with rotary high-speed instrument. (B) Final toilet of the wound with saline solution. (C) Flap returned and mattress suture used to evert the flap.

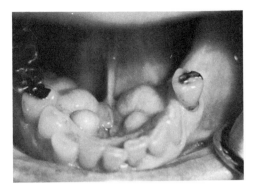

Fig. 13-54. Multiple mandibular tori.

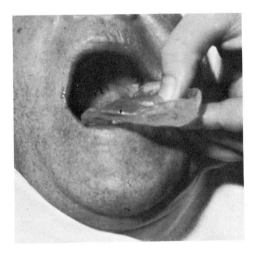

Fig. 13-52. A full arch acrylic splint inserted for postoperative comfort and protection to the wound.

wise, sectioning—as described previously—is the safest surgical approach.

The major complicating aspect of this procedure is that of access: a sufficiently long incision must be made to provide good vision and surgical access. This may include an incision from the molar area to the midline (Fig. 13-55). There is less

space for hematoma formation if the mylohyoid muscle is not stripped away and the excess flap is removed from the incised margin and sutured firmly. A previously constructed acrylic splint is the best way to ensure tissue adaptation and to limit edema and hematoma formation (Fig. 13-56). The presence of the salivary ducts and the lingual nerve, and the ease with which postoperative edema and infection occur in the floor of the mouth, add to the concern regarding any surgery in this area.

The surgical removal of multiple exos-

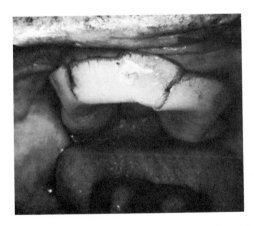

Fig. 13-53. Oral bandage (Squibb) used in place of splint.

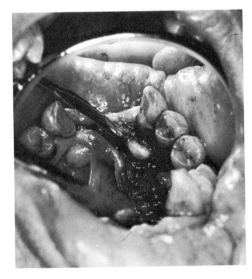

Fig. 13-55. Surgical removal of mandibular tori (mirror image). Note incision length.

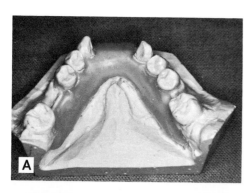

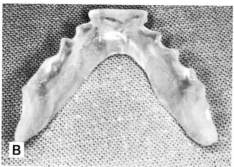

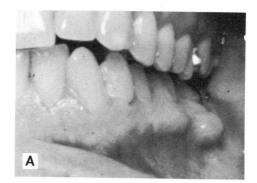

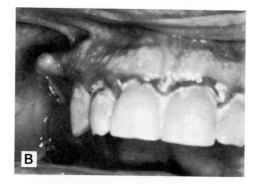

Fig. 13-56. (A) Model showing reduction of tori and wax-up for splint construction. (B) The acrylic splint.

toses is basically no different than that for tori, except that exostoses occur with no uniformity as to location. They also may appear singularly around the arch or in multiple formation (Fig. 13-57). The relationship of osteomas as a part of Gardner's syndrome* should be considered, particularly if supernumerary teeth are present.[12] The term "enostosis" appears in the literature, which in contrast to exostosis is a

* Multiple osteomas, fibrous and fatty tumors of the skin and mesentery, epidermoid inclusion cysts of skin, and multiple intestinal polyposis that may undergo malignant degeneration. (Gorlin, S. R., and Pindborg, J. J.: *Syndromes of the Head and Neck.* New York, McGraw-Hill, 1964.)

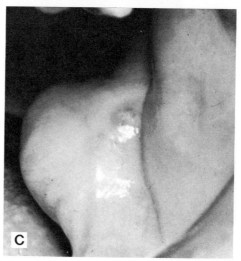

Fig. 13-57. (A) Multiple mandibular exostoses. (B) Maxillary buccal exostoses. (C) Large lingual exostosis in edentulous patient opposite the third molar area.

similarly dense radiopaque ossification except that it is confined within the cortical walls and is not palpable (Fig. 13-58).

The bony maxillary tuberosity is reduced in order to increase the vertical space between the arches and to remove undercut in preprosthetic surgery (Fig. 13-59). The bone of this area is usually very cancellous and can be reduced easily by rongeurs or files. An excess mucoperiosteal flap may be present, necessitating a wedge excision for appropriate closure.

The mylohyoid ridge, or the internal oblique line, is a bony prominence that frequently interferes with the prosthesis (Fig. 13-60). Its removal is somewhat more difficult and the tissues must be handled with delicacy. The mucoperiosteal flap is reflected with a horizontal incision on the crest of the ridge. When the muscle fibers come into view, they can be sectioned with the scissors or stripped with the periosteal elevator. The bony

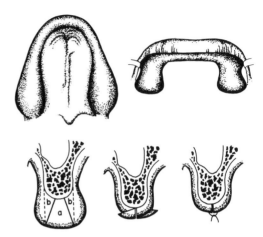

Fig. 13-59. Tuberosity—buccal undercut—demonstrating the wedge resection method for surgical correction.

prominence is then reduced by means of the chisel or the file until the sharpness and/or undercut is removed.

The term "endoalveolar crest" is not often used, but refers to the bony prominence lingual to the mandibular third molar (Fig. 13-60). This bony balcony is not the same as the mylohyoid ridge.

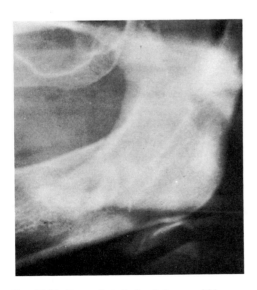

Fig. 13-58. Enostosis in body of the mandible.

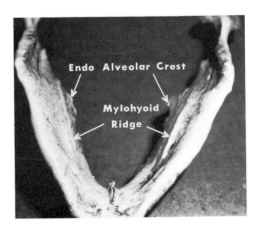

Fig. 13-60. Mylohyoid ridge and endoalveolar crest.

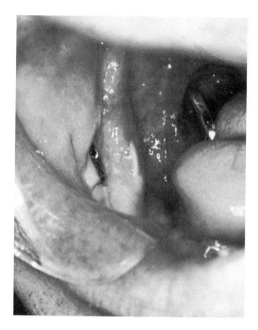

Fig. 13-61. Ulceration of the lingual mucosa due to sharp endoalveolar crest not reduced at time of surgery.

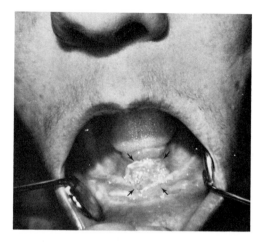

Fig. 13-63. Need for genial tubercle reduction and muscle lowering.

There is no muscle attachment to it, and it should be reduced at the time of third molar removal. When this is not done, the bony projection may become sharp and irritate the tongue, as well as interfere with the prosthesis (Fig. 13-61).

The genial tubercle is a normal ana-

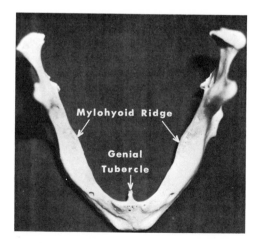

Fig. 13-62. Mandible showing mylohyoid ridge and genial tubercle.

tomic protuberance on the lingual symphysis of the mandible for the attachment of the genioglossus and the geniohyoid muscles. During the process of ridge atrophy or alveolar bone resorption these bony prominences and their muscle attachments may appear entirely on the crest of the ridge (Fig. 13-62). They may interfere with the prosthesis, and will have to be removed and the muscle attachment lowered (Figs. 13-63 and 13-64).

A sharp, spiny, knife-like ridge may be a painful condition for a patient (Fig. 13-65), but the temptation to perform surgery on it should be avoided. Any surgery may result in total loss of the ridge, making prosthodontic construction more difficult. Denture adjustment or special prosthetic construction may be indicated to provide patient comfort.

References

1. Shapiro, H. H.: Maxillofacial Anatomy, Philadelphia, J. B. Lippincott Co., 1954.

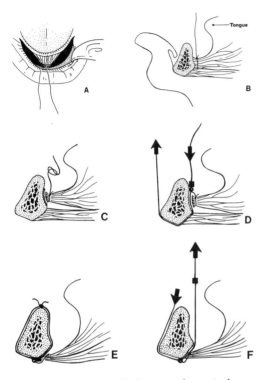

Fig. 13-64. Technique for lowering the genioglossus muscle. (A and B) Genioglossus muscle is isolated. (C) The muscle is cut free. (D) A circumferential nonabsorbable suture is passed with a stop knot (■). The suture around the muscle is tied beneath the stop knot. (E) The muscle is repositioned. (F) Ten days later, the circumferential suture is removed in a reverse manner.

2. Obwegeser, H.: Surgical preparation of the maxilla for prosthesis. J. Oral Surg., 22:127,1964.
3. Thiersch, K.: Uber die feineren Anatomischen veranderungen bei aufheilung von haut auf granulationen. Arch. Klin. Chir., 17:318–324, 1874.
4. Moszkowicz, L.: Uber Verpflanzung Thiersch' scher Epidermislappchen in die Mundhohle. Arch. Klin. Chir., 108:216–220, 1916.
5. Esser, J. F. S.: Studies in plastic surgery of the face. Ann. Surg., 65:297–315, 1917.
6. Pichler, H., and Trauner, R.: Die Alveolarkammplastik. F. Stomat., 28:675, 1930.
7. Gillies, H. D.: Plastic Surgery of the Face. London, Oxford University Press, 1920.
8. Steinhauser, E. W.: Free transplantation of oral mucosa for improvement of denture retention. J. Oral Surg., 27:955, 1969.
9. Boyne, P. J.: New Concepts in Facial Bone Healing and Grafting Procedures. J. Oral Surg., 27:557–559, 1969.
10. Shafer, W. G., Hine, M. K., and Levy, B. M.: Oral Pathology, ed. 2. Philadelphia, W. B. Saunders Co., 1963.
11. Kolas, S., et al.: The occurrence of torus palatinus and torus mandibularis in 2478 dental patients. Oral. Surg., 6:1134, 1953.
12. Suzuki, M., and Sakai, T.: A familial study of torus palatinus and torus mandibularis. Am. J. Phys. Anthrop., 18:263, 1960.

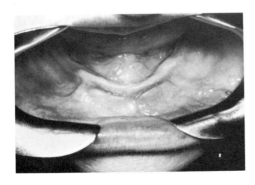

Fig. 13-65. Knife-like mandibular ridge.

14 Biopsy Technique

DANIEL E. WAITE

Biopsy is the removal of tissue from a living patient for microscopic examination. The biopsy procedure is a technique which every dentist must be competent to perform. Prior to the biopsy, an adequate history and examination, including the inspection and palpation of presenting lesions, are most essential. The same principles outlined in Chapter 3 should be followed. The examination should also include an evaluation for lymphadenopathy. If positive, the location of the lymph nodes and their character should be described (i.e., fixed or movable, painful or nonpainful, and estimation of size). A clinical impression can then be formed which can be confirmed only by the biopsy procedure. All persons who assume the obligations relating to either diagnosis and/or the treatment of patients must be prepared to obtain additional information from appropriate biopsies and arrange immediate referrals when indicated.

If the word "biopsy" is used in front of a patient, he may become concerned. Biopsy is a terrifying term and to most people indicates the possibility of cancer. In each instance the clinician should be cautious of the emphasis he places upon it. The great majority of biopsy specimens will be benign, but we must continue to be vigilant in our search to establish the etiology and diagnosis of any unknown lesion within the oral cavity (Fig. 14-1).

There are several types of biopsy procedures: The *incisional biopsy* is the removal of a portion of the lesion along with some normal tissue for identification (Fig. 14-2). The *excisional biopsy* is the complete removal of the lesion in question by circumscribing it in such a way that it is totally excised (Fig. 14-3). The *aspiration biopsy* is ideal for cysts, nonulcerated tumors, and lesions of bone as well as for cervical nodes; obviously, the material obtained by aspiration is the material in question and can be cultured or examined microscopically as well as grossly by inspection (Fig. 14-4). The *punch biopsy* uses special punch-type forceps for the removal of a portion of the lesion (Fig. 14-5). The electrocautery unit generally is not used for taking biopsy specimens because of the additional destruction of tissues caused by this instrument, which makes histologic interpretation more difficult. Oringer reports that biopsy specimens obtained by electrosection with fully rectified electronic current are comparable in all respects to the best obtainable by other surgical methods for histopathologic interpretation.[1]

In each instance, the biopsy material should be submitted immediately to a

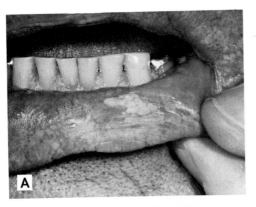

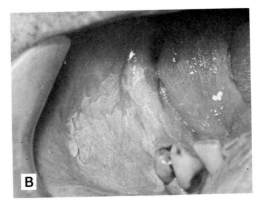

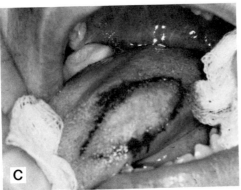

Fig. 14-1. Lesions amenable to biopsy. (A) White lesion on lower lip. (B) White lesion on buccal mucosa of snuff chewer. (C) White lesion on tongue outlined for limits of excisional biopsy.

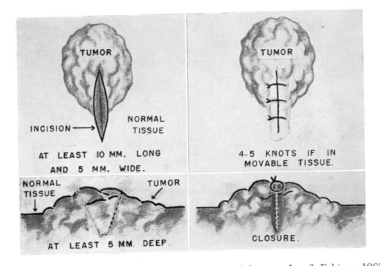

Fig. 14-2. Technique for incisional biopsy. (Clark, *Practical Oral Surgery*, Lea & Febiger, 1965)

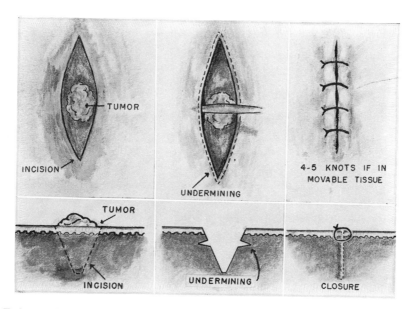

Fig. 14-3. Technique for excisional biopsy. (Clark, *Practical Oral Surgery*, Lea & Febiger, 1965)

clinical pathology laboratory for evaluation. The specimens should be placed in 10 per cent formalin and accompanied by appropriate information pertaining to the case. This includes the name and age of the patient, the clinical history which may include a previous history of treatment,

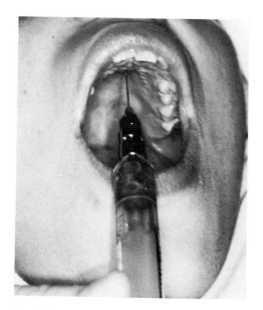

Fig. 14-4. Aspiration biopsy of nasopalatine cyst.

and the clinician's impression or clinical diagnosis. A careful description of the lesion and its location should be included, noting in particular its color, mobility, attachment, ulceration, induration, or any descriptive term that adds to the clinical impression. The size of the lesion in millimeters may be extremely important in final differential diagnosis. Many pathologists provide a specific form for giving information on the lesion and reporting (Fig. 14-6). Often, a simple sketch showing the location from which the tissue was removed will help the pathologist. If more than one biopsy specimen is taken from a given lesion, each should be placed in a separate bottle and marked accordingly, on both the diagram and the bottle. If x-ray films are valuable, as in the case of bony lesions, they should also accompany the specimen.[2]

Frozen section technique may be provided by some laboratories; it provides immediate information to the clinician, permitting appropriate treatment. When frozen sections are intended, the pathologist should be alerted of the incoming specimen and the specimen should be

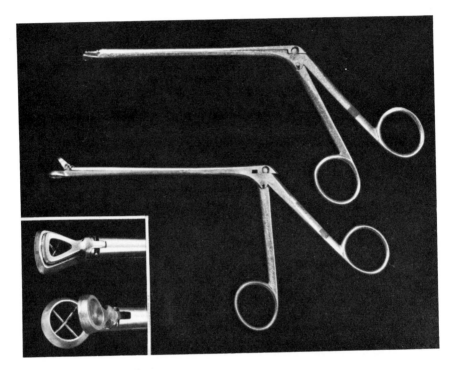

Fig. 14-5. Punch biopsy forceps.

immediately transported to the laboratory in saline or Ringer's solution. However, conventional biopsy techniques will be utilized in most instances, requiring time for reporting, and the patient should be advised as to the length of time necessary for the return information. Reassure the patient not to be unduly concerned until all information is available; he should be given the benefit of complete understanding and compassion on the part of the doctor and office personnel. As soon as the information regarding the diagnosis is available, notify the patient immediately or have him return to discuss the results and whatever treatment, if any, is indicated. Whenever malignant disease is found,

the patient must be referred to the appropriate specialist. Such referrals must be agreeable to all three parties and a specific appointment should then be made. The clinician has the responsibility to follow through and to see that, in fact, the patient did keep the appointment. The doctor to whom the patient is referred should be carefully selected to meet both the needs of the patient relative to his specific disease and, in addition, the possible psychologic needs arising from the diagnosis, which would require compassionate and sympathetic care.

In regard to the significance of a negative biopsy report, it is entirely possible that a biopsy specimen will be reported to be

069-D1131		
ORAL PATHOLOGY #		DENTAL SCHOOL REGISTRATION #

PATIENT   C.S.

ADDRESS

      U.H. #1109774

DATE   11-11-69   SEX   M

AGE   80   RACE   Cau

CLINICAL FINDINGS

(Description, Location, Duration, and Other Pertinent Data)

Patient had pain in mandibular alveolar and tongue areas, clinically noticeable since August, 1969. He was treated with cortisone for TMJ problem. Currently, there was a question of salivary stones of submandibular area. No lymphadenopathy. Specimen removed from ventral posterior tongue, approximately 0.5 x 0.5 cm. Patient unaware of lesion. Excised and submitted for frozen section.

Lesion

CONTRIBUTOR   Daniel E. Waite, D.D.S.

ADDRESS   University Hospital Dental Clinic

CLINICAL DIAGNOSIS

1. Traumatic ulcer.
2. Squamous cell carcinoma.

For Laboratory Use Only:

DATE RECEIVED   11-11-69

REPORT

Gross: The specimen is a superficially ulcerated mucosal ellipse measuring 1.1 x 0.5 x 0.4 cm. The cut surface shows an epithelial thickening.

Frozen diagnosis: Squamous cell carcinoma, grade 2, ventral tongue.

Microscopic: Hematoxylin and eosin sections confirm the frozen diagnosis. The squamous cell carcinoma noted previously is seen originating from covering lingual epithelium. The neoplastic proliferation of cells is located superficially in the examined portions but is characterized by active invasion into underlying, chronically inflamed, connective tissues. Individual cells within these invasive proliferations manifest the usual histopathologic features of malignancy such as increased numbers of mitotic figures, nuclear pleomorphism, anaplasia, and so forth. While occasional signs of differentiation such as epithelial pearls may be observed, the mitotic activity and anaplasia suggest that the entirety is less differentiated. A blood vessel within the superficial submucosa manifests tumor cells within the lumen. The lesion has been incisionally biopsied as tumor extends to and includes borders of the specimen.

Robert A. Vickers, D.D.S., M.S.D.

Division of Oral Pathology
University of Minnesota
School of Dentistry
Minneapolis, Minnesota 55455

DIAGNOSIS   Squamous cell carcinoma, grade 2, ventral tongue.

Fig. 14-6. Pathology form with complete write-up and histopathologic evaluations.

nonmalignant in the face of a serious and positive lesion. In such instances, the biopsy specimen may have been inadequately acquired, or laboratory problems may have arisen in its preparation. Therefore, be on guard for the negative biopsy report and be prepared to follow through with an additional specimen when any element of doubt exists.

As a matter of habit, the dentist should submit all tissue removed during regular surgical procedures to the pathologist for evaluation. Granulomatous masses near the apices of teeth, follicular sacs around impacted teeth, and white or red lesions of the mucosae cannot consistently be identified without microscopic evaluation (Fig. 14-7).

The incisional biopsy should be done when the lesion is entirely too large for removal and when there is a high degree of suspicion relative to the type of tumor. Leaving a portion of it to confirm its location enhances further diagnosis and ultimate treatment. Often, retaining the sutures in the biopsy site until the report has been obtained is helpful. For example, if the biopsy report indicates that the lesion is highly radiosensitive, the radiotherapist can then concentrate the radiotherapy at the exact location from which the original tissue was taken.

Excisional biopsy should certainly be utilized in lesions near the apices of teeth and where the ease of total excision is obvious. Partial excisional or incisional biopsy is contraindicated in instances of suspected hemangioma or malignant melanoma. Wide surgical excision is probably the treatment of choice in these cases to avoid serious bleeding or widespread metastasis. Biopsy in the presence of acute infection may be unwise and result in

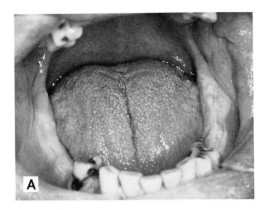

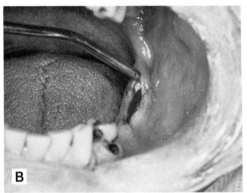

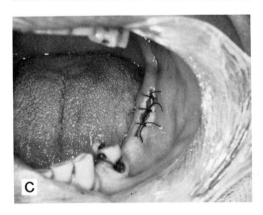

Fig. 14-7. (A) White lesion on alveolar ridge. (B) Incision. (C) Adequate suture by undermining.

spreading the infection, although this does not exclude using the biopsy technique to diagnose fungi and dermatologic lesions.

The role of exfoliative cytologic examination in oral cancer detection has caused considerable discussion, but it has not proved to be an accurate source of information for oral cancer. In this technique, cells are scraped from the surface of the lesion, spread upon a slide, fixed, and stained, and suspicious cells may be identified. The technique has achieved its reputation from the reliability of the Papanicolaou stain technique (referred to as the Pap smear) in cervical biopsy, but no such accuracy has been available for lesions of the oral cavity. Oral exfoliative cytologic examination may be of value when a patient refuses permission for surgical biopsy, or following postradiation treatment of a lesion, when repeated surgical biopsies would not be indicated.[3] It has the advantage of not requiring anesthesia to obtain the specimens. In an elderly patient or one unable to withstand even the insult of a surgical biopsy, information probably could be obtained from the cytology technique.[4] However, it must be stressed that, for final diagnosis, a surgical specimen undoubtedly will be needed.

Since most biopsy procedures will be done utilizing local anesthesia, attention should be given to the placement of the anesthetic. Whenever possible, the regular

nerve block should be administered, permitting complete and painless manipulation of the biopsy site. However, if infiltration anesthetic is used, a ring block is advisable. In such instances, place the anesthetic in such a way as to circumscribe the lesion to be sampled by biopsy examination (Fig. 14-8), but at an adequate distance to avoid any architectural change or distention of the tissues during the procedure. Too much anesthetic in close proximity to the lesion will distort the tissue, making the biopsy technique more difficult, and possibly causing an artifact in the biopsy specimen.

The technique of the biopsy follows:

1. Establish anesthesia.
2. Immobilize the tissue and make elliptical incisions. The depth of the incision is determined by the amount of tissue desired. In excisional biopsy, the lesion should be carefully palpated, its depth determined, and the initial incisions gauged to slightly exceed the total depth of the lesion. In incisional biopsy, any depth into the lesion that will obtain sufficient material for evaluation is adequate. The incision should include a significant portion of the suspected tissue while excluding necrotic tissue, which would be difficult to diagnose microscopically. Some portion of normal tissue approximating the lesion must also be included.
3. A traction suture, hook, or tissue forceps may be used to immobilize the tissue to be excised (Fig. 14-9). The traction suture, when left with the specimen, has the advantage of orienting at least one surface of the lesion for the pathologist. It also provides considerable ease in surgical removal, and avoids

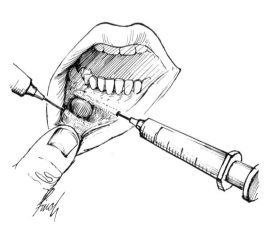

Fig. 14-8. Technique of administering an anesthetic ring block.

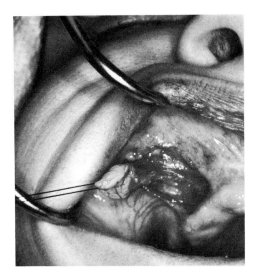

Fig. 14-9. Traction suture to remove biopsy specimen.

compressing or destroying the specimen tissues, as occurs with sharp pinching instruments.

4. Sever the base of the specimen with curved scissors or a blade. Place the specimen in 10 per cent formalin solution. Undermine the wound edges, control hemorrhage, and close the incision with interrupted sutures. When performing a biopsy on the cheek or the tongue, consider additional sutures and their placement, since the movement and manipulation of these structures may cause early loss of sutures.

5. When the biopsy specimen has been taken from the gingivae or palate and the incision is difficult to close, leave it open for healing by secondary intention and epithelization, or apply a surgical dressing.

Bone biopsy may be more difficult and will require the use of soft tissue flap design and a surgical approach to the lesion (Fig. 14-10). Careful attention must be given to obtaining adequate material in both quantity and quality for examination. After obtaining the specimen, return the flap and give the usual postoperative care as for any similar surgical procedure. The patient should be advised that considerably more time may be needed by the laboratory in preparing the biopsy specimen because of the necessary decalcification process.

Watchful waiting has no place in the evaluation of suspicious lesions. Although many clinical impressions support the diagnosis of cancer, such as induration, painless swelling, and bleeding, cancer may still be evident without these symptoms. If in doubt, biopsy. Figure 14-11 shows two lesions very similar in appearance, both of which occurred in similar locations in women of middle age. Both women wear dentures, and the lesions appeared as a response to trauma or irritation from the prosthesis. The induration and ulceration are obvious in both lesions; both lesions were painless. One was cancerous, the other, not (see legend for details). A cancerous surface lesion may be small in appearance, however, the tendency for infiltration and spread of the lesion may be extensive (Fig. 14-12).

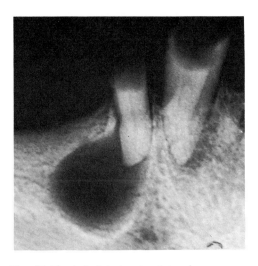

Fig. 14-10. Apical lesion involving bone; access gained through socket of extracted tooth.

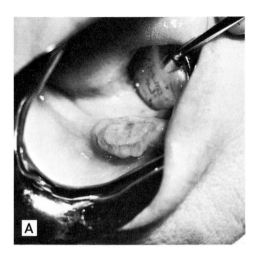
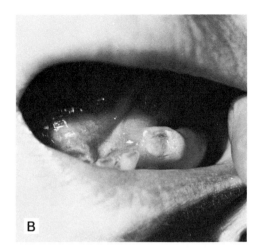

Fig. 14-11. (A) Traumatic lesion on alveolar ridge; biopsy results, negative. (B) Similar appearing lesion on floor of mouth; biopsy result, squamous cell carcinoma.

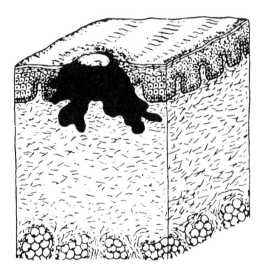
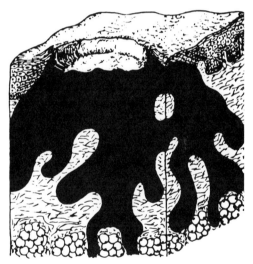

Fig. 14-12. Diagram illustrating the tendency of cancer to infiltrate.

References

1. Oringer, M. J.: Electrosurgery in Dentistry. Philadelphia, W. B. Saunders Co., 1962.
2. Shira, R. B.: Biopsy in oral diagnosis and treatment planning. Dent. Clin. North Am., 41–54, March, 1963.
3. Armstrong, S.: The relative value of oral cytology and biopsy as an adjunct to the diagnosis of oral lesions. J. Kentucky Dental Assoc., 17:19–23, 1965.
4. Rovin, S.: The role of biopsy and cytology in oral diagnosis. Dent. Clin. North Am., 429–434, July, 1965.

15 Inflammation, Repair, and Infection

DANIEL E. WAITE

Inflammation and Repair

Inflammation and repair comprise a standard physiologic process that occurs secondary to injury. Whether this injury is traumatic, or whether it is infectious, in which case it may be local or systemic, the basic process of inflammation and repair remains the same.

By definition, inflammation is the reaction to injury. The purpose of inflammation is to initiate repair. Leukocytes and antibodies infiltrate the area. Capillary dilatation increases the blood flow to the wounded part, which increases oxygen to the area, dilutes and eliminates toxic products, and stimulates phagocytosis and the complicated and lengthy process of repair. The work of Menkin has contributed much to our understanding of the inflammatory process.[1] The isolation of such substances as leukotaxin, pyrexin, and the leukocytosis-promoting factor has led to a clearer definition of inflammation and repair.

All wounds heal in a similar manner. The difference between healing by primary and by secondary intention is a matter of time and degree. In an uncomplicated wound healing process, there is an initial hemorrhage into the wound, covering it with blood, which coagulates. Inflammatory cells infiltrate the area, and the clot becomes organized. This forms a rich granulation tissue that initially bleeds easily if manipulated, but which ultimately diminishes its inflammatory response. The granulation tissue slowly transforms into fibrous connective tissue. If the wound involves bone, this tissue gives rise to osteoblasts, and the remodeling of the bone takes place.

Many factors influence the process of repair. The location of the wound is significant, and when the wound occurs in an area where there is a good vascular bed, as in the oral cavity, one can expect rapid healing. An increased temperature is advantageous to a healing wound and increases tissue metabolism. The inflammatory products of pyrexin and the leukocytosis-promoting factors are important in this stage of inflammation to increase local and systemic temperature and therefore metabolism and to increase the production of white blood cells. Certainly the oral cavity by natural habitat provides this warm moist environment to facilitate wound healing. Nutritional factors are important, especially protein and vitamins along with other well-established dietary requirements. Wounds in younger patients heal more rapidly than those in elderly persons, which probably relates directly to metabolism.

Some examples of diseases that may delay healing are the anemias and diabetes mellitus. Simple dehydration may also be a limiting factor, as is poor nutrition. Moreover, wounds of the oral cavity are constantly irritated by the tongue through talking and eating, so that the general mobility of the area and its uncleanliness may also deter healing.

Infection

Wound infection is probably the most common deterrent to normal wound healing because it produces additional injury and delays the entire healing process. The infection may be due to bacterial invasion or the decomposition of necrotic tissues. Both may be present at the same time, and if either process goes unnoticed or unchecked, the therapy may be inadequate.

If phagocytosis of bacteria present in the infected area is successful, we can apply the term *resolution* to the process; from that point on the wound will repair basically as a clean wound. However, if the leukocytes attracted to the site of the injury are unable to reverse the infectious process, it will continue to spread locally, causing a systemic response. This is reflected in an increase in body temperature, redness of the local part, and pain and swelling. An evaluation of the circulating blood will show an increase in the white blood cells, especially immature forms.

If neither resolution nor spread of the infection occurs, it is then referred to as a *localized* or *walled-off* infection. In this instance, there is a central area of necrosis as a result of the inflammation product necrosin, which acts upon the bacteria to form liquid pus. This can be referred to as an *abscess*, which will probably require

intervention by incision and drainage (Fig. 15-1).

From a practical standpoint, the locale of the environment in which the oral surgeon works presents many problems relative to infections. Since no mouth can be truly sterile, all our work takes place in a potentially infectious area. Any incision made in the oral cavity is susceptible to bacterial invasion; therefore, it is our responsibility as oral surgeons to keep pathogenic bacteria to a minimum. This can be achieved by the following: (1) do not operate on patients who give evidence of systemic or local infection; (2) prepare the mouth with oral rinses and meticulous oral hygiene prior to surgical intervention; and (3) emphasize special postoperative instructions relative to cleanliness.

Natural factors in the oral cavity help to prevent infections. The epithelium, by its constant desquamative activity, tends to rid itself of bacteria in addition to being resistant to direct bacterial penetration. The excellent vascularity of the mucosae permits a rapid turnover of nutrient materials in the oral cavity, which is a tremendous aid to the healing process and in minimizing infection. Although excessive saliva hinders good surgical management of oral tissues, saliva does seem to have an antibacterial quality, which aids in the control of infection.[2]

The natural defenses of the body certainly can be weakened when the surgeon neglects to handle tissue carefully and ignores basic surgical principles. This would include unnecessary trauma, poorly designed mucoperiosteal flaps that do not permit a broad-based blood supply, or operating in the presence of an acute cold or a sore throat. Also important is the psychologic adjustment of the patient in

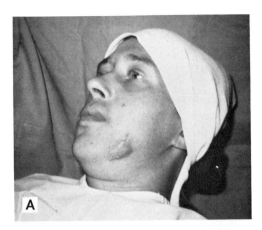

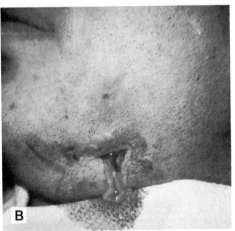

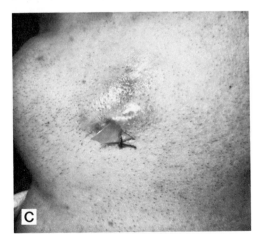

accepting his problems and having confidence in his doctor prior to a surgical procedure. The mental attitude of the patient and the chairside manner of the dentist will do much to influence the healing process.

The extraction of a tooth—no matter how carefully executed—creates a wound. Complete knowledge of how these wounds react to this form of injury is expected of every clinician. Other wounds that may occur in and around the oral cavity are lacerations, contusions, abrasions, and punctures. The incised wound usually results from a planned procedure, done under clean conditions, with an understanding of the blood supply and the intent of a good closure. This may not be the case with either lacerations or contusions, which require a special effort in postinjury cleanliness and improving the local environment for healing. The puncture wound is probably the most underestimated of all wounds, primarily because the ratio of the depth is not in proportion to the surface opening. Therefore, a wound that looks harmless on the surface may involve deep injury to structures below the surface; at the same time, large amounts of bacteria may have been inoculated deep within the tissues in a small and concentrated area.

The management of an intraoral wound is essentially the same as that of any wound. Immediate attention should be given to cleansing the wound with soap

Fig. 15-1. (A) Swelling and fluctuance near the inferior border of the mandible. (B) Extraoral incision and drainage. Etiologic factor is the second bicuspid. Note pus exuding from the incision. (C) Drain has been inserted to enhance drainage, dependent to the fluctuant area.

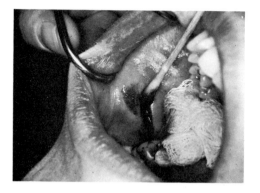

Fig. 15-2. Cleansing of oral wound. Debridement with hydrogen peroxide and saline solution.

and removing all foreign bodies (Fig. 15-2). Debridement and irrigation should be done. A primary closure is ideal, and the surgeon must allow for the obliteration of dead space as well as for drainage.

Treatment

The type of tissue involved in infection, as well as its anatomic location, is important in treatment. For example, an infection of the lateral pharyngeal space can seriously threaten life and must be treated expertly and efficiently. An infection of soft tissue would require an approach entirely different from an infection of bone, such as osteomyelitis (Fig. 15-3). After he thoroughly understands the anatomy of the tissues involved, the clinician can treat his patient with confidence and observe more capably the progress of the infectious process.

For the successful treatment of acute oral infections, the following outline can be used as a guide:

1. The bacteria are combated with chemotherapy.
2. The tissues are treated by:
   a. incision and drainage.
   b. removal of diseased teeth and necrotic bone.
3. Supportive therapy includes:
   a. rest
   b. fluids

c. analgesics
d. nourishment
e. physical therapy

The identification of the specific type of bacteria causing the infection and the an-

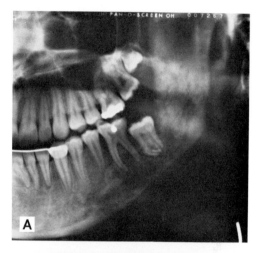

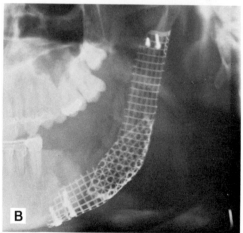

Fig. 15-3. (A) Severe osteomyelitis in a 19-year-old patient. Note bony destruction of ramus and body of the mandible. (B) Rebuilding was done with Vitallium mesh and bone marrow graft after mandibular resection and sequestrectomy. (Courtesy of R. G. Ogle)

tibiotic to which it is sensitive is desirable. This information is obtained only through laboratory testing with a culture; however, at least 48 hours are necessary to obtain culture results. To obtain the material for a culture, use a sterile swab to contact a small amount of the pus or exudate and submit it to the bacteriologist. A request should be made for (1) the identification of the organism, and (2) the antibiotics to which it is sensitive (Fig. 15-4).

Since time is a factor in the treatment of infections, the doctor must have a complete knowledge of the various sensitive and resistant strains of bacteria and the numerous chemotherapeutic agents in order to evaluate the infection clinically if he cannot wait for the results of a culture (see p. 548). The great majority of oral infections are caused by staphylococci and streptococci. The nature of the exudate

and the apparent ability of the infection to spread can also help the clinician make a diagnosis. The patient's systemic reaction frequently gives an indication to the virulence of the organism.

Choosing the proper antibiotics has become a difficult and somewhat complicated procedure because of the indiscriminate use of antibiotics, which promotes the development of sensitivity to the drugs by patients and resistance by the microorganisms. Inadequate antibiotic therapy in terms of size of dose or duration of treatment may also favor the development of resistant bacterial strains. Sensitivity of the patient to an antibiotic must be carefully considered each time a drug is used. Some patients now are sensitive to many of the antibiotics currently available; such sensitivity has resulted in serious illness and even death. Any his-

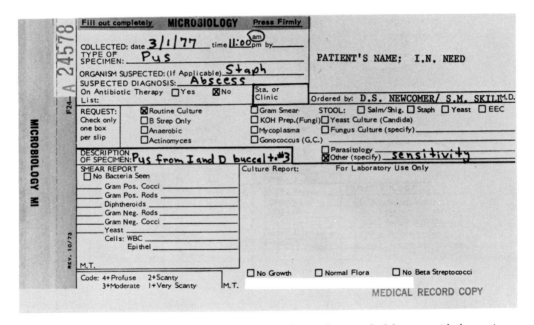

Fig. 15-4. An appropriate microbiology request form is filled out and sent to the laboratory with the specimen.

tory of pruritus, hives, rash, cough, or gastrointestinal upset following the use of an antibiotic contraindicates further administration of the drug. It is my opinion that one should not resort to antibiotics for every little flare-up, but give a patient the opportunity to build his own resistance and reserve the antibiotics for more serious infections.

Treatment of the tissues most certainly must not be overlooked. It is not uncommon to see a patient who has been treated with systemic antibiotics for several days with no local treatment showing no improvement. In this instance, the antibiotic has only served to mask the infection and to allow the microorganism to become more resistant (Fig. 15-5). In such cases, incision and drainage are important adjuncts to treatment. When purulent material is formed in an infectious site, it must be drained. Hot moist applications may well increase local metabolism and increase resolution when an egress for drainage has been provided. This form of therapy can only be carried out with a proper understanding of the anatomy involved (see discussions on fascial spaces, p. 219). When incising for drainage, it is important to know when the time is "right," which is best determined if the infection has been fluctuating. Make the incision to bone and through the periosteum. Insert a blunt instrument or hemostat and spread the tissues to create accurate and dependent drainage. However, remember that minimal tissue manipulation is a cardinal principle in acute infection.

The removal of diseased teeth, foreign bodies, and necrotic bone is important because it removes the cause of the infection or factors contributing to delayed healing. However, there is a difference of opinion regarding the proper time for removal of an involved tooth during an acute infection. Some believe that a tooth is never too "hot" to extract, in that the cause of the infection (the tooth) should

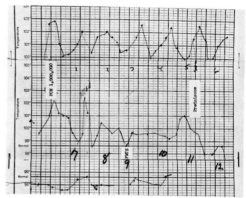

Fig. 15-5. Temperature chart of a patient who was admitted to the hospital with gross oral infection from teeth. Temperature on day of hospital admission (day 1) was 102.8° F. Penicillin was administered, but temperature continued to spike. Prednisone was added to regimen on day 5. The febrile course continued until day 9, when it was decided to proceed with the removal of all remaining teeth. In three days (day 12), the temperature returned to normal and the patient was discharged from the hospital on day 16.

be removed immediately. However, extraction in such instances is an insult to the involved tissues and may open new routes for the infection to spread, especially to the medullary portion of bone. A proper sequence of treatment would be to provide adequate drainage of the infected tissue and to remove the tooth when the infection has been controlled (Fig. 15-6).

The resistance of the patient cannot be minimized, and its importance increases with the severity and duration of the infection. It depends upon many factors, for which the doctor can provide guidance. Obviously, the age, general health, and physical condition of the patient are factors already existent. However, the doctor

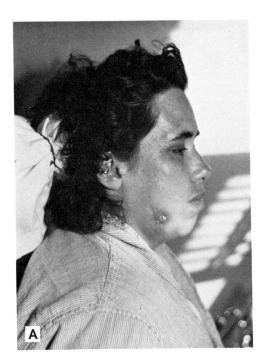 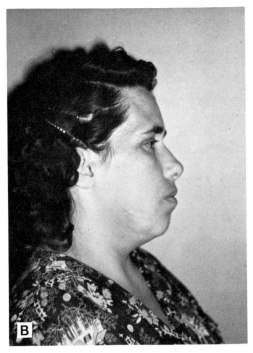

Fig. 15-6. (A) First molar infection draining extraorally. (B) The chronic drainage tract was excised one month after extraction of the tooth.

can emphasize certain measures, such as adequate rest, which is frequently disregarded as an important requisite in the supportive therapy of infection. Unfortunately, dental problems are too often minimized by the public. A patient will frequently be unconcerned when he has a swollen face as a result of "only" an ulcerated tooth, whereas he may become quite alarmed over a headache or sore throat. It is important that the entire body is rested in order to increase the total physiologic response to infection; rest or immobilization of the infected part is also important.

The doctor should know whether his patient is adequately hydrated and has a normal fluid intake; the fluid intake should be increased during infection, particularly when the body temperature is elevated. Intravenous fluids may have to be administered if the oral intake is impaired.

The diet during infection should not be neglected, as it definitely has an influence on the course and final outcome of the infectious process. Depending on the location of the infection and the ability of the patient to masticate, a liquid or soft diet high in nutritional value may be indicated. In some cases, forced food diets may be necessary, and the food and fluid intake carefully recorded in order to ensure adequate nutrition.

Analgesics for the control of pain and discomfort may be needed, as they will increase the cooperation of the patient. By careful selection of these and other medications, a patient may remain comfortable and ambulatory during the surgical and postoperative period.

Physical therapy is important in the various facets of infection control. The toxic substances produced by infectious processes frequently cause muscles to go into spasm and cause trismus. Exercise and massage are helpful; however, mechanical pressures on infected tissues prior to incision and drainage can contribute to the direct spread of the infection.

The proper therapeutic use of heat and cold seems constantly to be misinterpreted. In general, cold is used only to minimize immediate postsurgical trauma, and heat is used to treat infection. Properly used intraorally or extraorally, heat will substantially speed up the localization of infection by increasing the metabolism and thus the inflammatory response. Conversely, cold will retard the inflammatory process. Moist heat, in the form of moist compresses or irrigations, seems to be better than dry heat. Heat can also be used effectively after surgical intervention. It dilates the capillaries, thereby allowing a constant exchange of the accumulating toxic materials and the nutrient supply to the tissues.

The induction of satisfactory anesthesia during the treatment of oral infection is frequently complicated. One may proceed with incision and drainage if local anesthesia can be obtained without injecting into the inflamed tissues. However, if this cannot be done, a general anesthetic should be considered.

The Fascial Spaces

When considering infection of the mandibular and maxillofacial regions, one must have an understanding of the anatomic compartments that become involved. No one should be more familiar with the anatomy of the face and, more specifically, the mouth and related structures than the dentist.

The areas where infections might localize are determined by the fascial spaces. Fascial spaces are potential areas between planes of fascia. When the loose connective tissue that normally binds fascial planes together is destroyed by invading infection, the compartments thus established between the planes are referred to as fascial spaces.

Fascial spaces may be occupied by relatively loose connective tissue which lies between organs and layers of more dense connective tissue. The clinical significance of fascial spaces is that when infection develops and extends within these spaces they offer little resistance to the spread of infections, and it is frequently necessary to establish surgical drainage. For these reasons, a knowledge of location and extent of fascial spaces is important to their appropriate management.

Most of the fascial spaces to be discussed are formed by the superficial layer of the deep cervical fascia as it envelops bone, muscle, and vessels. These spaces are known by several synonyms, and we have attempted to use nomenclature that is both anatomically correct and understood by all.

For full understanding of the fascial spaces a knowledge of dental anatomy and a review of the local anatomy become very important. Infection spreads buccally or lingually from infected teeth and may remain subperiosteal or break through above or below muscle attachments to enter the fascial spaces (Fig. 15-7).

The buccal space may become involved from infection of either the maxillary or mandibular bicuspid or molar teeth. This

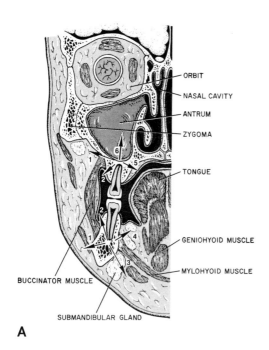

A

BUCCINATOR MUSCLE

SUBMANDIBULAR GLAND

ORBIT

NASAL CAVITY

ANTRUM

ZYGOMA

TONGUE

GENIOHYOID MUSCLE

MYLOHYOID MUSCLE

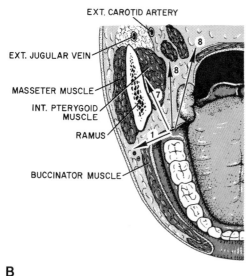

EXT. CAROTID ARTERY

EXT. JUGULAR VEIN

MASSETER MUSCLE

INT. PTERYGOID MUSCLE

RAMUS

BUCCINATOR MUSCLE

B

Fig. 15-7. Fascial spaces. (A) Sagittal section. (B) Horizontal section. Buccal (1); vestibular (2); submandibular (3); sublingual (4); palatal (5); maxillary antrum (6); masticator (7); lateral pharyngeal (8).

space contains loose connective tissue and is lateral to the buccinator muscle. It is in communication posteriorly with the masticator space. Infections in this space may extend from the mandible inferiorly to the orbital region superiorly and are best treated early when the infection is still limited to the vestibule or within the periosteal tissues. When a true buccal space infection spreads, dependent drainage may need to be extraoral with consideration of the location of the facial artery and nerve. If drained intraorally, the location of the parotid duct must be considered.

The space of the body of the mandible is formed as the superficial layer of the deep cervical fascia splits around the lower surface of the mandible, forming a potential space around the mandible. This is essentially a subperiosteal space from which infections can spread in several directions. Buccally, infection may enter the buccal space or the vestibule, whereas lingually the extension may be into the sublingual or submandibular spaces (Fig. 15-7A). Note the relationship of the mandibular teeth to the mylohyoid muscle (Fig. 15-8). The space of the body of the mandible extends from the symphysis to the third molar area. Infections of this

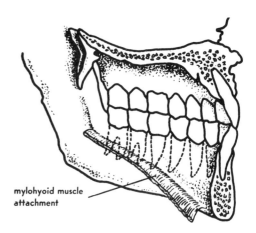

mylohyoid muscle attachment

Fig. 15-8. Schematic drawing of mylohyoid muscle attachment in relation to the apices of mandibular teeth.

region are often drained adequately by an incision in the depth of the buccal vestibule through periosteum to bone (Fig. 15-9). Extraoral drainage can be established when necessary by a 1 to 2-cm. incision parallel to the inferior border of the mandible, noting the location of the facial artery and seventh cranial nerve. A curved hemostat can then be inserted through the incision to bone to improve the drainage (Fig. 15-10).

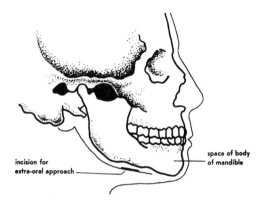

Fig. 15-10. Extraoral incision and drainage of infection involving space of the body of mandible. (Waite: Infections of dental etiology in the mandibular and maxillofacial region. J.O.S. Anes. Hosp. Dent. Service, *18*, July, 1960.)

The submental space lies in the midline of the neck between the hyoid bone and the symphysis of the mandible. The lateral borders are the anterior bellys of the digastric muscles, the roof is the mylohyoid muscle, and the floor is the superficial layer of the deep cervical fascia. This space becomes involved mainly from anterior mandibular teeth. Drainage is obtained through a stab incision over the area of tenderness and fluctuance.

The submandibular space is that area bounded by the mylohyoid muscle above and between the anterior and posterior digastric muscles. It contains the submandibular gland and lymph nodes. This space is continuous with the sublingual space posterior to the mylohyoid muscle. Infections of this space are of dental origin when space of the body of the mandible infections extend through the lingual plate of the mandible and below the level of the mylohyoid muscle. The molar and premolar teeth are usually involved but infection of the submandibular gland can

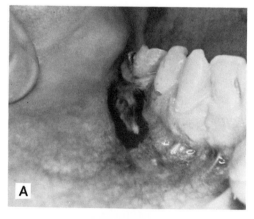

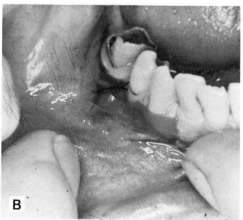

Fig. 15-9. (A) Intraoral incision and drainage of second molar infection. (B) Rubber drain is left in place for 24 hours.

also involve the space. Surgical drainage is obtained in a manner similar to that for a space of the body of the mandible infection.

The sublingual space is like a box, bounded by the mucosae of the floor of the mouth superiorly, the mylohyoid muscle inferiorly, the mandibular body laterally, and the mandibular symphysis anteriorly, and communicates to the submandibular space. This space is entered by infections above the mylohyoid muscle, mainly from anterior teeth. A sublingual space infection can raise the floor of the mouth and displaces the tongue, obstructing the oral cavity. If the sublingual, submandibular, and submental spaces are involved bilaterally, it is known as Ludwig's angina.

The masticator space is formed by the division of the superficial layer of the deep cervical fascia as a posterior extension of the space of the body of the mandible. These layers encompass the masseter and temporalis and pterygoid muscles and the ramus of the mandible and attach superiorly to the sphenoid bone. This space can be compartmentalized into subspaces, the superficial and deep temporal spaces. Infection of this space usually occurs by extension from the space of the body of the mandible. Infection from lower third molars is the usual course of involvement of this space.

The usual symptoms are pain, swelling, temperature, and trismus (Fig. 15-11), and occasionally dysphagia. Physical examination will generally show both an internal and external swelling. Over the ramus and angle of the mandible, the swelling may be indurated and brawny. Intraorally, the swelling may displace the anterior tonsillar pillar medially. Trismus often makes examination difficult and

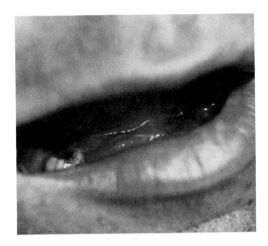

Fig. 15-11. Trismus due to masticator space involvement.

painful for the patient. Many authors believe infections in this space tend to become localized. Intraoral drainage may occur spontaneously. In most cases, the suppurative process will necessitate surgical intervention. This may be done intraorally by an incision parallel to the anterior border of the masseter muscle extending to bone. A curved hemostat can be inserted medial or lateral to the mandible to break up suppurative loculations. For extraoral drainage, an incision is made inferior and posterior to the angle of the mandible, as noted in Figure 15-12, through periosteum to bone.

Anatomically, the lateral pharyngeal space is considered the bilateral extension of the retropharyngeal space. The boundaries are the base of the skull superiorly, the hyoid bone inferiorly, the superior constrictor muscle of the pharynx medially, the masticator space laterally, the pterygomandibular raphe anteriorly, and the retropharyngeal space posteriorly. Extension of infection into this space may

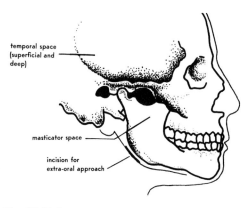

Fig. 15-12. Point of extraoral incision for drainage of masticator space infection. (Waite: Infections of dental etiology in the mandibular and maxillofacial region. J.O.S. Anes. Hosp. Dent. Service, *18*, July, 1960.)

occur from the tonsils, the floor of the mouth, the masticator space, or the space of the body of the mandible. Infections in this space are serious. This space contains the carotid artery and internal jugular vein, and can be a pathway for extension into the chest by way of the retropharyngeal space. Mandibular third molar infection is the most frequent contaminaton of the space. Symptoms include pain, trismus, high temperature, and dysphagia. Patients are often dehydrated as a result of an inability to eat or drink fluids secondary to the dysphagia and trismus. Considerable clinical judgment is necessary in these cases relative to hospitalization, intravenous fluids, antibiotics, and appropriate incision and drainage. The incision and drainage may need to be done in the operating room under general anesthesia. The internal jugular vein and internal carotid artery, being in this space, make the drainage particularly hazardous. Intraoral drainage is achieved by an incision medial and parallel to the pterygomandibular raphe, with the exploration being carried posteriorly and medially into the space.

Infections of the anterior facial triangle are those involving the base of the upper lip to the canine fossa (Fig. 15-13). Ana-

tomically, the venous drainage of this area is valveless and can flow retrograde superiorly to the facial vein to the angular vein and pass posteriorly by way of the superior ophthalmic vein to enter the cavernous sinus. The usual cause is the anterior maxillary teeth. Once an infection reaches the cavernous sinus it can be life threatening even with intravenous antibiotics. A case of anterior triangle involvement with superior spread is shown in Figure 15-14. Symptoms of high temperature, headache, and swelling of the eye were present. Note the cranial nerves and vascular contents of the cavernous sinus in Figure 15-14D. Infection of the anterior triangle of the face should be treated early by an incision placed in the depth of the mucobuccal fold over the involved area for drainage.

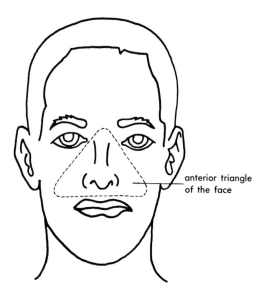

Fig. 15-13. Schematic drawing of space for potential infection referred to as the "anterior triangle of the face." (Waite: Infections of dental etiology in the mandibular and maxillofacial region. J.O.S. Anes. Hosp. Dent. Service, *18*, July, 1960).

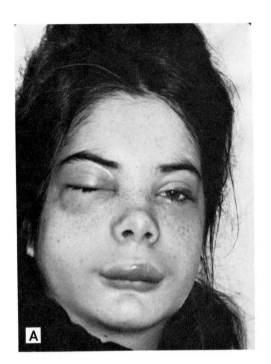

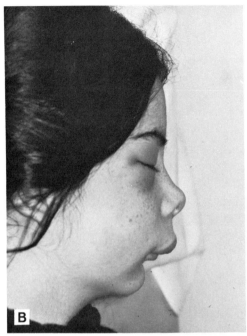

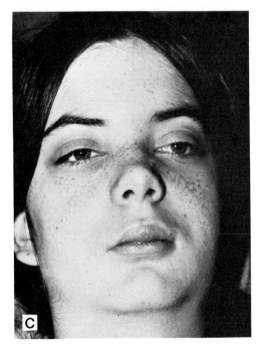

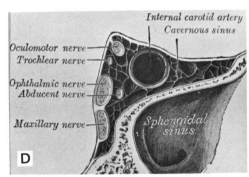

Fig. 15-14. (A) Frontal view of patient with postoperative infection 48 hours after root canal treatment of right maxillary incisor. (B) Lateral view. Note involvement of the anterior triangle of the face and periorbital edema. (C) Four days later, after treatment by incision and drainage and intravenous administration of antibiotics. (D) Cross section of the cavernous sinus and related structures. Involvement of the cavernous sinus is a severe threat to life. Infections easily contaminate this area.

Special Oral Infections

Apart from the general principles of infection and its process, a few special problems relating to the oral cavity need emphasis.

CHRONIC CYST, GRANULOMA, OR PERIAPICAL ABSCESS. A radiolucency at the apex of the tooth may be the only evidence of a previous infectious problem. The tooth may be nonvital as recorded by ice or electric pulp testing and otherwise may be asymptomatic. The exact diagnosis of cyst, granuloma, or periapical abscess can be known following biopsy and histologic evaluation. The clinical significance of these chronic problems is that, even though they have been asymptomatic for long periods, they may flare into an acute inflammatory process at any time. A quiescent periapical infection may retain its chronicity by draining into the oral cavity or through a sinus tract to the skin surface (Fig. 15-15).

Treatment involves removal of the offending tooth and the chronic abscess, granuloma, or cyst by curettage. Conservative management would be to remove the pulp canal contents and provide a root

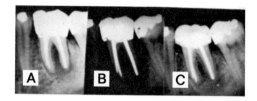

Fig. 15-16. Root canal with apicoectomy. (A) Note bifurcation involvement. (B and C) Note good bone fill two years later.

canal filling (Fig. 15-16). Apicoectomy would then be necessary to remove the apical lesion. However, if the apical lesion is a granuloma, root section and apical curettage are not necessary; the appropriate root canal reaming, sterilization, and filling are adequate.

CHRONIC PERIODONTAL DISEASE. Periodontal disease, as the acute form of local or general gingival inflammation or infection, also has its chronic counterpart. Long-standing chronic periodontal disease results in severe alveolar bone loss, creating deep gingival pockets (Fig. 15-17). The conservative corrective treatment of these long-standing problems lies largely within the field of periodontology. Some of these seemingly chronic and simple

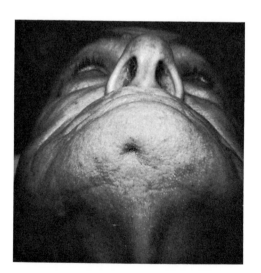

Fig. 15-15. Long-standing periapical infection of lower central incisors draining through sinus tract onto face.

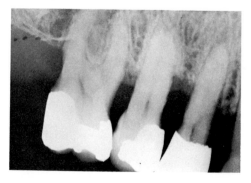

Fig. 15-17. Alveolar bone resorption with deep pocket formation.

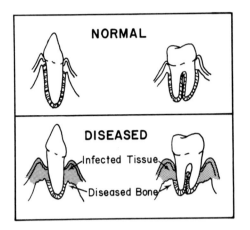

Fig. 15-18. Periodontally involved teeth. Schematic drawing of single and multirooted teeth showing normal and diseased tissue. Note bifurcation involvement of infected molar roots. (Waite and Bradley: Oral infection. J.A.D.A., 71, 1965)

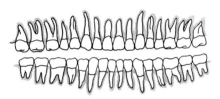

Fig. 15-19. Maximal diseased surface tissue when teeth are periodontally involved. Total diseased surface area of tissue is that quantity of tissue involved in entire root surfaces of all teeth. (Waite and Bradley: Oral infection. J.A.D.A., 71, 1965)

dental problems can become debilitating to the patient, often because of the tissue surface area involved.

"Consider the surface area of the tissues involved while doing a full-mouth extraction of teeth and alveolectomy procedures or the potential tissue involved in generalized periodontal disease. This is a large area of soft tissue and bony involvement (Figs. 15-18 and 15-19). This problem concerns the total tissues around the root or roots of the teeth involved.

"It is this maximal surface area of diseased periodontal tissues that may seriously contribute to a patient's systemic illness. This same surface area, however, compounds to considerable dimensions when full-mouth extraction of teeth is anticipated (Fig. 15-20).

"Analogously, the surface area of surgical exposures which represents that in full-mouth extraction procedures can be transferred to the inner aspect of the arm

to indicate graphically a comparable dimension of injury to tissue (Fig. 15-21). The black line on the arm represents the length of an incision that would be necessary to afford reflection of the flap in extraction procedures throughout the entire maxilla and mandible. The length of this incision approximates 12.25 inches. Added to this length would be the entire surface of tissue exposed in the reflection of labial and buccal mucoperiosteal flaps in a full-mouth extraction procedure."*

* From Waite, D. E., and Bradley, R. E.: Oral infection. J.A.D.A., 71:587–592, 1965.

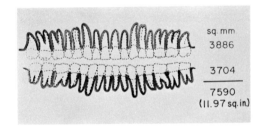

Fig. 15-20. Socket surface after full-mouth tooth extraction (FMTE) showing amount of surface area of sockets after extraction of teeth. Amount is based on dimensions of root surfaces. Surface area is same as area of total infected tissue in periodontal disease. (Waite and Bradley: Oral infection. J.A.D.A., 71, 1965)

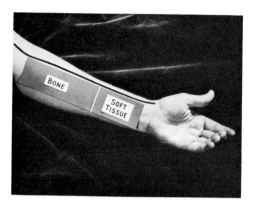

Fig. 15-21. Pictorial estimate used to establish amount of soft tissue and bone exposed in a full-mouth extraction of teeth. The black line represents the incision length. (Waite and Bradley: Oral infection. J.A.D.A., *71*, 1965)

Sialadenitis is inflammation of the salivary glands; any or all of the glands can be involved. Duct blockage by a salivary stone or a mucous plug may be attended by swelling, infection, and pain (Fig. 15-22). Dilatation of the ducts to locate and remove blockage is indicated, and in many instances antibiotics may be necessary. Chronic infection and neoplasm of the glands are also potential problems, although acute conditions are usually related to infection or blockage.

Maxillary sinusitis may be totally unrelated or much related to dental disease. A patient with a chronic case of maxillary sinusitis has nasal discharge, nasal obstruction, and dull intermittent pain. Roentgen examination in the Waters' position may reveal a fluid level, cloudy antra, or a thick antral membrane[4] (Fig. 15-23). The cause of such problems is usually a cold, complicated by structural defects of the nasal system, turbinates, and the like. Unfavorable drainage and ventilation also interfere and make the patient prone to additional infection. The acute form of sinusitis develops suddenly, with much pain and often accompanied by fever, chills, and malaise. The teeth proximating the antral cavity may be tender and even ache, making the diagno-

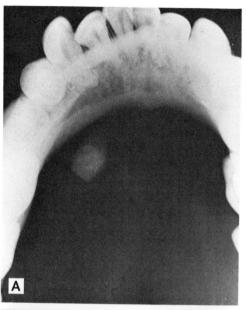

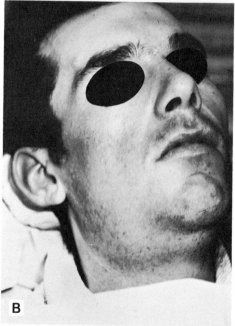

Fig. 15-22. (A) Occlusal plane film showing submaxillary calculus. (B) Swelling, pain, and infection due to salivary stone blockage.

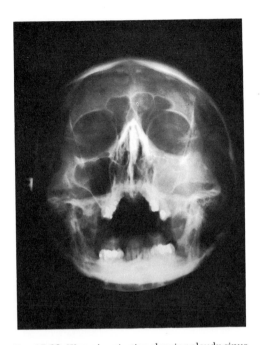

Fig. 15-23. Waters' projection showing cloudy sinus.

sis of maxillary sinusitis versus an acute pulpitis difficult.

Acute sinusitis of dental origin usually has its inception with an attempted extraction of a maxillary molar or bicuspid tooth. A perforation may occur as a result of the extraction, particularly if the root projected into the sinus. If such an opening occurs and the sinus is grossly contaminated with oral contents and is improperly cared for, an antral–oral fistula and maxillary sinusitis may develop. The care of such a condition requires careful management of tissue flaps, debridement, and the judicious use of antibiotics. Details of the surgical closure of antral–oral fistulas appear on page 239.

Pericoronitis is an inflammatory condition occurring around the coronal portion of a tooth. It occurs most frequently in

and around the flap or operculum of a partially erupted third molar (Fig. 15-24). The area can be painful and often additionally traumatized by the opposing tooth. Extension of this infection can involve deep fascial planes and spaces. Avoid undue manipulation of the tissues in conditions of acute pericoronitis. Pericoronitis can best be treated by cleansing the pocket with hydrogen peroxide and mechanical debridement. If there is a systemic response to the infection, antibiotics are indicated. Recurring pericoronitis may necessitate extraction of the tooth or operculectomy.

DELAYED EXTRACTION WOUND HEALING. There are several synonyms for this condition: localized osteitis, alveolar osteitis, postextraction alveolitis, alveolitis sicca dolorosa, and fibrinolytic alveolitis. Each of these names refers to some of the characteristics of this complication to extraction of teeth. Crawford first used the term *dry socket* in 1896, probably because of the lack of exudate and the loss of blood clot in the socket as noted in this condition.[6] A number of synonyms for dry socket refer to the consistent histologic

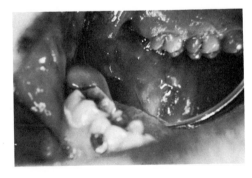

Fig. 15-24. Pericoronitis showing edematous operculum of third molar area. Inflammatory and painful.

picture, which is that of acute or subacute osteomyelitis with thrombosed vessels and heavy infiltration with inflammatory cells. The typical clinical picture of dry socket is that of excruciating, irradiating pain beginning two to four days postoperatively, an extraction wound with partial to complete clot loss, sensitive bone surfaces covered by a grayish-yellow layer of necrotic tissue, and a fetid odor.

Extensive clinical studies have shown that dry socket develops in 0.9 per cent to 4.4 per cent after all extractions with an average of 3 per cent. Dry socket most frequently occurs in the mandible after extraction of first and second molars, whereas it is rarely present after extraction of incisors. It is well known that it more often occurs after removal of impacted teeth, according to most investigators in about 20 per cent of all mandibular third molar cases. The majority of third molar surgery is done in the age group 20 to 40 years; therefore, this may explain why as many as 80 per cent of all cases of dry socket are found in this age group.

Until recently it has not been possible to establish a sound scientifically proved cause for this postextraction condition, even though numerous research studies have been reported. Most investigators believe the cause is closely related to surgical trauma and local inflammation. According to the investigations made by Birn, it may be explained by fibrinolytic activity in the postextraction socket.

The components of the fibrinolytic system are shown in Figure 15-25. The fibrinolytic activity in dry socket (fibrinolytic alveolitis) seems to be linked with a stable protein bound tissue kinase, an activator released from the alveolar bone due to inflammation caused by trauma and/or infection. This activator stimulates the transformation of plasminogen to plasmin (fibrinolysin, a proteolytic enzyme), which causes the lysis of fibrin and the dissolution of the blood clot. Birn demonstrated that the fibrinolytic activity in dry socket

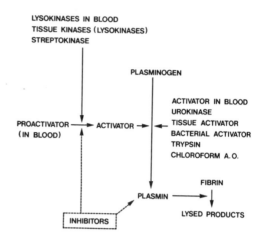

Fig. 15-25. The components of the fibrinolytic system and their relations. (Birn, H.: Etiology and pathogenesis of fibrinolytic alveolitis ("dry socket"). Int. J. Oral Surg., 2:211–267, 1973)

is high as compared to that in normally healing extraction wounds and is closely connected to the course of the disease. The amount of fibrinolytic activity increases steeply during the first days of the condition. Furthermore, it was shown that the intensity of the fibrinolytic activity is proportional to the clinical course and could cause dissolution of the blood clot in the socket. In this way, one of the most characteristic features in dry socket, the dissolution of the blood clot, may be explained.

The other characteristic feature, excruciating pain, may also be explained by the action of plasmin. One of the strongest known pain-producing agents is a polypeptide called kinin. Kinins are normally not found free in the human organism because they are instantaneously inactivated by kininases. The pain produced by kinin is characterized by violent burning, smarting, and pricking, and may be irradiating. Kinin is produced by transformation from kininogen by the action of

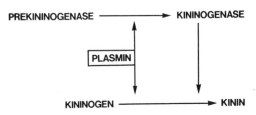

Fig. 15-26. The main components of the kinin-forming system and the function of plasmin as an activator. (Birn, H.: Etiology and pathogenesis of fibrinolytic alveolitis ("dry socket"). Int. J. Oral Surg., 2:211–267, 1973)

plasmin (Fig. 15-26), and kinin is present in dry socket.

The development of dry socket may be explained schematically (Fig. 15-27). Trauma and/or infection due to extraction causes inflammation of the bone marrow adjacent to the socket, which releases an activator. This activator causes the transformation of plasminogen to plasmin. Plasmin is responsible for the lysis of fibrin, leading to clot dissolution and the formation of the pain-producing kinin from kininogen.

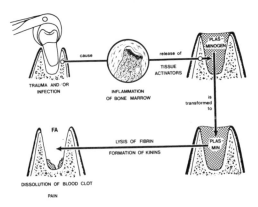

Fig. 15-27. Etiology and pathogenesis of fibrinolytic alveolitis. (Birn, H.: Etiology and pathogenesis of fibrinolytic alveolitis ("dry socket"). Int. J. Oral Surg. 2:211–267, 1973)

As seen in the diagram of the fibrinolytic system, it is possible to inhibit the lysis of fibrin (Fig. 15-25). The inhibitors may work in different stages in the system. The propylic ester of p-hydroxybenzoic acid is known to be a strong antifibrinolytic agent, which inhibits both the activator activity and the plasmin activity.[7] In a double blind study including 45 patients who had impacted mandibular third molars removed, propylic ester of p-hydroxybenzoic acid was inserted in the socket after the extraction. In the experimental group receiving the antifibrinolytic active propylic ester of p-hydroxybenzoic acid, none of the patients developed dry socket compared to 24 per cent in the placebo group. Thus, the prophylactic effect in this study using an antifibrinolytic substance was 100 per cent and statistically significant. However, the development of a safe prophylactic measure against dry socket is still on the experimental level, and only future studies may give a final solution.

Once this condition is established, the extraction wound is slow to heal, regardless of treatment, and healing generally continues through 10 to 14 days. During this period, discomfort is often unbearable unless the unprotected walls of the socket are covered with a prepared gauze dressing. The treatment is purely palliative and directed toward correction of the discomfort, prevention of further infection, and promotion of healing. Research studies in the prevention and treatment of dry socket have involved cortisone, antihistamines, antibiotics, analgesics, enzymes, vitamins, and a host of proprietary medications.

After proper diagnosis, the wound is carefully irrigated with saline solution and cleansed of all debris and necrotic tissue. The area of the socket is isolated and carefully dried with cotton pellets. If pain has been intense, a wiping of the socket walls with a topical anodyne will be helpful (Fig. 15-28). The gentle insertion of the medicated gauze dressing com-

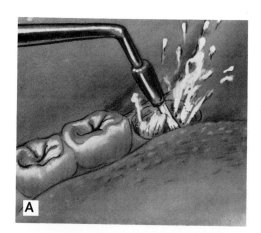

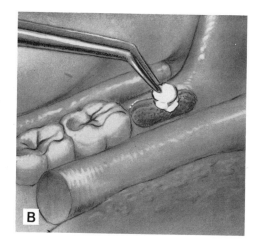

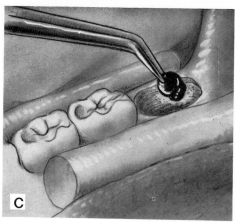

Fig. 15-28. (A) Irrigation. (B) Isolation. (C) Medication. (Waite, *Dry Socket, Practical Dental Monographs*, Year Book Publishers, Inc., 1957)

pletes the treatment. The socket should not be packed with the dressing, rather it should be placed loosely in the socket, attempting to seal the wound from oral contaminants (Fig. 15-29). If a socket is packed too firmly, healing with granulation tissue may be delayed, and pressure from the dressing may cause pain. The dressing should be changed as often as necessary to control the pain, and no individual dressing should be left in place longer than five days. To facilitate the cleaning of the socket after dressings have been discontinued, the patient can be given an irrigation syringe for home care (Fig. 15-30). This will greatly improve the postoperative course and avoid further complications by keeping the healing socket clean. (Contribution by Dr. Martin Ritzau)

References

1. Menkin, V.: Newer Concepts of Inflammation. Springfield, Ill., Charles C Thomas, 1950.
2. Green, G. E.: Properties of a salivary bacteriolysin and comparison with serum beta lysin. J. Dent. Res., 45:880–882, 1966.

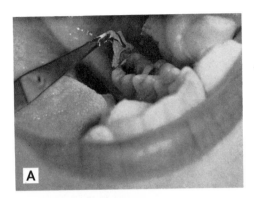

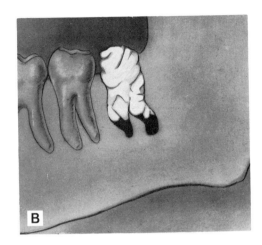

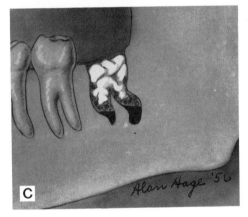

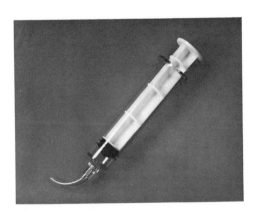

Fig. 15-29. (A) Insertion of dressing. (B) Wrong method of placing the dressing (overpacked). (C) Right method of placing the dressing, leaving room for granulations and providing a sealing effect at the periphery. (Waite, *Dry Socket, Practical Dental Monographs,* Year Book Publishers, Inc., 1957)

Fig. 15-30. Disposable irrigating syringe.

3. Crawford, J. Y.: Dry sockets. Items of Interest, *19*:22–23, 1897.

4. Merrell, R. A., Jr., Yanagisawa, E., Smith, H. W., and Thaler, S.: Radiographic Anatomy of the Paranasal Sinuses. Rochester, Minn., Custom Printing, Inc. (Reprinted from Arch. Otolaryng., *87*, 1968.)

5. Birn, H.: Etiology and pathogenesis of fibrinolytic alveolitis ("dry socket"). Int. J. Oral Surg., *2*:211–267, 1973.

6. Crawford, J. Y.: Dry socket. Dental Cosmos, *38*:929–931, 1896.

7. Ritzau, M., and Swangisilpa, K.: The prophylactic use of propylic ester of p-hydrobenzoic acid on alveolitis sicca dolorosa. A preliminary report. Oral Surg., *43*:32–37, 1977.

16 The Maxillary Sinus

DANIEL E. WAITE

The maxillary sinus at birth consists of a small tubular sac on the inner side of the orbit. The major portion of the maxilla is almost entirely filled with developing teeth (Fig. 16-1). The growth and development of the maxillary sinus proceed slowly during childhood until the seventh year, then the expansion progresses rapidly and pneumatization of the maxilla continues until the fifteenth year, when it is practically completed. The boundaries of the maxillary sinus are the orbital plate of the maxillary bone above, the external surface of the maxilla, and the posterior

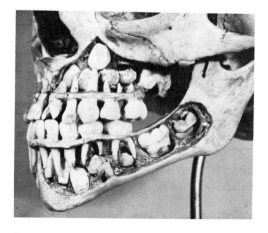

Fig. 16-1. The infant skull demonstrates the dentition essentially occupying the place of the maxillary sinus.

wall of the maxilla adjacent to the ptery-gomaxillary fossa.[1]

The nasal wall contains the sole outlet from the sinus; this is called the hiatus semilunaris. Its location is unfavorable for natural drainage from the antrum; therefore, the nasoantral wall, at its lower extremity, provides a simple approach beneath the inferior turbinate when surgical drainage must be instituted. Terminal branches of the infraorbital artery, a branch of the maxillary artery, provide the major blood supply to the maxillary sinus. Venous return is accomplished primarily through the anterior facial vein. The angular vein, which proceeds to the inferior ophthalmic vein and ultimately into the cavernous sinus, is also responsible for a portion of the venous drainage. The lymphatic channels are numerous in this area, providing drainage chiefly toward the submandibular lymph nodes. The innervation of the antrum is from the infraorbital nerve (Fig. 16-2).

It has been alleged that the function of the sinuses is to improve resonance, to warm inspired air, and to decrease the weight of the skull. Ballenger indicates that the sinuses may be nothing more than residual olfactory surfaces much more necessary for primitive man when finding food depended on sharp olfaction.[2]

233

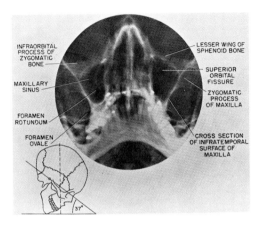

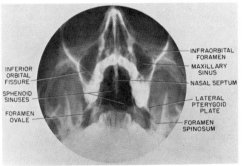

Fig. 16-2. Radiographs of normal maxillary sinus and related anatomy.

Pneumatization of the maxillary sinus, though generally complete in adolescence, may still increase during adulthood with further development into the alveolar process, especially when posterior maxillary teeth are lost prematurely (Fig. 16-3). In such instances, the antral cavity may be near the crest of the ridge. Great variations may also be seen in dentulous mouths, where the antral cavity may dip low between the maxillary roots and in other instances not appear at all on the dental x-ray films (Fig. 16-4). It is essentially the close proximity of the sinus to the dentition that involves the dentist in differential diagnostic problems arising from dental or sinus disease. The roots of the maxillary second bicuspid and the first and the second molars are most frequently involved. Reading studied 138 cases of antral-oral perforations and reported that 48 per cent were associated with the removal of maxillary first molars, 26 per cent with second molars, and 3 per cent with bicuspids.[3] Killey and Kay reported 250 cases of oral–antral fistula secondary to dental extraction, and found 61.2 per cent related to first molars, 25.2 per cent to second molars, and 6 per cent to third molars.[4] The remaining 13.6 per cent were associated with maxillary bicuspids.

Several anatomic and physiologic features obstruct the flow of drainage from the sinuses, thus precipitating infection. These are the inadequate anatomic openings mentioned earlier, obstructive polyps, septal deviation, hyperplasia of the turbinate, and inadequate ciliary action. A

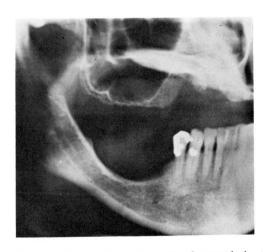

Fig. 16-3. The maxillary sinus may enlarge with the patient's age, and in the patient shown, pneumatization has extended into the edentulous alveolus.

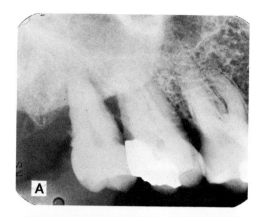

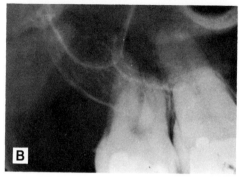

Fig. 16-4. (A) X-ray film showing no evidence of maxillary sinus dipping between roots of teeth. (B) X-ray film showing maxillary sinus dipping between roots of teeth.

x-ray films may be helpful in locating root tips or other foreign bodies that approximate the antral floor. However, because only a portion of the maxillary sinus can be radiographed intraorally, the usefulness of these x-ray views is limited. Intraoral radiographs of the antrum do not often reveal all aspects of the lining membrane or bony septa, and more important, both sinuses cannot be depicted together on the same radiograph by intraoral techniques. Comparison of the radiologic appearance of the sinuses on the same film is helpful from a diagnostic standpoint. For these reasons, the radiographic examination of the maxillary sinus should include extraoral techniques.

The panoramic radiograph is valuable for diagnostically viewing the maxillary sinuses (Fig. 16-5). If the practitioner has

covering, or blanket, of mucus is essential to normal ciliary action. It is like a conveyor belt in which cilia propel the mucous sheets toward the drainage areas. This mechanism destroys bacteria and ensnarls foreign bodies and debris, providing an excellent cleansing action. Air pollution and smoking assuredly impair this action. The sinus membrane does not tear easily and varies greatly in thickness depending on anatomic location, even in the normal sinus. In disease states, the thickness may be 10 to 15 times the normal, which is about 1 mm.

Roentgenology is an essential diagnostic aid to the practitioner for the study of pathologic conditions of the maxillary sinus. The routine maxillary bicuspid and molar periapicals, and maxillary occlusal

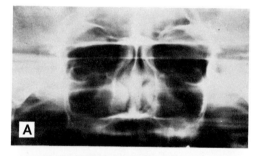

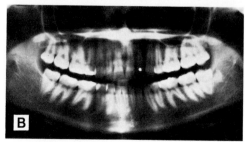

Fig. 16-5. (A) Special panoramic view of the maxillary sinus. (B) The conventional panogram demonstrates a good view of the maxillary sinus.

the special equipment, this radiograph is simple to take, and it depicts both sinuses on the same film. The panoramic view, however, does not always include the sinuses in their entirety, and they often appear distorted.

The paranasal sinuses are probably best reproduced radiologically by Waters' projection. This view can be obtained using the standard dental x-ray equipment and an x-ray plate. The patient's chin is placed on the plate with the nose 1.0 to 1.5 cm. above the plate, and the central ray is directed perpendicular to the film through the vertex of the skull and the symphysis of the mandible. Waters' projection provides a view of the maxillary and ethmoid sinuses unobstructed by the petrous portion of the temporal bone, and permits simultaneous comparison of both sinuses on the same radiograph to aid in the detection of abnormalities[5] (Fig. 16-6).

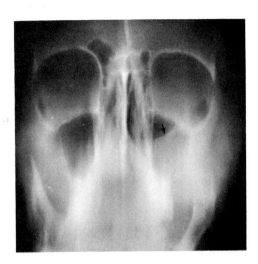

Fig. 16-7. Tomogram showing partial infiltration of left maxillary antrum by neoplastic process.

The tomogram is also a useful diagnostic x-ray technique (Fig. 16-7). The x-ray beam is focused at a predetermined depth in the structure being radiographed, so that all surrounding anatomy appears blurred. The success of this technique depends upon maximal blurring of nonessential structures plus sharpness at the focal plane level.[6] Because this method is well suited to detecting early bone erosion, it can be helpful in diagnosing antral neoplasia.

The normal antrum appears dark radiographically because it is filled with air, and a thin, radiopaque line of cortical bone is usually traceable at the periphery. In cases of sinus infection or neoplasm, the chief radiologic change is a cloudiness of the involved sinus. Cysts and polyps also appear as cloudy, gray entities within the antrum, although they may be more definite in outline.

Never attempt to diagnose a possible sinus pathologic lesion on the basis of a

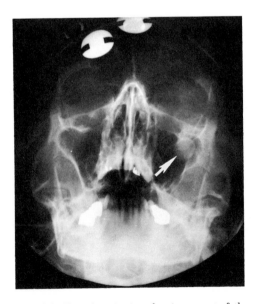

Fig. 16-6. Waters' projection showing a cyst of the left antrum.

radiograph alone. Any radiographic appearances must be correlated with the clinical findings. Taking a proper patient history is essential to the diagnostic procedure. Listening to the patient discuss his symptoms and relate the course of the disease with the aid of appropriate questioning by the practitioner may contribute significantly to the diagnosis. Palpation and percussion are other clinical methods that may be useful in interpreting maxillary sinus disorders. Any drainage from the sinuses should be recognized, and the type of secretions noted (e.g., mucous, serous, purulent, or sanguineous).

The transillumination technique may also prove a valuable diagnostic adjunct for detecting maxillary sinus disorders, especially infection. With the patient seated in a dark room, a special light is placed in the patient's mouth and his lips closed around it. Normally, the light should pass through the sinus and produce a considerable brilliance in the infraorbital and canine fossa areas. There will also be a pupillary reaction to the light. Usually this light is not transmitted in the presence of sinus inflammation. Both sides should be noted simultaneously for comparison.

Infection of the maxillary sinus can certainly result from an infected tooth or teeth (Fig. 16-8). An apical infection may perforate the wall of the antrum. The release of pressure and drainage into the antral cavity may never implicate the tooth, and only occur as a discharge of the sinus through the nose, creating a chronic maxillary sinusitis. Extensive periodontal lesions, which reach the sinus by trifurcation involvement of the maxillary molar teeth, may also produce an antral infection. These lesions frequently go undetected because there are no symptoms referable to the involved teeth.[7]

The maxillary sinus may become inflamed and acutely infected as a result of a cold, trauma, foreign body, or some infectious problem. Pain is the most im-

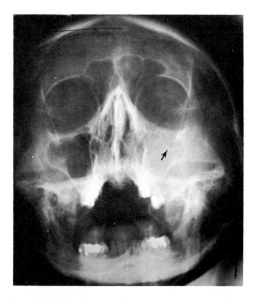

Fig. 16-8. Cloudy maxillary sinus from dental infection. Waters' projection.

mediate subjective symptom and is usually referable to the specific sinus area involved. The area may be sensitive to touch; this is best demonstrated in frontal sinusitis when finger pressure is applied to the frontal bone over the sinus. Headache is more common when the ethmoid sinus is involved.[8] Interference with smell may also be a symptom, and since all sinuses may be involved at one time, many overlapping complaints may be evident.

Pain referring to the teeth may be most confusing. A generalized posterior quadrant toothache may be evident, or if neuritis has resulted from the sinus infection, a specific tooth may respond to the painful stimulus. The tooth or teeth may feel elongated, be painful on chewing, sensitive to percussion, and be hypersensitive. Vitality testing by cold stimulation will probably reveal hypersensitivity, not only of one tooth, but of an entire group of maxillary teeth. Increased pain while walking or bending over both bring additional pressure to bear on the sinus, and may further implicate sinusitis.

Acute sinusitis can be stressful to the patient, and requires careful medical management. The condition is usually best treated with analgesics to relieve pain, antihistamines and decongestants to shrink the mucous membranes to promote drainage, the application of heat, and on occasion, the use of antibiotics. The inability to prove actual dental disease, by either x-ray study or history, should serve to implicate sinus disease unrelated to dental problems; in such cases, the patient should be referred to an otolaryngologist.

Exposure of the maxillary sinus as a result of a tooth extraction or the loss of a root into the sinus cavity may provide a nucleus for severe infection. Basic principles of management must be adhered to if these events occur, although prevention is the better course.

If a small opening into the antrum is noted during the extraction of a clean tooth and the curettement of the socket, immediate steps for a firm closure should be instituted: (1) Place a small amount of Gelfoam, Surgicel, or similar material into the apex near the opening. (2) Remove a small portion of alveolar bone on the lingual and buccal cortical plates to permit more complete flap closure. (3) Create a relaxing incision of the buccal and lingual mucosae and try to get an edge-to-edge mucosal closure over the socket (Fig. 16-9). In some cases, after the Gelfoam has been placed, a criss-cross suture will adequately ensure protection during primary healing.

It is important to realize that the best results are derived from the formation of a normal blood clot (if this can be expected to occur) rather than from surgical intervention. However, when sinus drainage is evident, no matter how small the antral tear, the foregoing measures may prove the best solution. Normal healing is less likely to occur if the perforation is larger than 4 mm. in diameter and when the vertical length of the socket is short. This is probably due to an inability to nourish the clot in the limited alveolar bone segment when the antral surface and the mucosal surface are close together.

In instances of sinus exposure from the

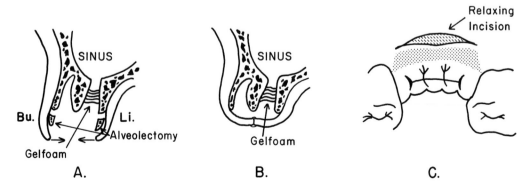

Fig. 16-9. Antral perforation over lingual root.

oral cavity, the patient should receive antibiotic coverage and sometimes antihistamine for nasal decongestion. In addition, instruction on limited chewing, tongue manipulation, blowing of the nose, and sneezing should be given.

If the exposure is large as a result of considerable bone having been removed with the tooth during extraction (Fig. 16-10), a different surgical technique is indicated. The surgical closure to consider first with this type of problem or with a chronic antra-oral fistula is the sliding

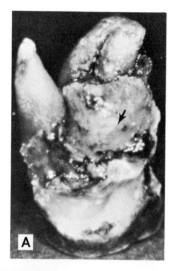

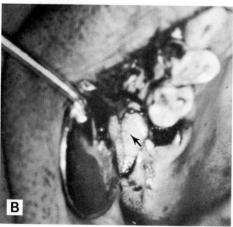

Fig. 16-10. (A) Molar tooth removed with alveolar bone. (B) A portion of antral floor. Note antral membrane.

buccal flap. The sliding flap referred to here is essentially the same as that described by Berger,[9] with the addition of denuding a portion of the palatal mucosa for overlapping and suturing the buccal flap into position (Fig. 16-11). A circular incision is made around the opening of the fistula in preparation for dissection of the epithelialized tract. Necrotic granulation tissue lying within the fistula or the antrum and any protruding polyps of sinus lining are removed. Two divergent cuts through the periosteum are made, extending from the alveolar socket area into the vestibule. The base of the flap will now be broad and, after reflection of the undersurface, the taut periosteal surface is incised, releasing the flap to be extended into the cheek by undermining. The surface epithelium on the palatal surface just beyond the fistula opening is denuded. The freely advanced buccal flap is then positioned over the opening and sutured first on the palatal side (Fig. 16-12). Additional sutures are then placed along the incision line, attempting to gain a watertight seal as nearly as possible. Buccal vestibular height will appear to be shortened at first, but eventually the vestibule regains its normal tissue elasticity. The sutures can be removed in seven to ten days (Fig. 16-13).

Additional methods of closure are the palatal pedicle flap (Fig. 16-14) and the sliding double-suturing envelope technique (Fig. 16-15). A 36-gauge, 24-karat gold plate may be used in antra-oral fistula closure by burnishing the plate to the alveolar bone contour and sliding it beneath the periosteum.[10] Granulation tissue proliferates on the sinus side of the plate, and when complete, usually in 10 to 14 days, the plate is removed.

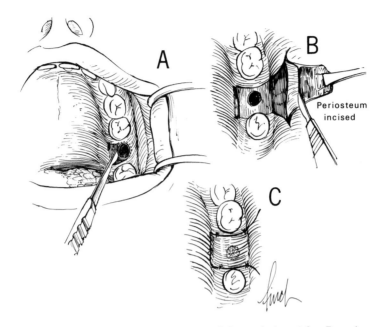

Fig. 16-11. Schematic drawing of buccal flap technique (after Berger).

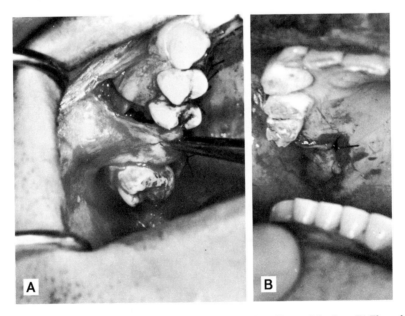

Fig. 16-12. (A) Buccal flap technique. Note relaxation of tissue and broad base of the flap. (B) Flap advanced and sutured to the de-epithelialized surface of palate.

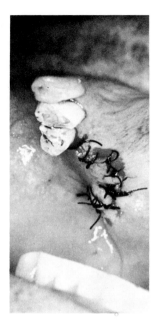

Fig. 16-13. Additional sutures in place.

A fistula must not be closed before an existing sinusitis has been cured. If a long-standing fistula exists, the antrum is usually infected as well, and this must be treated before closure of the antra-oral fistula. Remember that the longer the treatment is deferred in suspected antral perforations, the greater the risk of infection to the maxillary and associated sinuses. The techniques for closure of antra-oral fistulas are numerous, but the principles remain the same:[13]

1. Elimination and control of maxillary sinus disease including all other paranasal sinus disease.

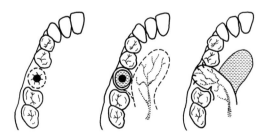

Fig. 16-14. Antral-oral fistula closed by pedicle flap from palate.

2. Adequate intranasal drainage.
3. Complete excision of epithelial lining of the fistula.
4. Elimination of all necrotic tissue.
5. Flaps designed in a manner to ensure adequate nutrition.
6. Sharp, clean incision and intact reflection of periosteal flap.
7. Approximation of raw surface to raw surface.
8. Minimal tension to the flaps.
9. Aseptic procedures during the conduct of the surgery.

Repair under such conditions should occur without undue complication.

If a root tip has been freshly fractured and lost between the antral membrane and the alveolar bone, or pushed into the antrum but still visible, it might be recovered through the socket. Conservative attempts should be made with the curette and suction. On occasion, the gentle threading of gauze into the opening and slowly removing it may entangle the root tip and bring it out. Do not attempt to increase the size of the socket opening if these techniques are unsuccessful.

When these steps are not successful, or when the root, tooth, or other foreign body is known to lie totally within the sinus, a more direct surgical approach is indicated. A window may be cut in the canine fossa or over the apices of the bicuspid teeth. Important anatomic landmarks to be concerned with are the roots of the teeth and their blood supply and innervation (Fig. 16-16).

The incision over the bicuspid teeth is made high enough to permit the reflection of the flap and entry into the antrum through the thin overlying wall. The opening through the bone should be made

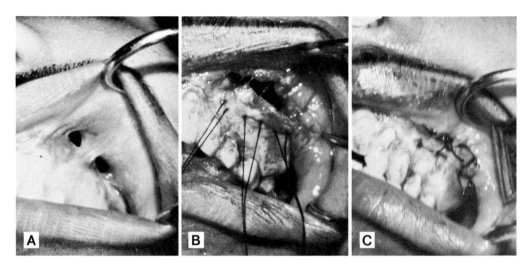

Fig. 16-15. (A) Antra-oral fistula closed by sliding envelope flap. (B) Envelope of tissue created on the alveolar bone surface with mattress suture placed for sliding the superior mucosal flap beneath it. (C) Suture placed. Lower row is composed of mattress sutures and the upper row of interrupted sutures closing the overlying mucosa.

high enough under the flap so that the major portion of the flap covers it upon closure, and that the closure of the incision occurs well beneath the bone cavity and over a solid bone table. The opening may be made with a bone chisel and enlarged by rongeur forceps. The Kerrison punch also works well for this purpose.

Once entry has been gained, a portion of the antral membrane may have to be in-

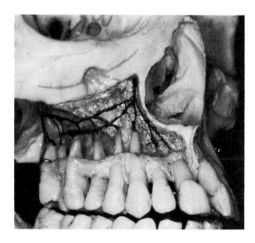

Fig. 16-16. Maxillary dentition in relation to the antrum and innervation.

cised. With good suction, light, and sometimes irrigation, the root or foreign body can be located. The tip may be lying on the bony wall but outside the sinus membrane. The antral curette may be of special help in exploring the antral floor and in scooping up the root. If bleeding is excessive, the placement of a firm, temporary antral pack of iodoform or petrolatum gauze will help to control it. The alveolar socket at the extraction site is then closed in a manner similar to that described previously; the mucosal flap over the antral wall is closed in a routine manner. A nasoantral window is not generally necessary (Fig. 16-17).

In maxillary sinus disease, the first line of treatment is conservative. Appropriate antibiotics are administered as determined by culture and sensitivity tests. In chronic maxillary sinus infection, drainage may have to be established, which is provided through the inferior meatus (Fig. 16-18). Nasoantral irrigation with warm saline solution may also be initiated. If this procedure fails to resolve the infection, or if polypoid tissue or septic disease is a complication, a Caldwell-Luc opera-

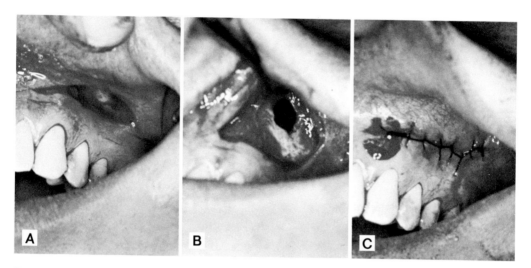

Fig. 16-17. (A) Antral opening for third molar root recovery over bicuspid apices. (B) Flap reflected; bony entry made. (C) Flap returned and sutured.

tion may be considered. This gives the otolaryngologist much greater access and improved anterior-posterior observation of the sinus for detailed antral surgery (Fig. 16-19).

A discussion of maxillary sinus pathology would not be complete without mention of the occurrence of related malignant tumors. The tumors that most frequently occur are sarcomas, usually in young patients, and carcinomas, usually in patients over 40. Early detection and treatment are essential, but unfortunately the symptoms may not be sufficient to motivate the patient to seek care until the disease has hopelessly progressed. According to Zange, the initial symptoms of carcinoma of the oral cavity or the nasopharynx may include increased difficulties in mastication, swallowing, and nose breathing, otitis media causing deafness and closure of the eustachian tube, cervical adenopathy, and unilateral trigeminal neuralgia.[11]

Radiographic examination may indicate a cloudy sinus, thickened mucosae, polyp formation, and/or an increased density of the sinus as a result of the growth of malignant tissue within the cavity (Fig. 16-20). Discontinuity and erosion of the bony antral wall may appear radiographically as the process advances. According to Stafne, any destruction of the antral wall revealed radiologically should be suspected as being caused by a neoplasm.[7] Naturally, a biopsy and tissue examination by a pathologist are necessary to arrive at a conclusive diagnosis.

A study by Badib and associates revealed that 88 per cent of 344 cases of paranasal sinus cancer originated in the maxillary sinus, 80 per cent occurred in persons over 50 years of age, and the five-year cure rate was only 14 per cent.[12] This illustrates the severe nature of the disease and should impress upon the practitioner the need for early detection.

Antral malignancies are usually treated

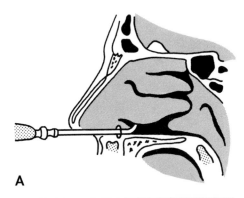

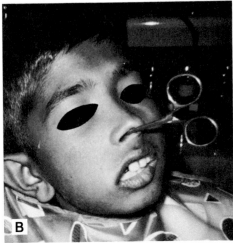

Fig. 16-18. (A) Nasal antrostomy (after Ballenger). (B) Hemostat showing nasal–antral communication after antrostomy.

by a combination of irradiation followed by radical surgery. Preoperative x-ray therapy may decrease the size of the tumor and minimize regional lymphatic spread, thereby providing a more favorable surgical prognosis.

In conclusion, the general practitioner need not be hesitant or fearful of maxillary sinus disorders if he is cognizant of their symptoms and manifestations and familiar with the treatment procedures.

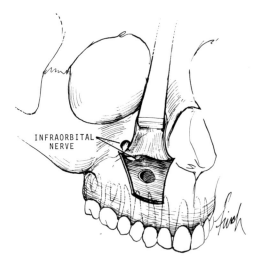

Fig. 16-19. Caldwell-Luc approach for access to maxillary sinus.

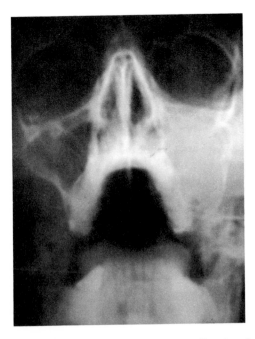

Fig. 16-20. Waters' projection showing infiltration of the left antrum by neoplastic disease.

Complications can be avoided by careful history-taking, a detailed examination that includes diagnostic intraoral and extraoral radiographs, and well-planned and controlled surgical techniques. Consultation with the appropriate medical specialty, including definitive treatment, may also be indicated. Nevertheless, there are instances when, even though all precautions have been taken, sinus complications related to dental disease may arise. In these cases, the practitioner who has taken the time to familiarize himself with all aspects of such problems, including the diagnosis, treatment, and postoperative management, will react calmly and be able to provide a vital health service for his patient.

References

1. Thoma, K. H.: Oral Surgery, 3rd ed. St. Louis, C. V. Mosby, 1958.
2. Ballenger, J. J.: Diseases of the Nose, Throat and Ear, 12th ed. Philadelphia, Lea & Febiger, 1977.
3. Reading, P.: Common Diseases of the Ear, Nose, and Throat, 4th ed. Boston, Little, Brown & Co., 1966.
4. Killey, H. C., and Kay, L. W.: An analysis of 250 cases of oro-antral fistula treated by the buccal flap operation. Oral Surg., 24:726–39, 1967.
5. Merrell, R. A., Jr., et al.: Radiographic anatomy of the paranasal sinuses. Arch. Otolaryngol., 87:184–195, 1968.
6. Pendergrass, E. P., et al.: The Head and Neck in Roentgen Diagnosis, Vol. 1, 2nd ed. Springfield, Ill., Charles C Thomas, 1956.
7. Stafne, E. C.: Oral Roentgenographic Diagnosis. Philadelphia, W. B. Saunders Co., 1958.
8. Wolff, H. G.: Headache and Other Head Pain. New York, Oxford University Press, 1963.
9. Berger, A.: Oroantral openings and their surgical correction. Arch. Otolaryngol., 30:400–10, 1939.
10. Fredrics, H. J., et al.: Closure of oroantral fistula with gold plate: Report of case. J. Oral Surg., 23:650–654, 1965.
11. Zange, J.: Malignant tumors of the oral cavity and the nasopharynx, Münch. Med. Wochenschr., 99:1936–1938, 1957. (From Dental Abstracts, 4:34–35, 1959.)
12. Badib, A. O., et al.: Treatment of cancer of the paranasal sinuses. Cancer, 23:533–37, 1969.
13. Waite, D. E.: Maxillary sinus. Dent. Clin. North Am., 15:349–368, 1971.

17 Hemorrhage and Shock

RICHARD G. OGLE

The shedding of blood is of concern to every surgical patient, and it is necessary for the operating dentist to convey his ability to cope with hemorrhage. This includes preoperative prevention, intraoperative technical control, and postoperative hemostasis.

Frequently, patients report that they bleed excessively from tooth extractions. A brief investigation usually reveals that this is either a misinterpretation by the patient or was caused by inadequate technical hemostatic procedures.

One must never become oblivious to the fact, however, that abnormal coagulation mechanisms occasionally are present in patients requiring oral surgical procedures.

Coagulation Mechanism

A careful medical history is the single most important method of ruling out hemorrhagic problems. Few persons with a hemorrhagic diathesis will survive many years without having first-hand knowledge of abnormal bleeding. Pertinent questions to a patient who is suspected of having a positive bleeding history include bleeding following other surgical procedures such as tonsillectomy or bleeding of unusual nature following minor trauma.

Any patient who has experienced spontaneous bleeding into a joint space or body cavity should be considered a "bleeder" until proved otherwise. In the event of a positive history, laboratory studies for screening purposes should be done, including a prothrombin time (PT), a partial thromboplastin time (PTT), and a peripheral blood smear for the platelet number adequacy. If either the history or the laboratory screening profile is abnormal, the patient should be referred to a hematologist for definitive diagnosis.

Normal coagulation is dependent upon vessel integrity, normally functioning platelets in adequate numbers, and an intact coagulation mechanism. A defect in any segment of the system can be reflected in clinically abnormal bleeding. The successive phases in normal coagulation are shown schematically in Figure 17-1,[2] and the plasma factors related to coagulation in Figure 17-2.

Disease States

Hemophilia is an inherited coagulopathy and is one of the most common and complicated congenital bleeding disorders with which the dentist will become involved.

The disorder is transmitted as an x-linked recessive mendelian trait passed

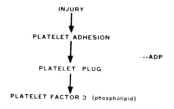

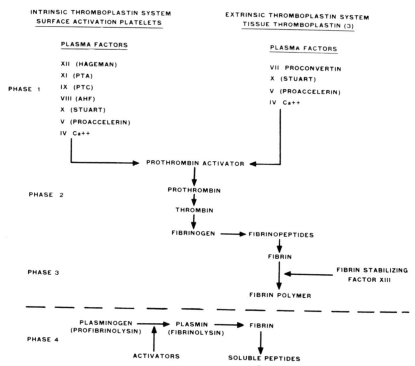

Fig. 17-1. Blood coagulation mechanism. (Gustafson, S. R., and Coursin, D. B.: *The Pediatric Patient 1966.* Philadelphia, J. B. Lippincott, 1966)

from mother to sons and, for all intents and purposes, is seen as a clinical bleeding disorder, therefore only in males.[1] In the past it was not unusual for individuals with hemophilia to be denied dental care because of fear of bleeding, and as such, many times dental extractions became necessary due to carious destruction of teeth.

The disorder is due to malfunction of the intrinsic portion of phase one of coagulation subsequent to lack of or an abnormal function of factor VIII. Because of functional integrity of the patient's vessels and platelets, his bleeding time is normal. Coagulation time, as monitored by the partial thromboplastin time, however, is abnormally prolonged.

Treatment involves replacement of factor VIII pre-, intra-, and postoperatively, usually with cryoprecipitated factor VIII, and importantly, the stabilization of clot integrity with orally administered epsilon amino caproic acid (EACA).[4]

There are many other diseases in which bleeding is a primary problem. Factor IX deficiency (hemophilia B, Christmas disease) is clinically indistinguishable from hemophilia with a similar pattern of inheritance. The treatment is replacement therapy with factor IX following laboratory profile by a hematologist.

Coagulation Factors

FACTOR	COMMON SYMPTOMS	ROLE IN COAGULATION
I	Fibrinogen	Precursor of fibrin
II*	Prothrombin	Proenzyme, activated by thromboplastin
III	Tissue prothromboplastin	Formed when enzymes released by damaged tissues enter the blood and activate factors X, VII and V in the presence of Ca^{++}
IV	Calcium	Necessary for all stages
V†	Proaccelerin (Labile factor: AC globulin)	Required for formation of both thromboplastins. Disappears on heating or storing of oxalated plasma; consumed in coagulation
VI	No longer considered a specifically different factor	Thought to be a product of the activation of factor V
VII*	Stable factor (Proconvertin)	Necessary for conversion of prothrombin to thrombin. An alpha globulin; is stable on storage and is not consumed in coagulation
VIII	Antihemophilic factor or globulin (AHF, AHG)	Necessary for thromboplastin formation—surface activation of platelets; deficient in classical hemophilia A
IX	Plasma thromboplastin component (PTC)	Necessary for thromboplastin formation; absent in Christmas disease (hemophilia B). Found in alpha globulin fraction
X	Stuart-Prower factor	Required for thromboplastin formation and conversion of prothrombin to thrombin. Present in prealbumin fraction; stable on storage and not consumed in coagulation
XI	Plasma thromboplastin antecedent (PTA)	Necessary for thromboplastin formation
XII	Hageman (Activation or Contact factor)	Initiates intrinsic thromboplastin system
XIII	Fibrin stabilizing factor	Fibrin $\rightarrow$ Fibrin polymer

* If congenitally deficient is not affected by Vitamin K administration.
† Vitamin K not necessary for its production.

Fig. 17-2. Coagulation factors. (Gustafson, S. R., and Coursin, D. B.: *The Pediatric Patient 1966*. Philadelphia, J. B. Lippincott, 1966)

Von Willebrand's disease, an auto-somal dominant hemostatic disorder, is therefore seen in females as well as in males, and is characterized by a deficiency in factor VIII function and platelet dys-functions, resulting in prolonged bleeding times and extended PTT values.

In addition, there are a variety of quan-titative and qualitative platelet disorders which result in clinical bleeding states. These conditions all come under the broad classification of thrombopathy and are characterized by purpura and petechia and abnormal bleeding times.

Many patients seen for dental surgery will have, by contrast to the previous dis-cussion, acquired disorders of hemostasis.

In leukemia, the initial symptom is manifested by enlarged, congested, and bleeding gingivae (Fig. 17-3). Surgical in-tervention by removal of teeth or gingi-vectomy results in serious prolonged bleeding. Agranulocytosis is a frequently fatal disease in which there is a severe reduction in the number of neutrophils in the circulating blood. Ulcers develop on the mucous membranes of the throat and mouth, and general resistance to infection is reduced.

Vitamin K deficiency can be caused by malabsorption of lipids and is treated with a preparation of vitamin K by oral admin-istration or parenteral injection. There-fore, bleeding due to lack of vitamin K can be expected in biliary obstruction, dis-eases of the gastrointestinal tract, and pa-tients receiving anticoagulant therapy for prevention of intravascular thrombi. It is not always necessary to withhold antico-agulants prior to tooth extraction, al-though there is some risk in returning the prothrombin time to a normal level once it has been prolonged. This is an area in which close cooperation of the dentist and the physician is necessary.

Because of the increased number of pa-tients receiving anticoagulant therapy, potential dental management of such pa-

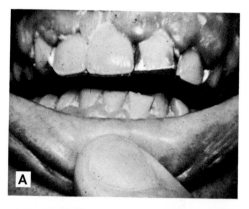

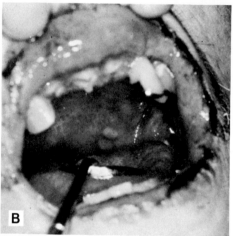

Fig. 17-3. (A) Acute leukemia. (Courtesy of Dr. Paul Morgan) (B) Chronic leukemia; note ulceration of lips and soft palate.

tients by the dentist is likely. In many instances, patients receiving these medi-cations will not have to be removed from them for minimal surgical procedures. The decision is based upon a comparison of the patient's prothrombin level with normal levels, and the extent of surgery to be done. Within the range of one and a half times the normal prothrombin level, certain limited surgery can be performed.

Should it become necessary to control the increased bleeding due to anticoagulants, vitamin K may be used to reverse the hypoprothrombinemia.

Treatment

Postoperative hemorrhage has been classified as primary, intermediate, or secondary, which indicates the time in which the bleeding occurs. Continued bleeding during and immediately following the surgery is referred to as primary hemorrhage. Bleeding that occurs soon after the surgery when there initially had been evidence of having the hemorrhage under control is intermediate hemorrhage. This usually indicates an inability to control the bleeding mechanically for a sufficient length of time following surgery. Secondary hemorrhage is of a greater concern and occurs after the initial clot has been organized, from 24 hours to 10 days postsurgery. Management of all three types of hemorrhage is essentially the same. The initial effort should be directed at controlling emotional and psychic factors. Persons who are bleeding become apprehensive and need to be reassured and made comfortable in a semisupine position. The use of sedatives may be indicated, as well as a local anesthetic with a vasoconstrictor. A moistened pressure pack is placed over the bleeding site. This initial procedure will usually control the problem and permit careful evaluation. Good suction is also helpful.

Arterial bleeding produces a spurting of bright red blood, whereas venous bleeding is characterized by a slow but continuous oozing of blood of a darker quality. If the bleeder is a spurting vessel from soft tissue, it may be clamped with a hemostat, or it may be necessary to insert a stitch tie or a figure-8 suture. If blood wells up from within the socket, a pressure gauze strip may be packed in the socket. Gelfoam or Oxycel placed into the socket will often control hemorrhage. Bovine thrombin may be used by direct application or by soaking a small portion of Gelfoam sponge in the thrombin solution. Burnishing a bone bleeder with a smooth instrument or applying bone wax may be helpful in con-

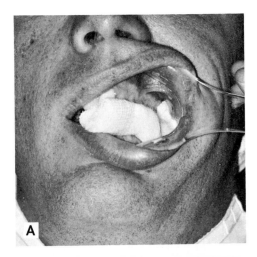

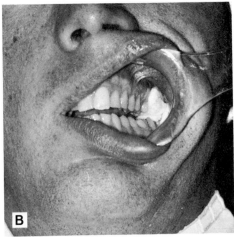

Fig. 17-4. (A) Improper placement of pressure gauze following third molar removal; gauze too far forward. (B) Proper placement of pressure gauze.

trolling this type of bleeding. Firm approximation of the tissues with additional sutures and placement of an adequate postoperative pressure pack should be sufficient to control most hemorrhages (Fig. 17-4). If bleeding persists after these measures have been instituted, a bleeding disorder should be considered and screening tests ordered. An emergency tray setup with the necessary instruments and medications should always be readily available to control hemorrhage; this would include (1) good suction; (2) adequate light; (3) local anesthetic; and (4) the appropriate instruments, such as hemostats, scissors, and pick-up forceps. The appropriate medications include 1:1000 epinephrine, Oxycel, Gelfoam, gauze strips and sponges, bovine thrombin, sedatives, and analgesic drugs. An electrocoagulation unit may also be helpful.

In all bleeding problems, careful evaluation of the patient is essential, as is an attitude of confidence on the part of the dentist.

Shock and Syncope

In the office or the hospital, or during a natural disaster or any traumatic situation, the dentist may be called upon to take charge of an emergency because of his knowledge of shock and other medical problems. For the purposes of this discussion, shock will be considered as a state of systemic circulation in which cardiac output is too low to supply the normal nutritional needs of the body's tissues, even when the subject is at rest. In fact, the one feature that appears to be common to all cases of shock is inadequate tissue perfusion. The clinical manifestations of shock vary widely, but may include:

1. Hypotension
2. Increased rate of breathing
3. Limited consciousness
4. Cyanosis of lips and nail beds

5. Cold sweat
6. Thirst
7. Restlessness and inability to communicate
8. Weak and rapid pulse

The etiologic factors of shock cause a decrease in arterial pressure and systemic blood flow, thereby diminishing the nutrition of the tissues. The result is a decreased venous return to the heart and then a decreased cardiac output. This cycle becomes progressively worse unless measures are instituted to reverse the process of deterioration. Therefore, the treatment of shock should be aimed at correcting the cause and helping the physiologic compensatory mechanisms to restore an adequate level of tissue perfusion.

The diagnosis of shock involves having and being able to use a sphygmomanometer and stethoscope. In addition, the use of oxygen and the equipment to deliver it under pressure are essential. The dentist should also have a working knowledge of the technique for cardiac and respiratory resuscitation. In general, the following procedures should be implemented upon recognizing the symptoms of shock:

1. Remove, prevent, or control causative factors
2. Record and continuously monitor blood pressure and pulse rate
3. Place the patient in the supine position (Fig. 17-5)
4. Maintain an adequate airway
5. Provide adequate oxygenation (Fig. 17-6)
6. Keep the patient comfortably warm at room temperature or slightly above

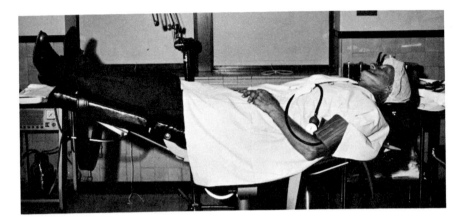

Fig. 17-5. Patient in supine position.

7. Support the circulation by administering fluids and/or vasopressor agents
8. Administer analgesic agents when pain or psychologic stress is a precipitating factor, but use them with caution

If these measures have been applied and the state of shock has not been resolved or the patient does not respond in a satisfactory manner, additional consultation is indicated.

Syncope, or fainting, is the manifestation of neurogenic shock most frequently encountered by the dentist. Many of the etiologic factors of neurogenic shock can be resolved by establishing rapport with the patient to allay fear and apprehension and to instill confidence. The use of premedication in the form of sedatives to reduce nervousness, analgesics and narcotics to elevate the pain threshold, and ataractics to relieve anxiety and fear will aid in alleviating the etiologic factors in neurogenic shock.

From the preceding discussion it should be obvious that the dental practitioner must know the physical and mental status of his patients. To accomplish this, the dentist should perform the following steps prior to instituting any dental procedures:

1. Observe and inspect the patient in regard to physical or behavioral deviations
2. Take and record an adequate medical history
3. Ascertain and record the blood pressure and pulse rate

This background information will not only equip the dentist with a tool to prevent episodes of shock in his office, but it will also prepare him to recognize changes in the patient's physiology that might require emergency measures.

Finally, the word shock itself connotes an event that is spontaneous and instantaneous. Therefore, it is the wise dentist who prepares for this emergency ahead of time by equipping his operatory with a special tray containing the necessary drugs and equipment needed to adequately discharge his responsibility in the care of his patient during such an emergency. In addition, a prepared staff is in-

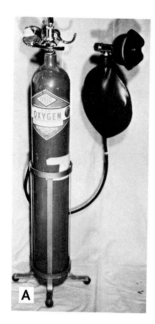

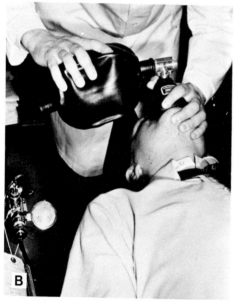

Fig. 17-6. (A) Oxygen for resuscitation; note reducing valve, bag, and mask. (B) AMBU bag used for resuscitation; it can also be connected to oxygen supply, if available.

dispensable for life-threatening emergencies such as shock. Each person should be assigned a given responsibility; these include obtaining the emergency kit, administering oxygen, monitoring the pulse and blood pressure, as well as calling an ambulance and/or physician when necessary. All responsibilities are performed without alarm or undue haste, but most important, each person must know how the assignment is to be performed and why, as well as the physical signs indicating improvement or worsening of the patient's condition.

An office staff coordinated for emergencies will have reviewed and discussed pertinent literature, recorded emergency telephone listings, made emergency equipment available, and have a working knowledge of this information. Periodically this knowledge should be put to a rehearsal. Always ensure the preparedness of your staff; the emergency might be you!

References

1. Krivitt, W., and White, J. G.: A simplified approach for the detection of coagulation disorders. Lancet, 1:381–384, 1965.
2. Gustafson, S. R., and Coursin, D. B.: The Pediatric Patient. Philadelphia, J. B. Lippincott, 1966.
3. Pool, J. G., and Shannon, A. E.: Production of high-potency concentrates of antihemolytic globulin in a closed-bag system. N. Engl. J. Med., 273:1443–1447, 1965.
4. Short, S., and Ogle, R. G.: The use of E.A.C.A. in the treatment of hemophiliacs. Minn. Med. 57:77–80, 1974.

18 Hospital Dental Practice and Operating Room Protocol

DANIEL E. WAITE

Hospital Dental Practice

The hospital is a health care institution for the community. Therefore, everyone who works in the hospital contributes to the community through patients with whom he comes into contact. The dentist, like other health care professionals, has an important role in the hospital in providing dental care for hospitalized patients. The dentist who wants to have hospital privileges should apply through the office of the hospital administrator and should review the constitution and bylaws of the hospital to which he wishes to make application. There are several categories of staff membership: active staff, associate staff, courtesy staff, honorary staff, and consultant staff.

The traditional role of the oral surgeon in the hospital is quite well established. However, involvement of the general dentist, pedodontist, prosthodontist, endodontist, and periodontist is increasing. The dentist who works in a hospital must work closely with the physician for good patient care, and he should become familiar with hospital protocol and environment.

All hospitals have operating rooms and emergency rooms where at least minimal dental care may be rendered. If a dental clinic is also available within the hospital, the dentist will be able to provide even better care for dental patients. In some clinics, general anesthesia for outpatients is available to facilitate service for a variety of minor dental problems. Special training and additional experience, however, are necessary before these procedures can be undertaken.

In the hospital, dentists may be called upon to function as diagnosticians, consultants, and restorative dentists, and to perform dental surgery.

Since tooth extraction is the oral surgical procedure which most frequently requires the dentist to operate in the hospital, the steps that must be followed in rendering this service will be described in detail. It may be necessary or desirable to extract teeth in the hospital for:

1. Patients who are already in the hospital.
2. Patients who desire to enter the hospital for their surgery.
3. Patients requiring general anesthesia.

254

4. Patients with systemic diseases that make them unacceptable for office care.

The dentist must have admitting privileges in the hospital where he plans to render his service. The admission must include a physical examination performed by a physician who is also on the staff of the hospital. The date and hour of the admission must be prearranged and the operation scheduled with the appropriate operating room personnel. The patient should be advised of the approximate cost of hospitalization, and often a "financial interview" is advisable with the admission department prior to admission.

The operating room has many facilities, and auxiliary assistance is provided. A complete aseptic routine is necessary. Since variations in routines exist in different hospitals, one should inquire about the policy of the specific hospital regarding such procedures as scrubbing technique and patient draping.

The dentist must determine the special equipment and instruments needed to provide dental care and bring them with him or have the hospital sufficiently aware of these needs that it will provide them. Dental radiographs must also be available at the time of surgery.

The operating room nurses may not be familiar with dental instruments and dental procedures. It is helpful to have lists, outlines, or photographs on file with the supervisor outlining the procedures and listing the instruments and equipment required. This will help to make the case go smoothly, and at the same time will be educational for the nurses and auxiliary personnel.

Hospital Instrument List for Multiple Extractions

Nos. 872 and 874 McKesson mouth props tied together with 6″ cord
Suction aspirator, two tips
Cleaning wire for suction tip
1 ⅝″, 25-gauge needle and syringe for local anesthesia
3″ × 3″ gauze squares
2″ roll bandage for pharyngeal pack
Sterile saline solution
½ pt. or 1 pt. S.S. cup, for irrigation solution
Two irrigating syringes
Headlight
No. 1 Woodson periosteal elevator
No. 9 periosteal elevator
Double-ended curette
Dental mouth mirror
University of Minnesota retractor
Bard Parker scalpel handle and no. 15 blade
Two single bevel chisels, Gardner (Hu-Friedy no. 2), for bone cutting
One bi-bevel chisel for splitting teeth
Mallet
Gilmore probe
6 ½″ nasal dressing forceps, bayonet
Side-cutting bone forceps (Clev-Dent no. 5)
Round-nose rongeur forceps (Clev-Dent no. 4A)
Double-ended bone file (rasp)
Two straight mosquito hemostats
Two straight Kelly hemostats
Two curved Rankin hemostats
Two Carmault forceps for prepping
Two towel clips
6″ Hegar-Mayo needle holder
Needles: cutting edge, Anchor Brand 1822-18 (large) and 1822-20 (small)

Deknatel type B (000) suture material
Dental engine and straight handpiece
Four no. 560 burs for straight handpiece
Suture and tissue scissors

Preoperative Period

MEDICAL RECORD. The medical record is important for medical-legal purposes, as well as for good patient care. Many abbreviations are used to conserve time in writing the history, orders, or other reports (Table 18-1). There has been increased use of the problem oriented medical record (P.O.M.R.) system. The problem oriented medical record system has four elements: data base, problem list, initial plan, and progress note (Fig. 18-1).

The data base as a part of admission note includes the patient profile, medical history, and physical examination (Fig. 18-2). The problem list sheet should be placed on the first page of the record as an index, and the problem(s) drawn from the data base and numbered and listed on the problem list (Fig. 18-3). The initial plan should be listed by number for each problem on the problem list. The progress notes consist of the narrative note, flow sheet, and discharge summary. The narrative note is written utilizing the abbreviation "SOAP"—, subjective (S), objective (O), assessment (A), and plan (P), for accurate recording of information.

ADMISSION ORDERS. The dentist must have admitting privileges in the hospital. The dental patient may be admitted in either of two ways: he may be admitted to a dental service or to the service of the family physician with the dentist treating the patient in consultation.

The newly admitted patient will receive no food, medication, or any care without specific orders. Hospital orders are written on the order sheet and are to be signed by the doctor. In case of telephone orders, all orders must be signed within 24 hours. Admission orders include such items as diet, the admission chest radiograph, and other routine laboratory procedures (Fig. 18-4).

PREOPERATIVE ORDERS AND PREOPERATIVE NOTES. The preoperative orders are distinct from the admission orders (Fig. 18-5). Preoperative orders refer to the specific management of the patient for the operation and include the appropriate medications. Admission orders are more general in nature than preoperative orders and are meant to provide care of the patient until the time of his pending operation when the preoperative orders are written. The consent form must be signed by the patient and confirmation of it made by the doctor (Fig. 18-6). The night before surgery, a preoperative note should be written (Fig. 18-7).

Day of Operation

The operator must be on time. A patient cannot be placed under general anesthesia until the doctor is present and ready to proceed with the patient's care. Every effort should be made during the operation to use the same techniques that are commonly employed in the office. Some modifications are inevitable due to the supine position of the patient, the anesthesia, and the general environment. Improvisations cause delay and should be planned beforehand.

Immediately after the operation, the dentist must accompany the patient to the recovery room. He then writes the postoperative orders and a brief operative note (Fig. 18-8). The formal operative report should be dictated for typing (Fig. 18-9).

Table 18-1. Abbreviations Commonly Used on Orders and Reports

ABBREVIATION	DEFINITION	ABBREVIATION	DEFINITION
a.c.	before meals	LMD	local medical doctor
ad lib.	at pleasure	Lt.	left
AHG	antihemophilic globulin	M	male
alvcty	alveolectomy	M	murmur
AMB	ambulatory	Mal.	malposed
Ant.	anterior	mg.	milligram
A.P.	anteroposterior	neg.	negative
apico	apicoectomy	#	number
ASHD	arteriosclerotic heart disease	OB or OBS	obstetric department
b.i.d.	twice daily	OPD	outpatient department
B.M.	bowel movement	O.R.	operating room
B.M.R.	basal metabolic rate	O.S.	oral surgery
b.p.	blood pressure	P.A.	posteroanterior
B.S.S.	black silk sutures	para	number of births, (para I, para II, etc.)
c̄	with	Path	pathology
C.C.	chief complaint	p.c.	after meals
CBC	complete blood count	Pdcl	periodontoclasia
C.H.D.	congenital heart disease	P.H.	past history
C.I.	color index	P.M.H.	previous (past) medical history
C.N.S.	central nervous system	P.O.	per os (by mouth)
C.O.D.	cause of death	post., posteri.	posterior
CV	cardiovascular	POT	postoperative treatment
CVA	cardiovascular accident	P.R.	pulse rate
CVD	cardiovascular disease	p.r.n.	as occasion requires
Drs.	dressing	Pt.	patient
ECG, EKG	electrocardiogram	q3h	every 3 hours
E.N.T.	ear, nose, and throat department	q.i.d.	4 times a day
E.S.R.	erythrocyte sedimentation rate	q.s.	quantity sufficient
F.H.	family history	q.n.s.	quantity not sufficient
FME	full-mouth extractions	RBC	red blood cell
FMS	full-mouth series of radiographs	r/c	root canal
Fx	fracture	R.H.D.	rheumatic heart disease
G.A.	general anesthesia	Rt.	right
G.I.	gastrointestinal	s̄	without
gr.	grains	S.O.B.	shortness of breath
gravida	pregnancies	Sub Q, S.C.	subcutaneous
G/S	glucose and saline	TBC (or TB)	tuberculosis
G.U.	genitourinary	TE	tooth extraction
G/W	glucose and water	Temp.	temperature
Hb	hemoglobin	t.i.d.	3 times a day
HCT	hematocrit	T & A	tonsillectomy and adenoidectomy
H.P.I.	history of present illness	UCHD	usual childhood disease
hs	at bedtime	WBC	white blood cell
I & D	incision and drainage	W/D	well-developed
I.M.	intramuscular	W/F (W+)	white female
Imp	impaction, impressions	W/M (or W)	white male
I.V.	intravenous	N/F	black female
LDDS	local dentist	N/M	black male

Before leaving the hospital or starting another case, the dentist should advise the relatives that the operation is completed and when they can expect the patient to return to his room. The doctor must see the patient the same evening and twice daily thereafter throughout the patient's hospital stay.

Postoperative Period

After the surgery, the patient may experience some postoperative effects, such as nausea, edema, or pain. During this post-

(*Text continues on page 276.*)

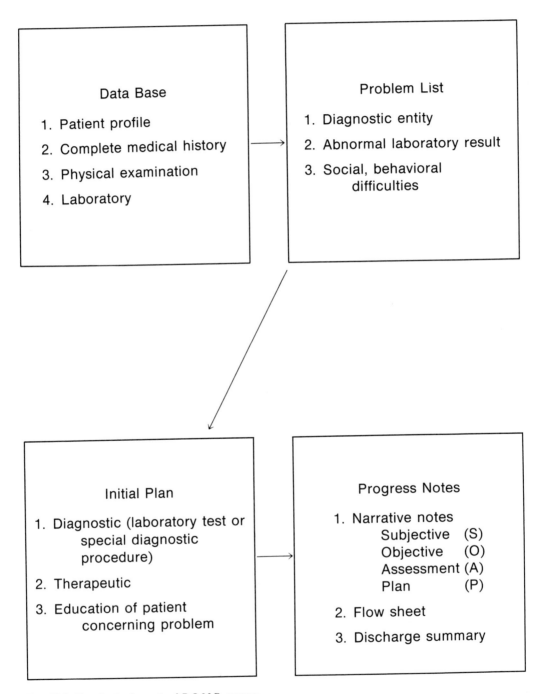

Fig. 18-1. Four basic elements of P.O.M.R. system.

ᘮᓐ PROGRESS NOTES UNIVERSITY OF HOSPITALS S—Subjective O—Objective A—Assessment P—Plan	Name: I. N. Need	
	Age: Hospital Number:	
	Date:	

DATE	Problem Number	
8-24-76		Dental Service Admission Note
		This is the first University of Minnesota hospital admission for this
		41 year old white male, admitted to the dental service for
		removal of all remaining teeth.
		cc = soreness in the mouth
		HPI = patient has been suffering from generalized periodontal
		disease and multiple dental caries since 1965. The
		patient complains of soreness of his mouth, generally
		all of his upper and lower teeth and constant draining
		of septic material from his gingiva and causing discomfort.
		P.M.H.
		Illness
		UCHD without sequelae
		denies rheumatic fever, diabetes mellitus, heart disease,
		hypertension, hepatitis, blood dyscrasia.
		Hospitalization and surgery
		1) T & A; age 6
		2) appendectomy; age 13
		3) Psychiatric Tx (depression); 1965
		allergies - none
		meds - none
		ROS
		HEENT
		Head: denies trauma, headache
		Eyes: wears glasses, denies diplopia
		Ears: denies hearing loss, otalgia, tinnitus
		Nose: denies chronic sinusitis, epistaxis

MR Form 28, JUL 74

Fig. 18-2. Example of physical examination form.

DATE	Problem Number	S—Subjective O—Objective A—Assessment P—Plan
		Mouth: see oral examination
		Throat: denies tonsilitis, dysphagia
		C.V. (cardiovascular):
		denies heart murmur, rheumatic fever, SOB,
		hypertension
		Pulmonary:
		denies pneumonia, bronchitis, asthma, cough
		G.I. (GASTROINTESTINAL)
		appetite = good. B.M. (Bowel Movement)
		Regular in Occurrence
		denies diarrhea, constipation, nausea
		G.U. (Genitourinary)
		denies kidney disease, polyuria, V.D.
		Neuromuscular
		denies decreased coordination, seizures,
		limitation of motion, change of sensation.
		Skin:
		denies skin disease, rashes
		Psychiatric:
		Hx. of psychiatric treatment 1965 (depression)
		Family History:
		Parents: father age 62 hypertension
		mother age 58 A & W
		Sibs: brother age 38 A & W
		sister age 35 A & W
		Social History:
		Marital status
		married 21 years
		children: 2
		Occupation: salesman

Fig. 18-2. (*Continued*)

UM UNIVERSITY OF HOSPITALS **PROGRESS NOTES** S—Subjective O—Objective A—Assessment P—Plan	Name: I. N. Need	
	Age:	Hospital Number:
	Date:	

DATE	Problem Number	
		Habits: alcohol: socially
		smoke: 1 pkg. per day/20 years
		Oral Examination:
		a) Extraoral exam
		face - symmetry, normal T.M. joint function, no
		adenopathy, no swelling of face or neck.
		b) Intraoral exam
		Poor oral hygiene with multiple dental caries &
		generalized gingivitis, non-restorable teeth with
		dental caries and chronic periodontal disease
		which will be extracted are teeth #'s: 2,3,7,8,9,
		10,11,12,13,14,15,18,20,21,22,23,24,25,26,27,28,29.
		Impression:
		1) 41 year old healthy male by history
		2) dental caries and periodontal disease
		Plan:
		1) physical exam by LMD
		2) Routine admission workup
		3) Removal of all remaining teeth under general
		anesthesia in O.R. in A.M.
		S.M. Skill

MR Form 28, JUL 74

Fig. 18-2. (*Continued*)

DATE	Problem Number	S—Subjective O—Objective A—Assessment P—Plan

Fig. 18-2. (*Continued*)

LM UNIVERSITY HOSPITALS **PROGRESS NOTES** S—Subjective O—Objective A—Assessment P—Plan	Name: I. N. Need	
	Age:	Hospital Number:
	Date:	

DATE	Problem Number	
8-24-76		Physical Examination

Vital signs

    P. 80, BP. 120/80 (R) arm sitting

    R. 16, Temp. 98, 6°F.

General

    This is a 41 year old healthy, pleasant, cooperative

    white male with poor oral hygiene.

HEENT

    Head - normocephalic

    Eyes: PERRLA, fundi benign, EOM's intact

    Ears: T.M. intact, External auditory canals clear

    Nose: Mucosa WNL, septum in middle

    Mouth: Multiple dental caries, moderate hyperplastic

           gingiva

    Throat: Normal

    Neck: Supple, no lymphadenopathy, Thyroid WNL.

    Chest: Chest - clear to A & P

           Heart - NSR without murmur

    Abdomen: Soft, flat without tenderness or organomegaly

    Extremities: Full range of motion

              strong, equal peripheral pulses bilaterally

    Neurological: Cranial Nerve II-XII intact

           motor & sensory intact.

    Impression:

        1) 41 year old healthy white male

        2) dental caries and periodontal disease

                  J.S. Skill

MR Form 28, JUL 74

Fig. 18-2. (*Continued*)

DATE	Problem Number	S—Subjective O—Objective A—Assessment P—Plan

Fig. 18-2. *(Continued)*

Problem Number	PROBLEM	DATE OF ONSET	DATE PROBLEM RECORDED	DATE PROBLEM INACTIVATED
1	Depression	1965	1976	
2	Dental caries, periodontal disease	1966	1976	

UNIVERSITY HOSPITALS
PROBLEM LIST
I. D. PLATE

I. Need

UH FORM 1005, MAR 74

Fig. 18-3. Example of problem list sheet.

Problem Number	PROBLEM	DATE OF ONSET	DATE PROBLEM RECORDED	DATE PROBLEM INACTIVATED

Fig. 18-3. (Continued)

University **Hospitals**	Name:	I. N. Need
DOCTOR'S ORDER SHEET	Age:	Hospital Number:
	Date:	

FORM 56

NCR PAPER. PRESS FIRMLY—USE BALL POINT PEN ONLY   (Addressograph Plate)

Date-Time	Doctors Orders	
8-24-76	Admission Orders	
9:00 A.M.	1) Admit to Station 51, Dental Service	
	2) Dx. = Multiple Dental Caries & Chronic Periodontal Disease	
	3) Condition - Satisfactory	
	4) Vital Signs = Routine	
	5) Activity = Up ad Lib	
	6) Diet = Regular	
	7) Admission CXR: PA, Lat.	
	8) Labs: C.B.C. $\bar{c}$ diff., P.T., P.T.T.,	
	U/A, E.K.G.	
	9) Physical Examination by LMD	
	S.M. Skill	

Fig. 18-4. Example of admission orders.

University Hospitals	Name: I. N. Need
DOCTOR'S ORDER SHEET	Age: Hospital Number:
	Date:

FORM 56   NCR PAPER. PRESS FIRMLY—USE BALL POINT PEN ONLY   (Addressograph Plate)

Date-Time	Doctors Orders	
8-24-76	Pre-op Orders	
7:00 PM	1) NPO after midnight	
	2) Void on call to O.R. PRN	
	3) Chart and labs to O.R. with patient	
	4) Seconal 100 mg. P.O. h.s. PRN sleep	
	5) Pre-anesthetic meds	
	Demerol 50 mg. I.M.	
	Vistaril 50 mg. on call to O.R.	
	Atropine 0.4 mg.	
	6) Consent - signed	
	S.M. Skill	

Fig. 18-5. Example of preoperative orders.

UNIVERSITY OF MINNESOTA HOSPITALS

MINNEAPOLIS, MINNESOTA

I. N. Need

Authorization for Surgical Treatment

Date_____ August 24, _____, 19 76

Time_____ 8:10 _____ a.m. / p.m.

I, the undersigned, a patient in University Hospitals, hereby authorize Dr._____ S.M. Skill _____ and/or whomever he may designate to perform or to participate in the following operation or procedure

_____ Removal of all remaining teeth _____ and such additional operations or pro-

(Name of Operation and/or Procedures)

cedures as are considered therapeutically necessary on the basis of findings during the course of said operation. Any tissues or parts surgically removed may be disposed of by the hospital in accordance with customary practice.

I also consent to the administration of such anesthetics as are necessary.

I hereby certify that I have read and fully understand the above Authorization for Surgical Treatment. I also understand the reasons why the above-named surgery is considered necessary, its advantages and possible complications, if any, as well as possible alternative modes of treatment, which were explained to me

by Dr._____ S.M. Skill _____. I also certify that no guarantee or assurance has been made as to the results that may be obtained.

Witness_____ *S. M. Skill* _____ Signed_____ *I. N. Need* _____

(Patient or nearest relative)

_____

(Relationship if other than patient)

If permission is given by a monitored telephone call, the authorization should be read to the person giving the permission, and the following completed:

_____ Name of person giving permission

_____ Relationship to patient

_____ Signature of person requesting authorization

_____ Signature of person monitoring authorization

Hosp. Form No. 33 — 5M
Rev. 1-69 0-151

Fig. 18-6. Example of consent form.

UM UNIVERSITY OF HOSPITALS **PROGRESS NOTES** S—Subjective O—Objective A—Assessment P—Plan	Name:	I. N. Need
	Age:	Hospital Number:
	Date:	

DATE	Problem Number	
8-24-76		Pre-op Note
8:20 PM		Pre-op Dx. Multiple, non-restorable teeth
		PMH - WNL, Psychiatric Tx. 1965
		Allergies - none Medication - none
		Labs:
		Hgb 13.3 HCT 38
		WBC 5500, PT 10.1 PTT 35.5
		E.K.G. WNL
		Consent Form: signed and on chart
		Imp. Healthy male with non-restorable teeth
		Plan: Full mouth extractions in O.R. under general anesthesia
		S.M. Skill

MR Form 28, JUL 74

Fig. 18-7. Example of preoperative note.

DATE	Problem Number	S—Subjective O—Objective A—Assessment P—Plan

Fig. 18-7. (*Continued*)

University Hospitals	Name: I. N. Need
DOCTOR'S ORDER SHEET	Age: Hospital Number:
	Date:

FORM 56   NCR PAPER. PRESS FIRMLY—USE BALL POINT PEN ONLY   (Addressograph Plate)

Date-Time	Doctors Orders	
8-25-76	Post-op orders	
9:00 AM	1) Patient had general N.T. anesthesia for full mouth extraction.	
	2) V.S: q 15 mins. until stable, then q 1 h x 4, then routine	
	3) I.V. Orders: Complete present I.V. at 100 cc/hour, then	
	$D_{5/w}$ 1000 cc. at 100 cc/hr.	
	4) Diet = NPO until fully awake, then clear liquid diet.	
	5) Meds =	
	a) Demerol 50 mg. I.M. q 4 h prn pain	
	b) Tigan 200 mg. I.M. q 6 h prn nausea	
	6) Elevate head of bed 30°	
	7) I & O while on I.V.	
	8) BRP with assistance until stable	
	9) Remove gauze packs from mouth at 10:00 A.M.	
	10) Gauze packs orally prn hemostasis	
	11) Ice packs to R & L side of face x 8 hrs.	
	12) Vaseline to lips	
	S.M. Skill	

Fig. 18-8. (A) Example of postoperative orders.

UNIVERSITY OF MINNESOTA HOSPITALS	Name:	I. N. Need
PROGRESS NOTES		
S—Subjective O—Objective A—Assessment P—Plan	Age:	Hospital Number:
	Date:	

DATE	Problem Number	
8-25-76		Brief Operative Note
		Pre-op & Post-op Dx: Dental caries & periodontal disease
		Surgeons: Drs. S.M. Skill and D.S. Newcomer
		Anesthesia: general anesthesia with nasoendotracheal intubation
		Procedures: multiple dental extractions and alveoloplasty
		under general anesthesia, removal of all
		remaining teeth #2,3, 7-15, 18, 20-29
		(total 22 teeth).
		Conservative alveoloplasty was performed. 3-0
		Black silk sutures were placed.
		E.B.L. = 150 cc. without replace
		fluid replacement = 500 cc. $D_{5/w}$
		complication = none
		The patient tolerated the procedures and anesthesia well
		and taken to the PAR in satisfactory condition.
		S.M. Skill

MR Form 28, JUL 74

Fig. 18-8. (B) Example of operative note.

DATE	Problem Number	S—Subjective O—Objective A—Assessment P—Plan

Fig. 18-8. (*Continued*)

UNIVERSITY OF MINNESOTA HOSPITALS
OPERATIVE REPORT

TO:		NAME: I. N. Need	
		AGE: 41	HOSPITAL NUMBER: 110 92 76
		DATE: 25 August 1976	

Operating Time: 7:30 AM - 8:45 AM

Preoperative Diagnosis:
Dental caries & periodontitis involved teeth #2, 3, 7 through 15, 18, 20 through 29 (total 22 teeth)

Preoperative Status:
The patient was seen in the outpatient oral surgery clinic where examination and radiographs revealed the presence of a non-restorable dentition, and it was decided that he should be admitted and his remaining teeth be removed under general anesthesia. Preoperative workup consisting of CBC, urinalysis, PT, PTT, chest x-ray, E.K.G. revealed no contraindication to general anesthesia or the intended procedure.

Name of Operation:
Multiple dental extractions and alveoloplasty.

Operative Procedure:
After the induction of satisfactory general anesthesia with nasoendotracheal tube, the patient was prepped and draped in the usual manner for an intraoral surgical procedure. A total of 8 cc. of 2% xylocaine with 1:100,000 epinephrine was infiltrated in the four quadrants of the mouth. Moist throat pack was then placed in the oropharynx. Incision was made around the necks of the remaining teeth of the maxillary (L) quadrant. A mucoperiosteal flap was elevated to the buccal and removed teeth #9, 10, 11, 12, 13, 14, 15 in the usual manner with elevators and forceps. A minimal alveoloplasty procedure was carried out with the Rongeur and file. The surgical site was irrigated with normal saline. Closure was then carried out in the usual fashion, utilizing continuous 3-0 black silk suture. Attention was then turned to the other quadrants and removed teeth #2, 3, 7, 8, 18, 20-29. Following completion of the procedure, the oral cavity was copiously irrigated with normal saline. The previously placed throat pack was then removed from the oropharynx and suctioned clean. Bacitracin was applied to the lips and gauze packs were applied bilaterally for hemostasis. Estimated blood loss was 150 cc., none of which was replaced. The patient was then extubated in the Operating Room; having tolerated the procedure well, the patient was then taken to the PAR in good condition.

Postoperative Diagnosis:
Same as preoperative

S.M. Skill, DDS
D.B. Newcomer, DDS

RO:dm
Dict. 8/25/
Transcribed: 8/26/

O
P
E
R
A
T
I
V
E

R
E
P
O
R
T

Fig. 18-9. Example of operative report.

operative period, the dentist should be particularly alert to manage the patient with professional skills and competence. At the time of each postoperative visit, a quick review of nursing notes, temperature chart, fluid intake and output records, and medications should be done to assess the patient adequately. New orders may be written or others adjusted according to the patient's needs; this includes directions regarding diet, antibiotics, analgesics, sedatives, hot packs, ice bags, mouthwashes, and dressings. A progress note should then be entered on the chart and signed by the doctor (Fig. 18-10). When the patient is afebrile and making satisfactory progress, an order for discharge should be written (Fig. 18-11). The discharge summary should be typed (Fig. 18-12). After discharge, the dentist must enter the properly worded diagnosis and name of operation on the face of the chart (Fig. 18-13).

Operating Room Protocol

Aseptic surgery began in 1867 with the publication of Lister's paper on the elimination of pathogenic bacteria from surgical wounds. Lister's use of a carbolic acid spray was an attempt to eliminate all bacteria from the operating room and the surgeon's and patient's body surfaces. A goal of modern surgery is to exclude, inhibit, or destroy microorganisms that might contaminate a wound. This exclusion of pathogenic bacteria is known as asepsis. Maintenance of an aseptic technique is a fundamental discipline in any surgical specialty, providing protection to both the patient and the surgeon and to his assistants.

In routine dental work, the dentist often feels that it is impractical to maintain asepsis in the office as strict as that in the operating room of a hospital, for several reasons: (1) Asepsis in and about the oral cavity is difficult to maintain because the oral cavity is the natural habitat of many kinds of bacteria. (2) Many more patients are seen in the office than in the operating room. Moreover, these patients enter the office directly off the street wearing street clothes, and they often come for treatment with mild upper respiratory infections or colds. (3) High-speed air rotary instruments and irrigation sprays tend to disperse saliva and bacteria, thereby increasing the contamination of equipment and persons close to the operative field. (4) Many dental materials cannot be rendered sterile, such as filling material, and not all handpieces of high-speed instruments used in the general dental office can tolerate repeated autoclaving. (5) The cost factor in maintaining sterile technique is quite significant. Rubber gloves, gowns and masks would have to be laundered and autoclaved unless disposable items were used, which are also costly. Therefore, the general dentist in routine dental work frequently uses a less sterile approach, which could not be permitted for oral surgery. Despite these problems, every patient deserves protection from bacterial and viral contamination at all times. Of special concern is cross-contamination, that is, contamination from one patient to another or from operator to patient. Usually a person tolerates his own organisms, but often cannot tolerate extraneous bacteria.

Every effort should be made to keep the level of asepsis high, whether in the office, clinic, or hospital. Surgery in the hospital operating room involves the purest form

(*Text continues on page 283.*)

	UNIVERSITY OF MINNESOTA HOSPITALS **PROGRESS NOTES** S—Subjective O—Objective A—Assessment P—Plan	Name: I. N. Need
		Age: Hospital Number:
		Date:

DATE	Problem Number	
8-25-76 6:00 PM	#2	Multiple Dental Caries and Periodontal Disease
		S = without complaints
		O = patient doing well, afebril, vital signs stable
		Moderate oozing from oral wound. No chest pain
		Chest clear to auscultation.
		Voided this P.M. (500 cc.), good fluid intake
		fluid intake (400 cc. P.O.)
		A = Normal post-op Progress
		P = 1) D/c I.V. tomorrow A.M.
		2) Possible discharge tomorrow
		S.M. Skill

MR Form 28, JUL 74

Fig. 18-10. Example of progress note.

DATE	Problem Number		S—Subjective	O—Objective	A—Assessment	P—Plan

Fig. 18-10. (*Continued*)

University **Hospitals**	Name:	I. N. Need
DOCTOR'S ORDER SHEET	Age:	Hospital Number:
	Date:	

FORM 56

NCR PAPER. PRESS FIRMLY—USE BALL POINT PEN ONLY

(Addressograph Plate)

Date-Time	Doctors Orders	
8-26-76	Discharge Orders	
9:00 A.M.	1) Discharge today	
	2) D/C. I.V.	
	3) Discharge Medication	
	tylenol #3 x 12 tabs; take one q 4 h, P.O. prn pain	
	4) Rinse Mouth c̄ warm salt water	
	5) R.T.C: out-patient oral surgery clinic	
	Sept. 1, 1976, 1:00 P.M.	
	S.M. Skill	

Fig. 18-11. Example of discharge orders.

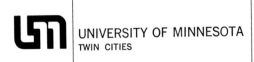

UNIVERSITY OF MINNESOTA | University Hospitals
TWIN CITIES | Minneapolis, Minnesota 55455

ADM.   8-24-76
DIS.   8-26-76

DISCHARGE SUMMARY

PRIMARY DIAGNOSIS: Dental caries, periodontal disease.

OPERATION PERFORMED: Full mouth extraction and alveoloplasty.

REASON FOR ADMISSION: This is the first UMH admission for this
41 year old white male for a full mouth extraction.

PAST MEDICAL HISTORY: The patient had psychiatric treatment for
depression at 1965. Hospitalizations: tonsilectomy and adenoid-
ectomy, age 6. Appendectomy, age 13. The patient denied any
rheumatic fever, diabetes mellitus, coagulopathies, lung, liver,
or kidney disease.

REVIEW OF SYSTEMS: Essentially non-contributory.

PHYSICAL EXAMINATION: Significant findings include mouth: poor
oral hygiene with multiple caries and periodontitis. The chest
to be clear to auscultation and palpation, and a cardiac exam showed
normal sinus rhythm without murmur.

LABORATORY STUDY: Laboratory data on admission was hemoglobin 13.3,
WBC 5500, PT 10.1, PTT 35.5, urinalysis, E.K.G. within normal limits.
Panorex showed deep periodontal pockets and multiple radiolucent
lesions on apex of teeth.

HOSPITAL COURSE - on 8-25-76 the patient was taken to the Operating
Room where, under general anesthesia, all remaining teeth were
removed. The remaining hospital course was uneventful.

CONDITION ON DISCHARGE: Improved, the patient was alert, fully
ambulatory, and able to care for himself.

DISCHARGE MEDICATIONS AND INSTRUCTIONS: Tylenol #3 q 3-4 h prn for
pain. The patient was instructed to use warm salt water for mouth
rinse and to return for postoperative followup on 9/1/76, 1:00 P.M.

Dict: D.B. Newcomer
      8-26-76, 5:00

                              S.M. Skill, DDS

Fig. 18-12. Example of discharge summary.

UNIVERSITY OF MINNESOTA HOSPITALS

Code Sheet

NAME_____

UH #_____

	Adm. #	Date Adm.	Date Disch.	Service	Classifi-cation	Responsible Physician	Date Letter Dictated
Admitted Transferred	1	8-24-76	8-26-76	Dentistry			
Admitted Transferred							
Admitted Transferred							
Admitted Transferred							
Admitted Transferred							
Admitted Transferred							

Admission Date	Code Number	ABBREVIATIONS ARE NOT TO BE USED ON THE CODE SHEET
	521.0	PRIMARY DX: Dental caries and periodontal disease
RECORD ABSTRACTED	523.9	
1803_____		OTHER DX:
1804_____		
	23.1	OPERATIONS and PROCEDURES: Full mouth extractions and alveoloplasty
	24.4	

Signature: ___S.M. Skill___ M.D.

University of Minnesota
Hosp. Form 481B (Revised)

Fig. 18-13. Example of code sheet.

Code Sheet Continued

Admission Date	Code Number	ABBREVIATIONS ARE NOT TO BE USED ON THE CODE SHEET
		PRIMARY DX:
RECORD ABSTRACTED		
1803_____		OTHER DX:
1804_____		
		OPERATIONS and PROCEDURES:
		Signature:_____M.D.

Admission Date	Code Number	ABBREVIATIONS ARE NOT TO BE USED ON THE CODE SHEET
		PRIMARY DX:
RECORD ABSTRACTED		
1803_____		OTHER DX:
1804_____		
		OPERATIONS and PROCEDURES:
		Signature:_____M.D.

Fig. 18-13. (Continued)

of aseptic technique, and since the dentist performs an increasing number of procedures in this environment, he must be familiar with the details of aseptic technique. Habit is the best teacher in establishing hospital operating room routine, and because dental experience in this area is limited, considerable emphasis is placed on it here. The chain of sterility must be maintained in the operating room to prevent postoperative complications and to provide initial, uncomplicated, primary healing. Each step is based on sound principles, and the neglect of one small detail will nullify all succeeding steps.

The Operating Room Suite

The operating room suite is designed to provide certain advantages:

1. Geographic isolation. Operating rooms are usually located in an isolated portion of the hospital, thereby providing a private, clean place with limited traffic in which to perform surgery.
2. Bacterial isolation. Special clothing and footwear must be used while performing duties within the area. These measures further attempt to reduce the introduction of pathogens into the operating room suite.
3. Centralization of equipment. The operating room suite is an integrated unit, the sole function of which is to provide an atmosphere for safe and effective surgery. By virtue of its isolation from other parts of the hospital, it is possible to maintain all the equipment and supplies in an adequate quantity and in their best condition.
4. Centralization of trained personnel. Modern surgery demands the combined talents of many groups of trained specialists, who, by working together in the operating room, acquire a great deal of efficiency, cooperation, and skill.

Within such an environment, it is possible to provide a patient with the best possible surgical care, which is the fundamental responsibility of all persons who work in the operating room area.

The walls, floor, and ceiling of the operating room are built as soundproof as possible and of a material that is easily cleaned. The floor is covered with a material that conducts static electricity. Most operating rooms have two doors: a main door to admit the patient on his litter from an adjacent anesthesia-induction area, and a door leading to a scrub and sterilization area. These doors should be kept closed at all times and should be used only by personnel involved in the management of the case. Air circulating in the operating room is thoroughly filtered to reduce the possibility of introducing pathogens. Each operating room contains a flexible and versatile operating table (Fig. 18-14). A main overhead operating light may be supplemented by portable spotlights. Oxygen, anesthetic gases, and suction apparatus may be mounted on the wall or ceiling.

Scrub areas are adjacent to the operating room with access through a separate door. One scrub area usually serves two operating rooms. Each area consists of sinks with foot or elbow valves. Soap dispensing units are found at each sink along with sterile brush dispensers and nail files (see p. 285).

The recovery room is a separate area fully equipped and staffed to provide patient care during the immediate postoperative recovery period (Fig. 18-15).

In the instrument room, the surgical instruments are cleaned, sorted, and packaged after they have been used (Fig. 18-16). Packs of instruments are then

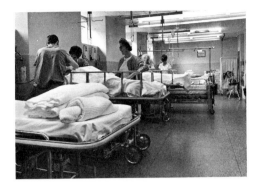

Fig. 18-15. The recovery room.

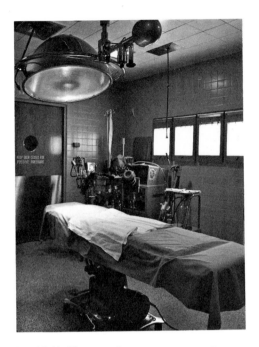

Fig. 18-14. The operating room.

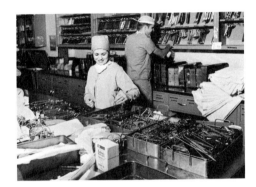

Fig. 18-16. The instrument room.

sterilized in a main sterilization area and stored in a supply room near the operating rooms where they will be readily available.

Operating Room Conduct

A fundamental goal of surgery is to prevent wound infection as much as possible. Therefore, the introduction of pathogens into the operating room must be reduced to a minimum. For this reason, personnel must be properly dressed before entering the operating room suite. Street clothes or clothes worn elsewhere in the hospital should never be worn into the operating area. In addition, anyone participating in an operation in a septic field or on a patient who has an infection should shower and change to clean clothes before re-entering the operating room area. Before leaving the operating room after an infected case, all personnel should leave their gloves, masks, operating gowns, and shoe covers in the special containers provided.

Street clothes are worn into the doctor's dressing room, where the conventional attire of a short-sleeved cotton suit is donned after removing all clothing except underwear and socks. The cotton shirt is tucked into the trousers and not allowed to hang loosely (Fig. 18-17). Underwear worn into the operating room should be made of cotton, because wool, silk, and synthetics such as nylon, Dacron, Orlon, and rayon tend to generate static electricity and retain a charge for a long period of time. In the presence of inflammable anesthetic agents, a spark can be dangerous.

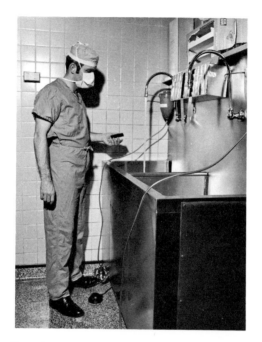

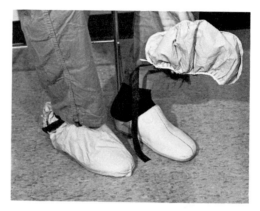

Fig. 18-18. Shoe covers with conductive strip.

Fig. 18-17. The doctor in special scrub shirt and pants.

Specially made conductive-soled shoes or shoe covers must be worn if the floor is conductive (Fig. 18-18). Shoes should be tested for conductivity on an apparatus intended for this purpose at the operating room entrance. Rings and watches can be conveniently pinned to the scrub suit with a safety pin or hung on the pants' drawstring.

Before entering the operating room, a cap and mask must be in place. They may be either reusable cotton or disposables of paper or other synthetics. Persons who wear glasses will be troubled by fogging after placing on the mask. This can be reduced by the use of specially prepared lens sprays (although coating the glasses with soap and polishing them after it dries works just as well and is less expensive).

Under no circumstances are relatives of a patient to be allowed into the operating room. Emotional stress is great and often unexpected. If prime attention is to be given to the patient, extraneous conversation and attention to others cannot be afforded. When visitors are present, there exists a certain tension that might preclude the routine measures to assure good patient care.

Entering the Operating Room Suite

After donning the appropriate operating room attire, the surgeon should go to the operating room before the patient is asleep. This allows the patient the opportunity to ask any last-minute questions and likewise allows the surgeon to give any necessary reassurance which may be needed. One should be thorough in covering all aspects of an upcoming surgical procedure with the patient; this must include a consent to operate.

Operating Room Personnel

It is important that the surgeon introduce himself to the operating room personnel who will be working with and assisting him throughout the case. These persons include the scrub nurse, the circulating nurse, and the anesthesiologist.

Before beginning, it is also wise to discuss any expected changes in routine with the operating room personnel.

The personnel in the operating room represent a team whose coordination is essential if the surgery is to be performed smoothly and efficiently. Each of these persons has a definite responsibility during the surgery. The circulating nurse is usually the most experienced nurse in the operating room. She is the only member of the surgical team who neither scrubs nor wears sterile gown and gloves; this leaves her free to function as an intermediary between the surgical team and other departments within the hospital as well as giving her freedom of movement so she can obtain additional sterile supplies as needed. In general, she supervises activities in her assigned room (Fig. 18-19).

The scrub nurse is the surgeon's "other pair of hands." During an operation, she hands instruments to the surgeon and in general tries to anticipate his needs (Fig. 18-20). The scrub nurse selects the instruments and supplies before the case and should be consulted if the surgeon anticipates any changes from routine.

The anesthesiologist relieves the surgeon of much of the responsibility for the well-being of the patient in the operating room so that the surgeon can concentrate on the technical aspects of the operation. His basic duties include the administration of the anesthetic agent(s) and other drugs as required, the transfusion of blood and other fluids, alerting the surgeon to any changes in the patient's status or to impending problems and the treatment of these as they arise, and the supervision of recovery room management of the patient.

During an operative procedure these personnel assume positions around the

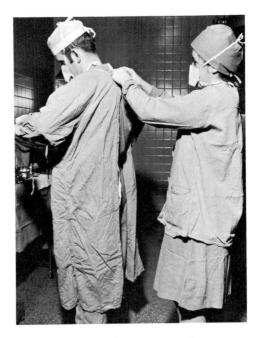

Fig. 18-19. The circulating nurse is free to move throughout the operating room suite.

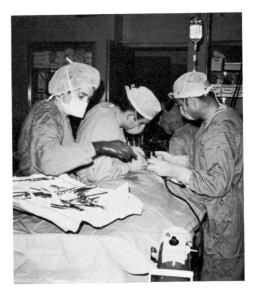

Fig. 18-20. The scrub nurse is prepared to participate directly in the surgery.

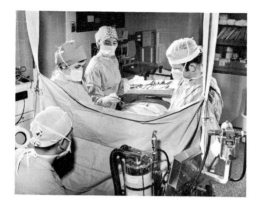

Fig. 18-21. Anesthesiologist administering the anesthetic. The doctor, the assistant, and the scrub nurse are in appropriate positions.

patient that allow the operation to proceed quickly and efficiently. The surgeon chooses the side from which he prefers to operate. In most cases, especially dental operations, this is the right side of the patient. The first assistant usually stands opposite the surgeon, and a second assistant, if present, is usually on the same side of the table as the surgeon. The scrub nurse can be on either side of the table (usually the same as the surgeon), but is always between the operating table and the back instrument table. The circulating nurse or orderlies move as needed throughout the operating room, bringing additional supplies to the suite or running errands outside the operating room. The anesthesiologist is usually at the head of the table, often walled off by drapes (Fig. 18-21).

Scrubbing

Scrubbing is done in the scrub room which adjoins the operating room. Deep sinks with elbow and/or knee controls for the faucets allow control of water flow and temperature without touching the handles with one's hands (see Fig. 18-17). If the surgeon is going to wear a headlight, it must be placed and properly adjusted before he begins the scrub. Instruc-

tions and variations in scrub procedures are usually posted above the scrub sink. Scrub techniques using conventional bar soap, liquid soap (tincture of green), and soaps containing hexachlorophene or povidone-iodine* are as follows:

A. *Conventional bar soap*
   1. Wash hands and arms to above the elbows for approximately one minute to remove gross bacteria and dirt.
   2. Clean the nails with a sterile nail file or orangewood stick under running water. This should be discarded into the sink after use. (Some hospitals autoclave a sterile file and brush together in the same package or dispenser.)
   3. Take a sterile brush and scrub to above the elbow. Once picked up at this point the soap should not be discarded until the scrub is complete. When not in use, palm the soap between the hand and the brush handle. Complete the 10-minute scrub as follows:
      a. After developing a stiff lather, follow a definite system to assure even scrubbing of all surfaces, especially the hands, nails, knuckles, and between the fingers (Fig. 18-22).
      b. Keep the hands higher than the elbows and rinse at intervals, allowing the water to run off at the elbows.
      c. At the end of five minutes of scrubbing, discard the brush but not the soap. Using a second

---

*Betadine, Purdue-Frederick Co., Inc.

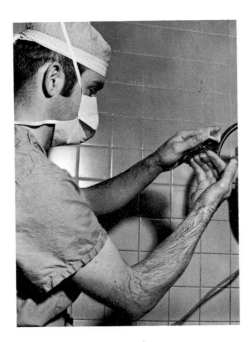

Fig. 18-22. The surgical scrub.

sterile brush, continue the scrub to just below the elbow for an additional five minutes. This avoids contamination of the forearms, hands, and fingers. Discard the brush and rinse completely, remembering to keep the elbow flexed so that the hands and forearms remain higher than the elbows.

    d. Immerse the hands and forearms in 70% ethyl alcohol for one minute (surgeon's choice).

B. *Use of liquid soap* (tincture of green soap). The scrub routine is unchanged except that the soap is dispensed from a foot-operated container.

C. *Use of soaps containing hexachlorophene or povidone-iodine.* The 10-min-

ute portion of the scrub is unchanged except that only one brush is used. Rinse hands and forearms often, adding sufficient soap to maintain a good lather. No alcohol rinse should be used following the scrub because it nullifies the effect of hexachlorophene or povidone-iodine.

Hexachlorophene enters the pores of the skin and is slowly exuded, thereby providing bacteriostatic activity for several hours. Povidone-iodine is a powerful bacteriocide which is most effective when it has had a long exposure (five to ten minutes) with the skin.

Drying the Hands and Gowning

After the scrub the doctor enters the operating room with the elbows flexed to prevent water from running down onto the hands and forearms. Upon entering the room the doctor is handed a folded sterile towel by the scrub nurse. The folded towel is grasped with the fingers of both hands and the doctor steps away from the table and other persons or objects. After opening the towel, one end is placed over one hand and it is used to blot the free hand and wrist. It is not necessary to dry the elbows. The unused, sterile portion of the towel is used to dry the opposite hand and wrist. The towel is then discarded into the proper receptacle. If the hands are still moist, powder or special hand cream is used to make it easier to put on the tight-fitting rubber gloves. The doctor is now ready for gowning. It may be necessary for him to gown himself or he may have assistance.

A. *Gowning and gloving with assistance*
    1. The scrub nurse unfolds the sterile gown and holds it in a position so the doctor can insert his arms (Fig. 18-23).
    2. The surgeon inserts his arms into the sleeves, being careful that the

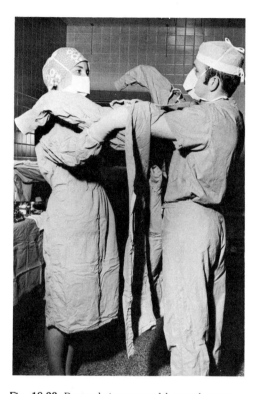

Fig. 18-23. Doctor being gowned by scrub nurse.

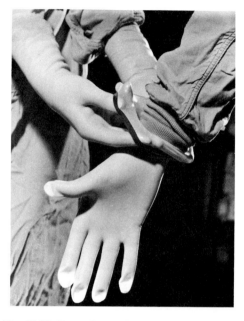

Fig. 18-24. Doctor being gloved by scrub nurse.

ungloved hands touch neither the nurse's gown or gloves, nor the outside of the gown being put on.

3. The circulating nurse or orderly pulls the gown into position and ties it in back (see Fig. 18-19). (The back of the gown is not considered sterile.)

4. The scrub nurse holds the cuff portion of the glove open widely and pulls the glove onto the surgeon's hand so that it covers the cuffs of the gown (Fig. 18-24). The doctor creates a counterforce by driving his hand firmly into the outstretched glove.

B. *Gowning without assistance*

1. When the gown is packaged for sterilization, it is folded inside out. The surgeon picks up the folded gown from the open sterile pack, holds it out at shoulder level, and carefully lets it unfold. The outside of the gown must not touch the body or any other object.

2. The surgeon places his hands and arms in the sleeves and holds them above his head.

3. The circulating nurse or orderly pulls the gown into position and ties it in back.

C. *Gloving without assistance.* Occasionally it is necessary to glove oneself without the aid of a scrub nurse, e.g., when an operating room is shorthanded or when prepping a patient:

1. A sterile glove pack is opened on a table. This contains a towel for drying the hands, glove powder, and gloves.
2. The hands are dried and powdered.
3. The gloves are already folded so that they are cuffed. The surgeon carefully lifts one glove by its cuff out of the pack with the forefingers and thumb of the opposite hand. He partially pulls the glove onto the hand, covering the fingers and palm (Fig. 18-25). The cuff is retained.
4. He places the gloved fingers under the cuff of the other glove, which is pulled into correct position (Fig. 18-26).
5. He places the fully gloved hand under the cuff of the other glove and pulls it into correct position.

At no point do bare fingers touch the outside of either glove.

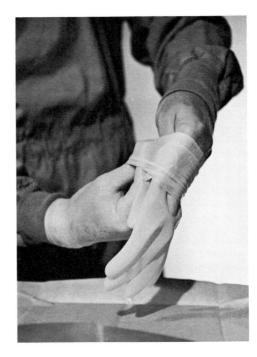

Fig. 18-26. Doctor gloving himself. Putting on the second glove.

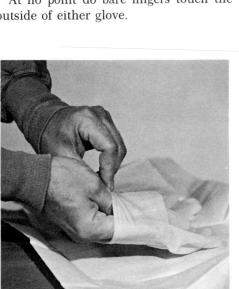

Fig. 18-25. Doctor gloving himself. Picking up the first glove by the cuff.

Preparation ("Prepping") of the Patient

Prepping of a patient is done prior to draping, usually by the surgeon's assistant. The primary aim of a surgical prep is to reduce the local bacterial flora on the operative site. On the skin the important bacteria found are gram-positive, coagulase-negative staphylococci, corynebacteria, and micrococci. Gram-negative bacteria are rare because they usually require a fluid medium in which to live. Skin bacteria are found mainly in the hair follicles, the upper layers of keratin, deep furrows and cracks in the skin, and the ducts of sebaceous glands.

Advise female patients that they should wear no makeup of any kind to the operating room. Likewise, male patients should be clean shaven. Full and partial dentures should also be left behind unless they will be needed during the operation. Two methods of skin preparation are described: one using conventional tincture of green soap and the other using soap containing povidone-iodine.

A. *Skin prep using tincture of green soap*
  1. Scrub the area of the incision for 10 minutes with soap and water, using gauze sponges held with a sponge forceps. Use fresh gauze sponges frequently. Start the prep at the point of the incision and gradually extend it to include a larger and larger area, being careful not to return to the initial point with the same piece of gauze. A much larger area should be scrubbed than will be exposed (Fig. 18-27).
  2. Remove soap with sterile water.
  3. With a new sponge forceps, sponge the area with 70% ethyl alcohol.
  4. Apply ether with a fresh sponge, using the sponge forceps just used with the alcohol.
  5. With a third sponge forceps, sponge the area with the antiseptic used by the hospital (e.g., tincture of benzalkonium chloride, tincture of Metaphen, tincture of Merthiolate).

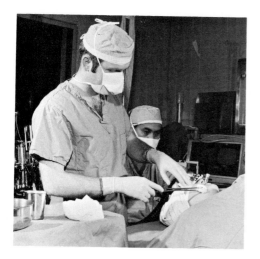

Fig. 18-27. The assistant preps the patient.

B. *Skin prep using soap containing povidone-iodine*
  1. Scrub the area of the incision for 10 minutes with the soap.
  2. Blot the area dry with a sterile towel or rinse it off with povidone-iodine solution. The color of the solution after it dries helps to demarcate the extent of the prep.

Preparation of the oral cavity prior to surgery presents a difficult situation: one can only attempt to reduce the resident bacterial flora. Preoperative oral prophylaxis to remove gross calculus deposits and the practice of good oral hygiene will greatly reduce oral flora, as will the use of mouthwashes containing either benzalkonium chloride (Cepacol) or povidone-iodine (Betadine). The patient should brush his teeth and use a mouthwash on the morning of surgery. Once he is in the operating room and asleep, the patient's mouth should be dried with gauze sponges and sponged with an antiseptic. The lips and skin around the mouth are then prepared in the manner described previously.

Draping The Patient

After the skin prep, the patient is draped by either the surgeon, his assistant, or both. Sterile draping assures that during an operation no contact occurs between the operative site and nonsterile items in the operating room. The following method is recommended for draping the head:

1. Place a sterile towel and half sheet beneath the patient's head, which is elevated by an assistant. The half sheet lies beneath the towel and covers the head of the table.

2. Place a second towel over the patient's face so that it runs from beneath the nose to cover both earlobes.

3. Holding this second towel in place over the face, cross opposite corners of the first towel over the patient's face and secure them with towel clips (Fig. 18-28).

4. Then place two towels to drape off the chin and neck region and secure with three towel clips.

5. Use a sheet drape, thyroid drape, or head and extremities drape to cover the remainder of the patient and the operating table.

6. Place a wall drape (also a half sheet), suspended by two intravenous (IV) stands, between the anesthetist and the patient's operative site (see Fig. 18-21).

This method can be easily modified if the mouth is not to be included in the operative site (e.g., for an extraoral surgical approach to the jaw). An adhesive-edged plastic drape running from the earlobes across the patient's lower lip will provide good isolation of the mouth from the operative site. Prior to placement of this adhesive drape, the skin must be dry. In some instances, drapes can also be sewn to the patient's skin to prevent their migration during the operation.

Sterilization

Sterilization may be defined as the destruction or removal of all forms of life, with particular reference to microorganisms. The usual limiting factors in sterilization are bacterial and fungal spores and viruses; methods capable of destroying these will also destroy vegetative forms. Methods of sterilization for instruments and supplies used in oral surgery include:

A. Physical Agents
   1. Steam under pressure
   2. Dry heat
B. Chemical Agents
   1. Ethylene oxide
   2. Glutaraldehyde solution (Cidex)
   3. Radiation

Steam Under Pressure

Moist heat is the most widely applicable and practical method of sterilization for most items (Fig. 18-29). In the form of saturated steam under pressure (autoclaving), moist heat has great penetrating power which enables it to rapidly denaturate vital microbial proteins.

All that is required to produce saturated steam is an airtight vessel or autoclave capable of heating water to the necessary temperature (Fig. 18-30). Under ordinary circumstances, a temperature of 121° C. applied for 15 minutes is sufficient to destroy all forms of life. At higher temperatures, sterilization is more rapid, requir-

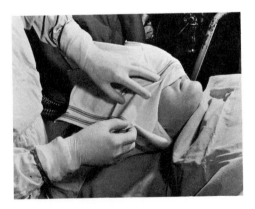

Fig. 18-28. Draping the patient.

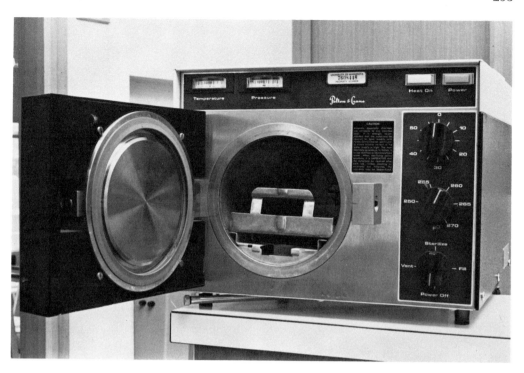

Fig. 18-29. The Sentry Sterilizer for office use requires no plumbing and utilizes distilled water.

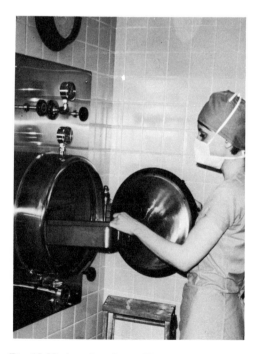

Fig. 18-30. Autoclave in sterilization room.

ing only 10 minutes at 126° C., 3 minutes at 134° C., and only a few seconds at 150° C. In practice, additional time is required to allow this temperature to be reached in the center of thick packages of dressings or containers of liquids. The operation of an autoclave needs to be governed only by its thermometer because pressure rises ahead of the temperature and 121° C. corresponds to 15 pounds pressure at sea level.

The primary disadvantage of steam under pressure is its effect on the surface of metals. Sharp instruments become dull and also stained after repeated passages through an autoclave. Therefore, instruments with cutting edges are often sterilized by other methods.

To prolong instrument life and achieve the best results using an autoclave, it is imperative to properly clean, lubricate, and package items prior to their sterilization. Surgical instruments should be cleaned as soon as possible after use, ei-

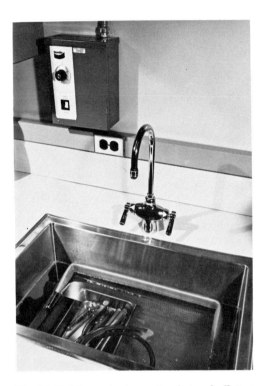

Fig. 18-31. Ultrasonic cleaner is a fast and efficient method to remove initial debris from instruments before autoclaving.

ther by handwashing or with an ultrasonic cleaner, to prevent blood and other debris from drying on their surface (Fig. 18-31). All box-lock instruments (e.g., needle holders, hemostats, rongeurs, forceps) must be opened to their fullest extent to assure complete removal of debris. Soil that is allowed to remain on instruments is difficult to remove if it bakes on during sterilization. Use a soft brush to scrub all instruments. If it is not possible to wash instruments immediately after their use, they should be soaked in a warm, noncorrosive, free-rinsing neutral detergent. Once cleaned, instruments

should be dried before sterilization because trapped moisture can cause corrosion.

Ultrasonic cleaning removes all traces of lubrication, so that instruments cleaned by this method must be relubricated before sterilization. Use only water-soluble lubricants.* Continuous improper cleaning and lubrication (as with mineral oil, machine oil, or silicones) will leave a gumlike or hard residue that may inhibit sterilization.

To protect instruments and other items during and after sterilization, it is imperative that strict aseptic methods be applied to packaging (Fig. 18-32). Cloth wrappers are usually used because they

* Instrument Milk. Snowden-Pencer Corp., Los Gatos, Calif.

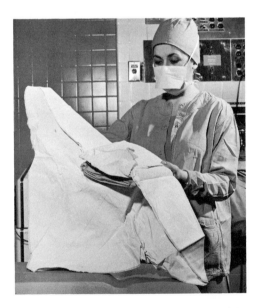

Fig. 18-32. Item properly wrapped for sterile delivery.

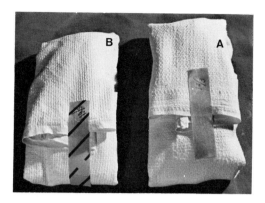

Fig. 18-33. Thermosensitive tape. (A) Before autoclaving there are no black lines visible on tape. (B) After autoclaving, black lines have appeared on the tape.

are readily reuseable, inexpensive, and allow free passage of steam. Specially prepared nylon film and paper packaging materials allow steam to pass freely at sterilization temperatures but block the entrance of microorganisms when cooled to room temperature. Sharp or delicate instruments may be protected by wrapping them in gauze or covering them with a dental cotton roll. This not only protects the instruments, but decreases the possibility of perforating the packaging material. Packages are best secured by a thermosensitive tape* which changes color after autoclaving (Fig. 18-33). Include a piece of this tape in the center of bulky or large packs of instruments or dressings as a test of satisfactory sterilization.

Dry Heat

As proteins dry, their resistance to denaturation increases, so that dry heat sterilizes less effectively than moist heat at a given temperature. Dry heat sterilization is usually done in ovens. Since hot air is a poor conductor of heat, large packages are slow to reach sterilizing temperatures.

*Autoclave Tape. The 3M Co., St. Paul, Minn.

The recommended temperature is 160° C. for not less than two hours. At this temperature, fabrics and rubber are weakened, ruined, or discolored. However, dry heat is a satisfactory method of sterilizing instruments when it is essential to preserve a cutting edge.

Ethylene Oxide

Gas sterilization using ethylene oxide offers another method for sterilizing items that cannot be readily steam-sterilized. This method depends on the toxicity of ethylene oxide to microorganisms. Ethylene oxide probably destroys microorganisms by alkylation, that is, replacement of the available hydrogen atom with its hydroxyethyl radical in some susceptible chemical groups in a protein molecule. The resultant interference with cell metabolism is irreversible and consequently bacteriocidal.

The use of ethylene oxide is generally restricted to hospitals because the equipment is expensive and usually bulky. While completely effective, ethylene oxide presents a number of problems: sterilization takes 4 to 12 hours, must occur in a vacuum, requires a temperature greater than 70° F., and must be used with the correct humidity. In addition, many materials (e.g., rubber and plastics) readily absorb ethylene oxide and considerable time is required for the elution of the gas before these items are safe to use without burning tissues with the highly reactive gas. Despite its limitations, ethylene oxide provides a highly effective additional means of sterilization, that is especially suited for cutting and delicate instruments.

References

1. Asp, D. S., and Brashear, J. M.: Problem oriented medical records in a private hospital. Minnesota Medicine, 56:12–18, 1973.
2. Bjorn, J. C., and Cross, H. D.: The Problem Oriented Private Practice of Medicine. Chicago, Modern Hospital Press, McGraw-Hill Publication Co., 1970.
3. Costich, E. R., and White, R. P.: Fundamentals of Oral Surgery. Philadelphia, W. B. Saunders Co., 1971, pp. 209–229.
4. Douglas, B., and Casey, G.: A Guide to Hospital Dental Procedure. Chicago, American Dental Association, 1964.
5. Hayward, J. R.: Oral Surgery. Springfield, Ill., Charles C Thomas, 1976, pp. 355–366.
6. Lowbury, E. J. L.: Skin disinfection. J. Clin. Pathol., 14:85–90, 1961.
7. Rendell-Baker, L., and Roberts, R. B.: Gas versus steam sterilization; when to use which. Med. Surg. Rev., 5:10–14, 1969.
8. Weed, L. L.: Medical Records, Medical Education and Patient Care. Cleveland, Case, Western Reserve University Press, 1969.
9. Weed, L. L.: Medical records that guide and teach. N. Engl. J. Med., 278:593–599 and 652–657, 1968.

19 Fractures of the Jaws

M. L. HALE

Oral surgery, as the surgical specialty of the dental profession, has contributed immeasurably to the improved knowledge and surgical capabilities in the diagnosis and management of trauma to the face and jaws. The most significant advancements in professional knowledge and surgical capabilities in the diagnosis and treatment of traumatic injuries to the facial structures have developed during periods of mass conflicts. The increased incidence of such injuries and the interprofessional cooperation needed for the management of these patients undoubtedly are the reasons for the improved total patient care in this area.

Skeletal Anatomy and Facial Trauma

A broken bone is a serious injury for any patient, but a fractured jaw can be a major catastrophe. Life's normal activities and pleasures, such as eating, speaking, drinking, maintaining good oral hygiene, and even the ability to breathe comfortably, make this type of traumatic injury one of great concern to most patients.

Rapid vehicular transportation has made serious injuries to the face and jaws a fairly commonplace incident today. Abrupt deceleration may cause severe injury to the head, face, and jaws when the pas-

senger is unable to maintain his normal position within the vehicle.[1]

Fractures of the jaws are basically similar to other fractures except that they are complicated by the close anatomic association of the mandible and maxilla to the mouth, nose, orbits, and sinuses, and by the presence or absence of teeth in the jaw fragments. Although this chapter does not present a detailed anatomic review of the mandible, maxilla, and associated structures, certain points of applied anatomy should be reviewed in brief as an aid in the diagnosis and management of such facial trauma. By understanding the anatomy, structural areas of weakness, and displacement actions of the muscles, the clinical findings of the patient will frequently lead the clinician to a proper diagnosis.[2]

Certain protective anatomic features exist in the jaws and adjacent structures. The thin bone at the angles of the mandible and in the surgical necks of the condyles permits a fracture to occur there under certain forceful stresses and thus tends to minimize an otherwise more serious head or brain injury. Such structures as the zygomatic arch, nasal bones, maxillary antra, and orbital rims all tend to cushion and absorb some of the direct forces and, in so doing, may actually serve as a protection to the head and brain from more severe trauma (Fig. 19-1). From the standpoint of frequency of injury in civilian life, the nasal bones are most frequently fractured, followed by the mandible, zygomatic arch, and maxilla in descending order. Statistics reveal that the head is the most frequent site of major injury in modern-day accidents, and some studies place the incidence rate about 70 per cent as compared to other anatomic sites.

The etiologic factor of fractures of the upper jaw is usually a direct impact over the anterior or lateral aspect of the maxilla. As might be expected, the maxillary fracture line tends to pass through the site of least resistance, and for this reason, most fractures of the maxilla tend to involve the maxillary sinus. Often the impact to the upper jaw will be transmitted through the occluding teeth from the mandible to maxilla. Because of the anatomic design of the maxilla, with the thinner bone structure located superior to the teeth and overlying the maxillary sinuses, it has been observed that the maxillary fracture lines most frequently occur in the horizontal plane and superiorly to the apices of the upper teeth. This type of fracture is frequently referred to as a Le Fort I fracture, or horizontal maxillary fracture (Fig. 19-2). In contrast, trauma to the mandibular arch, especially if the dentition is present, often follows the long axes of the teeth in

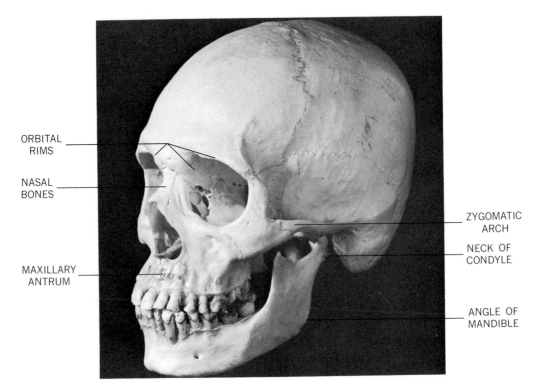

ORBITAL RIMS

NASAL BONES

ZYGOMATIC ARCH

NECK OF CONDYLE

MAXILLARY ANTRUM

ANGLE OF MANDIBLE

Fig. 19-1. Protective skeletal structures that tend to minimize the effects of trauma to the head.

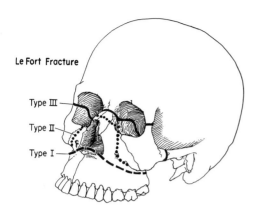

Le Fort Fracture

Type III
Type II
Type I

Fig. 19-2. Mid-third fracture classifications.

the area of stress. Therefore, since the fracture lines tend to pass through or along the tooth sockets, most mandibular fractures are considered compound fractures, in that the gingival mucosa has been lacerated intraorally even though there may not be an extraoral wound communication.[1-4]

Fracture forces applied to the maxilla are delivered against a solid, immobile bone structure, and usually the fracture is created at the site of impact. The mandible is a mobile bone structure and it consists of a horizontal portion termed the body and two vertical extensions known as the rami which articulate with the skull bilaterally. If the impact to the mandible is a solid, continuous force, the flow of force tends to be transmitted between the point of impact and the point of articulation in the glenoid fossa; thus, an angle fracture is perhaps the most frequent type of fracture in the mandible (Fig. 19-3). If a fracture occurs in the body of the mandible, it is quite possible that an indirect force may also have been transmitted to the condylar region, and a condylar neck fracture may have been produced on the side opposite the point of impact. Most condylar fractures are extra-articular, owing to the thin anatomic design of the surgical neck of the condyle. Fractures of the coronoid process are rare and usually require no treatment (Fig. 19-4). Fractures of the mandible

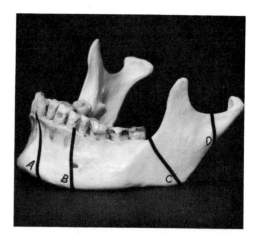

Fig. 19-3. The most frequent fracture sites in the mandible. (A) Symphysis fracture. (B) Parasymphysis fracture. (C) Angle fracture. (D) Ramus fracture.

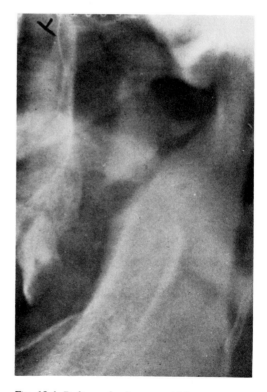

Fig. 19-4. Radiograph of a coronoid fracture.

usually produce malocclusion and jaw dysfunction, so that these are distinguishing clinical features. The presence of impacted teeth or unerupted teeth may leave the body of the mandible weakened and much more susceptible to fractures from trauma.

Fracture Displacement Factors

Fractures may be displaced primarily by the violence of the force creating the fracture, but more often than not, displacement results from the distraction forces of the muscles and ligaments attached to the fragments. If the muscle pull tends to hold the fracture fragments together at the line of fracture, this makes the fracture easier to control in most instances, and the fracture line is described as favorable (Fig. 19-5). If the fracture is such that the mus-

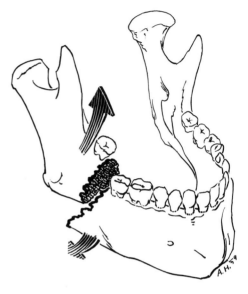

Fig. 19-6. An "unfavorable" fracture line. Muscle actions tend to displace the fragments.

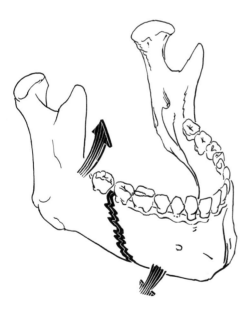

Fig. 19-5. A "favorable" fracture line. Muscle actions help to splint the injury site.

cle pull is a distracting force that causes displacement, then the fracture line is described as unfavorable (Fig. 19-6). In the mandible, in addition to the muscles of mastication (Fig. 19-7), the suprahyoid muscles also tend to exert a considerable influence on the displacement of mandibular fragments, and they must be given careful attention in the overall planning of the treatment for the fracture (Fig. 19-8). There are primarily three groups of muscles that have positive displacement tendencies on certain types of fractures. Group 1 consists of the masseter, temporalis, and medial pterygoid muscles, which tend to displace the proximal fragment superiorly, posteriorly, and medially. Group 2 consists of the suprahyoid muscles, especially the digastric, mylohyoid, and geniohyoid, which tend to displace the distal fragment or body of the mandible in an inferior and

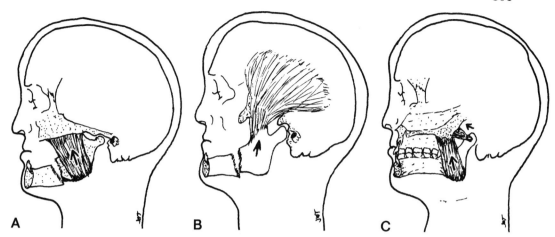

Fig. 19-7. (A, B, and C) Displacement forces exerted by the muscles of mastication (masseter, temporalis, and the medial and lateral pterygoids).

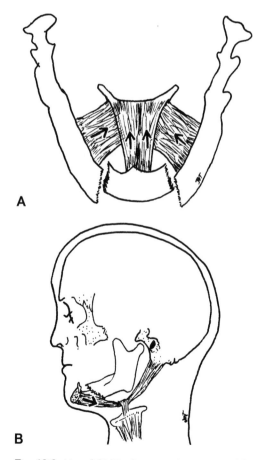

Fig. 19-8. (A and B) Displacement forces exerted by geniohyoid, mylohyoid, and digastric muscles of the suprahyoid group.

posterior direction. Group 3 consists of the lateral pterygoid muscles, which tend to displace the condylar heads anteriorly and medially.[1-4]

Patient Evaluation and Emergency Treatment

Patients who receive trauma to the jaws obviously require a thorough physical evaluation. One of the greatest threats to life for the patient with jaw injuries is the lack of an adequate airway. A fractured mandible may allow the tongue to be displaced posteriorly so that the airway may be obstructed. Blood, teeth, bone, denture material, and other foreign bodies within the oral pharynx must be removed and an adequate airway established and protected. Hemorrhage must be controlled. Bleeding from most oral wounds can be controlled temporarily by pressure dressings. Direct ligation or coagulation may also be advantageous in controlling minor points of hemorrhage under proper surgical conditions (Table 19-1).

Sometimes jaw fractures are associated with severe craniocerebral trauma, and in such instances, the traumatized jaw may be of secondary importance in overall patient management (Fig. 19-9). An axiom

Table 19-1. Basic Principles in the Early Treatment of Fractures

1. Establish and maintain a patent airway.
2. Control hemorrhage.
3. Be aware of the patient's respirations, pulse, and blood pressure.
4. Keep in mind the need for antibiotics and tetanus antitoxin.
5. Secure clearance for cranial injuries.
6. Be alert to legal responsibilities and liabilities.
7. Always treat the patient "first" and the fracture "second."

that must be kept in mind is that one treats the patient first and the fracture second. Therefore, the neurologic and hemodynamic status of the patient should be immediately evaluated and proper measures should be taken to minimize or correct shock. Once the patient's overall status has been determined and stabilized, the clinical examination can be directed toward the management of the fractured jaws and facial injuries.

In the presence of any of the following findings, the reduction and fixation of fractures should be delayed until such signs have been satisfactorily evaluated and the patient has been stabilized: loss of consciousness, diplopia, altered pupillary movements, irregular respirations, hemorrhage from an ear, abnormalities in blood pressure or pulse, vomiting, headache, dizziness, loss of spinal fluid, and partial or complete paralysis. To proceed to reduce and immobilize a jaw fracture in the face of such unexplained findings is poor clinical judgment and may be an open invitation to subsequent legal action in the event of a questionable end result or fatality.

The emergency administration of nar-

cotics prior to a definitive diagnosis may only hinder and delay patient evaluation. Narcotics given to a patient with a probable head injury (1) stimulate the oculomotor nucleus, causing miosis which masks the development of neurologic eye signs vital to the recognition of cerebral hemorrhage, (2) may depress respirations, and (3) may stimulate nausea and vomiting.

Record-keeping for accident cases is extremely important and must not be neglected in the total management of the patient's problem. A detailed history should be taken of the injury as to time, place, and persons involved. Frequently, severe injuries result in medicolegal decisions and, therefore, it is most important that records accurately relate the details pertaining to the injury (Fig. 19-10; see also Figs. 3-1 and 3-13). The records should show whether or not the patient has

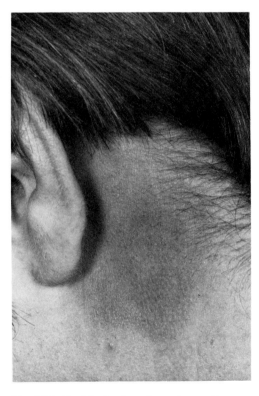

Fig. 19-9. Battle's sign is ecchymosis near the mastoid process and implicates a fracture of the base of the skull.

TRAUMA RECORD
(Oral Surgery)

Date

Name

Address

Age

Etiology of Injury:

Treatment before this examination:

Has patient lost consciousness? (Yes   No) Describe:

General oral hygiene: Physical Condition: Attitude:

X-ray findings:

Diagnosis:

Method of Treatment:

Oral Surgeon   Assistant:

Dates of: Injury: Admission to Hospital:

    Reduction and Fixation: Other Surgery:

Diagram of Injury:

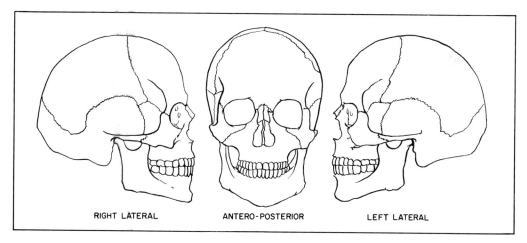

RIGHT LATERAL   ANTERO-POSTERIOR   LEFT LATERAL

Condition at Discharge:

Remarks:

Postoperative Record

Date							
Weight							
End of	1st week	2nd	3rd	4th	5th	6th	Extended Period

UNIVERSITY HOSPITALS

Fig. 19-10.

received other treatment prior to the time of the reduction and fixation of the fractures.

Extraoral examination should include a general inspection of the patient, palpation of the suspected areas of injury, and an evaluation for neurologic injury related to the injured area. The intraoral examination should include inspection of both soft and hard tissues, the alignment of teeth, and a digital appraisal of the teeth and alveolar structures. Some significant clinical findings that would aid in diagnosing a fractured jaw are malocclusion of teeth and jaws, mobility at the fracture site, disability or dysfunction, crepitus, swelling, ecchymosis, trismus, and pain.

Good diagnostic x-ray films are extremely important in studying and evaluating any fracture. However, clinical interpretation at the time of surgery still is the most significant way of understanding the nature of the fracture. Skull films, especially of the middle third of the face, may be indistinct and misleading, and even intraoral films in children with bony crypts around erupting teeth may make a linear fracture line with little or no displacement extremely difficult to diagnose on roentgenographs alone. Radiographic examination should include more than one view of the skeletal structures of concern. Most head and neck injuries can be covered by a combination of the following: Panorex, lateral-oblique, occlusal, posterior-anterior, modified Towne's, Waters' view, temporomandibular joint films, and intraoral dental films. Remember that the closer the film can be placed to the site to be x-rayed, the better the bone definition will be; therefore, intraoral films are often particularly helpful in the final decision regarding the extent of the injury.[1-4]

In considering the cause of jaw fractures, it is important to consider indirect as well as direct causes. The indirect, or predisposing, causes might result from local or generalized bone disease. Existing pathologic conditions, such as cysts, infections, or benign or malignant tumors, could produce local or general changes in the skeletal structures that could predispose to a fracture. Such existing pathologic lesions could also make surgical management of the problem more difficult. The direct causes usually involve high-speed vehicle accidents, firearms, falls, or physical violence.

Emergency treatment may necessitate temporary support of the injured structures until definitive care can be instituted. Intraorally, such wiring techniques as the Essig (Fig. 19-11), Risdon (Fig. 19-12), or Gilmer (Fig. 19-13) can be readily accomplished and should provide the necessary support required. If *extraoral* support is also desired, the application of a modified Barton head bandage using an elastic wrap from 2- or 3-inch wide roller bandage reinforced with adhesive strips may provide adequate support on a temporary basis until final reduction and fixation measures can be instituted (Fig. 19-14).

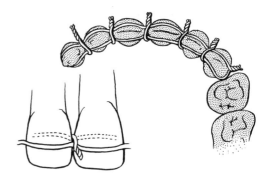

Fig. 19-11. The Essig type of splinting.

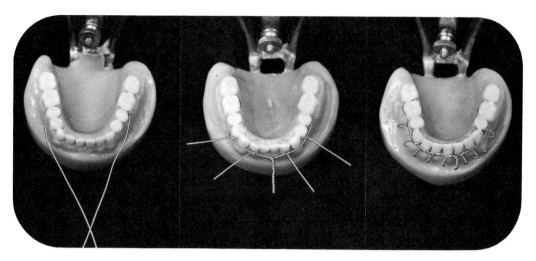

Fig. 19-12. The Risdon type of splinting is useful for emergency situations until more effective immobilization can be provided after patient's condition has been stabilized.

Reduction and Fixation Procedures

The major objectives in the treatment of fractures of the jaws include the following:

1. To re-establish functional occlusion and interarch relationships.
2. To preserve and protect the dentition.
3. To accomplish reduction and fixation of the fracture as soon as surgical judgment will permit.

4. To keep surgical trauma at a minimum.
5. To keep the aesthetic qualities, the general welfare, and the comfort of the patient in mind.

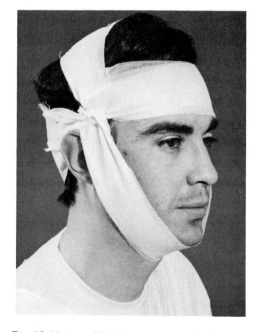

Fig. 19-14. A modified Barton support bandage is a useful method of supporting some trauma patients during transportation to treatment centers. The roller bandage may be reinforced, if necessary, with adhesive tape strips.

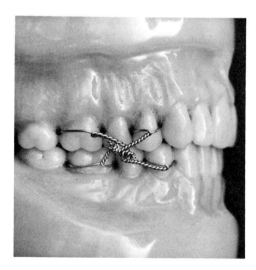

Fig. 19-13. The Gilmer type of splinting may be helpful in emergency situations, especially in cases with "favorable" lines of fracture.

The final decision regarding the treatment for any fractured jaw depends upon a thorough workup of the patient and the type of fracture involved. Some important matters to consider when deciding how the fracture can best be managed include the following:

1. The age and cooperation of the patient.
2. The dentition present:
   a. Deciduous dentition (note extent of root resorption).
   b. Permanent dentition (note extent of root development).
   c. Edentulous areas.
   d. Teeth in line of fracture.
   e. Fractured teeth with or without pulp involvement.
3. Extent of bone injury (alveolar and/or basilar bone):
   a. Single or multiple fractures.
   b. Simple, compound, or comminuted fractures.
   c. Loss of bone substance.
4. Control of bone fragments by:
   a. Closed vs. open reductions.
   b. Skeletal fixation.
      (1) Extraoral skeletal pin procedures (precision vs. frictional pins).
      (2) Circumferential wiring of splints or dentures.
      (3) Intraosseous pins.
      (4) Bone plates.
   c. Craniofacial techniques.

The information presented here is not to be considered a "how to do it" or "surgical primer." It is intended only to serve as a helpful guide for those special trauma cases that may be considered to fall within the professional skills and judgment of the doctor or in other special situations such as those occurring in remote or iso-lated locations where urgent treatment can provide no alternative treatment plan due to time and distance.

Under usual circumstances, treatment for complex trauma cases involving the head and face is not advocated to be undertaken by those in the health professions without formal training in advanced oral surgery procedures. However, in some carefully selected instances it may be determined by prudent professional judgment that closed reduction procedures are adequate to reduce and immobilize some fractures. In such special cases the following closed fixation techniques could be helpful in the treatment of such identified surgical problems. Practical closed reduction procedures should require minimal treatment time and be kept as uncomplicated as possible.

If an intra-arch splinting plan only is indicated, Figures 19-11 and 19-12 provide two methods for adapting such treatment plans to single arches, assuming that teeth are present for such ligation methods and that the type of fracture can be adequately controlled by such procedures. Sometimes a segment of an arch (e.g., an Erich fracture bar) may be ligated to the secure teeth on either side of an alveolar-type fracture, and this method of supporting and splinting an alveolar fracture may be sufficient immobilization.

When it is necessary to splint the mandibular dentition to the maxillary dentition, such treatment may be managed by several methods. Figure 19-13 illustrates a direct interarch wiring method termed the Gilmer splinting technique. Separate wire ligatures (approx. 22-gauge stainless steel wires) are passed around the cervical necks of teeth on either side of the fracture site. The long ends of the wire thus positioned are braided together by a twisting action until the wire ligature is secure in its position on the tooth. In the opposing arch, wire ligatures are placed similarly on teeth as nearly opposite to the first arch locations as possible.

Similar teeth on the opposite side of the mouth in both arches are located and the same wire ligature applications are completed. All teeth to be ligated should have the braided wires placed on them before bringing the teeth into the interarch occlusal relations and securing the two arches together by this direct wiring method.

Once the four braided wires are in position the most posterior braided wire on one side in either arch is braided with the most anterior one of the opposing arch. The two remaining wires are then brought together and braided in the form of a cross. This procedure is completed on the opposite side of the mouth. The interarch braided wires are twisted together and the extensions of the wires cut off. The double-wire-secured ligatures are then positioned as close to the interdental spaces as possible to minimize soft tissue irritation. Sometimes, soft dental carding wax can be molded over a sharp wire to protect the soft tissues of the cheek.

When direct wiring between the arches seems to be inadequate it may be helpful to ligate "ribbon-type" arch bars (e.g., Erich arch bar and the like) to each arch separately. By this method the arches can sometimes be held more securely in better dental occlusion. Figure 19-15 illustrates this type of immobilization between the arches.

Direct measurements from one posterior molar location around the outer aspect of that arch to the selected posterior tooth on the opposite side help in determining the necessary length of arch bar to prepare on each arch. The lengths of arch bars are curved to approximate the curvature of the arch to which they are to be ligated.

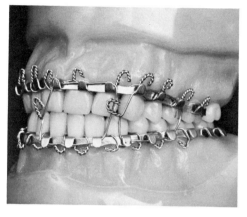

Fig. 19-15. Closed reduction secured by ligation of adaptable arch bars to each arch and then ligating the two arches together in a functional occlusal relationship. Secondary interarch wire ligatures are perhaps more hygienic once occlusal relationships have been attained.

Single wire ligatures are placed on "key teeth" on either side of the arch. The selected arch bar is then adapted to the outer surfaces of the teeth, and the ligature wires are passed around each tooth and secured to the arch bar as noted in the illustration. Additional ligature wires can be passed around other teeth, if necessary, to provide a better anchored arch splint.

A similar arch bar is now fashioned and secured to the dentition of the opposing arch. The ends of the ligature wires are clipped off, and the wire loops are positioned in the interdental spaces so as to minimize irritation to the soft tissues.

With the arch bars secured to the outer aspects of the dentition in either arch, the teeth are brought together into functional occlusal relations and secured by interarch elastic loops or direct secondary wire ligatures, depending upon the immediate occlusal relationships that are attainable. If the occlusion is immediately satisfactory, secondary wire ligatures can be placed. If the occlusion is at all questionable, interarch elastics can often be helpful in securing a more favorable occlusal relationship under elastic tension (see Fig. 19-22). Once good interarch dental occlusion is obtained, the secondary wire ligatures can be placed between the arches (Fig. 19-15). Better oral hygiene is possible usually with the secondary wire ties as opposed to interarch elastics. Also, the elastics should be carefully observed and changed frequently to maintain the desired occlusal relations. The elastics tend to lose their effective tension over extended periods and they usually result in poorer oral hygiene.

Oral hygiene is an important factor in the management of fractured jaw cases. The use of forceful dental sprays and professional assistance is routinely necessary. Patients can improve oral care in most instances by also using force sprays in effecting good home care (e.g., Water Pik).

It is a basic principle that, in multiple jaw injuries, the mandible should be restored first to anatomic contour and alignment. This is the foundation for restoring other facial structures to their proper relationship and is the cornerstone for reconstructing the entire facial bony complex (Table 19-2).

In the treatment of fractured jaws, the surgical procedures for repositioning and immobilizing the fractured segments are primarily closed or open techniques. *Closed techniques* suggest that the fractured ends of the bone structure can be manipulated, aligned, and maintained in proper relationships without surgically exposing the bone (Fig. 19-15). *Open reductions* are usually necessary for more complex or difficult reduction and immo-

Table 19-2. Major Objectives in Fracture Treatment

1. To re-establish functional occlusion and interarch relations.
2. To preserve and protect the dentition.
3. To secure reduction and fixation as soon as surgical judgment will permit.
4. To keep surgical trauma at a minimum.
5. To keep the aesthetic qualities, general welfare, and comfort of the patient in mind.

bilization cases (Fig. 19-16). Direct transosseous wiring techniques are effective, but occasionally it becomes necessary to combine such open procedures with additional surgical techniques such as intraosseous pins (Fig. 19-17), precision or friction skeletal pins (Fig. 19-18), bone plates (Fig. 19-19), or circumferential wiring with surgical splints or dentures (Figs. 19-20 and 19-21) to help immobilize the fractures. After the fractured segments have been repositioned and immobilized,

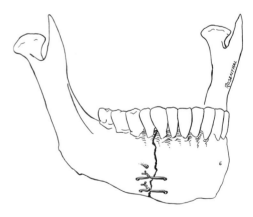

Fig. 19-16. Open reductions are usually immobilized by transosseous wiring at the site of injury. Double wiring and a figure-eight wiring that embraces the inferior border of the mandible are common surgical techniques.

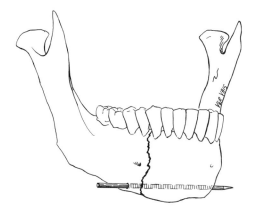

Fig. 19-17. Open reductions sometimes can be accomplished by proper placement of an intraosseous pin. Usually, this is also supported by interarch ligations.

it is often necessary to immobilize the dental arches in their normal approximating positions. The occlusal relations of the dentition can often be best secured if interarch elastic traction is applied initially (Fig. 19-22). Once functional occlusal relationships are established, secondary wire ties between the arches may provide a more stable immobilization and, in addition, will allow for better oral hygiene during the period of fixation (see Fig. 19-15).

Usually, a pliable type of arch bar can

be readily adapted to the dentition by lightweight stainless steel fracture wire. It is desirable to include as many teeth as possible in securing the arch bar to better distribute traction forces. Elastic traction, especially of single-rooted anterior teeth, may tend to cause extrusion of these teeth. Occasionally, double wire ligatures with dental floss leaders are used to secure arch bars (Fig. 19-23). Some oral surgeons prefer to pass only single wire ligations to secure the arch bars. It makes little difference which method is employed so long as gingival irritation is kept at a minimum.

More rigid arch bars are occasionally preferred in cases in which alignment of the fractured segments is difficult to control. Proper contouring of a rigid arch bar and ligation of this bar to the dentition may help considerably in maintaining good anatomic position of the fragments (Fig. 19-24).

Cast splints, especially lingual bracing splints for the mandible and the palate, provide excellent immobilization (Fig.

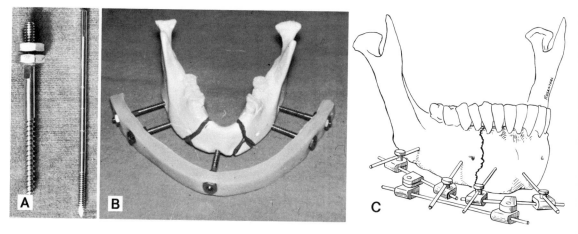

Fig. 19-18. (A) Precision skeletal pin (left), and friction skeletal pin (right). (B) Precision skeletal pin technique. (C) Friction skeletal pin technique.

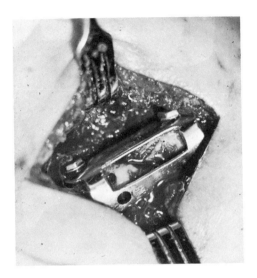

Fig. 19-19. Open reduction with a bone plate.

19-25). However, these techniques usually require more than one operating room procedure and additional laboratory facilities and procedures to fabricate such precision appliances.

Middle Third Facial Trauma

Middle third facial trauma is sometimes difficult to diagnose. The superimposition of other skeletal structures in the x-ray films often makes it difficult to get a good definition of the skeletal structures of concern to the surgeon.

Once the maxilla has been repositioned, there is little likehood of any forceful displacement tendency due to muscle pull. However, comminuted zygomas, nasal bones, blow-out fractures of the orbital regions, and craniofacial separations do present difficult surgical problems, and often such injuries require multidisciplinary professional care. It should be understood that, medicolegally, an oral sur-

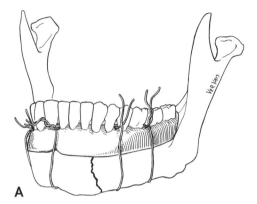

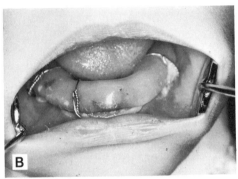

Fig. 19-20. (A) Circum-mandibular wiring utilizing patient's denture as the splint. (B) Circum-mandibular wiring with an acrylic splint adapted over a mixed dentition.

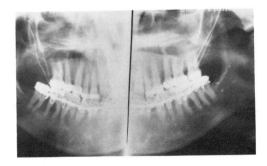

Fig. 19-21. Circumferential wires around the zygomatic arch immobilize the mandible and maxilla to firm cranial fixation.

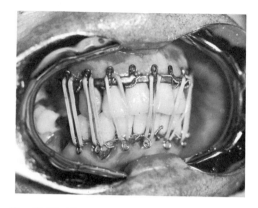

Fig. 19-22. Elastic traction may be necessary to secure the best possible occlusal relationship at time of surgery.

apices of the teeth and involves the maxillary antra. Le Fort Class II, pyramidal-type fractures, usually involve the nasal and ethmoid bones as well as the maxilla. Le Fort Class III represents a separation of the facial structures from the cranium. Usually, this involves separation at the frontal zygomatic sutures and fractures of the zygomatic arch (see Fig. 19-2).[1-5]

geon should not be held professionally responsible for such complications as postsurgical visual disturbances provided appropriate consultations have been initiated. Likewise, it should be clear that the surgical responsibilities related to the maxilla and mandible should be those of the oral surgeon.

Middle third facial trauma cases are usually classified as follows: In Le Fort Class I, horizontal maxillary fractures, the fracture line is usually superior to the

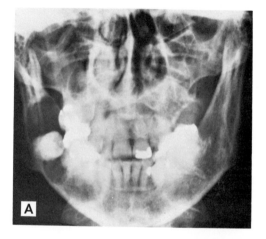

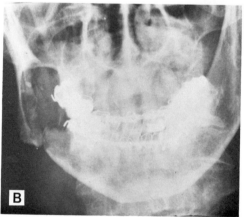

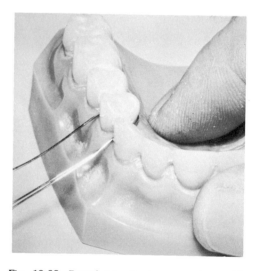

Fig. 19-23. Dental wire ligatures can be readily passed by use of a dental floss leader.

Fig. 19-24. (A) Odontogenic cyst and impacted third molar. (B) Fracture has occurred following surgical removal of the tooth. Note maxillary and mandibular arch bar in place with intermaxillary fixation.

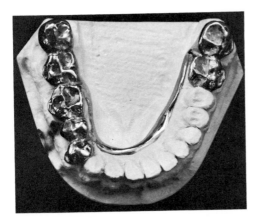

Fig. 19-25. Cast lingual bracing splints provide excellent stability for both lower and upper arch fractures. The additional laboratory requirements take more time and may necessitate a second surgical procedure to place the prepared splints.

Pediatric Jaw Fractures

Pediatric jaw fractures are usually more complex to diagnose and treat than similar injuries in adults. The deciduous or mixed dentitions together with the growth and development factors of this patient group, plus a frequently more apprehensive and less cooperative patient, are some of the additional complexities associated with such injuries.

One of the most important considerations in the management of pediatric fractures is that the surgeon must have a comprehensive knowledge of the growth and development of the jaws and their dentitions. Long-term growth and development studies based on cephalometric measurements have brought to light some important findings pertinent to the intelligent understanding of the growth and development patterns in the jaws of children.[6]

From cephalometric studies, we know that deficient arch length is the most frequently encountered type of malocclusion. It has also been established that there is no increase in arch length by growth from first molar to first molar positions after these permanent teeth have erupted. Actually, there may even be a slight dimensional decrease as the permanent incisors in the mandible erupt lingually to deciduous incisors over the symphysis. Therefore, fractures occurring in children anterior to erupted six-year molars are not as likely to result in injuries that might cause arch or facial disharmonies in these sites on the basis of interference with growth patterns. However, it should be apparent that, in this patient age group, severe trauma to or a fracture through the bony areas posterior to the six-year molars would necessitate a careful appraisal and evaluation to determine the necessary treatment and method of operation to minimize the surgical trauma to the developing structures and yet effect a satisfactory surgical result.

It has been determined cephalometrically that growth does not occur in a steady, gradual development; there are periods of slower growth followed by periods of more rapid growth. Therefore, in making a surgical appraisal of fractures involving centers of growth and development, it seems logical to predict that there would be fewer deforming results if the injury were incurred and treated successfully during the periods of "slow growth" as compared to the periods of proved "rapid growth"[6] (Table 19-3).

Several studies based on statistical research of cephalometric projects have been reviewed. The following facts appear to be well-documented as related to facial growth. In the first five years, 78 per cent of the height, 85 per cent of the width, and 82 per cent of the depth have been achieved. This means that, at the age of six years, approximately 20 per cent of the growth increment remains as an avenue of possible readjustment. Thus, it would

Table 19-3. Cephalometric Summaries–Growth of Jaws

RAPID GROWTH PERIOD	SLOW GROWTH PERIOD
From birth to 6 months (to provide anterior-posterior arch length to receive the deciduous dentition).	From 6 months to 4 years.
From 4 to 7 years (to permit the eruption of the six-year molars and development of space for the formation of the second molars).	From 7 to 15 years.
From 15 to 19 years (to provide space for the development and eruption of the third molars).	After 20 years—growth potential is almost negligible.

appear that after six years of age fractures anterior to the first molar positions in either jaw would not be likely to produce any injury to growth and development since, for all practical intents and purposes, these areas are already well developed. However, the trauma incurred by such injuries could conceivably result in injury to centers of growth elsewhere by the transmission of forces, with or without a fracture resulting to the growth centers.[6] Rowe and Killey report that in their experience a greenstick fracture of the condylar neck in children before the age of five years can be expected to heal rapidly with only minimal treatment, and it is not likely to interfere with condylar growth.[4] In contrast, they state that occasionally a severe fracture dislocation or a badly comminuted fracture of the ramus that is compounded externally will lead to an injury to the growth center by direct trauma or subsequent infection, and from these severe injuries an arrest of growth and development may result with ultimate facial deformity and asymmetry.

In summary, therefore, from the ages 6 to 20 years we are especially concerned with traumatic injuries to the four parallel suture lines related to growth centers connected with the maxilla, and to the hyaline cartilage region in the condyles of the mandible. Determining the severity of injuries to these important centers of growth and the extent of the growth potential already reached at the time of the injury should help establish the surgical evaluation and treatment procedure of choice for each patient.[7]

In a statistical study of 1,000 fractured jaw cases reported by Rowe and Killey[4] and a University of Iowa study,[8] it was observed that the frequency of such injuries to patients under 20 years of age as compared to those over 20 years was approximately 21 per cent. Therefore, one out of every five fractures, percentagewise, could conceivably require an awareness and a surgical evaluation of possible injury to centers of growth and development (Table 19-4).

MacLennan, reporting on a series of fractures in mandibles of children under six years, concluded that fractures in the condylar region are commonly of the greenstick variety.[7] These are extracapsular and do not, as a rule, give rise to any disturbances of mandibular development at a later date. Intracapsular fractures, on the other hand, are often associated with

Table 19-4. Fracture Frequencies by
Ages: Report of 1000 Fractures[4,6]

AGE (YEARS)	NUMBER OF FRACTURES	PERCENT OF TOTAL
0–5	6	1.2
6–11	18	3.6
12–19	81	16.2
20–29	189	37.8
30–39	78	15.6
40–60	97	19.4
Over 60	31	6.2

dislocation. The fracture dislocation of the condylar process in the young child must always be viewed with concern because of the likelihood of secondary growth anomalies from damage to the condylar growth center[7] (Table 19-5).

The emergency treatment of children with fractures of the jaws follows the same principles stated previously (see p. 301). Of primary importance in overall patient care are the following: to ensure a patent airway, to control hemorrhage, to combat or prevent shock, and to complete a neurologic examination.

In accomplishing the clinical and radiographic examination of children with

Table 19-5. Frequency of Occurrence of Fracture Sites in Mandibles Under Age of 6 Years[7]

1. Unilateral through body of mandible.
2. Unilateral of body with condylar process on opposite side.
3. Unilateral condyle.
4. Bilateral condyles with or without fracture in incisor region.
5. Bilateral body fractures.

traumatic injuries of the jaw, the age of the child and his willingness and ability to cooperate usually determine whether this workup can be completed preoperatively, or whether it can be only partially completed preoperatively, with the final examination of the extent of the injury delayed until a general anesthetic has been administered for the actual reduction and fixation procedure. Completion of as extensive a preoperative examination as the patient's general condition will permit relative to his head injury should be accomplished.

Fracture Healing and Bone Physiology

The process of bone repair in the jaws is similar to that in other bones of the body. Primarily a local phenomenon and not a systemic one, it depends upon the local tissue changes in the fracture area, and is not usually concerned with blood calcium, phosphorus levels, or other systemic metabolic processes. The phases of bone repair have been enumerated by many authors. A practical classification of these healing phases can be listed as follows:

1. Hematoma phase (24 to 72 hours after injury).
2. Fibrous repair phase (through first three weeks).
3. Final bone-forming phase (fourth through sixth weeks for mandible).

Interference by gross manipulation or unfavorable distraction stresses on the fracture site during the final bone-forming phase may result in non-union or malunion; therefore, this is considered a hazardous period and should be treated accordingly.

At the time of the injury, there occur coincidental laceration and contusion of the surrounding tissues. If the fracture is compounded intra- or extraorally, the problem may be complicated by contamination. If the fragments are displaced, the possibility of vascular impairment to the local fracture site must be considered and may influence the rate of healing.[9]

Summary Comments

Today, difficult fractures of the jaws and associated structures are managed more and more frequently by direct open reductions. The use of antibiotics to combat infections, improvements in general anesthetic agents and the techniques of their administration, and the improvement and intensification of graduate oral surgery training programs all contribute toward making such surgery safe and practical for both the patient and the surgeon. However, the practical methods that use extraoral traction to control some types of fractures in order to accomplish closed reductions should not become forgotten procedures (Fig. 19-26).

In the attempt to evaluate some of the differences in professional opinion regarding the management of jaw fractures, the primary contention appears to arise over the practice of frequent and sometimes extensive open approaches in the management of such fractures. Before a fracture is treated by either open or closed reduction, the following points should be taken into consideration: (1) The diagnosis and surgical management of such cases should be the responsibility of the surgeon who understands the growth and development of the jaws and the mixed and developing dentitions together with their related structures. (2) The gross stripping of periosteum from small bone fragments, especially in comminuted fractures of some thin membranous bones, to permit extensive open reductions may not necessarily be defensible surgical judgment. If satisfactory reposi-

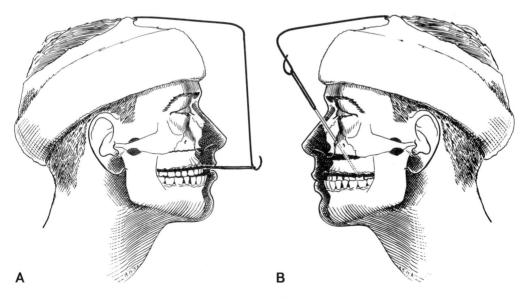

A **B**

Fig. 19-26. (A) Extraoral traction with head cap appliance. (B) Traction wire passed through cheek and attached to arch bar to improve fixation procedure.

tioning and alignment of fragments can be attained by closed reduction methods, the vascularity to these areas would be improved and the possibility of introducing infection and additional surgical trauma would be minimized. (3) Perhaps the most important factor to consider is the re-establishment of functional occlusion and satisfactory interarch relations.

The oral surgeon with his dental background should be the professional most adequately prepared to diagnose and treat such traumatic injuries of the jaws. However, patients with complicated facial injuries may also require additional medical consultation and care. In most dental and medical teaching centers where interprofessional teamwork is practiced, the management of such accident cases has taken on a reasonably routine aspect that tends toward improved patient care and better interprofessional respect and working relations. Improved intraprofessional as well as interprofessional communications are essential if we are to provide the best professional care available for patients with traumatic injuries to the face and jaws. It is generally recognized that in no other field is legal action so frequently taken as in the treatment of fractures. Fractures of the mandible and maxilla are no exception to this trend.

References

1. Kruger, G. O.: Oral Surgery. St. Louis, C. V. Mosby, 1969.
2. Major, G.: Fractures of the Jaws and Other Facial Bones. St. Louis, C. V. Mosby, 1940.
3. Irby, W. B., and Baldwin, K. H.: Emergencies and Urgent Complications in Dentistry. St. Louis, C. V. Mosby, 1968.
4. Rowe, N. L., and Killey, H. C.: Fractures of the Facial Skeleton. Baltimore, Williams & Wilkins, 1969.
5. Shires, G. S.: Care of the Trauma Patient. New York, McGraw-Hill, 1966.
6. Higley, L. B., Hixon, E. H., and Meredith, H. V.: Cephalometric growth study (1946–1960). University of Iowa, Department of Orthodontics. (More than 40 papers have been published on this research to date. Material is on file at the University of Iowa, in Child Behavior and Development. A follow-up study is still in progress.)
7. MacLennan, W. D.: Lecture delivered at the American Society of Oral Surgeons, Annual Scientific Session, Miami, Florida, 1957.
8. Hale, M. L.: Statistical research of 500 fractured jaw patients (1962). University of Iowa, University Hospitals.
9. Johnson, L.: Delivered at Armed Forces Institute of Pathology Seminar, Washington, D.C., 1957. (Unpublished)

20 Cysts of the Oral Cavity

DONALD R. MEHLISCH

A cyst is a pathologic space or sac usually containing fluid. Some have been found to be void; others contain soft tissue. Most lesions are uniform and consistent in their histologic features and are characterized by an epithelial lining of the lumen. Cysts of the oral regions may arise in any of the soft or hard tissues in the area of the mouth but are most frequently observed within the maxilla or mandible and quite commonly have several origins (Fig. 20-1). Some arise in association with the tooth or its primordium, the tooth germ. Others arise from the reduced enamel epithelium of a tooth crown, the epithelial rests of Malassez, or the remnants of the dental lamina. Still others arise from the extension of an inflammatory response in the pulpal tissues into the apical region and stimulate the residuals of Hertwig's sheath to proliferate. Another group may be due to embryonic inclusions and injury.

It is important for the clinician to have a working knowledge of basic principles of classification of benign cystic lesions in the oral cavity. Classifications originally were based upon clinical and roentgenographic features, but new findings and ideas regarding origin and growth have led to modifications. The classification devised by Killey and Kay, which has been modified after an example by Toller, will be used to guide our discussion.

I. Intraosseous cysts
   A. Odontogenic
      1. Apical
         a. Radicular
         b. Residual
         c. Lateral periodontal
      2. Follicular (dentigerous)
      3. Primordial
      4. Laminal (odontogenic keratocyst)
   B. Nonodontogenic
      1. Fissural
         a. Median alveolar
         b. Median mandibular
         c. Median palatal
         d. Globulomaxillary
      2. Vestigial
         a. Nasopalatine
   C. Nonepithelial bone cysts
      1. Solitary bone cyst
      2. Aneurysmal bone cyst
      3. Stafne's idiopathic bone cavity
II. Cysts of the soft tissues
   A. Salivary
   B. Gingival
   C. Dermoid
   D. Branchial
   E. Thyroglossal
   F. Nasolabial

317

Periodontal Cysts

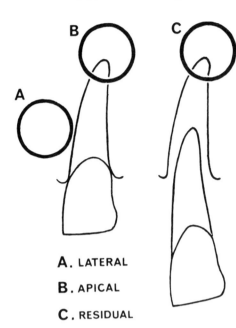

A. LATERAL

B. APICAL

C. RESIDUAL

Fissural Cysts

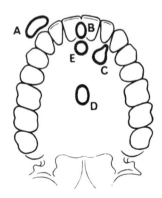

A. Nasolabial   C. Globulomaxillary
B. Median alveolar   D. Median palatal
E. Nasopalatine

DENTIGEROUS and PRIMORDIAL CYSTS

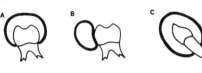

A. CORONAL
B. LATERAL
C. CIRCUMFERENTIAL
D. PRIMORDIAL

BONE CYSTS

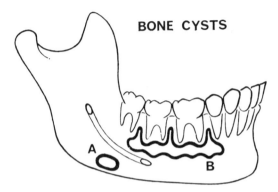

A. Stafne's Idiopathic Cavity

B. Solitary Bone Cyst

Fig. 20-1. Schematic drawings showing locations of cysts. (Killey, H. C., and Kay, L. W., courtesy of Int. Surg.)

and vary according to the particular stage at which the cystic change occurred. Inflammatory cysts result from infection extending from the pulp into surrounding periapical tissues.

Apical Cyst

RADICULAR CYST. *Incidence.* Of all cystic lesions in the jaws this is the most common and, therefore, the most common of all cysts of odontogenic origin. Males tend to be affected more than females, presumably because the latter are more conscious of appearance and seek attention sooner. This cyst is more frequently found in the maxilla than in the mandible (Fig. 20-2).

Intraosseous Cysts

Odontogenic Cysts

Odontogenic cysts originate developmentally or as a result of inflammation. The developmental cysts are those that form during the process of odontogenesis

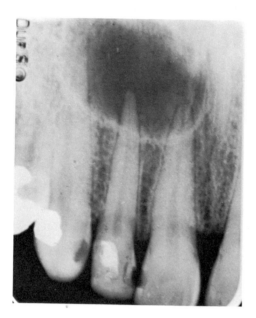

Fig. 20-2. Apical radicular cyst; lateral incisor does not respond to pulp testing. (Courtesy of Dr. D. E. Waite)

Etiology. Extension of inflammation into periapical tissues from the root canal forms a localized mass of chronic inflammatory granulation tissue, the apical granuloma. If the central cells degenerate due to inadequate blood supply, an epithelium-lined lumen results, the radicular cyst.

Features. Although often a painful condition initially as a result of inflammation, the cyst itself is frequently symptomless. The tooth in association with the cyst is nonvital. Generally, it does not grow to large dimensions and there is little if any expansion to the jaw. Radiographically, an area of translucency, which is often well circumscribed, exists at the root apex. The walls are of varying thickness, the lining of which may be smooth or

roughened. Contents consist of fluid or a rather thick cheese-like material. The cyst is lined by squamous epithelium with many processes penetrating into the underlying connective tissue. Chronic inflammatory infiltration of the cyst wall is usually well marked.

Treatment and Prognosis. The most commonly applied procedure is enucleation. Nonvital teeth that are associated should be treated by root canal and apicoectomy procedures or, if retention is not desirable, extracted. External sinus tracts must be excised. Marsupialization is indicated when there is a possibility of traumatic penetration of the maxillary sinus and the nose or involvement to some other structure such as the inferior alveolar nerve. Complete removal of the epithelial lining and elimination of the cause will be followed by bone deposition and resolution of the defect.

RESIDUAL CYST. When an apical cyst is overlooked after extraction of the causative tooth or root, it has the potential to enlarge and is called a residual cyst (Fig. 20-3).

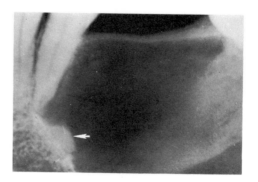

Fig. 20-3. Residual cyst originating from a root of a tooth previously extracted. (Courtesy of Dr. D. E. Waite)

Incidence. It is less common than the radicular cyst, as it most often is a missed radicular. Most patients are middle-aged or elderly and there is an equal sex predilection. The incidence is greater in the maxilla than in the mandible.

Etiology. The following causes have been given as probable ones:

1. It develops upon either a deciduous tooth or a retained root that later exfoliates or is extracted without knowledge of the underlying pathologic process.
2. If a tooth associated with a dentigerous cyst is removed but the cyst is unrecognized, the residual cyst will persist and increase in size.
3. Incomplete removal of a periapical cyst or granuloma.

Features. It is typically present in an edentulous area. The majority are asymptomatic and found on routine radiographic examination. Pathologic fracture or encroachment on associated structures may be the presenting symptoms. Histologically, it is like the underlying process that was initially present.

Treatment and Prognosis. The technique for removal is the same as that employed for an apical cyst, but it is important to preserve the contour of the edentulous ridge.

LATERAL PERIODONTAL CYST. These lateral inflammatory cysts must be distinguished from a minority of cysts which are developmental in character (Fig. 20-4).

Incidence. This is a rare but recognized entity. It is chiefly found in adults but is

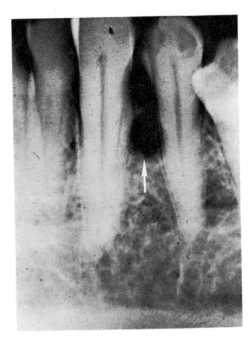

Fig. 20-4. Lateral periodontal cyst. (Courtesy of Dr. D. E. Waite)

of such rare occurrence that no significant conclusions can be drawn regarding specific age or sex. It occurs more often in the mandible than in the maxilla. Although found occasionally in the incisor region, it is most often related to the cuspid, bicuspid, or molar teeth.

Etiology. It appears to arise directly in the lateral periodontal membrane of an erupted tooth. Epithelial debris of Malassez in the periodontal membrane is suspected, but the stimulus for epithelial proliferation is undetermined.

Features. The majority of cases have no clinical signs or symptoms and, therefore, are discovered during routine roentgenographic examination. The associated teeth are vital. It may have a serous caseous content. This cyst usually has a wellformed stratified squamous epithelial lining, often keratinized. This is supported by a connective tissue wall that has a heavy inflammatory cell infiltration.

Treatment and Prognosis. Enucleation with preservation of the adjoining teeth is the procedure of choice. Diagnosis should be established due to similarity in appearance in an early stage between this cyst and other more serious lesions such as the ameloblastoma.

Follicular (Dentigerous) Cyst

DENTIGEROUS CYST. The occurrence of cystic change arising from the enamel organ after amelogenesis has been completed leads to the formation of a dentigerous cyst. There are three positional variations of cyst to tooth which are of much academic interest but little clinical significance. These include the *central or coronal type* which is most common. The *lateral type* is ascribed to activity in the lateral portion of the enamel organ. In the *circumferential dentigerous cyst*, the whole enamel organ around the neck of the tooth becomes cystic (Fig. 20-5).

Incidence. The dentigerous cyst is a far more common type of odontogenic cyst than the primordial but less common than the apical types. Incidence appears to be equal in the two sexes and the commonest age periods for diagnosis are childhood and adolescence, though sometimes they are found in adults. It occurs in the mandible more frequently than in the maxilla. Late erupting teeth are those frequently concerned in formation of a dentigerous cyst, and in descending order of importance are the lower third molar, upper cuspid, upper third molar, and lower bicuspid teeth.

Etiology. The cause is unknown, although two theories have been suggested

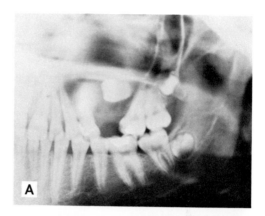

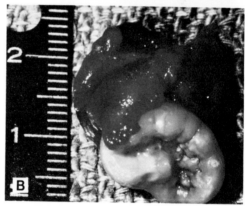

Fig. 20-5. (A) Radiograph of dentigerous cyst of maxilla. (B) Gross specimen of cyst with tooth.

which include perifollicular inflammation and retrograde changes in the stellate reticulum of the enamel organ. The cyst forms as a result of fluid collecting within the cell layers of the reduced enamel epithelium or between the crown and the enamel epithelium. Since the expanding cyst space is enveloped by a follicle, the term *follicular cyst* is sometimes substituted for its commoner counterpart.

Features. There is progressive enlargement of the jaw, though this is generally painless. Some degree of deformity may

along with the tooth of origin. It is widely held that ameloblastomas frequently arise in dentigerous cysts. Recurrence is a possibility if some epithelium remains.

Primordial Cyst

Cystic change that occurs in the enamel organ before the formation of calcified structures have developed results in the primordial cyst. Thus, this cyst is found in place of a tooth instead of associated with one (Fig. 20-6).

Incidence. This is the least common type of odontogenic cyst and perhaps accounts for 10 per cent of all epithelium-lined cysts of the jaws. The age of identification has ranged from the very young to the very old, but it is predominately found in the adolescent and young adult group with males and females affected equally. It is found most frequently in the mandibular third molar region but may arise elsewhere in the jaws.

Etiology. The stellate reticulum disintegrates to leave a cystic space bounded by the inner and outer enamel epithelium

result as the lesion is capable of much enlargement with concomitant destruction of the bone. Facial asymmetry may eventually induce the patient to request treatment. Pain may be a symptom if infection is superimposed. Those who wear dentures may have a sudden or gradual alteration in denture fit as the first intimation of the pathologic condition. Roentgenographic examination shows a well-defined translucency associated with the crown of an impacted or unerupted tooth. This is generally unilocular, but a multilocular effect can be present when the cyst is of irregular shape.

The cyst contents consist of clear yellowish fluid, in which cholesterol crystals may be present, or purulent material if infection has occurred. Mural thickenings may prove on microscopic investigation to be ameloblastic changes.

The cyst wall is composed of fibrous connective tissue in which the inflammatory infiltrate is usually minimal. The lining is stratified squamous epithelium, generally in a uniform thin layer, a few cells in depth. This cyst lining is seen to be continuous with the reduced enamel epithelium covering the crown. Occasionally, the epithelium is cornified.

Treatment and Prognosis. Treatment, to some degree, is dictated by the size of the lesion and whether or not it is desirable to save the involved tooth. If the tooth is to be maintained a Partsch-type procedure should be performed. Therefore, marsupialization as a method of treatment is strongly advocated in the child when the tooth and/or adjacent teeth are being prevented from assuming their normal positions in the arch. Alternatively, a dentigerous cyst should be carefully enucleated

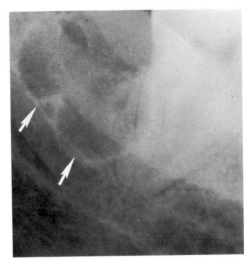

Fig. 20-6. Primordial cyst; no history of previous third molar removal. (Courtesy of Dr. D. E. Waite)

which becomes a stratified squamous epithelial lining. It may, therefore, take the place of a missing tooth or develop from the primordial cells of a supernumerary tooth.

Features. It is often asymptomatic until it reaches considerable size or becomes secondarily infected. There may be expansion of the jaw and displacement of neighboring teeth. Generally, the cyst does not reach as large or as expansile a size as does the dentigerous cyst, although it maintains the potential of displacing adjacent teeth by pressure.

A diagnostic feature of the primordial cyst observed at operation is the extreme thinness of the capsule when compared with other odontogenic cysts. The wall may be thickened by chronic infection.

It differs little in histologic appearance from the dentigerous cyst. Basal layers of the epithelium generally show a regular appearance without rete pegs or proliferation into the subjacent connective tissue. A thin layer of keratin is often present.

Treatment and Prognosis. Surgical removal by enucleation with thorough curettage of the bone and primary closure will render excellent long-term results and a recurrence rate that is negligible. Tendency to regrowth will follow marsupialization.

Laminal Cyst (Odontogenic Keratocyst)

Keratinization of the epithelial lining sometimes occurs in cysts of the jaws. For some time it was thought that this keratinization was not characteristic of any one particular type of odontogenic cyst, but rather it could be found in dental

cysts, either radicular, residual, dentigerous, and, indeed, in nonodontogenic inclusion cysts as well. It has now been well documented and proved that certain characteristic histologic features warrant consideration as a particular entity believed to be primordial in origin. This cyst is the odontogenic keratocyst.

Incidence. It comprises between 5 and 10 per cent of odontogenic cysts of the jaws. A relatively higher incidence in the second, third, and fourth decades of life is noted but it can occur in any age group. Slightly more males than females have been diagnosed. It has a strong predilection for the mandible and the most common site is the third molar region. In both the maxilla and mandible the majority of cysts occur posterior to the first bicuspids.

Etiology. Primordial cysts of the jaws are derived directly from the undifferentiated dental lamina. Thus, primordial cysts may develop from Serres' pearls, which are retained portions of the dental lamina, or from any suppressed tooth anlage, either from normal dentition or from a supernumerary tooth. Since almost all primordial cysts are keratinized, it has been assumed that keratocysts are actually primordial cysts.

Features. In approximately 50 per cent of cases there will be expansion of surrounding bone, not infrequently of both medial and lateral borders. Roentgenographic evidence of resorption of the roots of related teeth has also been shown. Recurrent inflammatory episodes in the region of a recently extracted tooth may be part of the clinical picture and help establish the diagnosis. Less common features include numbness of the lower lip on the related side. Other abnormalities may be associated and give consideration for the diagnosis of multiple basal cell nevi syndrome.

The cyst wall and lining are usually smooth and somewhat thinned. Occasional small projections of granulation tissue may be present. Not infrequently, bony septa divide the lining into loculations, and in multilocular lesions separate cyst cavities may be present. Cortical bone may be quite thin or perforated by the cyst.

Usually, the epithelium consists of five or ten rows of cells with an accentuated basal layer and occasionally vacuolated cells in the spinal cell layers. Rete pegs are rarely seen. Frank atypia (dysplasia) may characterize a basal cell hyperplasia, and increased mitotic activity may be seen.

Treatment and Prognosis. It is of surgical interest that keratocysts seem to have a pronounced tendency to recur. Recurrences may be over 50 per cent in some cases and there may be repeated recurrences. Recurrences may be due to daughter-cyst formation of the cyst wall or to the proliferation of the cyst epithelium into connective tissue that has been left behind after enucleation of the delicate cyst membrane. Treatment is by complete enucleation of the cyst and to be even more careful in removal of the cyst lining in keratocysts than in unkeratinized cysts. Aspiration of the cyst contents may prove to be an important aid in the diagnosis of the odontogenic keratocyst. The fluid removed shows a markedly reduced content of soluble protein when compared with serum from the patient. Therefore, electrophoresis of the cyst contents appears to be a valuable preoperative method of distinguishing the odontogenic keratocyst from other odontogenic cysts.

Nonodontogenic Cysts

Fissural Cyst

Cysts classified as fissural are believed to arise from remnants of the epithelium that covered the developing facial processes during the embryonic period of life. Various factors have been postulated suggesting the origin. These include epithelial entrapments in the lines of closure of the processes, which perhaps give rise to cleft palate and cleft lip as well.

MEDIAN ALVEOLAR CYST. *Incidence.* This cyst is relatively uncommon. However, it is more common in the maxilla than in the mandible. No conclusive statements can be made concerning incidence in males or females or in specific age groups. It is generally located in the midline of the maxilla just lingual and superior to the apices of the central incisor teeth.

Etiology. It arises from either vestigial epithelial structures or epithelial debris of embryogenesis which remains in suture lines.

Features. The median alveolar cyst is frequently asymptomatic until extremely large swelling causes expansion of bone or it becomes secondarily infected. Clinically, swelling may appear labially or immediately behind the palatal surfaces of the central incisors but the teeth remain vital.

As that of other cysts of this region, the character of the fibrous connective tissue wall varies with the age of the lesion and the amount of secondary infection.

The lumen of the cyst may be lined with either a stratified squamous epithelium or ciliated columnar epithelium (respiratory-type), depending upon whether the source of the enclaved epithelial remnants is oral or nasal in origin. On occasion, the epithelium may actively proliferate to produce bizarre patterns.

Treatment and Prognosis. Treatment of all fissural cysts is essentially the same, that is, enucleation of the cyst without disturbing the teeth in the area. Primary closure is used and a palatal splint may be helpful.

MEDIAN MANDIBULAR CYST. *Incidence.* This cyst is rare and only a few examples have been recorded. It is certainly less common than the other fissural cysts. There is no distinctive distribution between the sexes. It is found symmetrically in the midline of the mandible (Fig. 20-7).

Etiology. It arises from epithelial inclusions in the area of the symphysis, or from the enamel organ of supernumerary tooth germs. The epithelium proliferates and then becomes cystic. Inflammation and trauma may be considered as factors in the development of this lesion, as well as in all other fissural cysts.

Features. This cyst remains relatively small (1 to 3 cm. in size) and is therefore usually discovered on roentgenographic examination. There may be a detectable swelling in the labial sulcus. Although it appears to involve the apices of adjoining teeth, which may be in close relationship with the inclusion cyst, the lamina dura remains intact and the teeth are vital. It has a well-defined but variable shape, being ovoid, circular, or irregular. The cyst lining consists of stratified squamous epithelium. The wall is comprised of fibrous connective tissue which usually reveals little or no evidence of an inflammatory response.

Treatment and Prognosis. Treatment is careful enucleation without involvement of the apices of the incisors. Teeth that have had some divergence of the roots from the cyst may gradually improve their positions.

MEDIAN PALATAL CYST. *Incidence.* This cyst is rare and occurs mainly in adults of

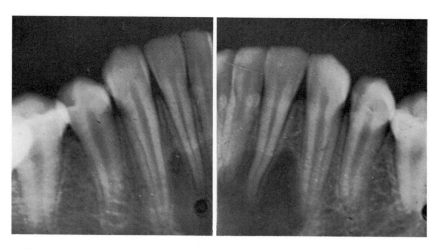

Fig. 20-7. Median mandibular cyst; all teeth are vital. (Courtesy of Dr. D. E. Waite)

either sex in the midline of the maxillary alveolus or the hard palate, between the lateral palatal processes. Generally it is present between the incisive fossa and the posterior border of the hard palate.

Etiology. It arises from the epithelial rests in the suture line, and is probably the result of inflammation or trauma. It has been suggested that this cyst is probably a nasopalatine cyst which has extended backward into the palate.

Features. There is no clinical evidence unless it becomes extremely large and causes expansion of surrounding bone with palpable swelling. It is well-defined, ovoid in outline, and essentially appears the same as the median alveolar cyst. The cyst is lined by stratified squamous or ciliated columnar epithelium. There may be some chronic inflammatory infiltration in the subepithelial connective tissue.

Treatment and Prognosis. Treatment and prognosis are the same as for median alveolar cysts.

GLOBULOMAXILLARY CYST. The term globulomaxillary cyst is really no longer appropriate, since the globular process is now referred to as the premaxillary process in embryologic terminology. However, the term lateral fissural cyst, which has been proposed as an alternative designation, has not gained general acceptance (Fig. 20-8).

Incidence. It is uncommon, appearing in adults of either sex. The cyst forms at the junction of the globular portion of the medial nasal process with the maxillary process (between lateral incisor and cuspid teeth).

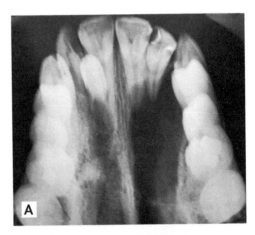
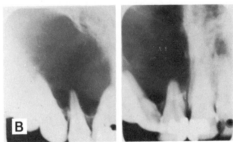

Fig. 20-8. Globulomaxillary cyst. (A) Occlusal view. (B) Periapical view. (Courtesy of Dr. D. E. Waite)

Etiology. The conventional view is that the cyst develops from residual epithelium in the areas of contact of the globular process of the frontonasal bone with the adjacent maxillary processes of palatine bones. These can be visualized as two upright triangular plates, which angulate posteriorly to join each other immediately behind the upper central incisor teeth.

Features. It is possible to make a presumptive diagnosis of the globulomaxillary cyst if the lateral and cuspid teeth are tilted together coronally, and each tooth gives a normal response to pulp testing. Roentgenographically, it appears as a

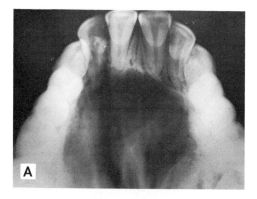

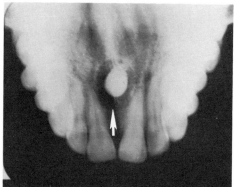

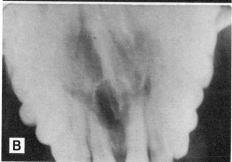

Fig. 20-9. Nasopalatine cyst. (A) Occlusal view. (B) Lipiodol indicates the internal cyst size and the thickness of the nasopalatine cyst wall. (Courtesy of Dr. D. E. Waite)

pear-shaped radiolucent lesion with a prominent cortical margin and with the lamina dura of adjoining teeth preserved.

When the cyst is small it is spherical in shape. With elongation, it ultimately resembles an inverted pear with the inferior, narrow V-shaped end extending into the interdental bone, and it may even reach the alveolar crest.

The epithelial lining of the cyst is more often from the nasal mucosa than from the oral covering; hence, it is pseudostratified columnar ciliated epithelium, or some modification thereof. The wall is usually thick with scattered lymphocytes and plasma cells concentrated along the lining.

Treatment and Prognosis. Enucleation, whenever possible, is the treatment of choice. However, if the lesion is extremely large, it may be prudent to perform a preliminary marsupialization to allow decompression and some bone regeneration. This should be followed by enucleation and primary closure to accelerate the healing process and reduce the risk of a residual defect.

Vestigial Cyst

NASOPALATINE CYST. The generic term nasopalatine cyst refers to both the cyst of the incisive canal and that designated the cyst of the palatine papilla. Distinction between these two is based on whether the lesion is intraosseous or located solely within the soft tissues in the region of the papilla. The nasopalatine duct connects the oral and nasal cavities in many mammals, and in the embryonic stage of the human. Cyst formation may occur from the epithelial remnants of the ducts that normally persist in the adult. Those cysts forming either within the palatine papilla or in the incisive canal will be considered together (Fig. 20-9).

Incidence. Asymptomatic cysts of this type have been found in 1 per cent of persons on roentgenographic survey. One out of every 66 cadaver specimens examined in another study had identifiable incisive canal cysts. This is the most common type of maxillary developmental or fissural cyst. It is predominantly found in adulthood with no apparent sex distribution. The cyst may arise at any point along the canal, but most originate in the lower portion of the maxilla between the apices of the central incisors.

Etiology. In the embryo, two wide tracts, the nasopalatine ducts, extend between the nasal and oral cavities. They do not normally persist as such into adult life, although some portion of these pathways may frequently remain. Cysts arise from the epithelial debris of these vestigial nasopalatine ducts.

Features. The majority remain asymptomatic and even those that demonstrate insidious symptoms follow no consistent pattern. The most frequent complaint is a lump in the midline of the palate anteriorly, and on palpation the cyst is usually fluctuant. Infection may be responsible for a pronounced swelling of the palatal soft tissues which occurs secondarily. There may be pain, which is either well localized or neuralgic in character, radiating to the side of the nose or the eyes. Adjacent teeth should be normal in color and nonsensitive to percussion, but a periapical condition should be ruled out with the aid of vitality testing.

There is a well-defined cyst outline situated apparently between or above the roots of the maxillary central incisor teeth and may be bilateral, giving the characteristic heart shape. However, it can be round or ovoid.

The presence of mucous glands in the walls of the cyst is highly indicative of their origin within the incisive canal. The cysts are usually lined with a modified-type or respiratory epithelium, although cysts of the papillae may be partly lined by squamous epithelium. Unexpected diversions from this descending pattern in epithelial type may be due to metaplastic transformation. Cartilage may also be identified in the wall of the cyst and incorporated as part of the specimen.

Treatment and Prognosis. When there is irrefutable clinical evidence of an incisive canal cyst with or without abnormal roentgenographic enlargement of the fossa, surgical removal should be instituted, which is usually adequate. Several cases of adenocystic carcinoma have been reported developing in the glands in the cyst wall and should be considered in the differential diagnosis.

Nonepithelial Bone Cysts

Solitary Bone Cyst

The solitary bone cyst occurs most often elsewhere in the body, principally the upper part of the diaphysis of the humerus and other long bones. It is an unusual lesion which appears with disturbing frequency and has been termed hemorrhagic bone cyst, extravasation cyst, and progressive bone cavity. The term "cyst" in relation to this lesion is controversial and probably a misnomer (Fig. 20-10).

Incidence. It is relatively common during the first two decades of life. The relative infrequence of this lesion in later decades of life has given speculation that the cavities tend to undergo a natural

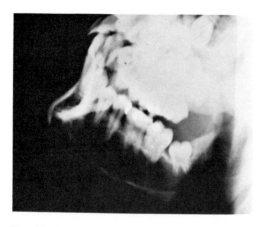

Fig. 20-10. Radiograph of solitary bone cyst.

cure. Lesions occur particularly in children and adolescents between 10 and 20 years of age. Males are affected more often than females, probably because of an increased exposure to traumatic injuries. The majority are located in the subapical region of the posterior portion of the mandible between the cuspid and the third molar. It is this area in which the marrow cavity of the jaw is situated in young persons. Occasionally, a lesion may develop in the incisor region.

Etiology. The cause and mode of formation of solitary bone cysts are still unknown, but a number of theories have been given. These include (1) trauma and hemorrhage with failure of organization, (2) spontaneous atrophy of the tissue in a central benign giant-cell lesion, (3) abnormal calcium metabolism, (4) chronic low-grade infection, and (5) necrosis of fatty marrow secondary to ischemia. There is little positive evidence to support these theories, and perhaps the best explanation is that, relative to cysts in all locations, it represents the results of an aberration in the development and growth of the local osseous tissue.

Features. The condition is usually symptomless and frequently discovered accidently on routine roentgenography.

There is often a history of trauma to the jaw though it is not always recent. Expansion of the bone is not common but may occur. Teeth that may be associated with the cyst retain their vitality and are not loosened despite extensions of the cyst into the surrounding bony spaces.

Surgical exploration reveals a space in the bone that contains a little clear or perhaps blood-stained fluid, shreds of necrotic blood clot, a thin connective tissue membrane lining, or nothing. Accordingly, the material available for pathologic examination comprises simply a mass of bone fragments, blood clot, and small scraps of soft tissue.

Treatment and Prognosis. Surgical exploration of the area is required for diagnosis and usually constitutes treatment. Any cyst lining should be enucleated and the area curetted. Curettage should stimulate hemorrhage which results in rapid obliteration of the defect and eventually healing by new bone formation.

Aneurysmal Bone Cyst

The aneurysmal bone cyst was first described and characterized as such by Jaffe and Lichtenstein in 1942. It occurs most often in long bones and the vertebral column. It may occur in other bones but is rare in the jaws. Previously, it has been described under such terms as hemorrhagic osteomyelitis, ossifying hematoma, osteitis fibrosa cystica, and aneurysmal giant-cell tumor.

Incidence. It is rare and reports of lesions in the jaws are limited but cases have been described. The abnormality occurs mainly in children, adolescents, or young adults with an overwhelming majority in those under 20 years of age. There is no marked sex predominance. The mandible is generally affected, but the lesion may also occur in the maxilla.

Etiology. Factors that may cause an aneurysmal bone cyst are still unknown. Even though a history of trauma is often obtained, it is not certain that it can be directly related to the development of this lesion. A possible relationship with the giant-cell lesion has been postulated. Another widely accepted theory is that the condition is caused by some variation in the hemodynamics or vascular supply of the area. This lesion has no relationship to the solitary bone cyst and it occurs in bone that has previously been apparently normal.

Features. Pain is not a feature with lesions in the mandible or maxilla, as is frequently the case in other bones that are involved. There is a firm enlargement of the jaw that may be tender. Characteristically, this benign solitary lesion causes local expansion, but the growth is not infiltrative and a thin layer of overlying subperiosteal new bone is preserved in most cases. The soap-bubble appearance seen roentgenographically in long bones is not evident in the jaw lesions. Instead, a radiolucent expansile lesion which may destroy the cortical plate is seen.

The lesion is soft, fusiform or round in shape, tender, of firm or springy consistency, and contains numerous blood-filled spaces. Resultant bleeding is a persistent ooze which may be difficult to control, rather than a sudden spurting or vigorous free hemorrhage.

The area involved by the lesion is honeycombed and consists of numerous blood-filled spaces lined by a single layer of compressed flattened cells and giant cells. The intervening septa and stroma consist of young fibroblasts, giant cells, blood vessels, and foci of hemosiderin. In general, it is similar to that of the peripheral and central giant-cell reparative granulomas.

Treatment and Prognosis. The lesion is amenable to treatment by curettage or surgical enucleation and this is the method of choice in a surgically accessible lesion. Recurrence may follow inadequate removal and require additional therapy.

Stafne's Idiopathic Bone Cavity

Stafne's idiopathic bone cavities can be mistaken for cysts in the mandible. Although not actually cysts of the jaw, they have been included because of their clinical and roentgenologic similarity to the cystic lesions that have been discussed. This similarity frequently presents a problem in differential diagnosis (Fig. 20-11).

Incidence. It is relatively uncommon, with the largest series of cases reported by the author for whom the lesion is named. Few defects have been observed in children and no sex distinction has been suggested. It is consistently situated beneath

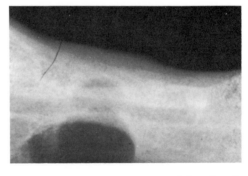

Fig. 20-11. Stafne's latent bone cyst, below the inferior alveolar canal. (Courtesy of Dr. D. E. Waite)

the mandibular canal and adjacent to the lower border of the jaw between the bicuspid region and the angle.

Etiology. The cause is unknown but several plausible theories have been suggested. Stafne believed that such cavities might arise during development of the jaws by failure of the normal deposition of bone in an area formerly occupied by cartilage or by failure of subperiosteal apposition at the lower border. Other theories suggest that the cavities might be constricted remains of solitary bone cysts, an eosinophilic granuloma, or embryonic defects.

Features. This is a symptomless lesion discovered during routine roentgenography in which it appears as a round or oval radiolucent defect. The area of rarefaction is well demarcated by a dense radiopaque line. Sometimes the lesion extends from cancellous tissue into cortical bone and may perforate the inferior margin of the body of the mandible. Cavities may vary between 1 and 3 cm. in diameter. Generally, there are constancy of position, uniform appearance, failure to change with time, and an occasional bilateral occurrence. All these factors strongly favor a developmental origin.

Since these are idiopathic bone cavities no diagnostic tissue can be mentioned. These cavities may, in fact, be empty. Contrary, they may contain normal salivary gland tissue, lymph node tissue, or abnormal glandular tissue. Published reports have stated that the outer plate was thin and that perforations had occurred along the inner cortical plate.

Treatment and Prognosis. In view of the fact that the lesions are symptomless and nonprogressive, surgical exploration is hard to justify. Apart from the diagnostic problem the lesions present, these idiopathic cavities are of no particular concern. They are nonpathogenic and require

essentially no treatment, although regular follow-up roentgenographs should be taken. This defect in the mandible may constitute a point of weakness and pathologic fracture may occur.

Cysts of the Soft Tissues

Salivary Gland Cyst

Salivary glands of the oral regions may give rise to small cysts in connection with the complex ductal system and may be found anywhere in the oral submucosa. Any disruption of the flow of salivary secretions may result in retention of fluid, which will produce the lesion.

Incidence. The salivary gland cyst is common in connection with the minor salivary glands, but has no predilection for age or sex. Common sites are the lips, cheeks, undersurface of the tip of the tongue, and the floor of the mouth (ranula). With the exception of the anterior half of the hard palate which is devoid of salivary glands, it can occur anywhere in the oral cavity.

Etiology. Origin is probably dual in nature. First, cyst formation may result from trauma to the ducts of mucous glands with escape of secretions into the surrounding connective tissue. Second, retention of the secretion results in dilatation of the duct system, and an epithelium-lined cyst.

Features. It appears as a small, circumscribed, usually elevated, translucent, bluish lesion on the mucosa. Spontaneous rupture often occurs, with the liberation of a viscous fluid. In the course of a few weeks or perhaps longer, additional fluid may accumulate and the lesion reappears. This cycle of rupture, collapse of the cyst, and refilling may continue for months.

Early lesions may not have a definite cystic cavity. A fully developed one consists of a cystic cavity filled with a lightly basophilic homogeneous material. The cyst-like space is lined by a thin layer of flattened cells that may resemble an epithelial lining, but which are in fact compressed connective tissue cells. In some cases only granulation tissue is present and no lining is seen.

Treatment and Prognosis. Salivary gland cysts are treated by surgical excision, together with the associated salivary tissue. If the cyst is due to a defect in the duct and close to the mucosal surface, a Partsch procedure may be indicated. Recurrence following excision is occasionally seen but becomes less likely if the associated salivary gland acini are also removed.

Gingival Cyst

Gingival cysts may not be deserving of a specific category and should not be confused with eruption cysts. The only specific criterion for the lesion is its location in the gingival tissues.

Incidence. It is relatively rare and of infrequent occurrence. It is found in infants and adults, with the largest incidence in the sixth decade. There is no sex predilection. It appears particularly in the cuspid and bicuspid areas of the mandible but occasionally in the anterior part of the jaw. Mandibular gingival tissues are involved twice as frequently as are the maxillary gingival tissues.

Etiology. Causation is obscure but the possible mechanisms by which the cyst may form are (1) traumatic implantation of epithelium, (2) surface epithelium that proliferates in a down-growing manner and undergoes cystic changes, or (3) dental lamina remnants, enamel organ or epithelial islands from the surface epithelium.

Features. It is a slowly growing and circumscribed swelling of the gingivae, which is usually radiolucent. Occasionally, large lesions occur and pressure may cause erosion of the adjacent cortical plate of bone. The lesion is lined by stratified squamous epithelium, the periepithelial collagen being free of inflammatory cells.

Treatment and Prognosis. Surgical excision is almost always curative.

Dermoid Cyst
(Dermoid Inclusion Cyst)

The dermoid cyst is similar to the epidermal or epidermoid cyst, but with the addition of skin appendages such as hair, sebaceous glands, or teeth. It is, therefore, a form of cystic teratoma. In the oral regions the term *dermoid inclusion cyst* is used to indicate a lesion derived from ectoderm only. Because of the differences in histogenesis and clinical significance, distinction between the dermoid cyst and dermoid inclusion cyst needs to be made (Fig. 20-12).

Incidence. The dermoid cyst is uncommon. The majority occur in young adulthood and show no sex predilection. The

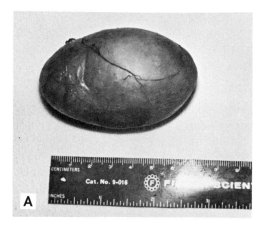

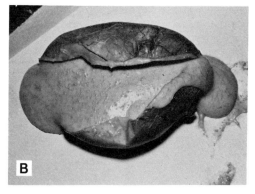

Fig. 20-12. (A) Gross specimen of dermoid inclusion cyst. (B) Gross specimen of dermoid inclusion cyst cut.

floor of the mouth and submandibular and sublingual regions are the most common sites.

Etiology. The dermoid cyst is thought to arise from epithelial rests persisting in the midline after fusion of the mandible and hyoid branchial arches. The dermoid inclusion cyst is derived from ectoderm only and capable of producing epidermoid tissue. The dermoid cyst, on the other hand, is derived from primordial germ cells and is comprised of a combination of ectodermal, mesodermal, and endodermal elements. In approximately 5 per cent of cases, one of the tissue elements in the dermoid cyst becomes malignant. The importance of the distinction between these two cysts, therefore, is significant.

Features. The typical lesion produces a bulge in the floor of the mouth if it is above the geniohyoid muscle and may become large enough to elevate the tongue, causing difficulty with mastication and speech. Cysts inferior to the geniohyoid muscle and above the mylohyoid muscle produce a submental swelling. This cyst may also arise below the mylohyoid muscle. Typically, there is a "dough-like" feel on palpation of the lesion. The cysts vary in size but generally approach several centimeters in diameter.

Microscopically, dermoid inclusion cysts are lined by keratinizing stratified squamous epithelium and contain keratin scales and sebaceous material. Sebaceous glands, sweat glands, and hair follicles may be found in the cyst wall and occasionally other structures are also present.

Treatment and Prognosis. Complete excision is curative treatment for such lesions.

Branchial Cleft Cyst

Branchial arch remnants may give rise to a lesion in the lateral aspect of the neck in the form of a fistula or cyst.

Incidence. This is not a common lesion overall; however, 10 to 15 per cent are seen at the angle of the mandible. Patients are most frequently young adults between 20 and 40 years of age. They do occur in children, but usually after sexual maturity. There is no known sex preference. It usually occurs on the lateral side of the neck, but some are seen at the angle of the mandible. Rarely, a branchial cyst may occur in the floor of the mouth.

Etiology. This cyst may arise from ectodermal or endodermal remnants associated with the branchial arches, usually between the second and third. It has also been shown to obtain histogenesis from residual cervical sinus epithelium or epithelial inclusions within lymph nodes in the region.

Features. It presents as a soft fluctuant mass that historically appears in the lateral aspects of the neck anterior to the sternocleidomastoid muscle or may involve the parotid region. It may slowly increase in size and may also develop a fistulous tract. The tract will drain externally in most cases; however, on rare instances it will drain intraorally.

Microscopic sections of superficial lesions reveal cysts that are usually lined by stratified squamous epithelium and contain a watery fluid. Lymphoid tissue may surround the cyst and show all the characteristics of a lymph node. Lesions located in the deeper structures of the neck are lined by pseudostratified columnar epithelium, and beneath the epithelium there is a dense infiltrate of lymphocytic cells which frequently contain well-developed germinal centers. In a deeper lesion the lumen may contain a great deal of mucus instead of the watery fluid.

Treatment and Prognosis. If these lesions are aspirated or drained, they will recur because the cyst itself has not been removed and will persist. The lesion is best treated by complete surgical removal.

Thyroglossal Duct Cyst

The thyroglossal duct cyst is an uncommon developmental cyst which can occur anywhere along the course of the embryonic thyroglossal duct, which extends from the foramen cecum of the tongue into the deep fascia near the thyroid isthmus.

Incidence. It is relatively rare and there are no significant data on age or sex predilection. As stated, it can occur anywhere along the course of the thyroglossal duct, the commonest area of involvement, however, being close to the hyoid bone in the midline. It may also be found beneath the foramen cecum in the musculature of the tongue.

Etiology. The thyroid gland rudiment appears during the fourth embryonic week between the derivatives of the first and second branchial arches that, in part, form the tongue. A hollow stalk, the thyroglossal duct, extends from the foramen cecum in the base of the tongue down through the neck to the thyroid gland. By about the tenth week this duct breaks up and disappears, but cysts may form from residues of this duct.

Features. It appears as a soft fluctuant mass unattached to the surrounding tissues unless fistulous tracts develop, which occurs in approximately 25 per cent of cases. Dysphagia may be the initial symptom but usually the cyst is painless and varies from 1 to 5 cm. in diameter.

Cysts occurring above the level of the hyoid bone are lined by stratified squamous epithelium and those below this level by ciliated respiratory-type or columnar epithelium. However, the histologic pattern is variable and a single cyst may show different types of epithelium from one area to another.

Treatment and Prognosis. Complete surgical removal of the cyst with its tract is essential to prevent recurrence. Because of the relationship to the hyoid bone this bone may need to be divided during surgery.

Nasolabial Cyst

The nasolabial cyst is strictly a soft tissue lesion and does not occur within bone. Its inclusion in certain classifications with fissural cysts of the jaws has been a convenient and accepted practice. Alternative designations of naso-extra-alveolar cyst, nasal vestibule cyst, nasal wing cyst, and mucoid cyst of the nose have been used (Fig. 20-13).

Incidence. The condition is uncommon with less than 200 cases reported in the literature. It is found in the young and the elderly but most are in persons in the third, fourth, and fifth decades. An overwhelming majority of cases reported have occurred in females, almost 80 per cent. Cysts of this type develop at the junction of the globular, the lateral nasal, and the maxillary processes. There is no predilection for one side of the midline or the other. In fact, 12 per cent of cases will be bilateral, and in these the female again is affected most frequently.

Etiology. These lesions are thought to arise from epithelium of the embryonal clefts of the face at the point where the maxillary, the median nasal, and the lateral nasal processes fuse. The frequency of bilateral cysts seems too high to be accounted for by possible external etiologic factors, and helps substantiate the theories advancing developmental disturbances as the cause of nasolabial cysts.

Features. This lesion produces a visible external swelling of the lip, can displace the ala cartilage, may distort the shape of the nose, and may obliterate the nasolabial fold. Swelling is mentioned as the chief complaint in 60 per cent of cases and upward extension into the nasal vestibule may cause eventual obstruction of the airway, interfering with breathing. Protrusion downward between the lip and alveolus may allow palpation of the lower border of the cyst in the labial vestibule. Since the cyst occurs in soft tissue only, it is not visible roentgenographically unless it has caused some resorption of the maxilla by pressure, as occasionally occurs.

The cyst usually lies just beneath the epithelium of a thin layer of condensed connective tissue that contains only a few vessels and fibroblasts. The connective tissue capsule is lined by stratified squamous or columnar epithelium and the cyst contains straw-colored mucinous fluid.

Treatment and Prognosis. Treatment of the nasolabial cyst is surgical removal from an intraoral approach. The operation can be complicated by perforation of the nasal mucosa and great care needs to be taken when separating the cyst lining from the surrounding mucosa. This will be more difficult if the cyst has previously drained into the nose, and sometimes the sac is firmly attached to the margin of the ala.

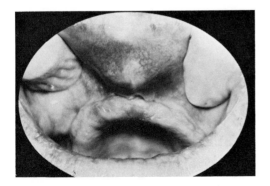

Fig. 20-13. Inflammatory (nasolabial) cyst.

General Principles of Treatment of Cysts of the Oral Cavity

Obvious reasons exist for treatment of benign cysts of the oral cavity. Foremost, cysts increase in size and have a tendency to become infected. Their location in the jaw also constitutes an area of weakness which may cause a pathologic fracture. Further, it is not possible to be certain of the benign nature of a cystic lesion until it has been explored surgically and examined histologically.

The treatment of benign cysts of the oral cavity is predominantly surgical, and there are two basic types of operative procedures: (1) enucleation and (2) marsupialization.

Enucleation

Enucleation allows for the opening to the cyst cavity to be covered by a mucoperiosteal flap and the space filled with blood clot which will eventually organize and form normal bone. Undoubtedly this is the most satisfactory method of treatment of a cyst. In many instances a window in the bone will already exist from expansion of the cyst. However, if the bone covering the cyst remains intact, a window will be necessary, and this can be made through the cortical plate using either mallet and chisel or bone burs. Rongeurs are helpful in enlargement of the opening and are less likely to puncture or tear the cyst wall, which should remain intact. The margins of the cyst are easier to define if the membrane is not ruptured, and enucleation is simplified because the lining can be separated more readily from the bony cavity if the fluid content re-

mains compressed. Curettes and small periosteal elevators can be used to thoroughly strip the cyst from its bony walls. After the cyst lining has been removed, the bony defect should be thoroughly inspected and the surface dried. The empty cyst cavity should then be gently irrigated with warm saline solution and the flap sutured back into position.

In some extensive lesions a biopsy may be indicated. At the time of opening, overlapping or excessive tissue is trimmed away from the buccal mucoperiosteal flap. The remainder of the flap is then turned into the cavity to cover part of the bare area of bone and packed with iodoform gauze dressing. This procedure will collapse the body of the cyst but permit filling of the cystic space by compression from the formation of new bone external to the cyst. When sufficient bone has formed, the entire cyst should be enucleated and primary closure effected.

Marsupialization (Partsch Operation)

Marsupialization of cysts consists of surgically producing a window by removing a generous section of the overlying mucoperiosteum, bone, and adjacent cyst wall to decrease intracystic tension. The border of the incised mucosa is then sutured to the border of the cyst wall that has been cut completely around its circumference. After this procedure, the cystic cavity should slowly decrease in size. Ideally the window should be as large as possible, because if the diameter of the opening is small, continuity of the cyst membrane may be re-established and the cyst will refill and expand again.

In general, marsupialization, or the Partsch operation, of cysts within the jaws should be avoided. The marsupialization method is indicated when a cyst is too large to enucleate with safety, to avoid devitalizing involved teeth, or if it is anticipated that unerupted teeth in a dentigerous cyst will erupt into position. In the case of fissural cysts, marsupialization is an unsatisfactory procedure because obliteration of the cavity does not occur. Another disadvantage to consider is that only a small portion of the cyst membrane can be submitted for biopsy examination, in contrast with the complete specimen that is obtained by extirpation.

Vitality of Teeth

Regardless of the method of treatment employed, it is essential to perform routine preoperative and postoperative vitality tests on all teeth related to the cyst.

Aspiration

Aspiration of a suspected cyst can be a valuable diagnostic aid, especially when doubt still exists about the nature of the lesion after careful clinical and roentgenographic examination. This investigation is helpful in distinguishing between a maxillary cyst and the maxillary sinus. If it is impossible to withdraw the plunger of the syringe during attempted aspiration, a solid lesion should be considered. The presence of blood under considerable pressure in a suspected cystic formation is probably indicative of the existence of an aneurysmal bone cyst, whereas in a central cavernous hemangioma the pressure of the blood is considerably less marked.

In the case of a solitary bone cyst, either a minute quantity of serous or sanguineous liquid is aspirated or the cavity is found to be devoid of fluid.

Infected cysts will usually contain pus as well as normal cyst fluid. After longstanding infection the cyst is likely to contain a thick, semisolid mass of pus together with cholesterol crystals which cannot be aspirated.

Complications

FRACTURE. Although relatively rare, a pathologic or spontaneous fracture can occur as a result of cyst formation. The presence of a cystic lesion in the mandible weakens the bone, and a fracture may occur from comparatively minor trauma. Occasionally, an undiagnosed cyst may become so large that a fracture may occur during normal mastication. When the traumatic fracture of a cystic area does occur management may become a problem. The cyst must be completely removed and the fracture parts reduced and immobilized. A small cyst of the mandible will usually leave sufficient bone on either side of the fracture line to ensure an area of contact sufficient for healing. However, when the cyst is extremely large, as it usually is in pathologic fractures, so much bone may have been destroyed that little remains in apposition across the fracture line after the fragments are reduced, and therefore satisfactory resolution is less likely to occur at the fracture site. Replacement of the missing portion of bone by a bone graft may be necessary.

INFECTION. Two-stage treatment of this problem may be necessary. First, control the infection, and second, render definitive surgery to eradicate the cyst. The infection will probably require establishment of drainage and use of antibiotics. Chronically infected cysts may be removed without initial drainage since localization of the infection exists. Antibiotic coverage is indicated. Postoperative infections should be controlled locally by irrigations, iodoform packing of the bone cavity, and use of systemic antibiotics. Bone cavities that remain open must be irrigated frequently to prevent accumulation of food and debris until healing by secondary intention is complete.

Selected Reading

Bhaskar, S. N.: Synopsis of Oral Pathology, 3rd ed. St. Louis, C. V. Mosby, 1969.

Browne, R. M.: The odontogenic keratocyst., Br. Dent. J., *128*:225–231, 1970

Colby, R. A., Kerr, D. A., and Robinson, H. G.: Color Atlas of Oral Pathology, 3rd ed. Philadelphia, J. B. Lippincott, 1971.

Dahlin, D. C.: Bone Tumors, 2nd ed. Springfield, Charles C Thomas, 1967.

Ferenczy, K.: The relationship of globulomaxillary cysts to the fusion of embryonal processes and to cleft palates. Oral Surg., *11*:1388, 1958.

Gorlin, R. J.: Potentialities of oral epithelium manifest by mandibular dentigerous cysts. Oral Surg., *10*:271–284, 1957.

Hayward, J. R.: Dentigerous cysts. Am. J. Orthod., *32*:140, 1946.

Jaffe, H. L.: Giant-cell reparative granuloma, traumatic bone cyst, and fibrous (fibro-osseous) dysplasia of the jawbones. Oral Surg., *6*:159, 1953.

Killey, H. C., and Kay, L. W.: An analysis of 471 benign cystic lesions of the jaws. Int. Surg., *46*:540–545, 1966.

Robinson, H. B. G.: Classification of cysts of the jaws. Am. J. Orthod., *31*:370, 1945.

Shafer, W. G., Hine, M. K., and Levy, B. M.: A Textbook of Oral Pathology, 2nd ed. Philadelphia, W. B. Saunders, 1963.

Thoma, K. H.: Diagnosis and treatment of odontogenic and fissural cysts. Oral Surg., *3*:961, 1950.

Thoma, K. H.: Oral Pathology, 4th ed. St. Louis, C V. Mosby Co., 1954.

Tiecke, R. W.: Oral Pathology. New York, McGraw-Hill, 1965.

21 Tumors of the Oral Cavity

DONALD R. MEHLISCH

This account of lesions of the oral tissues is directed especially to the student of dentistry and the general dental practitioner. For the most part, it is concerned with benign tumors involving tissues that are observed frequently in the course of care rendered to every patient seen in the dental office. Although the list of potential lesions that could be amassed is extensive, lesions discussed are considered essential from the standpoint of frequency, severity, potential for initial recognition, and differential diagnosis. Some tumors that occur in this location are similar to neoplasms found elsewhere, whereas others are peculiar to the head and neck area.

Naturally, the full assessment of each patient's malady depends on the integration of various sources of available information. These include clinical, roentgenographic, historical, and laboratory parameters that require consideration in arriving at a diagnosis. To provide a full description of all aspects that need to be taken into account in arriving at a diagnosis is beyond the scope of this chapter but the information is available in a number of excellent texts, for those who require a more comprehensive description.

Neoplasms of Epithelial Origin

Squamous Cell Papilloma

The squamous cell papilloma is a common tumor occurring at all ages and found anywhere in the oral cavity. Common sites are the mucosae of the cheeks, lips, palate, tongue, and gingivae. It may be attached to the underlying tissues by either a narrow or a broad pedicle and projects well above the adjacent mucosa in a cauliflower-like pattern. Irritation, infection, viral, and metabolic disturbances have been mentioned as causes for this lesion. Microscopically, there are papillary projections of stratified squamous epithelium covering a thin core of connective tissue. Treatment consists of excision and should include the pedicle and base. Recurrence is rare and these lesions do not undergo malignant change.

Malignant counterpart: squamous cell carcinoma

Papillomatosis (Pseudoepitheliomatous Hyperplasia, Inflammatory Papillary Hyperplasia)

Under the influence of a variety of conditions such as chronic inflammation, irritation, chronic ulcers, fungal or viral

339

infections, bony sequestra, poor oral hygiene, and poor-fitting dentures, there may arise several discrete tumors that will be scattered over the mucosae. The palate is the most commonly affected area but the lips, tongue, alveolar ridges, and occasionally, the cheeks are involved. Clinically, there are numerous papillary projections that microscopically consist of a core of connective tissue covered by acanthotic squamous epithelium. On rare occasions, inflammatory papillary hyperplasia may undergo malignant change. These lesions, which appear to occur in males more frequently than in females during the fourth to fifth decades, should be treated first by removal of the cause and then with surgical excision.

Malignant counterpart: squamous cell carcinoma

Pigmented Cellular Nevus (Pigmented Mole)

A tumor-like malformation that occurs on the skin and mucous membrane, the nevus may be congenital or developmental. *Intradermal, junctional, compound, juvenile,* and *blue* are the different types of recognized nevi. Pigmented moles are congenital, occurring generally after puberty. Histologically, nevus cells are large distinct cells situated within the connective tissue and separated from the overlying epithelium by a well-defined band, except in the junctional type. The fact that this zone is not present in the junctional nevus has serious implications—a tendency for this nevus to develop into a malignant lesion. For moles that require removal because of cosmetic or irritational considerations, surgical excision is indicated. Junctional nevi do require close follow-up care, because 10 per cent of all

malignant melanomas are believed to arise this way.

Malignant counterpart: malignant melanoma

Leukoplakia

The definition of leukoplakia is white plaque and unfortunately has been used loosely with various interpretations by clinicians and pathologists alike. The diagnosis of leukoplakia should be reserved for a microscopic examination demonstrating dyskeratosis and premalignancy. This lesion, like oral cancer, occurs more frequently in males than in females, and generally in patients over the age of 40 years. Causative factors are various forms of tissue irritations, chief of which is smoking. Primary sites are the lower lip, tongue, cheeks, and floor of the mouth (Fig. 21-1). Microscopic findings are those of varying degrees of hyperkeratosis, parakeratosis, acanthosis, and dyskeratosis, the latter being the important factor. Other white lesions which may appear similar include frictional keratosis, lichen planus, familial white dysplasia, monili-

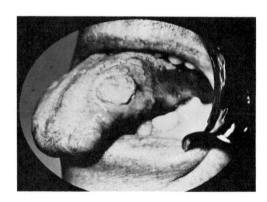

Fig. 21-1. Leukoplakia of the tongue.

asis, and stomatitis nicotina. Treatment is directed at elimination of recognizable irritating factors and *total* excision.

Malignant counterpart: squamous cell carcinoma

Squamous Cell Carcinoma
(Epidermoid Carcinoma)

The most common malignant neoplasm of the oral cavity, constituting 5 per cent of all malignant tumors in the body, the squamous cell carcinoma accounts for 90 per cent of oral malignant neoplasms. Tobacco, alcohol, syphilis, dental and oral infections, exposure to sunlight, ionizing radiation, occupational factors, as well as intraoral lesions such as leukoplakia, herpes simplex, lichen planus, median rhomboid glossitis, and Plummer-Vinson syndrome have been implicated as etiologic factors. Carcinoma of the oral cavity demonstrates a striking sex predilection, occurring much more frequently in men than in women with the peak age between 50 and 70 years. Location of the neoplasms has a strong influence on the clinical appearance, histology, and prognosis (Figs. 21-2 and 21-3). Papillary, ulcerative, nodular, or wart-like growths may be seen, and the microscopic findings can vary between a well-differentiated to highly invasive malignancy. Tumors of the lip have generally the more favorable

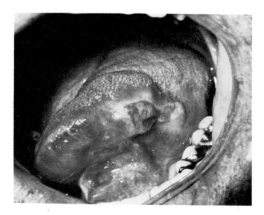

Fig. 21-3. Cancer of the tongue.

prognosis, for these metastasize to the regional lymph nodes much less frequently than those in other locations. Surgery, x-ray radiation, and chemotherapy have been used alone or in combination. Depending upon the location of the cancer, radiation can be hazardous because of the damaging effects of the x rays on the bone and potential osteoradionecrosis.

Basal Cell Carcinoma

Basal cell carcinoma occurs in the skin of the face and possibly in the oral mucosae (Figs. 21-4 and 21-5). Exposure to the ultraviolet rays in sunlight has been recognized for many years to be carcinogenic. It is probably the most common type of cancer that occurs in men, especially those exposed to the weather. This tumor will frequently begin as a small papule which ulcerates, heals, and then ulcerates again, giving foundation to the name "rodent ulcer" which it has been termed. Basal cell carcinoma exhibits essentially no tendency for metastasis, and good results can be anticipated from surgical excision or from x-ray radiation. Multiple

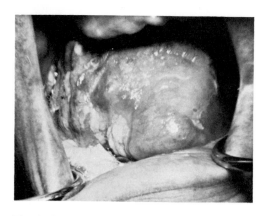

Fig. 21-2 Cancer of tongue and floor of the mouth.

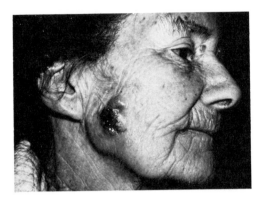

Fig. 21-4. Basal cell carcinoma of the face.

nevoid basal cell carcinomas, keratocysts of the jaws, vertebral and rib anomalies, most commonly bifid rib, comprise the *basal-cell syndrome* which was first reported in 1951. Lesions associated with this syndrome have malignant potentiality. The multiple nevoid basal cell carcinoma cannot be differentiated from the ordinary basal cell carcinoma.

Neoplasms of Connective Tissue Origin

Lesions of fibrous and connective tissue are common in soft tissues of the oral cavity. Most of these growths are probably

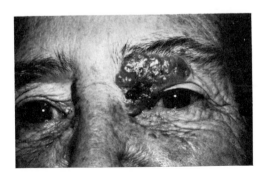

Fig. 21-5. Basal cell carcinoma of the eyelid.

hyperplasias although some may be true neoplasms. These tumors may also appear as central lesions within the jaws, but they are much less common than are their counterparts in the soft tissues.

Fibroma

Fibroma is the most common benign neoplasm of connective tissue that occurs in the oral cavity (Fig. 21-6). It is often related to some form of chronic irritation. They have been given a variety of designations such as fibrous hyperplasia, fibro-

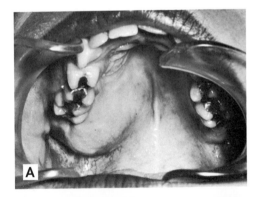

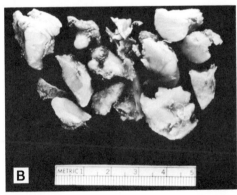

Fig. 21-6. (A) Fibroma of maxilla causing expansion of palate. (B) Gross specimen of fibroma. (Courtesy of Dr. D. E. Waite)

epithelial polyp, fibrous epulis, epulis fissuratum, epulis granulomatosa, and others. Fibrous growths occur at any site in the oral tissues appearing in all age groups and affecting both sexes equally. The gingivae are affected most often and in this location it is more common in women than in men. The major part of the lesion is composed of connective tissue, which ranges from highly cellular fibroblastic proliferation to masses of collagen. A slow-growing, deep or superficial, sessile or pedunculated lesion, it is not associated with any apparent single etiologic factor. Fibrous growths of the oral tissues are readily dealt with by simple excision but recurrence is not unusual if the entire lesion is not removed, together with any causal factors.

Malignant counterpart: fibrosarcoma (Fig. 21-7).

Peripheral Giant Cell Reparative Granuloma

Peripheral giant cell reparative granuloma is a not uncommon lesion of the oral tissues that has been described under a variety of terms denoting confusion relative to the true nature of the tumor. Although it occurs at any age, the average is between the third and fourth decades. Overall, females are affected several times

more frequently than are males. Characteristically of deep red or purple appearance, the cuspid and bicuspid regions are the preferred site of development. If the lesion is ulcerated, which is not uncommon, it is covered by fibrin. Microscopically, large numbers of giant cells in a stroma of collagen fibers and spindle cells with osteoid tissue, bone, and inflammatory infiltrate are the usual findings. Believed to be granulomatous and reparative in nature instead of neoplastic, the lesion is benign and unencapsulated. It does not recur if completely removed by surgical excision, but complete removal of deep lesions may not be possible. Similar lesions are *pyogenic granuloma* and *pregnancy tumor* (granuloma gravidarum).

Malignant counterpart: fibrosarcoma, osteogenic sarcoma

Myxoma (Fibromyxoma; Lipomyxoma)

The myxoma is a true neoplasm composed of tissue resembling primitive mesenchyme, but few examples have been recorded in the oral soft tissues. Some are sessile or pedunculated lesions having specific origin in the gingivae, lips, palate, or less frequently buccal mucosa (Figs. 21-8 to 21-10). Generally, they are thought to be myxomatous degeneration of a fibrous neoplasm, so it is difficult to discuss the nature of these growths on the basis of the few, incomplete reports available. Treatment is essentially surgical and in some cases wide excision. Myxomas have a tendency to infiltrate the surrounding bone tissue, and therefore, an adequate margin of normal tissue is necessary (Fig. 21-11).

Malignant counterpart: myxosarcoma, fibromyxosarcoma

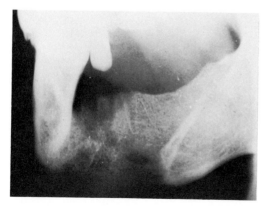

Fig. 21-7. Fibrosarcoma. Note discontinuity of bone at inferior border. (Courtesy of Dr. D. E. Waite)

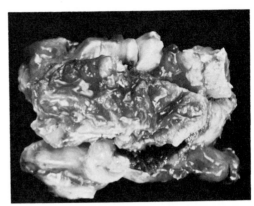

Fig. 21-9. Gross specimen of fibromyxoma.

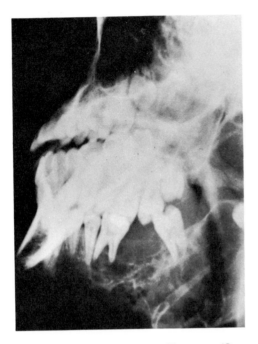

Fig. 21-8. Myxoma in a 20-year-old woman. (Courtesy of Dr. D. E. Waite)

Lipoma (Fibrolipoma; Myxolipoma)

Tumors of adipose tissue are uncommon in the oral tissues, although occurring with considerable frequency in other areas. A benign, slow-growing neoplasm that is usually solitary, the lipoma occurs generally in adults that are middle-aged. Congenital fatty lesions that have been reported in infants are probably developmental in nature. The tongue is frequently involved as is the buccal mucosa where the lesion appears as a lobulated tumor with thin overlying epithelium allowing the yellow color of fat to be seen. Microscopically, the tumor consists of lobules of mature fat cells, with a varying proportion of connective tissue. The fibrolipoma and myxolipoma have more fibrous or myxomatous tissue than the

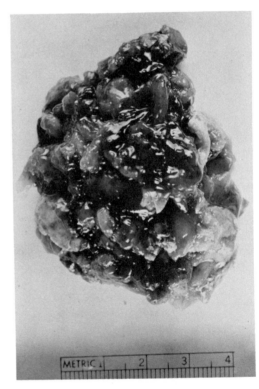

Fig. 21-10. Gross specimen of myxoma.

true lipoma but all are considered essentially the same tumor. Treatment of this pedunculated, encapsulated, elastic-type lesion is surgical excision and recurrences are rare. Slightly wider margins may be necessary for poorly encapsulated lesions.

Malignant counterpart: liposarcoma

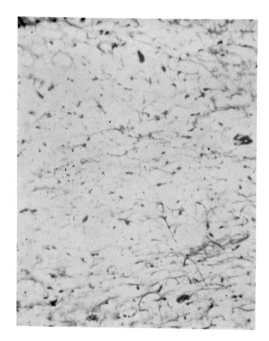

Fig. 21-11. Histologic section of myxoma.

Neoplasms of Vascular Tissue

Hemangioma

The hemangioma is characterized by proliferation of blood vessels and occurs more frequently in the head and neck region than in any other part of the body. There are several types of vascular lesions (capillary, cavernous, sclerosing, cellular), some of which are relatively aggressive but benign. These lesions are considered by many to be hamartomas or developmental malformations rather than true neoplasms. The majority of oral lesions are situated in soft tissues but also found in muscle and bone (Fig. 21-12). The vast majority are present at birth or arise at an early age. A history of recent rapid growth is not uncommon. Pain is usually not part of the clinical findings. These dark reddish blue or purple lesions are smooth and soft, frequently becoming traumatized and suffering ulceration and secondary infection. The central hemangioma located in the mandible or maxilla, although rare, deserves special attention, since patients can die from sudden massive hemorrhage if the lesion or the teeth associated with the lesion are manipulated. The honeycombed radiolucency, with fine fibrillar networks, is distinctive on the roentgenogram. Treatment for this lesion usually includes resection with carotid ligation. Aggressive surgery is also indicated for the *hemangiopericytoma* and possibly the *hemangioendothelioma*. The *sclerosing hemangioma, endothelioma,* and *nevus flammeus (port-wine stain)* are treated like the hemangioma, which is surgical resection, and perhaps sclerosing agents. It is important to know that many congenital hemangiomas have been found to undergo spontaneous regression.

Malignant counterpart: angiosarcoma, hemangiopericytoma, Kaposi's sarcoma

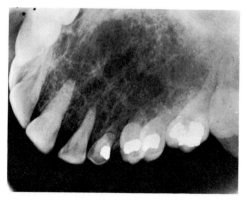

Fig. 21-12. Hemangioma of maxilla. (Courtesy of Mayo Clinic)

Lymphangioma

Lymphangioma is similar in many respects to the hemangioma and the two are considered essentially the same. A benign tumor of lymphatic vessels, it is far less common than its counterpart the hemangioma. The lips, cheeks, palate, and most especially the tongue are involved. The majority of lesions are present at birth, but are distributed equally in the sexes, which is different from the hemangioma in which the female develops the lesion more often than the male. Because they are superficial, they are circumscribed, rather diffuse, ill-defined masses consisting of lymph spaces and treated best with surgical excision. They will not respond to sclerosing solutions.

Malignant counterpart: malignant lymphoma (follicular lymphoma, reticulum-cell sarcoma, lymphosarcoma, Hodgkin's disease)

Tumors of Nerve Tissue

Neuroma

The neuroma is a tumor-like, irregularly shaped mass of nerve tissue that is not a true neoplasm but rather an exuberant attempt at repair of a damaged nerve trunk. It most commonly results from the accidental or planned sectioning of a nerve and is remarkably rare in the oral tissues considering the frequency with which teeth are extracted and nerves consequently severed. The lips, tongue, and mental foramen are common sites of involvement. The dominant feature is pain, and reflex neuralgia with distant radiation has been recorded. Because of the pain and progressive nature of the lesion,

it is best treated with surgical excision of the nodule.

Malignant counterpart: neurogenic sarcoma

Neurofibroma

Often referred to by a variety of names such as neurogenic fibroma, perineural fibroblastoma, and neurogenic fibroblastoma, the neurofibroma is a benign tumor of nerve tissue origin arising either from the fibrous connective tissue of the nerve sheath or from the sheath of Schwann. A circumscribed mass surrounded by a capsule, it usually occurs on the skin but is also found in the mouth with the tongue the most common site. On oral mucosae, they appear as small sessile, smooth-surfaced growths. Men are affected more than women with most lesions occurring in the first three decades. Multiple neurofibromas of the skin and other tissues in conjunction with café au lait spots and skeletal abnormalities are characterized in *multiple neurofibromatosis (von Recklinghausen's disease)*. Oral lesions in this disease occur in about 10 per cent of cases. Microscopic features of these lesions are the same as those of the solitary neurofibroma and nearly always that of a plexiform neuroma. Treatment for the single neurofibroma is excision but the great number in the multiple disease precludes a surgical cure. Malignant degeneration of a sarcomatous nature occurs in approximately 50 per cent of patients with von Recklinghausen's disease.

Malignant counterpart: neurofibrosarcoma

Neurilemmoma (Schwannoma; Neurinoma)

A tumor that may occur along any of the peripheral cranial or sympathetic nerve routes, the neurilemmoma is derived from the cells of Schwann in the nerve sheath and behaves like a benign neoplastic tumor (Fig. 21-13). Oral tumors

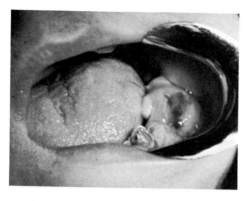

Fig. 21-13. Neurilemmoma. (Courtesy of Dr. D. E. Waite)

give rise to relatively few symptoms, aside from those caused by reason of their size or location. Generally of slow growth and long duration, they are soft on palpation and may be tender. All age groups and both sexes are involved with virtually any area of the head and neck being susceptible, including retropharyngeal, nasopharyngeal, and retrotonsillar. An encapsulated tumor, it consists microscopically of two parts which are interspersed yet discrete. The solid portion is made of cells which have elongated or spindle-shaped nuclei and a palisading pattern (Antoni type A), whereas the other areas (Antoni type B) do not exhibit palisading and have a rather unorganized arrangement of cells and fibers with the formation of microcysts. Treatment is surgical excision. The neurilemmoma does not undergo malignant transformation as does the neurofibroma.

Malignant counterpart: malignant Schwannoma

Neoplasms of Muscle Tissue

Leiomyoma

A true neoplasm arising from embryonic rests of smooth muscle cells, the leiomyoma is an extremely rare tumor of the oral cavity, much more rare than in other parts of the alimentary canal. When it

does occur, the posterior part of the tongue is the usual site, but it may involve the soft palate. It is a slow-growing circumscribed lesion that is painless, and it grossly resembles the ordinary fibroma. Histologically, it is composed of interlacing bundles of smooth muscle fibers supported by a delicate fibrous connective tissue stroma. Treatment is best accomplished by complete surgical excision.

Malignant counterpart: leiomyosarcoma

Rhabdomyoma

The rhabdomyoma is also a rare tumor in the oral cavity, and develops from skeletal muscle. It generally occurs in children and infants with the most frequent site being the tongue. Less commonly, it involves the uvula and palate. The microscopic picture is one of varying degrees of pleomorphism of the muscle cells. This slow-growing lesion is poorly encapsulated and owing to its aggressive histologic nature needs to be removed in its entirety with a wide margin of normal tissue.

Malignant counterpart: rhabdomyosarcoma

Myoblastoma (Granular Cell Myoblastoma)

An uncommon tumor of controversial origin, the myoblastoma occurs equally in males and females at all ages. The tongue is the commonest site but it has been reported in the lip, gingivae, soft palate, and uvula. It appears as a slowly growing nodule of the submucosal tissue, and is usually small (hardly exceeding 0.5 cm. in diameter), well circumscribed, and firm. A growth of similar structure, though not of similar nature, occurs as a congenital lesion in the gums of infants, the *congenital epulis of newborn*. The histogenesis of myoblastoma is still debatable, with several theories, including one of myogenous origin, one of histiocytic origin, and one of neural origin being advocated. Although the nature of the myoblastoma remains obscure, there is little doubt as to its behavior and treatment. The lesion is entirely benign and local excision effects a cure. Pseudoepitheliomatous hyperplasia may occur in the overlying epithelium in many tumors and may give the lesion the appearance of squamous cell carcinoma which does not develop.

Malignant counterpart: alveolar soft part sarcoma

Neoplasms and Dysplasias of Bone and Cartilage

Osteoma

Osteoma is a benign neoplasm characterized by slow growths of cancellous or compact bone that increase in size by continuous formation in an endosteal or periosteal location. It occurs as a circumscribed hard protuberance growing outward from the bone, or as a dense mass growing centrally within the bone, and is capable of causing facial asymmetry. The mandible is more often involved than is the maxilla (Fig. 21-14). All ages can be affected but it is more common in adults past the fourth decade. Roentgenographically, a dense radiopaque mass protruding from the bone is seen in the peripheral type, whereas a well-circumscribed sclerotic mass appears with the central lesion. Trabeculae of mature lamellar bone with varying amounts of intervening fatty or fibrous marrow are seen microscopically.

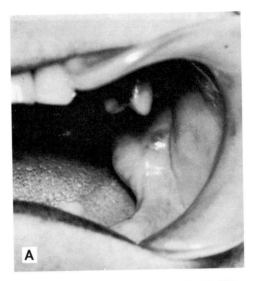

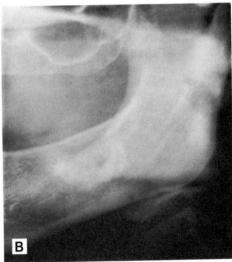

Fig. 21-14. Osteoma. (A) Osteoma projecting lingually from mandible. (B) Radiograph of osteoma. (Courtesy of Dr. D. E. Waite)

Surgical removal is indicated if the lesion produces symptoms or interferes with a prosthesis. Skeletal "osteomas" of various bones, but often prominently involving the skull and jaws, are associated with intestinal polyps, fibromatous and other connective tissue lesions, and epidermoid cysts in *Gardner's syndrome*.

Malignant counterpart: osteogenic sarcoma (Fig. 21-15)

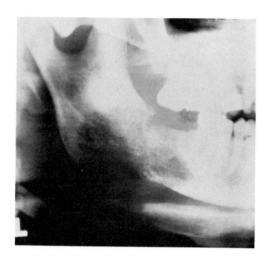

Fig. 21-15. Radiograph of osteogenic sarcoma of the left mandible.

Exostoses and Tori

Exostoses and tori, dense bony overgrowths, are non-neoplastic lesions of unknown origin occurring in the mandible and maxilla. The midline of the palate is the most frequent area of involvement, occurring there in about 20 per cent of the population, where it is termed *torus palatinus* (Fig. 21-16). Those of the man-

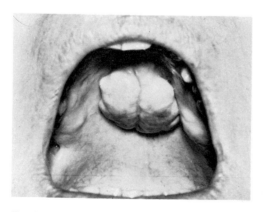

Fig. 21-16. Torus palatinus.

dible are termed, appropriately enough, *torus mandibularis,* and are seen in only 8 per cent of persons, but frequently they are bilateral on the lingual aspects of the jaw. Some studies indicate the palatal lesions are more common in females than in males but no sex incidence holds in the mandible. Formation in both jaws is generally before the age of 30 years, although frequently they are discovered quite late in life. Histologic sections show dense normal bone. Because the general rate of growth is slow, these lesions are not usually treated actively unless interfering with speech, or with fabrication of prosthetic appliance, or overlying mucosa demonstrates chronic irritation or ulceration. Exostoses occur on either side of the maxilla or mandible alveolar processes and deserve the same considerations as tori. Treatment, when indicated, is by excision, generally with a mallet and chisel or surgical bur.

Malignant counterpart: osteogenic sarcoma

Osteogenic Fibroma (Osteofibroma; Central Fibroma)

Osteogenic fibroma is a rare benign tumor in the jaws, composed of fibroblasts and collagen fibers without formation of bone or osteoid. If bone is being formed, then the tumor should be termed ossifying fibroma, although it will not be of any significance relative to treatment or behavior. It is reported so infrequently that little is known of the lesion. It causes few symptoms and is found during routine roentgenographic examination. It has well-defined margins and is encapsulated. Histologically, it may be difficult to decide whether the tumor is of odontogenic or osteogenic origin. Treatment is by simple excision.

Malignant counterpart: fibrosarcoma

Osteogenic Myxoma
(Fibro-osteogenic Myxoma)

Osteogenic myxoma may occur in any part of the skeleton but the jaws are the most common site. It is one of several unusual tumors occurring in the jaws and needs to be distinguished from its odontogenic counterpart, the odontogenic myxoma. There is neither a sex or an age preference, and it may involve either the maxilla or mandible equally. It is thought to arise from vestigial embryonic tissue within the jaw or from degeneration of a central fibroma. It is slow growing but capable of producing considerable facial deformity. A soap-bubble-like area of radiolucency is seen on the roentgenogram. Microscopic examination reveals a myxomatous structure containing few cells and

consisting mainly of mucus. The tumor is not encapsulated and infiltrates the marrow which is important. It is benign and does not metastasize but because of its infiltrative nature requires wide excision for treatment.

Malignant counterpart: myxosarcoma

Fibrous Dysplasia of Bone
and Ossifying Fibroma

There is a group of central lesions of the jaws included in the general category of fibrous dysplasia in which normal bone is replaced by fibrous tissue from which new calcified tissue subsequently forms by metaplasia (Fig. 21-17). These include the typical lesions of fibrous dysplasia, ossifying fibroma, fibro-osteoma, fibrocementoma, the familial condition of cherubism, and polyostotic fibrous dysplasia, or Albright's syndrome.

"Fibro-osseous dysplasia" is a term that is gaining acceptance for many of the de-

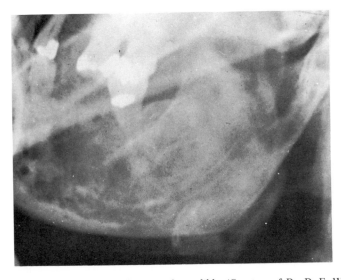

Fig. 21-17. Fibrous dysplasia of ramus of mandible. (Courtesy of Dr. D. E. Waite)

fects of this type that involve the jawbones. Here, these lesions are considered
separately, though their histology, roentgenographic features and treatment make
it convenient to group together (Figs.
21-18 and 21-19).

1. Ossifying fibroma (monostotic
   fibrous dysplasia) has an equal predilection for males and females, but
   is more common in children and
   young adults. Painless and nontender, it appears as a localized hard
   swelling of either jaw occurring in
   the mandible more frequently than
   in the maxilla. Growth is generally
   slow with gradually increasing facial
   deformity.

2. Polyostotic fibrous dysplasia (Albright's syndrome) often occurs in
   the bones of one limb, particularly a
   lower one. The skull bones and jaws
   are affected when the upper limb is
   affected most generally. Polyostotic
   disease affecting more than a few

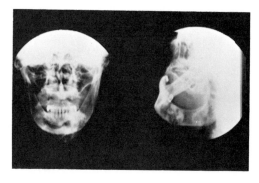

Fig. 21-19. Radiograph of fibro-osseous lesion of the mandible.

bones is almost always seen first
during childhood. The disease is relatively common and, if accompanied
by such manifestations as cutaneous
pigmentation, endocrine disorders,
precocious puberty, and premature
skeletal maturation, is termed Albright's syndrome, which is a relatively uncommon disease. The endocrine disturbances may alter the
time of eruption of the teeth.

3. Familial fibrous dysplasia (cherubism; disseminated juvenile fibrous
   dysplasia) affects children, who appear to be normal at birth. Males are
   affected twice as often as females
   and swellings are initially seen at
   about the ages of two and four years.
   The mandible is almost always affected and often also the maxilla,
   with bilateral occurrence the rule
   rather than the exception in both
   jaws. The deciduous and permanent
   dentitions show many abnormalities
   including premature exfoliation,
   lack of eruption owing to nondevel-
   opment of tooth germs, and irregularly spaced teeth as a result of the
   expanded bone. Of interest is the fact

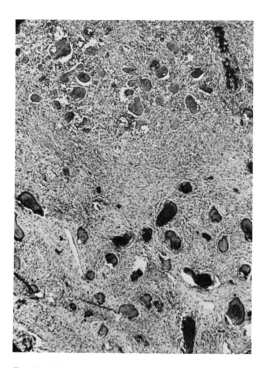

Fig. 21-18. Histologic section of fibro-osseous lesion.

that the lesions will increase in size quite rapidly to the age of about seven years and then enter a static phase until puberty. Facial deformity is the chief complaint.

Microscopically, the major feature is proliferation of fibroblasts that produce a dense collagenous matrix. Varying amounts of osteoid or bone trabeculae are seen and have no meaning relative to function. Mitotic figures may be seen.

Roentgenologically, the defects of fibrous dysplasia are well-defined zones of rarefaction. Expansion with thinning of the cortex is especially likely and those lesions with a large osseous component will be radiopaque in areas.

Treatment should be conservative since the lesions commonly stop growing at puberty. Primarily, therapy should be directed toward restoring normal configuration to the jawbones. The prognosis in fibrous dysplasia is generally good.

Malignant counterpart: osteogenic sarcoma, fibrogenic sarcoma

Central Giant Cell Tumor of Bone

Few lesions of bone have provoked the controversy that the central giant cell tumor has. It is considered to be a true neoplasm. Giant cell tumors occur almost exclusively between the ages of 20 and 40 years. The principal symptom is swelling, accompanied in some cases by pain. Slight to moderate swelling of the jaw due to expansion of the cortical plates may occur in the involved area. The tumor forms a maroon or reddish-brown mass that replaces bone, and microscopically, consists of numerous giant cells lying in a cellular matrix of spindled-shaped cells and

scanty collagen (Figs. 21-20 and 21-21). Roentgenographically, the appearance is not pathognomonic but does present several features suggestive of the diagnosis: the location of the radiolucent area, no periosteal new bone formation over the involved area, "soap-bubble" appearance, thinning of the cortex and expansion of the bone. Removal of the tumor by curettage is the most widely accepted type of therapy. There are recurrences, in rather high percentages, at times, and more radical surgery may be necessary for this, as well as for malignant change which can complicate the course in approximately 10 per cent of cases outside the jawbones.

Malignant counterpart: fibrosarcoma, osteogenic sarcoma

Giant Cell Reparative Granuloma

Giant cell reparative granuloma is peculiar to the jawbones. Understandably, it has been confused with the benign giant cell tumor of bone. The giant cell reparative granuloma occurs in adolescents and young adults between the ages of 10 and 25 years. Found in the female more than

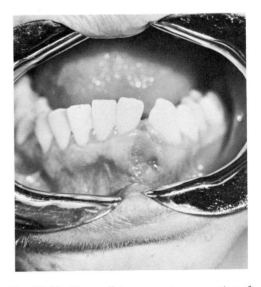

Fig. 21-20. Giant cell tumor causing separation of teeth. (Courtesy of Dr. D. E. Waite)

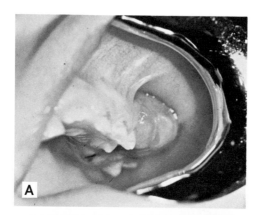

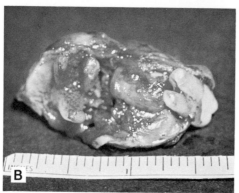

Fig. 21-21. (A) Giant cell tumor in an eight-year-old boy. (B) Gross specimen of giant cell tumor. (Courtesy of Dr. D. E. Waite)

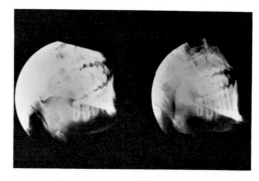

Fig. 21-22. Radiographs of giant cell reparative granuloma. (Courtesy of Mayo Clinic)

in the male, it occurs more frequently in the mandible than in the maxilla and is confined to the tooth-bearing area of the jaw (Fig. 21-22). Microscopically, the distinguishing features of the giant cell reparative granuloma are the scarcity and irregular distribution of the giant cells, compared to the giant cell tumor. A variable amount of vascularity and microcyst formation may be seen. Similar histologic findings are present in the *"brown tumor" of hyperparathyroidism.* A benign condition, the reparative granuloma can be treated satisfactorily by curettage and only rarely will there be a recurrence.

Malignant counterpart: fibrosarcoma, osteogenic sarcoma

Chondroma

Chondroma is a rare benign tumor of cartilaginous tissue occurring in the jaws. It may occur at any age with cases reported in infants and children. Commonest in the maxilla, where the anterior alveolar area is the usual site, the maximum incidence is in the fifth and sixth decades. Males are affected more often than females. The presenting symptom is usually the presence of a mass, as there is no pain in the initial stages. Roentgenographically, there is an area of irregular bone destruction, and resorption of roots can occur. Cartilaginous tumors vary considerably in histologic appearance from area to area. Hyaline cartilage, bone formation, myxomatous changes, and cystic degeneration may all be seen. Surrounded by a fibrous capsule, the tumor may break through indicating aggressive growth and, therefore, should be excised with a safe margin. In a number of cases chondromas

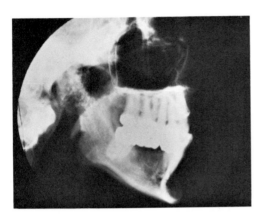

Fig. 21-23. Radiograph of chondrosarcoma of the neck of the mandible. (Courtesy of Mayo Clinic)

have been reported to gradually transform into malignant lesions.

Malignant counterpart: chondrosarcoma (Fig. 21-23)

General Principles Related to Tumors of the Oral Cavity

The study of tumors of the oral cavity, indeed of the head and neck region, is important to practitioners in several different fields. General surgeons, otolaryngologists, radiologists, plastic surgeons, dentists, oral surgeons, and at times, ophthalmologists and even neurosurgeons are included in this group. Tumors will be encountered in each of these specialties, either as a matter of diagnosis or during therapy. Surgical procedures may be complicated, demanding a wide range of technical ability. There can be no place for the occasional operator who may fail to provide uniformity of treatment or to seek out that therapeutic modality most likely to

succeed in a specific case. Many times, this is best achieved by a group approach. A dental contribution is of great importance. Dentists have an opportunity to recognize early lesions and to play a significant role in carrying out cytologic diagnostic techniques. The removal of decayed and infected teeth before surgery or prior to radiation therapy may also be required. The dentist can also provide responsibility for intraoral splints and prosthetic appliances.

SIGNS AND SYMPTOMS. The nature of the symptoms produced will vary according to the location of the lesion. Oral lesions in the asymptomatic stage may, in fact, be first recognized by the patient, especially tumors of the lip, anterior tongue, or floor of the mouth. An irregularity or abnormality of contour may be discovered while brushing the teeth, or bleeding may draw attention to impending trouble. Loosening of one or more teeth may occur if the alveolar ridge is involved. Tongue movement may be influenced and protrusion limited because of infiltration and fixation of the lesion in the floor of the mouth. Lesions arising from the palate, tonsillar fossa, or base of the tongue will usually first be manifested by the development of a persistent sore throat. Initially, pain may be intermittent, but become progressively more intense and prolonged.

Local pain eventually develops as the tumor invades adjacent structures, but is only rarely an early symptom. Pain is frequently referred to the ear from numerous primary sites, including tumors of the floor of the mouth, tongue, alveolar ridge, palate, tonsillar fossa, and hypopharynx.

The clinical characteristics of oral tumors are:

SIGN	BENIGN	MALIGNANT
History	Long	Short
Induration	Absent	Present
Ulceration	Rare	Frequent
Margin	Well-defined	Irregular
Mobility	Freely moveable	Fixed
Papillary outgrowth	Frequent	Infrequent
Regional adenopathy	Absent	Frequent

(Sharp, G. S., Bullock, W. K., and Hazlet, J. W.: *Oral Cancer and Tumors of the Jaws.* © 1965. McGraw-Hill Book Co. Used with permission of McGraw-Hill Book Co.)

EXAMINATION OF THE ORAL CAVITY. The examination must always be performed in a methodical manner to avoid the possibility of overlooking an area. Dentures, both partial and complete, are always removed first. Maximum illumination is essential. It should be from either a fixed light or headlight in order to leave the examiner's hands free for manipulation of tongue blades and palpation.

The examination should start with the lips and proceed to the mucous membrane of the cheek back to the anterior pillars. The mandibular gingiva is observed, then the floor of the mouth and tongue, which can be examined together. The tongue should be shifted back and forth to examine first one side and then the other, starting anteriorly and progressing posteriorly to the glossopalatine fold. The maxillary gingiva and hard palate follow, then the soft palate and uvula. Finally, the tonsillar fossa, anterior and posterior pillars, posterior pharyngeal wall, and hypopharynx are examined.

Palpation with a gloved finger must be a routine part of the oral examination. In the floor of the mouth attention to the submaxillary ducts is necessary, and these glands need to be felt and salivary flow determined. The parotid gland is similarly examined. Palpation is especially important for that part of the tongue behind the circumvallate papillae.

BIOPSY. A biopsy specimen of an accessible lesion in the oral cavity may be obtained with the use of local anesthesia. Areas of slough or obvious inflammation should be avoided. When the tumor underlies an intact mucosal surface, care should be taken that the specimen is removed at a deep enough level to include any malignant tissue. At times, with small lesions suspected of being cancerous, excisional biopsy may be undertaken, but in this instance, a wide margin of normal tissue must be removed.

Staging and grading are two methods of assessing cancers. The TNM method is useful in describing the anatomic involvement of the lesion. The letter T indicates a primary tumor, N implies regional lymph node involvement, and M indicates distant metastasis. Broder's grading method separates the histopathologic appearance of tumors into four groups:

Grade I: Tumors composed of 25 per cent or less abnormal cells.

Grade II: Tumors composed of 25 to 50 per cent abnormal cells.

Grade III: Tumors composed of 50 to 75 per cent abnormal cells.

Grade IV: Tumors composed of 75 per cent or more abnormal cells.

Odontogenic Tumors

Lesions that arise from the odontogenic apparatus or that are associated with it form a complex group. It is necessary to recognize the distinctive histologic features of these lesions and certain others hamartoma-like tumors such as the ameloblastic odontoma.

Ameloblastoma

A true neoplasm of enamel organ tissue, the ameloblastoma is the most common of the epithelial odontogenic tumors that does not undergo differentiation or induction of mesodermal derivatives. The now current term *ameloblastoma* was introduced by Ivy and Churchill in 1930, although first mention of the tumor can be dated back to 1868 and Broca's report. Baden found more than 50 terms associated with this tumor and greater diversity of opinion has existed concerning all aspects of this neoplasm than perhaps any other found anywhere in the body.

Incidence. This lesion comprises approximately 1 per cent of the tumors and cysts seen in the mandible and maxilla and is the most common of the epithelial odontogenic tumors. Sixty-five per cent occur in the 20 to 50 year age range, with nearly half in the third and fourth decades of life. Ages can vary from the young to the old. More males than females have generally been reported in the literature, although studies with a slight predominance of female patients at the time of histologic diagnosis have also been documented. An overwhelming majority occur in the mandible, with well over 75 per cent in the body and ramus regions. Maxillary tumors are generally in the posterior regions with possible antrum and/or floor of the nose involvement.

for which they may be mistaken. Some oral tumors develop from dental structures and may simulate neoplasms of osseous derivation. The basis for a clear interpretation of odontogenic tumors demands first a basic understanding of normal odontogenesis.

There is some question whether odontogenic tumors are true neoplasms. Many lesions of the oral tissues that appear clinically as tumors are not neoplasms but are non-neoplastic developmental anomalies or overgrowths of inflammatory or other causation.

In a discussion of odontogenic tumors and tumor-like lesions, a simple classification is offered. In 1969 the World Health Organization brought forth a much needed classification of odontogenic tumors, jaw cysts, and allied lesions. The first part of that classification deals with tumors and tumor-like lesions related to the odontogenic apparatus.

> Ameloblastoma
> Odontogenic adenomatoid tumor (adenoameloblastoma)
> Ameloblastic fibroma
> Ameloblastic odontoma (odontoameloblastoma)
> Complex composite odontoma
> Compound composite odontoma
> Odontogenic fibroma
> Odontogenic myxoma
> Calcifying epithelial odontogenic tumor
> Calcifying odontogenic cyst
> Cementoma
> Melanotic neuroectodermal tumor of infancy (melanotic progonoma, melanoameloblastoma)

Although dentinomas are included in many classifications, it seems likely that they are but variants of some of the

Etiology. Many theories have been advanced about causal factors, most of which have not been shown conclusively to be correct. Trauma, extraction of teeth, ill-fitting dentures or bridges, malocclusion, periodontal disease, loose teeth, rickets, oral infection, unerupted third molars, and supernumerary teeth have all been implicated. Whether these condi-

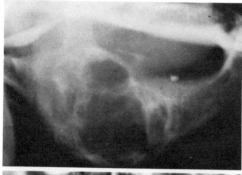

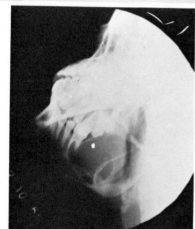

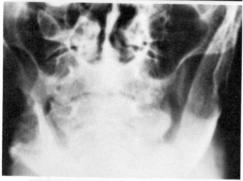

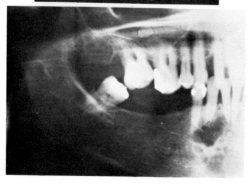

Fig. 21-24. Radiographs of ameloblastoma.

tions give rise to the tumor or only cause symptoms leading to its detection is debatable. The latter conclusion is probably more correct. They appear to arise from epithelium endowed with the potentiality of odontogenesis.

Features. Swelling is the single most common symptom, occurring in as many as 85 per cent of cases. Pain, while not a frequent symptom, has been found in 41 per cent of cases in some studies. The ameloblastoma is a tumor that grows slowly, and it is important to realize that patients may be asymptomatic in the early stages of the neoplasm. Panographic roentgenographs have been of great help in the discovery of this tumor in this early asymptomatic state during the routine dental examination. In maxillary tumors, sinus problems or nasal obstruction may be the first symptom. Draining sinuses, unhealed extraction sites usually associated with red granulation tissue within the tooth socket, bleeding, trismus, neural involvement, and other dental problems may be the chief complaint. Roentgenographic aspects typically show a coarsely trabeculated zone of osseous destruction that has the appearance of a multilocular cystic cavity. Bone will often appear to be replaced by a number of well-defined radiolucent areas that give the lesion a honeycomb or soap-bubble configuration. Maxillary tumors produce a monocystic cavity in most instances. Thickening of membranes, cloudiness, and destruction of the walls are usual findings when sinus involvement is present. The roentgenographic examination and diagnosis, as with any tumor, are nonspecific, and diagnosis cannot be made solely from the roentgenographic evidence (Fig. 21-24).

Although ameloblastomas have been described as solid or cystic, the degree of cyst formation is so variable as to preclude division on this basis. The tumor appears as a grayish-white or grayish-yellow mass replacing bone and containing no calcified tissue. A tumor will commonly contain solid areas with microcystic formations together with larger cysts. Partitions between cysts may be bone or, more frequently, soft connective tissue. Clear to straw-colored fluid or a gelatinous material is contained in the cystic spaces. Both the inner and outer cortical plates of the jaw are often thinned and expanded.

Essentially, the ameloblastoma is an epithelial tumor composed of irregularly anastomosing strands, nests, islands, and cords of epithelium separated by variable amounts of connective tissue. All tumors show a follicular, plexiform, or mixed follicular and plexiform pattern (Fig. 21-25). It appears to serve no useful purpose to separate "follicular" from "plexiform" ameloblastomas. Many tumors show at least some foci of squamous differentiation and are commonly called "acanthomatous," and such neoplasms have been mistaken for squamous carcinoma. Granular cells, which usually occur in large masses within the follicle, may replace part or all of the stellate reticulum and sometimes the basal layer of cells as well.

Behavior. The ameloblastoma is a neoplasm that causes expansion more than destruction of bone. However, there is a certain degree of local invasion of the surrounding bone. In the absence of proper treatment, this tumor can grow to a great size, but still remain localized. Recurrences are common, depending on the tumor's size, location, length of duration, and initial forms of treatment. Recurrent tumors demonstrate the same histologic pattern as that of the primary tumor and there is no correlation between histologic pattern and the clinical course.

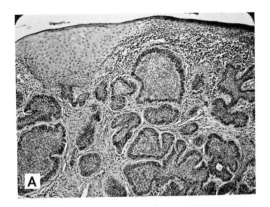

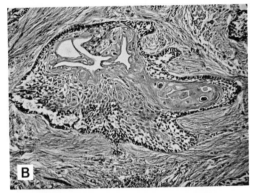

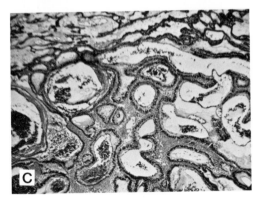

Fig. 21-25. Histologic sections of ameloblastoma. (A) Follicular pattern. (B) Acanthomatous pattern. (C) Plexiform pattern.

Metastasis is unlikely, and if it does occur it is probably a result of aspiration rather than of lymphatic or hematogenous dissemination.

Treatment and Prognosis. When the results of treatment of ameloblastomas are assessed, several factors are important.

First, long-term follow-up is essential. This neoplasm has the capacity for continued growth and extension beyond the margin of what appears to be normal tissue. The relationship between the type of treatment and the rate of recurrence is basic to much of the controversy concerning treatment of this tumor today. Excision, cautery, and curettement are forms of treatment generally considered conservative and are associated with the highest degrees of recurrence. However, when these forms of treatment are used in combination with each other, or with other modes of therapy, effectiveness is increased. Curettement is the least desirable form of therapy, whereas resection, whether en bloc or segmental, with an adequate margin of uninvolved tissue gives the best overall prognosis.

Odontogenic Adenomatoid Tumor (Adenoameloblastoma)

First recognized as an entity by Stafne at the Mayo Clinic in 1948, odontogenic adenomatoid tumor has been reported in the literature under varying designations. This neoplasm is a distinctive lesion with characteristic clinical and pathologic features apart from the ameloblastoma.

Incidence. Slightly more than 100 cases have been recorded in the literature denoting the uncommon occurrence of this tumor. Noteworthy is the fact that the adenoameloblastoma occurs in a young age group, over 75 per cent of patients being under 20 years of age and rarely beyond the third decade. Females are affected about twice as often as are males. Generally, adenoameloblastoma is situated in the lateral incisor, cuspid, or bi-cuspid region of the jaw. Well over half of these tumors are in the maxilla.

Etiology. The actual point of origin of the tumor remains a matter of considerable doubt. Columnar cells, which bear a close resemblance to ameloblasts, and the frequent association of the tumor with unerupted teeth suggest its origin from dental epithelium. Because the adenoameloblastoma is frequently associated with an impacted tooth or originates in a cyst wall, it could theoretically be derived from the enamel organ or its remnants, or from a dentigerous cyst.

Features. It is frequently, but by no means constantly, associated with unerupted teeth and may also occur in a normally erupted dentition. Few symptoms apart from swelling occur and pain is not a usual finding. There may be expansion of the bone from the gradually increasing swelling and fluctuation may be evident. Roentgenographically, the lesion reveals a destructive process that is poorly outlined in the jaw. While there is no characteristic roentgenographic finding, the tumor most commonly occurs as a single radiolucent area which varies considerably in size (Fig. 21-26).

Generally the tumors are small, measuring less than 3 cm. in diameter. A well-defined fibrous capsule exists, and on cut section small areas of hemorrhage in a grayish-white tissue are demonstrated. Cystic spaces of various sizes containing a yellowish gelatinous material may be present. Teeth may be embedded in the tumor or attached to it.

These tumors are composed of sheets and strands of epithelial cells which whorl and appear active. The characteris-

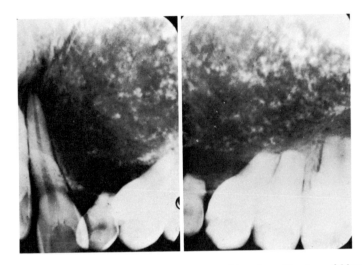

Fig. 21-26. Odontogenic adenomatoid tumor in 18-year-old patient. (Courtesy of Mayo Clinic)

tic feature of the adenoameloblastoma is columnar cells which appear to be similar to ameloblasts and form tubular spaces. These columnar cells are supported by a scant fibrous connective tissue stroma and have nuclei situated toward the ends of the cell body farthest from the central space. Small foci of calcification are scattered throughout the tumor.

Behavior. The tumor is benign and does not recur after enucleation. It has been noted to show continued growth and can attain a fairly large size before detection.

Treatment and Prognosis. Conservative surgical excision is indicated. Enucleation has also been used successfully in certain instances. Of great importance is the fact that this tumor lacks the propensity for recurrence, as does the ordinary ameloblastoma, and does not demand radical surgery.

Ameloblastic Fibroma

The ameloblastic fibroma contains both odontogenic epithelium and odontogenic mesenchymal tissue elements, the former deriving from the enamel organ and the latter from the dental papilla or the dental follicle.

Incidence. The ameloblastic fibroma is much less common than the ordinary type of ameloblastoma. Although it is a relatively uncommon neoplasm of odontogenic origin, it is the most common of the tumors that contain both ectodermal and mesodermal components. It occurs in patients of the younger age groups, typically 15 to 25 years. Males have been affected slightly more often than females in the reported cases. It arises most commonly in the bicuspid-molar region of the mandible. Overall, it is similar to the ameloblastoma in this respect.

Etiology. The ameloblastic fibroma is a slow-growing tumor often associated with disturbed odontogenesis or embedded teeth. Since no calcified substances are produced, its development from tissues representing the early stages of odontogenesis is indicated. It may well develop from the dental follicle after the onset of calcification of the tooth.

Features. The tumor grows slowly and painlessly, expanding the jaw. It exhibits a somewhat slower clinical growth than the ameloblastoma and it does not tend to infiltrate between trabeculae of bone. It enlarges by gradual expansion so that the periphery of the lesion often remains quite smooth. Unerupted teeth may at times be associated with the tumor. No significant difference exists roentgenographically between the appearance of the ameloblastoma and that of the ameloblastic fibroma. It produces a well-circumscribed cyst-like radiolucent zone with well-defined borders. Spreading of the roots of adjacent teeth may be noted occasionally in the roentgenogram (Fig. 21-27).

There may or may not be a definite capsule, but the growth is circumscribed and has a smooth surface. A cut section has the appearance and consistency of a soft fibroma, and grossly the tissue is a soft fibrous mass.

The ameloblastic fibroma is composed of strands and nests of proliferating odontogenic epithelium which seldom undergoes cystic degeneration. This epithelium tends to take on the physical characteristics, as well as the cellular features, of the

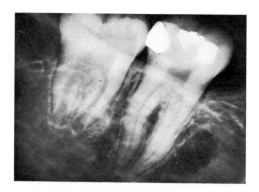

Fig. 21-27. Ameloblastic fibroma in a 20-year-old patient. (Courtesy of Dr. D. E. Waite)

dental lamina or enamel organ and resembles to some extent the strands and nests seen in the ameloblastoma. The connective tissue element generally takes the form of a cellular fibroblastic tissue that resembles the dental papilla in the developing tooth, though in some cases, thick collagen bands may be present.

Treatment and Prognosis. Its clinical behavior in most cases has been almost entirely benign. Therefore, treatment is somewhat more conservative than that of the ameloblastoma, as it does not appear actively to infiltrate the bone. Removal by curettage is usually adequate since the tendency for recurrence is limited. En bloc resection may be employed if the tumor recurs. The histologic pattern of the recurrent lesion is identical with that of the initial tumor.

Ameloblastic Odontoma (Odontoameloblastoma)

The ameloblastic odontoma occupies a place between the ameloblastic fibroma and compound composite odontomas. In fact, the ameloblastic odontoma has been regarded as an early stage of the complex or compound composite odontoma. The lesion is quite unusual in that a relatively undifferentiated neoplastic tissue is associated with a highly differentiated tissue, both of which may show recurrence following inadequate removal.

Incidence. The ameloblastic odontoma is less common than either the ameloblastoma or the composite odontomas. It is considered to be a rare clinical entity. The ameloblastic odontoma occurs at any age but is particularly prevalent during childhood. The majority of patients are younger than 11 years, but older persons are also affected. No sex predilection is known. Any part of either jaw may be affected but there is a predilection for the bicuspid and molar areas. It appears to occur in the maxilla more than in the mandible.

Etiology. Odontogenic epithelium and odontogenic connective tissue are both involved in this tumor, as in the ameloblastic fibroma. The mesenchymal and epithelial elements attain the capabilities for which they were intended and are able to produce calcified portions of a tooth. It should not be inferred that this tumor represents two separate neoplasms growing in unison; rather, there exists a peculiar proliferation of tissue of the odontogenic apparatus in an unrestrained pattern including complete morphodifferentiation, as well as apposition and even calcification.

Features. Most ameloblastic odontomas are larger than other odontogenic tumors, although this is not always the case. The tumor grows slowly and painlessly to form a hard, nontender mass in the jaw. It is an expanding lesion of bone which can produce facial deformity or asymmetry if left untreated. Since it is a central lesion, considerable destruction of bone may also occur. Roentgenographically, the tumor appears as a translucent area containing irregular radiopaque areas, some of which may be tooth-like in outline. The borders of the translucency are generally smooth but occasionally there may be indications of bone destruction. Associated teeth may be unerupted or impacted.

The tumor forms a firm, fibrous-appearing mass that contains a variable amount of calcified material and there may be a fibrous capsule. The dental tissues are produced in a fairly normal pattern.

The histologic pattern is striking, for all stages of development involving dental tissues can be seen. Proliferating odontogenic epithelium is present in nests, strands, or compact masses. Dentin and enamel, which are present in poorly organized states, differentiate it from the ameloblastoma and indicate its basically hamartomatous nature.

Treatment and Prognosis. Nearly all these well-circumscribed tumors are readily cured by conservative surgical means but a margin of normal tissue is indicated, as the tendency for recurrence is marked. Sometimes an en bloc removal or resection is necessary. Sarcomatous change in the connective tissue has been observed only on extremely rare occasions.

Composite Odontomas

The term "odontoma" refers to any tumor of odontogenic origin. This tumor is composed of more than one type of tissue and, for this reason, has been called a composite odontoma. Two types of composite odontoma are customarily described, the complex and the compound. The former consists of a mass of irregularly arranged dentin, enamel, cementum, and connective tissue. The latter has large numbers of small though morphologically recognizable teeth. The complex and compound odontomas are discussed together (Fig. 21-28).

Incidence. The odontoma is a common odontogenic tumor with the capability of its odontogenic epithelium and mesenchyme reaching a degree only slightly below that of normal odontogenesis. The odontomas may be discovered at any age in any location of the dental arch, maxil-

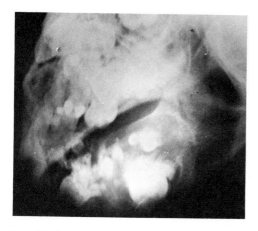

Fig. 21-28. Compound composite odontoma in eight-year-old patient. (Courtesy of Dr. D. E. Waite)

lary or mandibular. The complex odontoma is found most often in older children and in young adults. It is considered to be somewhat more common in females than in males. At least 60 per cent of the compound odontomas are diagnosed in the second to third decades and more often in females than in males. The complex odontoma has a predilection for the molar portion of the lower jaw, whereas compound odontomas tend to occur in the incisor-cuspid region most commonly.

Etiology. The origin of the odontoma is unknown. Local trauma and infection have been suggested as possible causes. They may also be developmental malformations of dental organs or of tissue with odontogenic potential. However, since the odontoma often replaces a missing tooth, this suggests that the dental organ gives rise to the malformation instead of to a normal tooth.

Features. Generally, the lesions are quite small and cause no symptoms though occasionally they may attain quite large dimensions. These tumors grow slowly often reaching a certain stage and becoming quiescent for many years. The lesion is usually an incidental roentgenographic finding that appears as an area of opacity similar to osteosclerosis. The mass of calcified dental tissues of which it is composed appears as an irregular dense area. The compound odontoma shows numerous small tooth-like structures, but a great variety of appearances can occur.

The complex odontoma is surrounded by a fibrous capsule which is partially separated by fluid. The compound odontoma is also generally enclosed in a fibrous capsule and consists of a number of separate small teeth or denticles embedded in fibrous tissue in which there may be some trabeculae of bone.

The complex odontoma consists of enamel, dentin, and cementum, forming an extensive mass arranged quite irregularly. Much of the enamel is fully calcified. These substances demonstrate a strong tendency to establish an interrelationship with each other similar to that in the normal development of the tooth. In the compound odontoma, enamel, dentin, and cementum are arranged into small separate teeth, most of which are oddly shaped. Each small tooth is an independent structure, and the number of teeth may vary from a few to many. They are bound together with a fibrous tissue capsule, and the entire mass is embedded in bone.

Treatment and Prognosis. Both the complex and compound odontomas are benign in spite of the size they sometimes attain. Surgical removal is indicated and there is little expectancy of recurrence.

Odontogenic Fibroma

The odontogenic fibroma is similar in many respects to the myxoma and is perhaps only a more cellular form of that lesion. Its great frequency has not been well recognized because it resembles or is identical to the dentigerous cyst on the roentgenograph.

Incidence. The odontogenic fibroma is probably one of the most common odontogenic tumors of the jaws but one that has been reported so infrequently that little is known of the characteristic clinical features. It occurs with equal frequency in both male and female and the majority are diagnosed during the second decade of life. The mandible is affected more frequently than is the maxilla, with the most common site being the third molar and the cuspid regions.

Etiology. The odontogenic fibroma is considered to arise from the mesenchymal dental tissue (periodontal membranes, dental papilla, or dental follicle) on the grounds of its proximity to the teeth and structural appearance. The protracted period during which odontogenesis takes place, from about the sixth week of intrauterine life to approximately the twenty-fifth year, one or more of the 52 teeth is being formed and therefore, this embryonic tissue persists in the jaws into adult life.

Features. Because of its origin, the odontogenic fibroma is in close proximity to the tooth, either the root, or in the case of an unerupted tooth, the crown. It grows slowly and painlessly and follows a benign course. There may be a slight enlargement of the area and it is most often associated with an impacted tooth. Being asymptomatic they may go unnoticed for years, only to be discovered on roentgenographic examination which reveals a ra-

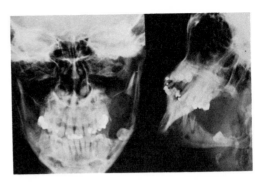

Fig. 21-29. Radiograph of odontogenic fibroma.

diolucent lesion of varying size associated with the crown of the tooth (Fig. 21-29).

A solid rather than a cystic lesion is usually found on histologic examination. The tumor forms a circumscribed mass that is moderately firm depending on the fibroblastic component. The cut surface of the tumor is pinkish-white.

The histologic pattern of the tumor, particularly the mesenchymal component, belies its clinical behavior and it should not be regarded as malignant. Primitive-appearing fibroblastic connective tissue similar to that of the developing dental pulp is seen. Collagen formation may be marked and distributed throughout the plump fibroblasts. Small clumps of epithelial cells that represent rests of dental epithelium are scattered in the tumor and emphasize the odontogenic origin of the growth (Fig. 21-30).

Treatment and Prognosis. The indicated treatment for this neoplasm is conserva-

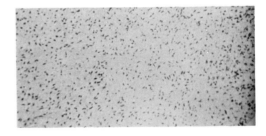

Fig. 21-30. Histologic section of odontogenic fibroma.

tive surgical removal or curettage and complete removal will effect a cure. Although it is true that failure to recur may be considered as evidence of adequate surgery, malignant tumors in this area show a marked tendency to recur and metastasize even after unusually extensive surgery.

Odontogenic Myxoma

Odontogenic myxoma of the jaws constitutes a definite clinical and pathologic entity. Myxomas of bone practically always occur in the jaws, which suggests that they are probably of odontogenic origin.

Incidence. The incidence of myxoma as a neoplasm of bone varies in different studies of bone tumors. The odontogenic myxoma is one of the rare odontogenic neoplasms, and it must be distinguished from the true myxoma. It has been reported to be one sixth as common as the ameloblastoma. Odontogenic myxomas of the jaws occur chiefly in children and young adults with the majority of patients being in the second decade and usually under 35 years of age. The sexes are equally affected. The upper and lower jaws appear to be affected about equally, but there are conflicting studies claiming that the mandible or maxilla to be the common site. The molar and bicuspid regions of either jaw are particularly involved.

Etiology. The fact that this tumor is generally associated with unerupted or missing teeth and in young people with abundant odontogenic epithelium support the theory that in most cases it arises from the mesenchymal portion of the tooth germ.

Features. It is a slowly growing, painless central lesion of the jaw. Expansion of the bone may cause destruction of the cortex as well as facial deformity. Roentgenographically, a radiolucent defect that is often multilocular due to occasional intraosseous septa of bone radiating throughout the tumor is seen. This finding is similar to that produced by other tumors such as the ameloblastoma and giant cell tumor.

The tumor is soft, semitranslucent, and appears as a fusiform swelling in the jaw that may be covered by a layer of thin bone. The cortex is only rarely perforated and the overlying mucosa is normal. The cut surface appears grayish or yellowish-white and has the characteristics of myxomatous tissue. Occasionally, a capsule will be found but it is usually lacking if the growth is infiltrative.

Loosely arranged triangular or spindle-shaped cells, many with long fibrillar processes that tend to intermesh, are found in a loose mucoid intercellular material. The intercellular substance may be somewhat granular and basophilic and mitotic figures are few.

Treatment and Prognosis. Current evidence suggests that myxomas of the jaws have a capacity to recur in a manner similar to the ameloblastoma, but do not metastasize. The goal of treatment, therefore, should be directed toward complete local removal. Conservative block resection should be used to minimize the possibility of recurrence. Curettage has seldom been found to be adequate.

Calcifying Epithelial Odontogenic Tumor

Prior to 1958 when Pindborg described it under its present designation, the calcifying epithelial odontogenic tumor was considered a type of ameloblastoma or odontoma. It has distinctive pathologic features.

Incidence. It is a rare lesion, with relatively few cases being reported in the literature. Men between the ages of 25 and 50 years have been affected primarily in the cases thus far reported. The bicuspid-molar region of the mandible has been predominantly involved and may be involved with an unerupted tooth.

Etiology. Its invariable occurrence in relation to an embedded tooth suggests its dental nature and it has been indicated to develop from the reduced enamel organ of the embedded tooth.

Features. The growth is symptomless, apart from progressive swelling of the jaw, and examination shows a hard tumor that may be diffuse or well defined. The roentgenogram shows an impacted tooth with radiolucency around the crown. This translucent zone has areas of radiopacity which may not be well demarcated from surrounding normal tissues.

The tumor is well circumscribed in most cases, and the apparent cystic spaces seen on the roentgenogram are filled with soft tumor tissue. This is an invasive tumor that destroys surrounding bone, a feature generally noted at operation.

Sheets of polyhedral epithelial cells tend to be closely packed in a connective tissue stroma. Calcification is the most striking feature of the tumor, as its name would suggest. The calcium is deposited in and around epithelial cells which appear to be undergoing degeneration.

Treatment and Prognosis. This neoplasm appears to behave in much the same manner as does the ameloblastoma,

recurring if not completely removed. Conservative therapy will most likely result in recurrence, and once the diagnosis of calcifying epithelial odontogenic tumor is made follow-up care is essential, with recurrent lesions receiving aggressive treatment.

Calcifying Odontogenic Cyst

The calcifying odontogenic cyst is an uncommon epithelial lesion characterized by unusual keratin production and dystrophic calcification, and it bears a marked similarity to the cutaneous calcifying epithelioma of Malherbe and may also be confused with a variety of cutaneous, odontogenic, and other tumors. Although the term calcifying odontogenic cyst may not be entirely accurate on a histomorphologic basis, the apparent limited growth potential and strictly benign behavior of the lesion make this designation reasonable on a clinical basis.

Incidence. The existence of this relatively rare new odontogenic lesion has only been described as a separate and distinct oral lesion within the past 12 years. Patients of any age may be affected, but a significant number of lesions have been reported in children and adolescents. There appears to be no sex predilection. Calcifying odontogenic cysts have been described in either jaw and no particular region shows a dominance.

Etiology. Although histogenesis has not been definitely established, there appears to be strong evidence suggesting an odontogenic origin. The occasional association of an unerupted tooth or odontoma, the ameloblastic basal-cell layer with areas resembling stellate reticulum, epithelial rests resembling remnants of dental lamina, and almost exclusive occurrence in the gingiva or alveolar processes of the maxilla or mandible support an odontogenic origin.

Features. A peripheral or intraosseous lesion causing nonspecific signs and symptoms is the usual feature, although resorption of adjacent teeth may occasionally be seen. Roentgenographic findings, while not distinctive, are the means to detecting most of these tumors. The appearance is a monoloculated radiolucency with variably defined borders that may or may not have perforated cortical bone. Small radiopacities can appear within the lesion, suggesting the possibilities of ossifying fibroma, odontogenic adenomatoid tumor (adenoameloblastoma), ameloblastic odontoma, and calcifying epithelial odontogenic tumor, among others.

There is a marked resemblance among cases and all have a cystic cavity lined by a stratified epithelium. The basal layer of cells is distinct and takes up more stain than that of the ordinary cyst. These cells are cuboidal to columnar resembling enamel epithelium and have big "ghost" epithelial cells scattered among them which appear to be aberrant keratinization. The presence of melanin in this lesion is not a unique finding.

Treatment and Prognosis. Calcifying odontogenic cysts seem to have a limited growth potential and surgical enucleation has been the preferred therapy. Some tendency toward recurrence has been noted and close follow-up care is indicated. More extensive surgery including resection may be necessary in cases of recurrence.

Cementoma and Cementifying Fibroma

Cementum is a calcified mesenchymal tissue formed in the late stage of odontogenesis and deposited on the roots of teeth continuously throughout life. The morphologic appearances of the proliferated cementum also vary, and terms such as benign cementoblastoma (true cementoma), cementifying fibroma, gigantiform cementoma, periapical cemental dysplasia (periapical fibrous dysplasis), and others have been used. Unfortunately, there is not yet a generally agreed nomenclature. All these will be considered as cementomas even though all are probably not of the same nature.

Incidence. Cementoma is classically described as a lesion of rather common occurrence, and incidence data are difficult to obtain because of the practice of grouping all types together. The commonest type of lesion occurs more often in women (almost ten times that of men) and the majority of patients are over 30 years of age. Over 90 per cent occurs in the mandible, usually in connection with the anterior teeth. The maxilla is rarely involved.

Etiology. The cause of the cementoma is unknown, although pulpal and periodontal infections, as well as abnormal occlusal forces, have been suggested as contributing factors. However, the lesions are often seen when these factors are not present. The cementifying fibroma (periapical fibrous dysplasia) derives from the specialized bone around the dental roots and thus is not strictly odontogenic.

Features. The condition generally produces no symptoms and is usually detected on roentgenographic examination. Lesions may be single or multiple and do not enlarge sufficiently to expand the jaw. Their evolution continues over a period of many years. Occasionally they are superficially situated where they are prone to become infected. The roentgenographic appearance depends on the stage of development of the tumor. Early, it will be radiolucent and similar to a dental granuloma or radicular cyst. Later, with the beginning of calcification in the radiolucent area of fibrosis, specks of radiopacity are seen which will appear as circumscribed areas of dense radiopacity with time and maturity of the lesion.

The microscopic features vary with the stages mentioned in the roentgenographic examination. The early stage demonstrates young fibroblasts and a moderate amount of collagen. As the lesion matures more cementum is produced and incorporated into the lesion. Eventually the entire lesion consists of deeply basophilic calcified masses of cementum. Cementum can be distinguished from surrounding bone, which it closely resembles, by the irregularity of incremental growth lines and the paucity of cementocytes. The lacunae tend to be oval rather than round and often extend only in one direction.

Treatment and Prognosis. Caution is urged in the interpretation and treatment of the early radiolucent area which may resemble a granuloma. The cementoma requires only recognition and periodic observation. It is *not* necessary to extract teeth or institute endodontic procedures. Lesions that can be diagnosed as cementifying fibroma may require removal, sometimes aggressive surgery, owing to expansion and involvement of large areas.

Melanotic Neuroectodermal Tumor of Infancy (Melanotic Progonoma, Melanoameloblastoma)

Although it has been a debatable point whether the melanotic neuroectodermal tumor is a retinal anlage tumor rather than an odontogenic one, the association of many of these tumors with disturbed odontogenesis or with displaced teeth seems to present some evidence of their odontogenic background. It appears appropriate to discuss them with the odontogenic lesions until more data are available to the contrary.

Incidence. It is a rare tumor, considerably less than 100 cases being reported in the literature. It occurs in infants younger than 12 months of age, and in most instances less than 6 months. Girls are affected about twice as often as boys. The maxilla is affected much more often than the mandible (more than 80 per cent of cases), and the anterior part is the preferred site.

Etiology. There is still considerable controversy as to the origin of the melano-ameloblastoma. The retinal anlage theory suggests that the tumor is derived from retinal elements that had been misplaced in the course of development. Another theory implies that the tumor derives from the vomeronasal organ or from misplaced sensory neuroectoderm. Too few cases of this tumor have been reported to be able to draw any definitive conclusions regarding its origin.

Features. The rate of growth is variable. The majority of reported cases have been rapidly growing non-ulcerated, darkly pigmented lesions, but some have been described as of slow growth. Roentgenographically, there may be a well-defined area of translucency suggesting a cyst, but often with margins demonstrating bone destruction and giving the appearance of an invasive malignant neoplasm. The basic features are those of bone enlargement, migration of teeth and tooth germs, and difficulty in sucking.

Generally the lesion separates quite readily from the bone though it is unencapsulated or has only a partial fibrous capsule. The cut surface has a character-istic slate-blue to grayish-black appearance with occasional grayish-white streaks.

The principal cells are small and round with large nuclei. They may be arranged in an alveolar pattern or drawn out into strands. The pigment they often contain has been identified as melanin.

Treatment and Prognosis. All tumors thus far reported have been benign. Conservative surgical excision is recommended, and provided the entire tumor is removed, there is little likelihood of recurrence. No case has ever been reported to metastasize.

Selected Reading

Albright, F., Butler, A. M., Hampton, A. O., and Smith, P.: Syndrome characterized by osteitis fibrosa disseminata, areas of pigmentation and endocrine dysfunction, with precocious puberty in females. Report of five cases. N. Engl. J. Med., *216*:727, 1937.

Anderson, W. A. D.: Pathology, 3rd ed. St. Louis, C. V. Mosby Co., 1957.

Broders, A. C.: The grading of carcinoma. Minn. Med., *8*:726, 1925.

Chaudhry, A. P., Robinovitch, M. R., Mitchell, D. F., and Vickers, R. A., Chondrogenic tumors of the jaws. Am. J. Surg., *102*:403, 1961.

Cook, T. J.: Oral tumors, benign and malignant. Oral Surg., *4*:2, 1951.

Geschickter, C. F.: Tumors of the jaws. Am. J. Cancer, *26*:90, 1935.

Morgan, G. A., and Morgan, P. R.: Periapical osteofibrosis—differential radiological interpretation. J. Ontario Dent. Assoc., *45*:532–534, 1968.

Robinson, H. B. G.: Oral malignancies—the dentist's responsibility. Dent. Radiogr. Photogr., *21*:1, 1948.

Sandler, H. C., and Stahl, S. S.: Exfoliative cytology as a diagnostic aid in the detection of oral neoplasms. J. Oral. Surg., *16*:414, 1958.

Silverman, S., Jr., and Chierici, G.: Radiation therapy of oral carcinoma effects on oral tissues and management of the periodontium. J. Periodontol., *36*:478–484, 1965.

Waite, D. E.: Inflammatory papillary hyperplasia. J. Oral Surg., *19*:211, 1961.

Wynder, E. L, and Bross, I. J.: Etiological factors in mouth cancer. Br. Med. J., *1*:1137, 1957.

Odontogenic Tumors

Aisenberg, M. S.: Histopathology of ameloblastomas. Oral Surg., *6*:1111–1128, 1953.

Bernier, J. L.: Tumors of the Odontogenic Apparatus and Jaws. Atlas of Tumor Pathology. Section IV, Fascicle 10a. Armed Forces Institute of Pathology, Washington, D.C., National Research Council, 1960, pp. 9–107.

Gorlin, R. J., Chaudhry, A. P., and Pindborg, J. J.: Odontogenic tumors: Classification, histopathology, and clinical behavior in man and domesticated animals. Cancer, *14*:73, 1961.

Guralnick, W. C.: Textbook of Oral Surgery. Boston, Little, Brown & Company, 1968.

Lucas, R. B.: Pathology of Tumors of the Oral Tissues. Boston, Little, Brown & Company, 1964.

Mehlisch, D. R., Dahlin, D. C., and Masson, J. K.: Ameloblastoma: A clinicopathologic report. J. Oral Surg., *30*:9–22, 1972.

Thoma, K. H., and Goldman, H. M.: Odontogenic tumors. A classification based on observations of the epithelial, mesenchymal, and mixed varieties. Am. J. Pathol., *22*:433, 1946.

Tratman, E. K.: Classification of odontomas. Br. Dent. J., *91*:167, 1951.

22 | Salivary Glands

MARK T. JASPERS

Gross Anatomy

Parotid Gland

The parotid gland is the largest of the three paired salivary glands(Fig. 22-1). It is shaped somewhat like an inverted pyramid, with an apex, a base, and lateral, anterior, and posterior surfaces. The gland's apex lies between the sternomastoid muscle and the mandibular angle.

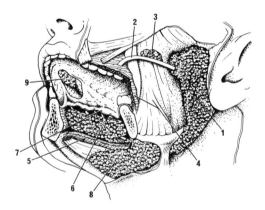

Fig. 22-1. The major salivary glands and surrounding structures. Parotid gland (1); Stensen's duct (2); accessory lobe of parotid (3); masseter and buccinator muscles (4); mylohyoid muscle (5); sublingual gland (6); plica sublingualis (7); submandibular gland (8); gland of Blandin-Nuhn (9). (Redrawn from H. Ferner (Ed.): Atlas of Topographical and Applied Human Anatomy. Philadelphia, W. B. Saunders Co., 1963)

The base lies near the zygomatic bone and the condylar neck of the mandible.

The anterior surface is grooved by the mandibular ramus and the masseter muscle. The posterior surface is grooved by the mastoid and styloid processes and the sternomastoid and digastric muscles. Laterally, the gland may have a detached portion known as the accessory parotid gland. Medially, the gland contacts the internal pterygoid muscle and approximates the lateral pharyngeal wall (Fig. 22-2).

The entire parotid gland is invested with a connective tissue capsule or sheath. This capsule is derived from portions of the deep cervical and masseteric fascia.

The facial nerve, having emerged from the stylomastoid foramen, enters the gland and courses ventrolaterally, forming the parotid plexus within the gland.

The parotid gland empties into the oral cavity by way of Stensen's duct. This duct emerges from the gland, passes anteriorly, lateral to the masseter muscle, and turns abruptly medially around the masseter's anterior border to pierce the buccal fat pad and the buccinator muscle. It terminates intraorally at the parotid or Stensen's papilla. This opening is located opposite the crown of the maxillary second molar. Stensen's duct has a relatively uni-

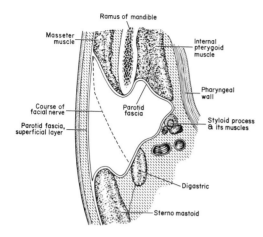

Fig. 22-2. Transverse section of parotid space and related structures. Note the close relationship between the parotid and the lateral pharyngeal wall. (Redrawn from J. P. Schaeffer (Ed.): Morris' Human Anatomy, 11th ed. New York, McGraw Hill Book Co., 1953)

form diameter of approximately 1.5 mm. throughout its course.

Each of the salivary glands is innervated by both parasympathetic and sympathetic fibers. The parotid gland receives its parasympathetic (secretory) fibers from the otic ganglion by way of the auriculotemporal nerve. Sympathetic innervation to all the salivary glands is probably entirely vasomotor.

The secretion of the adult parotid gland is purely serous. The proportion of the total volume of saliva secreted by all glands that is secreted by the parotid assumes an intermediate position. With an increase in stimulation, the relative proportion of the parotid contribution increases.[1]

Submandibular (Submaxillary) Gland

The submandibular gland is the second largest of the three main salivary glands (Figs. 22-1 and 22-3). This gland consists of a larger superficial part and a smaller deep process. The two parts are continuous with each other around the posterior border of the mylohyoid muscle.

The larger portion lies in the digastric triangle. It is bounded superficially by skin and platysma muscle, laterally by the mandible and medial pterygoid muscle, and inferiorly by the mylohyoid, stylohyoid, and digastric muscles.

The smaller, deep process of the gland is a tongue-like extension that passes around the posterior edge of the mylohyoid muscle. The deep process is bounded by the mylohyoid laterally, the hyoglossus medially, the lingual nerve superiorly, and the hypoglossal nerve inferiorly.

The entire submandibular gland is surrounded by a capsule similar to that which surrounds the parotid. This capsule is derived from portions of the external

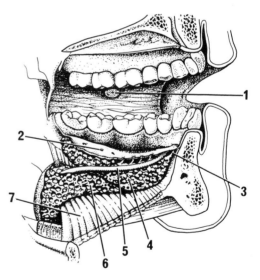

Fig. 22-3. The submandibular and sublingual salivary glands and surrounding structures. Stensen's papilla (1); plica sublingualis (2); sublingual duct (3); sublingual gland (4); Wharton's duct (5); submandibular gland (6); mylohyoid muscle (7). (Redrawn from H. Ferner (Ed.): Atlas of Topographical and Applied Human Anatomy. Philadelphia, W. B. Saunders Co., 1963)

cervical, digastric, and styloid muscle fascial layers.

The excretory duct of the submandibular gland is Wharton's duct. This duct arises from the junction of the superficial and deep processes, turns at a right angle superiorly, and courses under the oral mucosa to open at the sublingual caruncle. This sublingual caruncle, or papilla, is located at the side of the lingual frenulum. Wharton's duct has an average diameter of 1.5 to 3.5 mm.; occasionally, however, at the point of turn around the mylohyoid muscle, the ductal lumen may enlarge considerably.

Parasympathetic secretory fibers that supply the gland are derived mainly from the submandibular ganglion.

The submandibular gland secretes a mucous and serous saliva; the serous element predominates. This gland accounts for the largest fraction of the total salivary secretion in the unstimulated state; upon stimulation, this relative proportion decreases.[1]

Sublingual Gland

The sublingual gland is the smallest of the major salivary glands. This gland is in reality a group of glands forming an elongated mass in the floor of the mouth, lateral and inferior to the tongue (Figs. 22-1 and 22-3).

The superior border of this gland forms a distinct ridge called the plica sublingualis in the floor of the mouth. Inferiorly, the gland rests on the mylohyoid muscle; its lateral surface contacts the mandible and medially it is related to the genioglossus and the submandibular duct.

The connective tissue capsule surrounding the submandibular gland is ill defined. This gland lies rather independently within the general submandibular space.

The principal excretory duct, or Bartholin's duct, of the sublingual gland may fuse with the submandibular duct to share a common opening on the sublingual caruncle. More commonly, however, Bartholin's duct opens independently, also on the sublingual caruncle.

In addition to Bartholin's duct, from 5 to 30 additional smaller ducts, the ducts of Rivinus, drain the sublingual gland. These ducts open along the crest of the plica sublingualis at the superior border of the gland.

Parasympathetic innervation to the sublingual gland is similar to that to the submandibular gland; it is derived from the submandibular ganglion.

The secretion of the sublingual gland is mucous and serous, mucous being the predominate type. The sublingual gland accounts for the smallest fraction of total unstimulated salivary flow.

Minor Salivary Glands

In addition to the three major salivary glands outlined previously, there are numerous smaller salivary glands (450 to 750 in number) located within the mucosae throughout the oral cavity.[2] These glands, on an anatomic basis, are classified into the labial, buccal, glossopalatine, and palatine glands. Some secrete a mucoserous saliva (labial and buccal), whereas others (glossopalative and palatal) secrete only mucus.

The tongue also contains minor salivary glands. Near the apex on the inferior tongue surface is the gland of Blandin-Nuhn which secretes mucous and serous saliva (Fig. 22-1). The base of the tongue contains mucous glands. The glands of von Ebner, located near the valliate papillae, produce a serous secretion.

The minor salivary glands throughout the oral cavity contribute a variable amount of secretion to the total salivary flow. Their total relative contribution has been estimated from 8 per cent to 53 per cent of the total salivary volume.

Development and Microscopic Anatomy

Development

Salivary glands begin development through a proliferation of oral epithelium into the underlying connective tissue. This epithelial proliferation develops into an extensively branched system of cords of cells. As development proceeds, lumina form within the cords to form a system of ducts. The smallest, terminal branches of this system differentiate into the secretory portions of the gland.

Microscopic Anatomy

The secretory portions of a salivary gland, the acini, consist, in general, of a layer of secretory cells lining a narrow lumen. These secretory cells are of two types, mucous and serous.

The acini are connected to intercalated ducts which in turn connect with striated ducts. The striated ducts, so named because of cellular striations, empty into excretory or interlobular ducts and thence into the oral cavity.

Situated between the basement membrane and the ductal or glandular cells are spindle-shaped cells termed myoepithelial cells. These cells are believed to be contractile; their function is apparently to facilitate salivary flow.

Each major salivary gland is separated into segments called lobes by involutions of the surrounding connective tissue. Lobes, in turn, are further divided into lobules by connective tissue septa. These septa bind and support the salivary elements which comprise the lobule: acini, their intercalated ducts, myoepithelial cells, and the striated ducts.

Salivary Flow

The secretion of saliva is continuous, even at rest. The quantity of saliva secreted is subject to considerable variation, ultimately dependent upon the control exerted by the central nervous system. Secretion is subject to reflex stimulation: stimuli from touch and taste receptors of the oral cavity, or psychic stimuli from other sensory centers or body zones, all converge on the salivary nuclei in the medulla oblongata. Efferent pathways from this salivary center are the parasympathetic and sympathetic parts of the autonomic nervous system.

The total quantity of salivary secretion produced per day has been estimated at 500 to 1500 ml.[3] It is known that a large variation in flow rates occurs between individuals; it is therefore safe to assume that there will also be a large range for the normal salivary secretion volume.

The salivary flow rate is affected by a number of psychologic, physiologic, and environmental factors. Diet, age, body water balance, mental stress, anxiety, ambient air temperature, cigarette smoking, and certain drugs may influence the rate and type of salivary flow. Salivary flow rate is diminished by mental stress, systemic dehydration, and increased room temperature; it is increased by hyperhydration and cigarette smoking.

Epinephrine (Adrenalin) and ephedrine cause a stimulation of predominately serous secretion; mucous secretion is stimulated by acetylcholine, pilocarpine, and histamine.

The major salivary glands all secrete into the oral cavity and contribute to the mixed saliva which has several important functions. Saliva provides lubrication for, enhances the taste of, and begins the digestion of food. It also serves as a cleansing, buffering, and antibacterial agent.

Diagnostic Methods

Clinical Examination

Physical examination of the salivary glands involves an examination of a large portion of the cervicofacial region. The examination involves an assessment of the gland's size and consistency, the nature of the salivary flow, and if necessary, an exploration of the salivary duct and its orifice.

The initial step in this examination should consist of a face-to-face observation of the patient. The examiner should note any signs of facial asymmetry, discoloration, visible pulsation, or discharging sinuses. This inspection, especially when judging asymmetry and discoloration, should be conducted from a distance of 3 to 4 feet from the patient.

Following this initial general examination, the individual glands are examined.

Parotid Gland

A parotid gland enlargement usually appears as a diffuse swelling which, when viewed from the front, may overlap the tragus of the ear, giving the patient a full-cheeked appearance. This type of diffuse swelling may be quite obvious if it

is unilateral, but may be more difficult to detect if it is bilateral (Fig. 22-4).

Palpation of the parotid gland is accomplished using the fingertips with a circular, firm, but delicate pressure. The entire area occupied by the gland should be palpated (Fig. 22-5). The examiner should note any well-defined nodular or diffuse enlargements within the gland substance.

When the parotid gland is examined, it is important to bear in mind the "stylomandibular tunnel" and the parotid tissue it may contain. As will be recalled, a portion of the parotid gland approaches the lateral pharyngeal wall through a tunnel formed by the base of the skull, the internal pterygoid muscle, and the styloid process and its muscles. Occasionally, parotid tumors may assume a dumbbell configuration; the tumor may grow in a parapharyngeal direction to appear clinically as a mass in the lateral pharyngeal or the retromandibular fossa area. In consideration of this, a complete examination of the

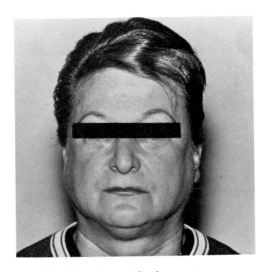

Fig. 22-4. Bilateral parotid enlargement.

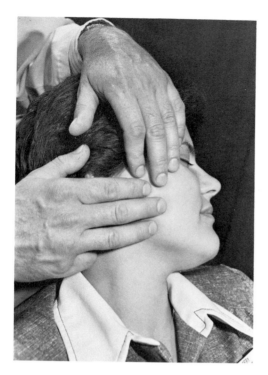

Fig. 22-5. Palpation of the parotid gland.

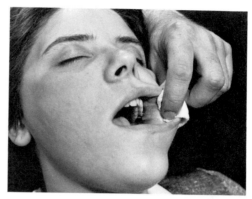

Fig. 22-6. Eversion of cheek to expose the orifice of Stensen's duct.

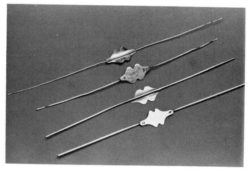

Fig. 22-7. Salivary duct or lacrimal probes.

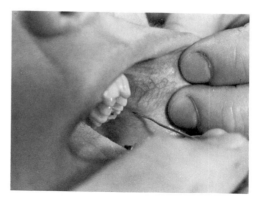

Fig. 22-8. Insertion of salivary duct probe into Stensen's duct.

parotid should include a visual examination for a medial protrusion from the lateral pharyngeal wall or into the retromolar fossa area.

The nature of the parotid flow may be examined by "milking" the gland. The patient's cheek is slightly everted, the duct orifice dried with gauze, and the saliva expressed by a gentle but firm forward pressure initiated immediately anterior to the ear and extending forward (Fig. 22-6). In this manner, saliva may be expressed, or milked, from the gland. A normal gland will easily yield watery clear saliva; in diseased states it may contain purulent material, debris, or thick mucus.

Occasionally, it may be necessary to probe the parotid duct to determine the presence of ductal obstructions or strictures. This procedure is best accomplished by everting the patient's cheek, which usually reveals the ductal orifice, and inserting a lacrimal probe (Figs. 22-7 and 22-8). By careful manipulation of this probe, Stensen's duct may be tactilely examined proximal to the point of its right-angle turn through the buccinator muscle.

Submandibular Gland

An enlargement of the submandibular gland may be diffuse, simply adding fullness to the submandibular region, or nodular. Like those of the parotid, unilateral enlargements are more easily detected owing to the resultant asymmetry.

The submandibular gland is best palpated bimanually, using both an intraoral and extraoral approach. With the patient's head inclined slightly downward (to flex the neck and relax the tissues in this area), the examining fingers are positioned as illustrated in Figure 22-9. With an upward pressure on the external finger (to raise the contents of the floor of the mouth), the submandibular gland may be palpated between the fingers.

The salivary flow from the submandibular gland should be evaluated. With the patient's tongue elevated as shown in Fig-

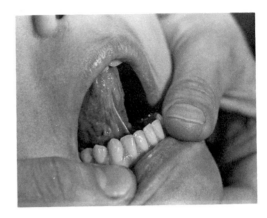

Fig. 22-10. Elevation of tongue; the sublingual caruncle is thus exposed.

ure 22-10, the sublingual papilla may be dried with gauze. Saliva may be milked from the gland by a gentle but firm upward pressure medial to the mandibular ramus with one or two fingers, beginning at the angle of the mandible and extending forward. Saliva thus expressed should be somewhat viscous and clear.

Not infrequently, Wharton's duct needs to be probed to examine the duct proper for obstructions or strictures and to determine accurately its course prior to minor surgical procedures on the floor of the mouth. The orifice of the submandibular duct may be located by expressing saliva as outlined previously. After the orifice is located, a thin lacrimal probe is carefully inserted and advanced along the duct. Caution should be exercised due to the thinness of the walls of the duct. This procedure is frequently difficult; several attempts may need to be made.

Sublingual Gland

Enlargements of the sublingual gland appear as elevations in the floor of the mouth. Again, unilateral enlargements are more easily detected.

The sublingual gland may be palpated bimanually; one finger exerts upward pressure in the submental region and the

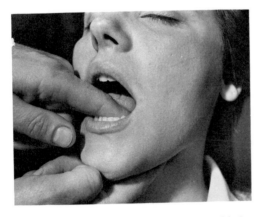

Fig. 22-9. Bidigital palpation of the submandibular gland.

second is placed intraorally as shown in Figure 22-11. Salivary flow from the sublingual gland is usually examined with the same procedure utilized in the examination of the submandibular flow. With careful drying and observation of the crest of the plica sublingualis, small drops of saliva may be seen. Owing to the small size, probing the sublingual gland's ducts is not possible.

Minor Glands

Enlargements of the minor salivary glands usually appear as discrete nodules within the substance of the submucosa.

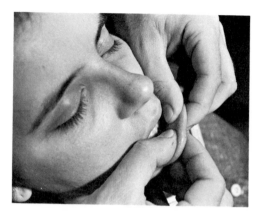

Fig. 22-12. Bidigital palpation of the minor salivary glands of the lower lip.

Palpation of the minor glands of the lips, cheeks, and other areas should always be done bidigitally whenever possible. With one examining finger intraorally and one extraorally, the cheeks, lips, and parts of the tongue may be examined (Fig. 22-12). The minor glands of the palate may be examined by compressing them against the palate. Examination of salivary flow and the ducts proper of minor salivary glands is usually not attempted in a routine physical examination of the oral regions.

Radiologic Examination

Radiologic examination is frequently useful in the diagnosis of calculi within Stensen's or Wharton's ducts.

Radiographic visualization of calculus within the distal portion of Stensen's duct is possible utilizing a periapical film which the patient holds against the buccal mucosa along the course of the duct. The patient's head is positioned vertically and the central ray directed through the cheek toward the first molar area (Fig. 22-13).

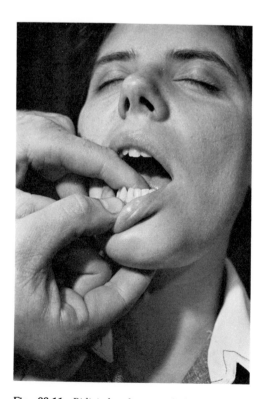

Fig. 22-11. Bidigital palpation of the sublingual gland.

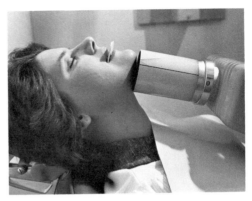

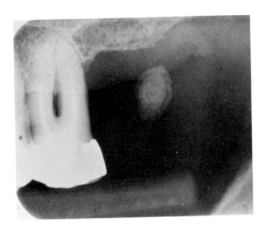

Fig. 22-13. Calcification in the region of Stenson's duct. This calculus is visualized on a routine periapical film of the second molar area. (Courtesy of Dr. D. E. Waite)

Fig. 22-14. Radiographic examination of Wharton's duct. The patient's head is inclined approximately 50° from the horizontal. The central ray is directed −20° in the midline.

Visualization of calculus within the distal portion of Wharton's duct or the sublingual gland is frequently possible. The patient's mandibular occlusal plane is inclined backward 45° to 50° to the horizontal. An occlusal film is centrally placed as far backward as possible and the central ray directed under and behind the chin so that it strikes the film at a right angle (Figs. 22-14 and 22-15).

Occasionally, it may be necessary to radiographically examine for a calculus within a minor salivary gland. The technique utilized is similar to that utilized for calculi within Stensen's duct. Obviously, this technique is only adaptable for the lip and cheek regions.

In order to prevent a "burnout" of a small or poorly calcified intraductal calculus, it is necessary to reduce the radiologic exposure time from one third to one half of the exposure utilized for dental and osseous tissues.

Intraductal calculus infrequently may

be exhibited on a routine panographic radiograph. Figure 22-16 illustrates a large calculus within Wharton's duct.

Sialographic Examination

Sialography is a roentgenographic visualization of the ductal system of two of the paired major salivary glands. (Because of its multiductal nature, the sublingual gland does not lend itself well to this examination method.) This visualization is made possible by means of a radiographic contrast solution which is introduced into the duct.

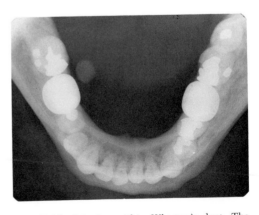

Fig. 22-15. Calculus within Wharton's duct. The patient experienced no symptoms; the calculus was clinically palpable. (Courtesy of Dr. R. Kuba)

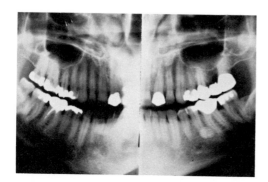

Fig. 22-16. Calculus within the left Wharton's duct at apex of second bicuspid (same patient as shown in Fig. 22-15). (Courtesy of Dr. R. Kuba)

A wide variety of contrast media is available; generally they may be classed into water-insoluble and water-soluble compounds.

Water-insoluble media:

Lipiodol and Iodochlorol are derivatives of poppyseed oil with iodine. These compounds exhibit a high viscosity and may cause adverse tissue reactions if retained within the gland.

Ethiodol, also a derivative of poppyseed oil, exhibits a lower viscosity than Lipiodol and Iodochlorol and produces no adverse tissue reactions.

Hytrast, a suspension of two organic iodides, may be diluted with saline solution to reduce its viscosity. It causes no tissue reaction.

Pantopaque (ethyl iodophenylundecylate) may be used in an emulsified aqueous form. This emulsion adheres to the mucous membrane surfaces, has a low surface tension, and is miscible with tissue fluids.

These compounds are all relatively viscous and are all water insoluble; they are thus more difficult to introduce into the gland and are slowly absorbed by tissue. They may tend to blot out subsequent sialographic examinations because of their sustained opacity.

Water-soluble media:

Urokon (sodium acetrizoate), *Hypaque* (sodium diatrizoate), *Conray* (meglumine iothalamate), *Renografin* (methylglucamine diatrizoate), and *Cholagrafin* (methylglucamine iodipamide) are common water-soluble compounds. None maintains opacity for long periods of time or causes adverse tissue reactions. These compounds are homogeneous, are miscible in body fluids and saliva, are rapidly eliminated, and have low viscosities. Major criticisms of these compounds include their rapid elimination, thus requiring ready accessibility of the radiographic apparatus, and their relative lesser degree of radiopacity.

Many factors must be considered when choosing a contrast medium. The status of the gland to be examined, the possibility of adverse tissue reaction, retention duration of the solution, the solution's viscosity, and the examiner's experience must be borne in mind. No one contrast medium meets all requirements; selected situations may require different media.

Sialography, as it has been traditionally practiced, involves the hand injection of a water-insoluble medium into the gland. The duct orifice is located, and dilated if necessary with graded lacrimal probes. An injection apparatus is assembled, including a thin, 14- to 18-gauge, soft plastic intravenous catheter approximately 25 cm. in length (Fig. 22-17). A stopcock

should be injected, the amount is entirely governed by the patient's reaction. Approximate amounts to be injected may vary from 0.5 to 6 cc. When the patient experiences pain, the stopcock is closed and suitable radiographs taken.

Recently, a hydrostatic sialographic technique has been developed. This procedure usually involves the use of the newer, water-soluble contrast media. An apparatus similar to that for injection sialography is prepared; a thin 14- to 18-gauge soft plastic intravenous catheter approximately 25 cm. in length is attached to a syringe barrel or similar calibrated reservoir with an intervening stopcock valve and connecting tubing (Fig. 22-18).

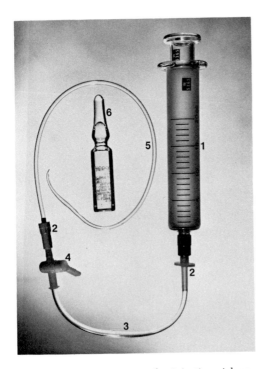

Fig. 22-17. Instrumentation for injection sialography. 20-cc glass syringe (1); adapter (2); plastic tubing approximately 20 cm. in length, (3); stopcock (4); plastic tubing approximately 25 cm. in length, one end of which has been tapered by drawing over a spirit flame (5); suitable oil-base contrast medium (6).

is positioned between this catheter and a Luer-Lok syringe which has been filled with suitable contrast medium. All air is removed from the system and the terminal end of the catheter is inserted 1.5 to 2.0 cm. into the duct. The soft tissues around the ductal orifice serve as a splinter to hold the catheter in position and prevent leakage. The catheter is anchored to the patient's cheek with tape. Contrast medium is injected into the gland until the patient begins to feel pain. No preconceived or predetermined amount of dye

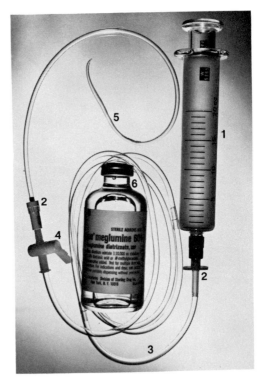

Fig. 22-18. Instrumentation for hydrostatic sialography. 20-cc glass syringe (syringe plunger is removed prior to filling) (1); adapter (2); plastic tubing approximately 100 cm. in length (3); stopcock (4); plastic tubing approximately 25 cm. in length, one end of which has been tapered by drawing over a spirit flame (5); suitable water-soluble contrast medium (6).

The contrast medium in the reservoir is positioned approximately 72 cm. above the orifice of the duct, and the medium is allowed to flow until the patient feels pain. The stopcock is closed and a suitable radiograph taken. The proponents of the hydrostatic method maintain that this method gives them more control over the amount of dye introduced.

For additional detailed information the reader is directed to several excellent articles covering the injection[4,5] and hydrostatic[3,6] methods of sialography.

Irrespective of the method of introduction of contrast medium, the goal is the same; a completely filled ductal system. The ideally filled gland shows filling of intercalary ducts with minimal delineation of the acini (Fig. 22-19). Excessive acinar filling, the so-called "cumulus cloud effect," "cloud-like shadow," or "sialo-acinar reflux," all refer to overfilling of the gland.[4]

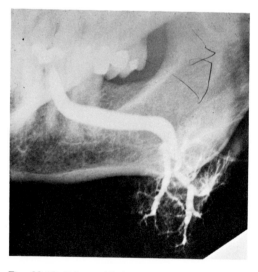

Fig. 22-19. Submandibular sialogram. (Courtesy of Dr. D. W. Waite)

When the gland has been filled and suitable radiographs exposed, the catheter is removed from the duct and the patient is given a strong sialagogue such as a slice of lemon to suck. This causes an emptying of the contrast dye from the ductal system. This emptying phase has contributed as much diagnostic information as has the filling phase.[4] A normal gland will show virtually complete elimination of the dye shortly after use of this sialagogue. Post-evacuation radiographic films are exposed 5 minutes and, if necessary, 24 hours following use of the sialagogue. Any dye remaining in glandular substance or ducts after 24 hours indicated the presence of an abnormality.[5]

Sialographs of the parotid gland usually include the true lateral and the anteroposterior projections. The submandibular gland is best examined with the lateral oblique and the true lateral projections. Occlusal projections and panoramic radiographs may also be used to advantage.[7]

Prior to the insertion of the catheter and the contrast medium, a "presialogram," or "scout film," should be taken. This film establishes a baseline appearance and may be useful in comparing with the filling and postevacuation films.

Sialography is but one procedure in the diagnostic repertoire for salivary gland problems. Determination of a pathologic condition requires weighing all available data: the history, physical examination, laboratory findings, dental findings, examination of the saliva, and other roentgenographic studies.

Sialography illustrates the presence of ductal strictures, cysts, and fistulas; it may identify a salivary duct obstruction which is too small or poorly calcified to be demonstrated with routine radiography

(Figs. 22-20 and 22-21). Sialography may be useful in determining the status of the gland proximal to an obstruction by depicting alterations in the diffusion pattern of the radiopaque solution within the gland proper. These findings aid in the diagnosis of intra- or extraglandular neoplasms; specifics will be mentioned later when these diseases and neoplasms are discussed.

Finally, sialography may be of some therapeutic benefit. The contrast solutions may dilate the duct or break up mucous or inflammatory plugs that impede salivary flow. Some solutions may exert an antiseptic effect through the liberation of iodine from the dye itself.

Most sialographic media derive their radiopacity from the presence of iodine. Uncommonly, a patient will have a his-

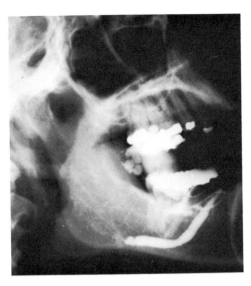

Fig. 22-21. Submandibular sialogram showing radiolucent total obstruction of Wharton's duct. Note ductal distention proximal to the obstruction and lack of glandular filling distally. (Courtesy of Drs. Vickers and Gorlin)

tory of hypersensitivity to this element; no serious adverse effects, except this hypersensitivity, have been noted in sialography. Sialography is also contraindicated in the presence of an acute glandular or ductal inflammation; its use is superfluous if a clinical diagnosis of malignant neoplasia, radiation damage, hypersensitivity, or metabolic disease has been made.[6]

If salivary glands are not examined during periods of acute inflammation, side effects will be few. Most patients exhibit some residual glandular edema for 24 hours. If this edema proves uncomfortable for the patient, a mild analgesic may be prescribed.

Scintigraphic Examination

Scintigraphic procedures allow the visualization of salivary gland activity. These procedures utilize a radioactive isotope which, following systemic administration, is actively concentrated by the salivary glands.

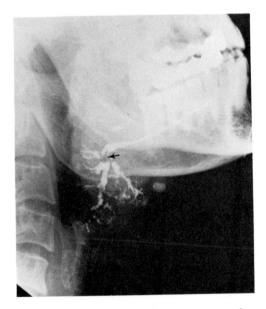

Fig. 22-20. Submandibular sialogram showing radiolucent partial obstruction (arrow) within Wharton's duct. (Courtesy of Dr. D. E. Waite)

The artificial radioactive element technetium, administered as ^{99m}Tc pertechnetate, is most widely used in these procedures. Following the intravenous administration of the technetium, the patient is placed under a scintillation scanner and the area involving the salivary glands is scanned.

Salivary scintigraphy involves the use of scintillation camera rather than scintiscanner. The uptake concentration and excretion of the isotope is detected and recorded with scintigrams taken at periodic intervals (Fig. 22-22). This method allows the visual sequential recording of glandular activity and provides a permanent record (Fig. 22-23).

At this time, scintigraphic examination must be considered only as a promising diagnostic tool. The equipment needed is costly and not available universally, and the tests themselves have not been used

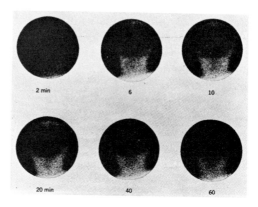

Fig. 22-23. Scintigrams of salivary glands severely involved with Sjögren's syndrome. There is complete absence of active concentration of the ^{99m}Tc pertechnetate. Glandular activity is no more than background. (Courtesy of Schall, G. L.: Xerostomia in Sjögren's syndrome. J.A.M.A., *216*:2109–2116, 1971. Copyright 1971, American Medical Association, reprinted by permission)

extensively enough in disease states to allow an accurate assessment of their value. Sufficient information is available, however, to allow some preliminary statements as to results that may be expected in certain disease states (see under the various conditions).

Biopsy

Surgical biospy of salivary glands is one diagnostic procedure that may give an accurate indication of the nature of the pathologic process. Biopsy of the major salivary glands, however, may be contraindicated. The close relationship of important neurovascular structures, the creation of salivary fistulas, and the possibility of "seeding" abnormal cells must be considered when a biopsy is contemplated. In addition, tissue repair at a previous biopsy site may make subsequent

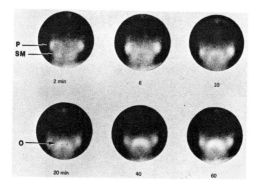

Fig. 22-22. Scintigrams of normal salivary glands. Uptake of ^{99m}Tc pertechnetate by the parotid (P) and submandibular (SM) glands occurs immediately after administration of the technetium and shows progressive increase in concentration. Oral uptake begins at 8 to 10 min. and also increases. (Courtesy of Schall, G. L.: Xerostomia in Sjogren's syndrome. J.A.M.A., *216*:2109–2116, 1971. Copyright 1971, American Medical Association, reprinted by permission)

biopsies or definitive surgery difficult. For these reasons, biopsy of the major salivary glands, especially the parotids, is rarely undertaken unless the lesion is superficial and a malignancy is suspected.[3]

Some work has been done in the area of aspiration biopsy of major salivary gland neoplasms in an attempt to avoid or minimize the problems listed previously. Eneroth and co-workers have reported a 92 per cent positive tumor diagnosis in 1000 cases using this technique.[8] Spiro and associates reported a somewhat lower success ratio of 62 per cent and an erroneous benign diagnosis in 17 per cent in their series of 125 cases.[9] Aspiration biopsy of major salivary gland neoplasms must therefore be considered unreliable.

Minor salivary gland biopsies are undertaken for two major reasons: the removal of a pathologically involved gland and for diagnostic purposes.

Excisional biopsies of the minor salivary glands, with few exceptions, present few of the problems noted concerning major salivary gland biopsy. This technique permits the total removal of a diseased gland and, in the case of certain systemic diseases, provides a safe and relatively easy collection of tissue to be used in laboratory studies.

The operative technique used in the removal of a minor salivary gland neoplasm will be described later.

Frequently the diagnosis of systemic diseases, such as Sjögren's syndrome or sarcoidosis, is aided by a microscopic examination of salivary gland tissue. The minor salivary glands of the lower lip lend themselves readily to this procedure.

The minor salivary glands lie immediately below the surface epithelium, above the muscle layer of the lower lip. They may be easily removed by means of an incision just through the epithelium on the inner surface of the lower lip. The incision need be no longer than 1 to 2 cm. If an eversion of the lip over the surgeon's fingertip does not expose several glands (which clinically appear as whitish-yellow globules), blunt dissection laterally and inferiorly may be necessary. The glands thus exposed should be lightly grasped at their bases with a cotton forceps and severed from the surrounding connective tissue with scalpel or scissors. Several glands should be thus secured, taking care that their microscopic anatomy is not distorted by the use of tissue clamps or forceps. The incision is closed with 4-0 or 3-0 black silk sutures. The sutures should be placed closely together and tied well; this tissue is mobile and relatively fragile, and it is not unusual for several sutures to be lost over a week's time. The patient should be supplied with a mild analgesic and instructed in methods of maintaining wound cleanliness. The salivary glands obtained should be submitted in a suitable fixative/preservative to a histopathology laboratory for diagnosis.

Laboratory Procedures

Several laboratory procedures may be helpful in the diagnosis of salivary gland disease states.

A complete blood count and a differential blood count may offer some help in determining the acuteness or chronicity of the disease. A blood examination may aid in distinguishing between several entities (mumps, infectious mononucleosis, and acute sialadenitis), which may resemble each other.

Microbiologic examinations of saliva or

purulent material from an affected gland are occasionally desirable. Fluid for these studies should not be collected from the oral cavity but from the cannulated duct of the gland in question. In this fashion, oral contamination of the sample is avoided. (See section on sialography for cannulization technique.)

Disorders of the Salivary Glands

Inflammatory Disorders

Inflammation of the salivary glands, or sialadenitis, may be acute or chronic. It is due to bacterial or viral infection or other specific causes.

Acute Bacterial Sialadenitis

Symptoms. This condition usually appears as a painful swelling of the gland accompanied by a decrease in its function. There may be a low-grade fever, malaise, and headache. The overlying skin appears reddened and tense due to glandular edema. A purulent discharge from the gland's duct may be evident spontaneously or with digital expression.

Etiology. The microorganisms involved represent a wide range of normal oral bacteria: *Staphylococcus aureus, Staphylococcus pyogenes, Streptococcus viridans,* and *pneumococci.* Occasionally, fungal forms may be identified. Infections involving mixed bacterial forms appear to ascend to the gland from the oral cavity; infections involving specific bacterial forms are more commonly blood borne.[10]

Diagnostic Aids. History, as related by the patient, and a febrile state point to the acute nature of the problem. The blood profile may show a leukocytosis. Bacterial culture of the purulent discharge may aid in determining bacterial type and antibiotic sensitivity.

Plain radiology is valueless except when an infection of the submandibular gland must be differentiated from an infection originating within the dental alveolus. Sialography, as mentioned previously, is contraindicated.

Treatment. The treatment plan involves rest, antibiotic therapy, and if necessary, surgical drainage. After the acute phase has subsided, the salivary duct may be dilated with graded salivary duct lacrimal probes to facilitate drainage. A salivary washing action should be instituted using a sialagogue such as citric acid or lemon extract. Throughout the treatment, the patient's hydration status must be maintained.

Prognosis. Once this condition has occurred, it tends to recur. Frequently, this recurrence takes the form of a subacute or chronic form of the disease.

Chronic Bacterial Sialadenitis

Symptoms. The symptoms of chronic sialadenitis are similar to those of the acute form; the degree of severity may be less. Salivary flow may be reduced and a purulent discharge noted at the duct orifice. There is usually no erythema of the overlying skin.

Etiology. The etiologic agents are generally similar to those of acute bacterial sialadenitis. This condition is almost exclusively a complication from an obstruction in the duct of the submandibular gland. This obstruction in the salivary duct causes ductal dilatation and salivary stasis followed by glandular atrophy and fibrosis. The gland becomes firm and hard. Bacteria move in a retrograde fashion into the duct, incubate, and form abscesses. The cause of this chronic condition in the parotid gland is less well known; low secretion rate is probably an important predisposing factor.

Diagnostic Aids. As with acute bacterial sialadenitis, the history is important. The patient may relate a prior episode of acute sialadenitis or glandular pain or swelling during meals. Bacterial culture of purulent material expressed from the gland aids in diagnosis. Plain radiology may show a calcified ductal obstruction.

Sialography may show a "pruned tree" appearance with lack of acinar filling (probably owing to acinar edema). With a long-standing problem, punctate dilatation of the peripheral ductules may be noted.[5] Sialography may aid in determining the status of the gland proximal to an obstruction, thereby determining optimal treatment. A diagnosis of severe chronic sialadenitis may be made from a sialogram; lesser degrees of inflammation are difficult to recognize sialographically.[11]

Treatment. Conservative treatment in the form of obstruction removal, ductal dilatation, antibiotic therapy, and therapeutic sialography may effect at least a temporary cure. Recurrence is common and surgical removal of the gland is often necessary.

Chronic Recurrent Parotitis in Children

Chronic recurrent parotitis in children differs from that which occurs in adults. This condition occurs approximately ten times less frequently in children than in adults.[3] The cause of this condition in children is, as in the adult, uncertain.

Although it can occur from the age of 1 month to 13 years, it is most common between 3 and 6 years of age.[10] The symptoms in children are similar to those in adults.

Sialography usually shows the parotid gland and ducts to be normal.[10] The course of chronic parotitis in children is characterized by spontaneous healing in the majority of the cases. A conservative approach to management and treatment is recommended.[3,10,12]

Differential Diagnosis. Epidemic parotitis (mumps) must be excluded in a differential diagnosis of chronic recurrent parotitis in children. Chronic parotitis is usually unilateral whereas mumps is bilateral. Purulent material is usually evident from the duct in chronic parotitis but not with mumps. Also, the mumps virus may be detected in saliva with the complement fixation test.

Sialectasia

There is some disagreement as to the true nature of sialectasis.

The symptoms of this condition as described by Prowler and co-workers are similar to those of chronic recurrent sialadenitis.[13] Prowler and associates state that the sialographic appearance of this condition is that of a gross enlargement of the secretory acini at the proximal end of the ductules, producing the "bunch of grapes" appearance (Fig. 22-24). They state that there may also be multiple ductal strictures with or without enlargement of acini, intraglandular abscesses, or both.[13]

Diamant states that this condition is not typical of any special disorder, but is a

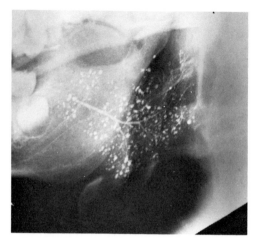

Fig. 22-24. Parotid sialogram illustrating the "bunch of grapes" appearance. (Courtesy of Dr. D. E. Waite)

sign of an inflammatory reaction, especially in the parotid; the typical "bunch of grapes" sialographic appearance is due to preformed cavities.[14]

Other explanations of sialectasis as visualized on sialograms include a phenomenon of ductal rupture in areas of inflammation owing to the injection of contrast media into weakened ducts[11] and congenital dysplasia of ducts.[4]

Mumps

Mumps, or epidemic parotitis, is a viral disease that primarily affects the salivary glands but also may affect other organs (pancreas, ovaries, testes) as well. It is the most common of all salivary gland diseases.

Symptoms. Fever, headache, and painful swelling of one or more salivary glands, most commonly the parotid, are the main symptoms. Usually one gland is affected followed by the other in three to six days. The onset of the symptoms is usually sudden. The swelling of the glands reaches a maximum within two days and diminishes over an additional week.[3] This clinical enlargement is due to

glandular inflammation precipitated by the virus.

Etiology. Mumps is caused by a virus which can be transmitted by droplets of saliva. The incubation period is two to three weeks.

Diagnostic Aids. Mumps is usually bilateral; it usually affects the parotids, but may also affect the submandibular glands. Purulent material cannot be expressed from the duct. The complement fixation test is probably the best diagnostic test for mumps virus antibodies.

Treatment. The treatment of mumps is usually symptomatic. Isolation of the patient for six to ten days is recommended to prevent contagion.

Salivary Gland Inclusion Disease

Salivary gland inclusion disease results from an infection by the deoxyribonucleic acid (DNA) cytomegalovirus; it may be acquired in utero or at any time postnatally. As many as 81 per cent of certain populations over the age of 35 years harbor the virus or have been exposed to it.[15]

Pathologic changes include the appearance of large intranuclear and less distinct cytoplasmatic inclusion bodies in grossly enlarged cells of many organs. The organs most often affected are the salivary glands, kidneys, liver, lungs, pancreas, and thyroid. The gross tissue changes are minimal; they consist chiefly of edema and slight enlargement of the organ. Occasionally, however, areas of focal necrosis and fibrosis may occur.[15]

Infection with the cytomegalovirus may cause subclinical infection or overt illness known as cytomegalic inclusion disease (C.I.D.). Most infections are subclinical, but serious diseases characterized by prematurity, microcephaly, intracranial calcifications, hepatosplenomegaly, and thrombocytopenia may occur in the unborn infant. Acquired infection characterized by fever, rash, pneumonitis, or hepatitis may occur in persons with generalized malignancies or leukemia, and in renal transplant patients.

Diagnosis depends upon the identification of the virus in saliva, urine, blood, or tissue. It is interesting to note the fact that the parotid gland is most often affected in the infant and child whereas the submandibular gland is more frequently involved in adults.[10]

Postirradiation Chronic Sialadenitis

Patients who have received therapeutic irradiation for malignancies of the head and neck region invariably complain of a dry mouth between two to six hours after treatment. Additionally, these patients develop pain and enlargement of the parotid and submandibular glands during the same period. This enlargement increases for 12 to 24 hours, then rapidly subsides without treatment. These symptoms are due to an acute inflammatory reaction within the salivary glands. From this reactive pattern, a progressive change in which continued degeneration and loss of acini, replacement of acute inflammatory cells by chronic inflammatory elements, and intralobular fibrosis may occur.[16] This degenerative change continues to frank atrophy of glandular and interstitial elements with consequent loss of function. Interestingly, there are no major alterations in the ductules within the gland.

The dry mouth, or xerostomia, following therapeutic irradiation may be transient or become permanent. Treatment for this condition is empirical at best (see Xerostomia).

Postsurgical Parotitis

So-called postoperative, or postsurgical, parotitis may occasionally occur following major surgery or lengthy dental and oral surgery procedures.

Symptoms. The symptoms of surgical parotitis are similar to those of acute sialadenitis: swelling, discomfort, and suppuration. The symptoms usually occur from four to six days following the surgical procedure, with the majority of patients manifesting them within two weeks postsurgery.[17]

Etiology. The causative organism is usually *Staphylococcus aureus.* The predisposing factor is diminished salivary flow which permits retrograde infection. This diminished salivary flow is probably due to dehydration, fever, and blood loss. Trauma to the glands from the prolonged pressure of the anesthesia mask has also been suggested as a contributing factor.[17]

Diagnostic Aids. The history of a recent major surgical procedure should lead to the correct diagnosis; certain other diagnostic procedures such as those discussed under acute sialadenitis are probably unnecessary. Bacterial culture of the purulent discharge is recommended to determine bacterial type and antibiotic sensitivity.

Treatment. Treatment of postoperative parotitis consists of adjustment of the pa-

tient's fluid balance, stimulation of salivary flow, and antibiotic therapy.

Obstructive Disorders

A salivary duct obstruction impedes or
halts salivary excretion into the oral cavity. At least for a time, the gland continues
the secretion of saliva. This damming
with consequent accumulation of saliva
under pressure produces pain, swelling,
and if the condition is long-standing,
glandular infection and atrophy.

Symptoms. A partial ductal obstruction
causes acute pain and swelling in the
gland region. These symptoms are especially evident immediately prior to, during, and immediately following meals because of the increased stimulation of the
salivary gland. The patient usually reports
that the swelling slowly diminishes between meals only to recur again at the
next mealtime. A partial obstruction
causes these symptoms by allowing some
saliva to leak past during periods of low
salivary secretion, but not enough during
periods of increased secretion to prevent
accumulation.

A partial obstruction may lead to glandular infection; bacteria may ascend the
duct until they reach the stagnant pool of
saliva proximal to the obstruction. This
condition may occur even if the degree of
obstruction is not enough to cause mealtime swelling.[18]

Alternatively, the patient may be unaware of the glandular swelling, but will
complain of dull pain following meals.
This pain may be poorly localized; it may
be described as originating in the throat,
molar tooth, or ear.[18]

Etiology. Ductal obstruction may be
caused by mucous plugs, calculi within
the duct (sialolithasis), ductal strictures or
ulcerations, or neoplasms.

Salivary calculi (sialoliths) are frequently the cause of ductal obstruction,
particularly in Wharton's duct. Calculi
are usually unilateral and may assume a
wide range of size. Rauch, Gorlin, and
Seifert have presented a review of the
various theories regarding the origin and
subsequent enlargement of sialoliths.[10]

Mucous plugs may cause ductal obstruction. They may be treated with the
administration of a strong sialagogue. The
contrast medium used in sialography may
also "break up" a mucous obstruction. If
both these methods fail, these obstructions
should be treated as a sialolith.

Parotid Obstruction

PAPILLARY OBSTRUCTION. Stensen's papilla and duct orifice may be traumatized
by the dentition, a faulty restoration, or a
dental prosthesis. Trauma to this area frequently occurs during eruption of the second and third molars.[18] The edema associated with this trauma (and possible
subsequent ulceration) may cause ductal
obstruction. If this trauma is of long duration, chronic fibrotic papillary stenosis
occurs: a partial or total closure of the
ductal orifice caused by scarring.

Diagnostic Aids. Stensen's duct may
resist the insertion of or feel rigid upon
the insertion of a lacrimal probe. Following milking of the gland, the tissue behind
the papilla may assume a bluish tone
owing to a pool of saliva.[18]

Sialography will demonstrate a narrowing of the duct in the papillary region and
a dilatation of the duct proximally.[3]

Treatment. The treatment of papillary
obstruction consists of removal of the
cause of trauma. If stenosis has occurred,
dilatation of the ductal orifice with graded

lacrimal probes or surgical removal of the papilla and distal duct portion may be necessary. If the surgical approach is necessary, care must be taken to suture the duct walls to the oral mucosae.

DUCT OBSTRUCTION. Parotid duct sialoliths are not as common as submandibular sialoliths; they account only for approximately 6 to 10 per cent of salivary calculi.[10] These calculi are usually smaller but more symptomatic than Wharton's duct calculi; patients therefore seek treatment earlier. Calculi in the parotid duct may be located in four areas: impacted at the papilla, in the submucous portion, in the extraglandular portion of the duct external to the buccinator, and in the intraglandular portion of the duct.[19]

Symptoms. The symptoms of parotid duct obstruction are acute pain and swelling associated with meals or recurrent infections of the gland.

Salivary calculi in Stensen's duct, because of their usual sharpness and pointedness, may cause pain during mastication and upon palpation.[10]

Diagnostic Aids. In some cases, the location of the calculus may be assessed by noting the area of swelling. If the accessory parotid is enlarged, the calculus lies distally in the duct; if the lower pole of the gland is involved, the calculus lies in the intraglandular portion of the duct.[19]

If the calculus is impacted near the ductal orifice, it may be visualized protruding from the papilla or as a hard, yellowish swelling immediately under the epithelium.

Plain radiography may be useful in establishing a diagnosis of a Stensen's duct calculus. A periapical film applied against the inner aspect of the cheek and exposed as previously described (see section on plain radiology) usually demonstrates the calculus. A calculus that lies in the intraglandular portion of the duct may be difficult to demonstrate with plain radiography.

Sialography may be useful in demonstrating a mucous or poorly calcified obstruction. Care must be exercised so that the calculus is not forced proximally by the pressure of the injection.

Treatment. If the calculus lies immediately subjacent to the ductal orifice, the orifice may be simply slit open with a surgical scissors. It may be necessary to milk the calculus out with salivary flow. The papilla and ductal orifice heal well without the use of sutures.

The removal of salivary calculi within the buccinator portion of the duct or more proximally can be surgically difficult; the technique involved is beyond the scope of this text. For further information, the reader is referred to several excellent reviews of this technique.[3,19,20]

Submandibular Obstruction

Frequently, following a surgical procedure (such as a biopsy) on the anterior floor of the mouth, symptoms of submandibular gland obstruction appear. They are usually due to a ductal stricture caused by healing of the adjacent tissue.

Sialoliths are the most frequent cause of obstructions of Wharton's duct. The most common site is just distal to the body of the gland.[10] Calculi in this posterior segment of the duct may not cause symptoms for some time owing to the relatively large size and elasticity of the duct. If the stone increases in size to the point where salivary flow is slowed considerably or if infection supervenes, the patient will experience symptoms.[21]

Symptoms. Symptoms of submandibular duct obstruction are acute pain and swelling or those of infection.

Diagnostic Aids. Most sialoliths within at least the distal portion of Wharton's duct may be palpated. With palpation it is possible to determine the location of the obstruction and to ascertain the status of the gland proper (a fibrosed gland feels firm and inelastic; a normal gland or one with little change feels elastic).[21]

Plain radiography is usually helpful; the film should be positioned and exposed as described previously (see section on plain radiography).

Sialography should be used with caution; there is a possibility that a sialolith may be forced proximally by pressure from injection of the contrast medium. Sialography may be used following the removal of the sialolith to aid in determining the status of the gland.

Treatment. If the obstructive calculus lies in the extraglandular portion of the duct and if the gland itself has suffered no irreparable damage, the calculus is removed surgically.

If the calculus lies in the intraglandular portion of the duct or if the gland has become fibrosed owing to long-standing obstruction or infection, the entire gland is removed.

The surgical removal of submandibular duct calculi which lie in the distal portion of the duct may be accomplished under local anesthesia (Fig. 22-25). A brief description follows: Anesthesia is achieved by a lingual nerve block. A suture is passed around the duct posterior to the calculus and tied gently; this prevents proximal displacement of the calculus

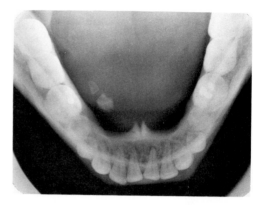

Fig. 22-25. Preoperative radiograph of calculus within Wharton's duct.

(Fig. 22-26). Wharton's duct is identified by means of blunt dissection in the floor of the mouth following an incision through the oral mucosae. The duct is stabilized by means of a distal suture and incised over the calculus (Fig. 22-27). The calculus is extirpated (Fig. 22-28), the duct irrigated, and the stabilization sutures removed. The mucosal incision only is sutured; at-

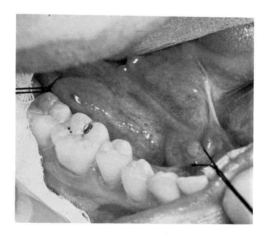

Fig. 22-26. Removal of Wharton's duct calculus. Isolation of calculus between posterior ligature and anterior traction suture. (Courtesy of Dr. D. E. Waite)

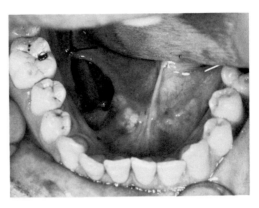

Fig. 22-29. Removal of Wharton's duct calculus. The ductal incision is not sutured; the overlying mucosa is sutured. Note the duct traversing the surgical opening. (Courtesy of Dr. D. E. Waite)

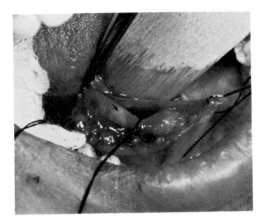

Fig. 22-27. Removal of Wharton's duct calculus. Wharton's duct with contained sialolith (arrow) is surgically isolated with blunt dissection. (Courtesy of Dr. D. E. Waite)

tempts to suture the duct itself may lead to stricture formation (Fig. 22-29).

Submandibular calculi that lie in the proximal portion of the duct are usually removed under general anesthesia; this surgical procedure and the procedure involved in the removal of the submandibu-

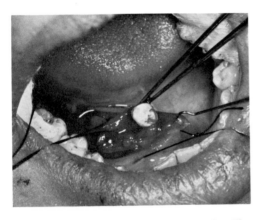

Fig. 22-28. Removal of Wharton's duct calculus. The duct has been stabilized with traction sutures. The sialolith is removed via a longitudinal incision. (Courtesy of Dr. D. E. Waite)

lar gland proper are beyond the scope of this text. For further information regarding these procedures, the reader is referred to several articles which have appeared in the literature.[3, 21-23]

Sublingual and Minor Gland Obstruction

Obstructions of the ducts of the sublingual and minor salivary glands are rare; there have been probably fewer than 30 reported cases of minor gland sialolithiasis. The buccal mucosa seems to be the most common site for minor gland sialolithiasis.

Symptoms. Localized sublingual edema coupled with a small concrement near Wharton's duct may indicate a sublingual duct sialolith.[10] Minor gland obstructions appear as hard swellings.

Diagnostic Aids. Glandular palpation will aid in localizing sialoliths in these locations. Plain radiography is useful in the diagnosis of a minor gland sialolith if located in the cheek or lip.

Treatment. If the sublingual sialolith is at the ductal orifice, treatment is afforded by a surgical enlargement of the orifice, similar to the treatment described for a calculus impacted immediately beneath Stensen's papilla.

Treatment of minor gland sialoliths consists of removal of the entire gland and duct. The surgical technique is identical to that which will be described for the removal of a mucocele (see section on Mucocele).

Sialadenosis

Sialadenosis is the noninflammatory, non-neoplastic bilateral swelling of the salivary glands. This clinical enlargement is accompanied by gland hypofunction. The disorder may affect all salivary glands, but usually only the parotids are involved.

The course of sialadenosis is chronic, undulating, recurrent, usually indolent, and patients are afebrile. Women, especially those in the age of hormonal alterations, are often more affected than men.[10] The glandular hypofunction associated with this condition may lead to chronic sialadenitis since the mechanism which acts to prevent retrograde infection (salivary flow) is impaired.

Symptoms. Sialadenosis is characterized by a slowly increasing, chronic, undulating multiglandular enlargement, usually bilateral, of the salivary glands, accompanied by a systemic disorder or hormonal imbalance which may be undiagnosed.

Etiology. Sialadenosis may be associated with hormonal disturbances such as diabetes mellitus, hypothyroidism, menopause, Cushing's syndrome, menstruation, and pregnancy. Hepatogenic sialadenosis has been associated with alcoholism with or without cirrhosis. This condition is common in certain nutritional deficiency states, especially in hypoproteinemia. Parotid gland enlargement has been noted in association with the intake of certain drugs such as phenylbutazone, certain norepinephrine derivatives, and catecholamine.

Diagnostic Aids. Diagnosis of this disorder may often be made by clinical history; pursuit of this diagnosis may lead to discovery of a previously unsuspected systemic condition.

Sialography reveals a normal ductal structure[3] or one exhibiting a thin, hairline architecture.[10]

With glandular milking salivary secretion presents as a scanty, whitish, viscous flow.

Clinical palpation reveals a gland that is doughy, painless, and poorly demarcated.[10]

Biopsy specimen of an involved gland reveals the nature of the enlargement: serous acinar cell hypertrophy, edema of the interstitial supporting tissues, and atrophy of the striated ducts.[3]

Treatment. The treatment of the associated systemic disturbance usually affects resolution of the associated sialadenosis. This has been especially noted when the sialadenosis is associated with alcoholic cirrhosis of the liver and with malnutrition.

Glandular Atrophy

Salivary gland atrophy may be a result of disease, ductal obstruction or ligation, radiation, or the aging process.

True atrophy results from wasting diseases (e.g., disseminated carcinoma) or following radiation therapy, with the decrease in both glandular and interstitial elements.

Benign atrophy shows an increase in the apparent gland size; actually this represents an increase only in the interstitial elements; the glandular component of the gland decreases. Two types of benign atrophy may be considered. (1) Fatty atrophy, the more common form, clinically appears as a uniform doughy gland without nodularity. Salivation is normal or decreased. (2) Fibrous atrophy clinically appears as a firm, finely glandular or nodular gland. Glandular atrophy following long-term ductal obstruction or radiation has been previously discussed.

Waterhouse and associates have shown that between childhood and old age approximately one quarter of the active parenchymal cell volume is lost.[24] Fat and connective tissue replace this cell volume and may even cause an increase in overall gland size. This loss of the active parenchymal cell volume with senescence probably accounts for the reduction of salivary flow volume seen in some older individuals.

Developmental Anomalies

The congenital absence of salivary glands (aplasia or agenesis) or the congenital occlusion or absence of salivary ducts (atresia) is rare. These conditions, when present, may give rise to xerostomia and its associated increased caries rate or retention cyst formation (see section on Xerostomia).

Salivary gland tissue at an abnormal anatomic site is termed aberrancy. Aber-

rant salivary gland tissue has been reported at the base of the neck, the hypophysis, sternoclavicular joint, and middle ear.[25]

In 1942, Stafne originally described a series of 34 cases of bone defects near the angle of the mandible below the inferior alveolar nerve canal.[26] Since that original report, the presence of this static bone cavity or defect has been described frequently. In most cases, these cyst-like cavities have been found to contain salivary gland tissue, probably representing ec-

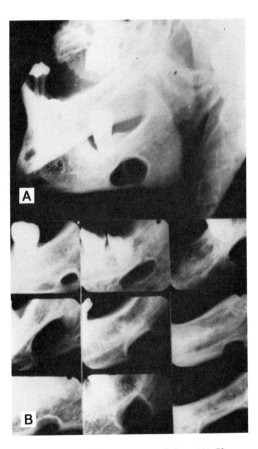

Fig. 22-30. Static bone cavity or defect. (A) Characteristic location of defect near mandibular angle and below inferior alveolar canal. (B) Other mandibular defects which may contain salivary tissue. (A, Courtesy of Dr. E. C. Stafne. B, Stafne, E. C.: Bone cavities situated near the angle of the mandible. J. Am. Dent. Assoc. 29:1969–1972, 1942. Copyright by the American Dental Association, reprinted by permission)

topic submandibular gland nests (Fig. 22-30). Occasionally, these nests may maintain a ductal connection with the submandibular gland proper; sialography, therefore, may be helpful in the diagnosis.

This condition has been considered congenital; a premature growth of the submandibular gland causing an accommodation by the osseous structure of the mandible. Evidence has been presented, however, that indicates formation of this defect may occur after middle age.[27]

The exact method of development of these salivary tissue enclaves is open to question; a probable explanation may be surface bone resorption by an unknown cause.

Aberrant, normal-appearing mixed salivary gland tissue has been described within bone in the incisor-premolar area of the mandible.[25] The occurrence of rests in this location must be considered rare.

These examples of aberrant salivary gland tissue represent simply variations from normal and should be recognized as such; no treatment is usually necessary. It is important to note, however, that any area of aberrant salivary gland tissue may be the site of neoplastic change.

Functional Disorders

Sialorrhea (Ptyalism)

Increased salivary flow, or sialorrhea, may result from many different causes. They may be grouped into two main categories: (1) factors affecting the higher central nervous system and (2) local factors that reflexly stimulate flow.

Sialorrhea may occur in mentally retarded individuals; it is also associated with deteriorated schizophrenia, epilepsy, parkinsonism, mercury poisoning, acrodynia, and other mental, psychiatric, and neurologic disturbances.

The most common causes of sialorrhea are acute inflammations of the oral cavity; these cause excessive salivary secretion through reflex stimulation. Sialorrhea is common with herpetic or aphthous ulceration and acute necrotizing gingival stomatitis. Sialorrhea may also accompany ill-fitting dentures and the eruption of teeth in young individuals.

Treatment. The underlying cause of the excessive salivary flow should be treated. Symptomatic relief may be frequently obtained with the antihistaminic drugs such as methantheline bromide (Banthine) (50 mg.) or atropine sulfate ($\frac{1}{150}$ grain).

Xerostomia

In 1868, A. G. Bartley wrote to the editor of London's *Medical Times and Gazette.* His question concerned treatment of dryness of the oral mucosae and dryness and soreness of the tongue in an elderly patient. In writing this letter, Bartley became the first individual of record to describe the symptoms associated with diminished salivary flow. Shortly afterward, in 1888, Hutchinson and Hadden termed this condition xerostomia.

Xerostomia may be defined as occurring when salivary secretion is equal to or less than 0 to 2 ml. per 15 minutes; this flow rate is less than 4 per cent of the average salivary flow rate for persons under 65 years of age.[28]

Symptoms. The patient with xerostomia will often complain of a dry mouth. Clinical examination may reveal pronounced reddening of the tongue coupled with total papillary atrophy, lobulation, or deep fissuring. Glossodynia, cheilosis of the lip commissures, dysphonia, dysphagia, taste disturbances, and denture difficulties may also be manifest. These signs and symptoms tend to increase in severity as the salivary secretion decreases.[28] Severe cases of xerostomia may be accompanied by an increased caries rate, especially in the cervical areas of the teeth. This increased caries rate is probably due to the loss of the cleansing properties of saliva.

Etiology. Xerostomia may be idiopathic or a manifestation of a local factor such as mouth breathing, inflammatory conditions of the salivary glands, irradiation, and degenerative or aging changes. Xerostomia may also be associated with systemic conditions such as anemias, certain syndromes (Sjögren's, Mikulicz's, Heerfordt's), lupus erythematosus, hormonal disturbances, drugs, emotional and anxiety states, and fluid loss.

Diagnostic Aids. The patient's medical history and clinical examination are of great importance. Approximately 80 per cent of patients with xerostomia show clinical manifestations within the oral cavity.[28] Clinical milking of the salivary glands may give some indication of the nature of the salivary flow. Plain radiography, sialography, and scintigraphy may be of assistance in the diagnosis of obstructive or systemic disorders. Bacterial cultures and blood studies may lead to the identification of infectious or hematologic disorders.

Treatment. The definitive treatment of xerostomia is the removal of the cause.

Since the majority of cases of xerostomia are due to idiopathic or obscure conditions, treatment must frequently be symptomatic.

Symptomatic treatments of xerostomia are several, but none has gained universal success or acceptance. A mouthwash containing citric acid (12.5 gm.), essence of lemon (20 ml.), and glycerine (q.s. 1 liter) is suggested by some.[3] Mouthwashes containing sodium chloride and sodium bicarbonate may be useful. Laskin recommended a 1 per cent methylcellulose mouthwash on an "as needed" basis, proper humidification of the ambient air, and avoidance of mouth breathing.[29]

Whichever method of symptomatic treatment is chosen, the patient should be monitored closely to prevent a serious infection with candidal organisms, should be encouraged to increase fluid intake, and should be instructed in meticulous oral and dental hygiene.

Cysts and Cyst-like Lesions

True Cysts

True cysts of the major salivary glands are rare if the branchiogenic cysts are not considered.[10] Cystic disorders of salivary glands may include congenital cysts, traumatic cysts, or far-advanced cavitary diseases secondary to chronic sialadenitis.

Cysts of the major salivary glands occur most frequently in the parotid and represent but a small percentage of surgical salivary gland problems.

Mucocele

The mucocele is a fluid-filled or semi-fluid-filled cavity surrounded by a capsule composed of compressed granulation tissue or epithelium. These abnormalities may be superficial or deep and may vary in size from a few millimeters to a centimeter or more in diameter. Superficial mucoceles have a bluish translucent color and rupture easily; those more deeply seated may assume the color of the surrounding oral mucosa.

Mucoceles may be found almost anywhere within the oral cavity; the majority occur on the lower lip. The buccal mucosa and the mouth floor may also be involved. A mucocele that involves the salivary gland tissue in the anterior ventral tongue area is termed a cyst of Blandin-Nuhn (Fig. 22-31). Mucoceles are rarely found on the upper lip.

Mucoceles are generally considered to be of two types, extravasation or retention. The extravasation mucocele is not a true cyst since the cavity is not lined by epithelium. This type consists of a mucous pool or eosinophilic hyaline material (with mucus-laden macrophages) surrounded by granulation tissue with macrophages and inflammatory cells. Extravasation mucoceles occur most frequently in the lower lip and in individuals below the age of 30 years.

Retention mucoceles, or mucous retention cysts, may be considered true cysts; they consist of a mucous pool surrounded by columnar, pseudostratified, or cuboidal epithelium. Retention mucoceles occur rarely in the lip; they are usually found elsewhere in the oral cavity. This type of mucocele is most frequently seen in individuals over the age of 50 years.

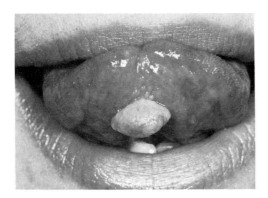

Fig. 22-31. Mucocele of the minor salivary glands of the ventral anterior tongue; the so-called cyst of Blandin-Nuhn. (Courtesy of Dr. R. Gorlin)

Symptoms. Mucoceles have a rather characteristic behavior pattern. The patient will report an increase in size of an area followed usually by a spontaneous shrinkage with a subsequent enlargement. This history of alternate enlargement and shrinkage is typical, especially of lesions located superficially on the lip or buccal mucosa. The obstructed salivary gland continues to secrete saliva which escapes into the connective tissue or distends the duct. This process continues until the expanded tissue ruptures from pressure, trauma, or surgical manipulation. The rupture heals in the now-collapsed lesion and the saliva again accumulates to repeat the enlargement. Patients may occasionally report a drainage of fluid from the expanded lesion; usually, however, this drainage goes unnoticed.

Etiology. The extravasation mucocele probably occurs as a result of trauma. Trauma, chiefly mechanical, causes a rupture of the duct of a minor salivary gland, resulting in secretion of saliva into the surrounding tissue. This saliva compresses the surrounding connective tissue and causes a variable degree of chronic inflammation.

The retention mucocele occurs following partial obstruction of a minor salivary gland duct. The gland continues to secrete saliva and an enlargement or ballooning of the duct results. This dilatation of the duct becomes a cystic lesion lined by epithelium.

Diagnostic Aids. The clinical appearance coupled with the history should lead to the correct diagnosis. If the lesion is superficial, the contained fluid may be frequently palpated.

Treatment. Successful treatment of small mucoceles located in the labial or buccal mucosa consists of total excision of the lesion and surrounding salivary tissue.

Figure 22-32 illustrates a mucocele of moderate diameter. Anesthesia is achieved by a series of submucosal injections surrounding the lesion, a so-called ring block (Fig. 22-33). Anesthesia administered in this fashion does not distort the subsequent microscopic interpretation of the tissue. Stabilization without distortion of the tissue is achieved by passing a suture under the lesion; tension may be applied to the tissue using this suture throughout the procedure (Fig. 22-34). A wedge-shaped elliptical incision is performed to include the mucocele; the tissue is separated from the underlying submucosa with sharp dissection (Fig. 22-35). Frequently, additional minor salivary glands are seen in the surgical site; these should be removed since, because of the trauma they have experienced, they may be the source of a recurrent mucocele. The surgical margins are undermined with

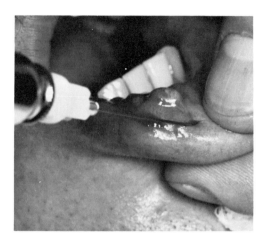

Fig. 22-33. Ring block anesthesia for removal of superficial mucocele.

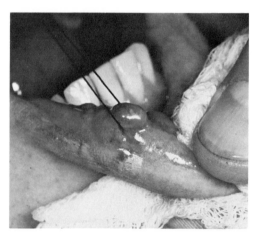

Fig. 22-34. Removal of superficial mucocele. Traction suture passed under and outside of the lesion.

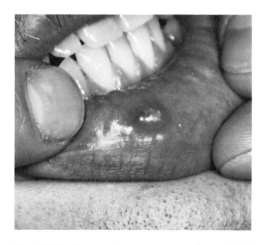

Fig. 22-32. Preoperative appearance of superficial mucocele.

blunt dissection (Fig. 22-36), and the wound sutured through the mucosa only so as to avoid trauma to any residual salivary tissue (Fig. 22-37). The sutures should remain in place for five to seven days. It is important to remember that the patient should be cautioned that this type of lesion may recur.

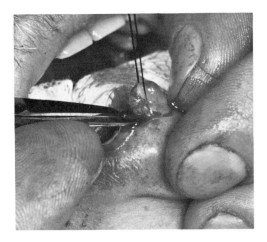

Fig. 22-35. Removal of superficial mucocele. A V-shaped elliptical incision to include all the lesion is accomplished with a scalpel. The lesion is separated from the underlying tissue with sharp dissection. Note traction suture.

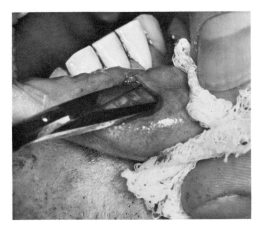

Fig. 22-36. Removal of superficial mucocele. As a preliminary to closure, the surrounding epithelium must be undermined with blunt dissection. A surgical scissors works well.

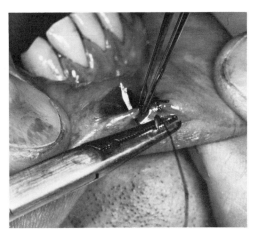

Fig. 22-37. Removal of superficial mucocele. Closure is achieved with sutures placed through the mucosa only. Note use of tissue forceps to avoid trauma.

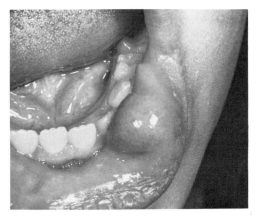

Fig. 22-38. Large mucocele of lower lip.

Treatment of large mucoceles and deep lesions involves a meticulous dissection of the mucocele from the surrounding tissue (Fig. 22-38). After complete removal, the overlying mucosa is sutured. As with smaller mucoceles, recurrence is possible.

It should be noted that surgical drainage of these lesions does not represent treatment. Although this procedure effects a shrinkage, healing soon occurs and the enlargement reappears.

Ranula

A mucocele occurring in the anterior floor of the mouth is rather arbitrarily termed a ranula. The name derives from the similarity of its color to that of the ventral surface of a frog (rana).

These lesions are usually unilateral and may be from 2 to 3 cm. in diameter. They are soft and fluctuant and usually have a blue-violet color. The walls are thin and do not pit with pressure. They are usually associated with the sublingual gland. Ranulas are usually relatively superficial lesions lying above the mylohyoid muscles; they may extend posteriorly.

Microscopically, ranulas are generally unilocular. The lumen contains a viscous, mucoserous fluid. The wall of a ranula is composed of compressed connective tissue which contains variable numbers of chronic inflammatory elements. Rarely, ranulas may contain an epithelial lining; in these cases the lining is usually similar to that found in an excretory duct (cuboidal epithelium).

Symptoms. Ranulas are generally painless; they may interfere with speech, mastication, and deglutition simply by their location or size.

Etiology. These lesions probably arise from the partial obstruction to salivary flow; they therefore share a common etiology with mucoceles elsewhere in the oral cavity.

Diagnostic Aids. The location, clinical appearance, and history of this lesion should lead to the correct diagnosis. Clinical palpation will reveal contained fluid. As with mucoceles elsewhere in the oral cavity, the patient may relate a history of periodic enlargement and shrinkage.

Treatment. Treatment is marsupialization or excision of the ranula; incision with drainage alone results in recurrence. Marsupialization involves the removal of the superior wall of the ranula and the suturing of the remaining lining to the mucous membrane of the mouth floor.

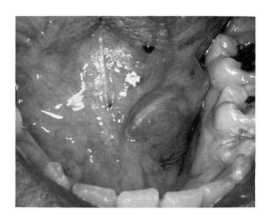

Fig. 22-39. Preoperative appearance of ranula. Anesthesia is achieved through a block of the lingual nerve or with the ring block technique.

After suitable anesthesia has been established (Fig. 22-39), a tissue scissors is used to remove the overlying mucosa and ranula lining around the greatest perimeter of the lesion (Fig. 22-40). Sutures are then passed through the oral mucosae and the lesion's lining and knotted (Fig. 22-41). Recurrence is possible; the patient should be so informed.

Total excision of the ranula is a difficult

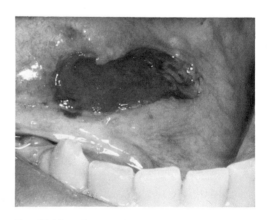

Fig. 22-40. Following the perimeter, the ranula may be readily de-roofed with a surgical scissors.

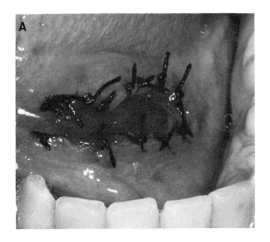

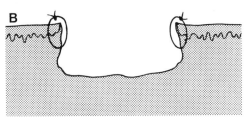

Fig. 22-41. Marsupialization of ranula. (A) The floor of the lesion is sutured to the overlying mucosa. Upon healing, the lining of the ranula will become continuous with the oral mucosa. (B) Diagrammatic cross-sectional view of clinical view in A. Note the sutures through the epithelium and the ranula's lining.

procedure because of the lesion's location and thin wall but may be indicated if it is made up of multiple compartments or is deeply located.

Salivary Gland Neoplasms

Tumors of the salivary glands are relatively rare, constituting from 1 to 4 per cent of all head and neck neoplasms.[10] The paragraphs to follow will include discussions of the most common benign and malignant salivary gland neoplasms and salivary gland problems as presented in children. For more detailed information concerning these entities, the reader is referred to a text of oral pathology or to the literature.

Benign Salivary Gland Neoplasms

Pleomorphic Adenoma (Benign Mixed Tumor)

The pleomorphic adenoma is the most common salivary gland tumor of the major or minor salivary glands. It has been estimated that this tumor accounts for approximately 90 per cent of all benign tumors of all the salivary glands,[30] and for over 50 per cent of all tumors (benign or malignant) of all salivary glands.[31]

Features. When only the major glands are considered, this tumor most frequently involves the parotid, especially the tail of the parotid, which lies below the earlobe. The least frequently involved of the major salivary glands is the sublingual. When considering minor salivary glands, those most frequently involved are the glands of the hard palate, and those least frequently involved are the glands of the lower lip.[30]

Most studies indicate that this tumor is somewhat more common in females than in males. The majority of these neoplasms are diagnosed in the fifth and sixth decades of life.

Pleomorphic adenomas usually begin as solitary, small, painless nodules that slowly and intermittently increase in size without fixation to superficial or deeper structures. The most frequent symptom is a mass that may have been present for greater than five years. Overlying skin and mucosa are seldom ulcerated even though some examples of these neoplasms are quite large.

The pleomorphic adenoma is aptly named; a diverse histologic pattern is the hallmark of this group of neoplasms. Cuboidal, stellate, polyhedral, spindle, or squamous cell elements may exhibit proliferation within a connective tissue stroma. This connective tissue stroma may show a variety of mucoid, myxoid, chondroid, or hyaline patterns. Ossification foci rarely may be observed (Fig. 22-42).

The tumor is surrounded by a connective tissue "pseudocapsule" so-named because of frequent viable tumor nests within the capsule wall. An additional characteristic of pleomorphic adenomas is their nodular outline; though most frequently rounded hummocks, the outgrowths may be pedunculated and form peninsulas with narrow necks.[32]

Treatment and Prognosis. The primary treatment of pleomorphic adenomas of the parotid is surgical excision. The extent of the surgical excision recommended ranges from careful local excision[3] to removal of at least the entire involved lobe.[30] Simple enucleation of these tumors cannot be recommended. There may be a well-marked plane of cleavage between the gland and tumor in most areas, but in at least some interface areas, the plane of cleavage may lie just below the surface of the tumor.[32] Additionally, the viable nests of tumor tissue within the capsule and the tumor's peninsular outgrowths may be surgically left behind.

Treatment of this neoplasm in the submandibular and sublingual glands is usually total glandular excision.

Pleomorphic adenomas of the minor salivary glands are usually treated somewhat more conservatively. The removal of

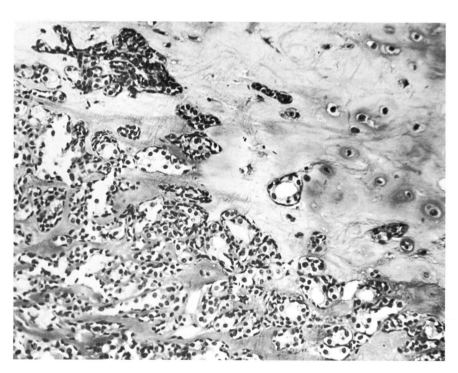

Fig. 22-42. Photomicrograph of pleomorphic adenoma. Note the "pseudocartilaginous," relatively acellular area and the duct-like structures. (Gorlin, R. J., and Vickers, R. A.: Lips, mouth, teeth, salivary glands, and neck. In Pathology, 6th ed. W. A. D. Anderson (Ed.) St. Louis, C. V. Mosby Co., 1971)

the neoplasm along with a margin of surrounding normal tissue is adequate.[30,33]

In the past, recurrences following "shelling out" of the tumor were frequent. With more radical surgical procedures, the recurrence rate has dropped to less than 1 per cent.[10] If the tumors do recur, they probably result from incomplete initial removal. Recurrent lesions are invariably multifocal; this apparently is caused by a seeding of some of the cells during removal or to leaving behind the nests that are contained within the capsule. The recurrences may arise as late as 47 years after initial treatment.[30] There seems to be no increased danger of malignant change with recurrence.[10]

This tumor is radioresistant; the use of irradiation in its treatment is therefore contraindicated.

Adenolymphoma (Warthin's Tumor, Cystadenoma Lymphomatosum)

The adenolymphoma is the most common of the monomorphic adenomas. (Monomorphic adenomas are distinguished from pleomorphic adenomas by their uniform cell structure and pattern.)

Features. This tumor is found most frequently in the parotid gland in a superficial location, especially at the lower pole.[3] It is the only salivary gland tumor to be frequently found bilaterally, with estimates ranging from 3 to 30 per cent.[10] It may also arise multifocally. This tumor has been reported in the submandibular and sublingual glands and in minor glands of the lips, buccal mucosa, palate, and maxillary sinus.[34]

Men over middle age are more commonly affected than women; this represents a departure from other salivary gland tumors which more often affect females.

Adenolymphomas are generally superficial and seldom attain a size exceeding 3 to 4 cm. in diameter. They are slowly growing, painless, and firm to palpation; as such, they may be clinically indistinguishable from other benign salivary neoplasms.

The adenolymphoma has a distinctive histologic appearance. There are two components, epithelial and lymphoid (Fig. 22-43). The epithelium usually takes the form of columnar or cuboidal cells, usually in two layers. This epithelium forms papillary projections into cystic spaces. The lymphoid component is usually abundant and is composed of mature and normally developing lymphocytes. Germinal centers are common. It seems likely that this tumor arises from residues of salivary duct epithelium included within lymph nodes. These nodes probably become entrapped in the parotid owing to the late encapsulation of the gland during development. The lymphoid component, therefore, may represent a passive element in the neoplastic process.

Treatment and Prognosis. Treatment of this neoplasm consists of surgical excision; the tumor does not tend to recur. Excision can usually be accomplished without damage to adjacent structures because of the tumor's superficial location and small size.

Oxyphilic Adenoma (Oncocytoma)

The oxyphilic adenoma is a rare salivary gland neoplasm. It constitutes less than 1 per cent of parotid gland neoplasms.[10]

Features. This neoplasm is a slow growing, small tumor which usually occurs in the parotid. Its presence in other locations has been documentated.[10]

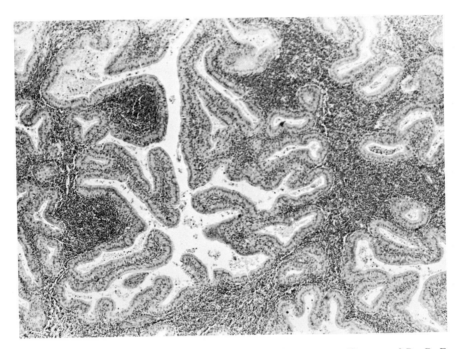

Fig. 22-43. Photomicrograph of adenolymphoma or Warthin's tumor. (Courtesy of Dr. D. E. Waite)

Women more often than men are affected with this tumor, usually within the seventh decade of life or later. It usually appears as a discrete, firm, freely mobile, small, encapsulated mass.

The name oncocytoma is derived from the resemblance of the tumor cells to oncocytes. (Oncocytes are cells normally found within the salivary ducts of elderly persons; they may be a normal consequence of the aging process.) The cells of the oxyphilic adenoma are uniformly large eosinophilic granular cells arranged in rows, cords, sheets, or an alveolar pattern.

Treatment and Prognosis. Treatment of oxyphilic adenoma is complete surgical removal. The tumor has exhibited no tendency to recur.

Necrotizing Sialometaplasia

Necrotizing sialometaplasia has been classed as a benign inflammatory condition of minor salivary glands. It is included here because of its close resemblance to more serious entities. The first report of this condition by Abrams and associates appeared in 1973.[35] Since that time, eight additional cases have been reported.[36,37] This entity must be considered unusual, but the consequences of its misdiagnosis warrant its discussion.

Features. This entity has only been described as occurring on the palate; the majority of the cases have been located at or anterior to the junction of the hard and soft palates. Of the 15 total cases reported, 11 were described in men, 4 in women.

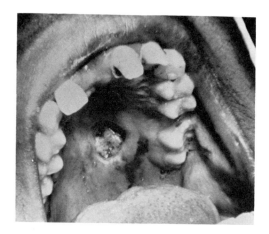

Fig. 22-44. Necrotizing sialometaplasia may clinically appear malignant. Note the deep ulceration and rolled borders. (Courtesy of Dr. A. M. Abrams and Dr. V. J. Castaldo)

All reported patients have been between the ages of 23 and 66 years.

This lesion usually appears as a painful ulceration which may have rolled borders and may measure 3 cm. in diameter (Fig. 22-44).

The associated epithelium exhibits hyperkeratosis and marked pseudoepitheliomatous hyperplasia. The underlying salivary gland ducts exhibit extensive squamous metaplasia. These underlying masses of squamous epithelium may be closely associated with or directly connected to the overlying epithelium. This may give the impression histologically of infiltration from a surface squamous cell carcinoma (Fig. 22-45). The underlying minor salivary gland regions may show areas of mucus escape and pooling with a subsequent foreign body reaction. Areas of this lesion may bear close resemblance to a mucoepidermoid carcinoma.

The cause of necrotizing sialometaplasia is unclear. The basic lesion seems to be a vascular infarction with subse-

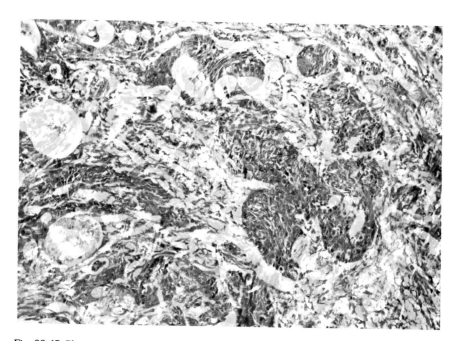

Fig. 22-45. Photomicrograph of necrotizing sialometaplasia. Epithelial islands represent salivary gland ducts in the connective tissue which have undergone extensive squamous metaplasia. These ductal changes bear strong resemblance to squamous cell carcinoma. (Courtesy of Dr. A. M. Abrams)

quent ulceration and repair. The basis for this vascular alteration is unknown.

Treatment and Prognosis. The treatment of this condition consists of recognizing its true benign nature. All reported cases have healed in 6 to 8 weeks without treatment. Recurrence has not been noted.

Malignant Salivary Gland Neoplasms

Malignant Mixed Tumor (Malignant Pleomorphic Adenoma)

The malignant mixed tumor is a rather ill-defined neoplasm. Because of a lack of precise criteria for establishing a diagnosis of this neoplasm, its frequency in surveys has varied considerably.[10] Estimates suggest that it comprises approximately 3 to 5 per cent of all salivary gland tumors and 7 to 20 per cent of all malignant salivary tumors.

There is some question whether these tumors represent originally benign neoplasms that have undergone transformation into malignant types or if they are malignant from the outset.

Features. The clinical differences between benign and malignant pleomorphic adenomas are slight. There may be fixation of the malignant tumor to overlying skin or mucosa or underlying structures. Surface ulceration and pain may be a more frequent complaint in the malignant than in the benign lesion.

Most of these neoplasms are found in the parotid; occasionally it manifests in the submandibular or minor salivary glands. Most of these tumors have been found in men between 40 and 50 years of age.

The histologic variations of this tumor are numerous. In some tumors, the benign component may predominate with only a small area demonstrating evidence of malignancy (nuclear hyperchromatism and pleomorphism, increased or abnormal mitosis, and increased nuclear/cytoplasmic ratio, focal necrosis, and invasion with destruction of normal tissue). In other tumors, the malignant component may almost completely overgrow the benign areas.

The microscopic criteria for malignant pleomorphic adenoma are essentially those utilized in the diagnosis of a benign pleomorphic adenoma coupled with the identification of malignant tumor regions.

Treatment and Prognosis. The treatment of malignant pleomorphic adenoma is surgical excision. These neoplasms exhibit a high rate of recurrence as well as regional lymph node involvement and distant metastases.

Mucoepidermoid Carcinoma

The mucoepidermoid carcinoma was originally considered a variant of pleomorphic adenoma. It has now come to be considered a separate entity. This tumor represents approximately 3 to 11 per cent of all salivary gland tumors.[10] In 1970, Eversole reviewed the English literature regarding this tumor.[38] Of 815 reported cases, approximately 70 per cent were found in the major glands.

The mucoepidermoid carcinoma represents the most common malignant tumor of the major salivary glands.

Clinical and histologic experience have led most investigators to separate these neoplasms into those of low-grade or those of high-grade malignancy. These degrees of malignancy represent differences in clinical behavior, recurrence, and histologic features.

Features. Of the major glands, the parotid is the most commonly involved. The most commonly involved minor glands are those of the palate.

These tumors are most frequently diagnosed in persons between the third and sixth decades of life. There is no significant difference between the sexes.

The tumor of low-grade malignancy usually appears as a soft, slowly growing, painless mass. This mass is usually small, rarely exceeding 5 cm. in diameter. The mass is frequently cystic, containing pools of viscid, mucoid material.

The tumor of high-grade malignancy may present a different clinical history. It grows rapidly and pain is more frequently an early symptom. On palpation, the high-grade tumor feels firm; cystic spaces are less frequent.

Low-grade mucoepidermoid carcinomas are characterized by mucous and epidermal cells whose architectural arrangement is characterized by duct and cyst formation (Fig. 22-46). An intermediate cell type has been described, which is thought to represent a transitional type.

High-grade mucoepidermoid carcinomas are characterized by epidermoid and intermediate cell types; the mucous cell is not prominent. Cysts and ductal elements are usually missing and frank histologic evidence of malignancy is present.

Neither of these variants exhibit encapsulation.

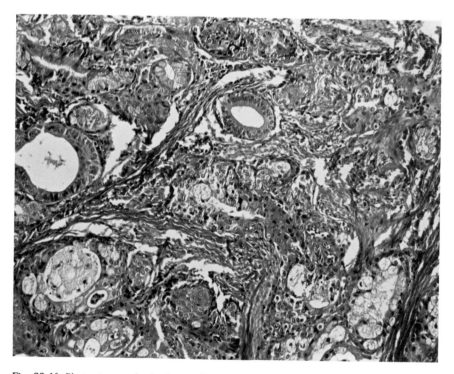

Fig. 22-46. Photomicrograph of a low-grade mucoepidermoid carcinoma. Note the epidermoid cells, the duct formation, and the mucus accumulation.

Treatment and Prognosis. Treatment of both the high-grade and the low-grade mucoepidermoid carcinoma is surgical excision. Local excision has proved adequate for those neoplasms of low-grade malignancy provided histologic confirmation of complete removal is obtained.[39] Adequate treatment of high-grade tumors includes wide excision of the tumor, overlying mucosa, and a margin of surrounding normal tissue.[33]

Generally, recurrences are much more common with tumors of high-grade malignancy.[10] Intraoral tumors (those of the accessory salivary glands) may generally show a poorer prognosis than those of the parotid.[38]

Because of the differing treatments and prognosis of these tumor types, the clinician must discuss individual cases of this neoplasm with the pathologist.

Acinic Cell Carcinoma

The acinic cell carcinoma is a moderately malignant tumor. It constitutes approximately 2 per cent of all salivary gland tumors. Prior to 1953, this tumor was considered benign; clinical experience regarding its recurrence rate and metastatic potential, however, demonstrates its malignancy.

Features. This tumor is almost exclusively limited to the parotid gland. It has been also reported in the sublingual gland and in the floor of the mouth. The acinic cell carcinoma usually occurs in persons at or over middle age. It has also been described in children. The clinical appearance resembles that of the pleomorphic adenoma, usually a small, round, encapsulated mass. Only rarely is there associated pain or facial nerve paralysis. On palpation, the tumor feels firm and may or may not exhibit fixation to surrounding tissue.

This tumor consists essentially of solid epithelial sheets of round or polygonal cells. Glandular structures are frequently present. Cellular cytoplasm is granular and usually basophilic, thus bearing a strong resemblance to the normal serous acinar cells (Fig. 22-47).

Treatment and Prognosis. The accepted treatment of acinic cell carcinoma is surgical excision; a margin of surrounding tissue should be included. The recurrence rate of this tumor may reach as high as 50 per cent.[10]

Adenoid Cystic Carcinoma (Cylindroma)

The adenoid cystic carcinoma was first described by Billroth in 1859. This tumor represents the second most common tumor of the minor salivary glands. (The pleomorphic adenoma is the most common.) The adenoid cystic carcinoma is the most common malignant tumor of the minor salivary glands. Totally, this tumor represents about 2 to 4 per cent of all salivary gland tumors.

Features. The adenoid cystic carcinoma is found over a wide distribution; the minor glands are involved in about 7 per cent of the cases and the major glands in about 28 per cent.[40,41] The palate is the most frequent site of tumor formation.

This tumor occurs somewhat more frequently in women than in men when the major glands are considered, but shows no sex predilection when minor gland frequency is considered.[40] The tumor most frequently arises in persons between 40 and 80 years of age.

The cylindroma tends to appear as a firm mass, thereby resembling the pleomorphic adenoma, but may be more adherent to surrounding tissues. Pain is a

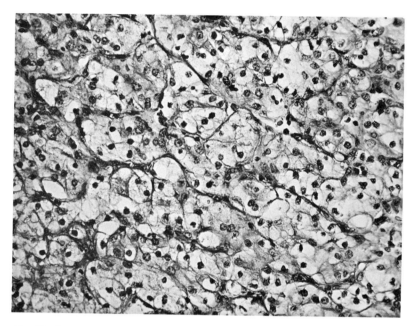

Fig. 22-47. Photomicrograph of acinic cell carcinoma. Note tumor cells with granular cytoplasm. Mucus is not produced by this tumor. (Courtesy of Dr. D. E. Waite)

prominent feature in the early stages.[40,42] Ulceration may be present.[40] The frequent and early association with pain has been attributed to this tumor's apparent tendency to perineural or intraneural invasion.[43] Eby and associates, however, found no correlation between pain and perineural extension.[42] Paresthesia has frequently been associated with this neoplasm.[44]

The adenoid cystic carcinoma is composed of small cells with darkly staining nuclei and scant cytoplasm (Fig. 22-48). These cells are usually arranged in a "swiss cheese" or cylindromatous pattern (hence the term "cylindroma"). Occasionally, the tumor cells may form solid sheets showing no cylindromatous pattern. This solid pattern may be associated with a poorer prognosis;[40,42] few pathologists, however, accept this correlation

without some qualifications.[44] The tumor cells are usually surrounded by varying amounts of connective tissue which itself may range from a hyaline to a myxoid composition.[41]

Treatment and Prognosis. The treatment of this tumor is surgical excision; radiation treatment has been successfully coupled with surgery. Conley and Dingman maintain that the most extensive surgical procedure that can be rationally developed is best; the inability to evaluate the perimeters of this tumor clinically dictates that a bold surgical approach should be the primary objective.[44]

Radical treatment notwithstanding, the prognosis of this tumor is poor. The adenoid cystic carcinoma exhibits a marked tendency to recur and metastasize to

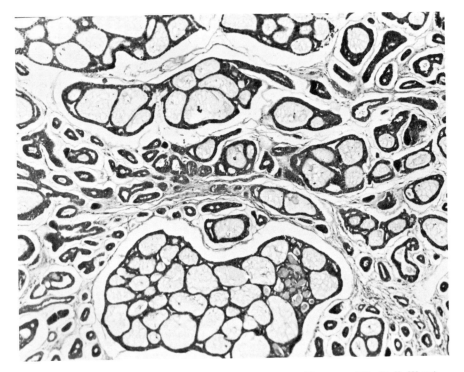

Fig. 22-48. Photomicrograph of adenoid cystic carcinoma. (Courtesy of Dr. D. E. Waite)

lymph nodes, lungs, bones, and liver. Metastasis seems to be a natural function of this neoplasm, which is slow in appearance and unpredictable in growth rate. Clinical experience seems to indicate that the prognosis depends somewhat upon the location of the original tumor site. When the primary tumor is on the palate the prognosis is best; when the submandibular gland is involved primarily, the prognosis is poorest.[45,46] The late appearance of metastatic spread becomes apparent when one examines the cure rate; one study showed a five-year cure rate of 6 per cent.[41]

Salivary Gland Neoplasms in Children

Salivary gland neoplasms are more uncommon in children than in adults. From 1 to 5 per cent of all salivary gland tumors are found in persons under 17 years of age.[10,47]

The most frequent salivary gland neoplasm of children is the hemangioma. The pleomorphic adenoma is the most frequent benign salivary gland tumor, and mucoepidermoid carcinoma is the most frequent malignant tumor.

Hemangioma

The hemangioma usually occurs superficially in the parotid region and is usually noted within the first six months of life. It more commonly affects girls than boys and enlarges rapidly.

Features. As is generally the case with hemangiomas, two microscopic forms are distinguishable in children: (1) the capillary type composed of numerous small blood channels and (2) the cavernous type composed of large endothelium-lined, blood-filled spaces. These blood-filled spaces exhibit a tendency to undergo spontaneous sclerosis and phlebolith formation. (A phlebolith is an organized coagulum which becomes calcified.)

Diagnostic Aids. Since these lesions are nearly always superficial, the diagnosis is easily made with a clinical examination and patient history. O'Riordan has recently published an excellent article dealing with the differential diagnosis between swellings from obstructive salivary gland disease and hemangiomas.[48]

Plain radiology is useful in the diagnosis of hemangioma; a soft tissue mass with contained calcifications (phleboliths) may be noted. Sialography may be useful to determine the extent of involvement of the glandular parenchyma.

Not infrequently, these phleboliths are the only residual sign in the adult of an early hemangioma; they are frequently misdiagnosed as sialoliths. Rauch and associates[10] and O'Riordan[48] have listed diagnostic criteria which aid in distinguishing between residual phleboliths and sialoliths.

Treatment. The treatment of choice has been surgical excision; recently, however, surgical excision has been recommended only if the lesion does not regress spontaneously by the age of five years or if the neoplasm arises late in childhood.[49]

Pleomorphic Adenoma and Mucoepidermoid Carcinoma

The incidence of pleomorphic adenomas in children appears to be lower than that in adults. Mucoepidermoid carcinomas appear five times more frequently in children than in adults, but their course is more benign.[10] In general, salivary gland tumors in children have a more benign course than those in adults.

The clinical and histologic descriptions as well as the treatment for these neoplasms have been discussed earlier and will not be repeated here.

General Comments

As a conclusion to this section on salivary gland neoplasms, several general considerations need to be presented.

Eneroth, in his study of over 2500 salivary gland tumors, found the most common sites of occurrence to be the parotid, submandibular, and the minor salivary glands of the palate; these locations account for 95 per cent of all salivary gland tumors. A palpable lesion in the parotid or submandibular gland is generally a true salivary gland tumor; in the parotid, this is true in 95 per cent and in the submandibular gland, 84 per cent of the cases.[45,46] In the palate, only 46 per cent of all tumors are true salivary gland tumors. Of this total number of salivary gland tumors, 20 to 25 per cent of parotid tumors are malignant and 40 to 60 per cent of submandibular and minor gland tumors are malignant.

Malignant salivary gland neoplasms in the submandibular gland deserve special mention. Malignant tumors in this gland behave more aggressively than in other salivary gland systems.[50] These tumors tend to invade the parapharyngeal space and related structures, the posterior one third of the tongue, and the pillars of the anterior fauces. Involvement of the soft palate and the palatal arches is also common.[2] Aggressive treatment of these neoplasms has been described, glandular resection with examination of a frozen section. If the neoplasm proves to be malignant, an augmented local resection and composite resection are recommended.[50]

Clinically, all salivary gland neoplasms most frequently are painless masses; ulceration is rarely present. The duration of symptoms prior to initial presentation may be lengthy; symptom duration of three years or more has been reported. Patients frequently appear for treatment following a recent increase in size of a long-standing swelling.

Sialography has a limited use in the diagnosis of tumors of the salivary glands. This examination method may show ductal displacement or a nonopacified area in glandular parenchyma caused by a space-occupying lesion. Amputation or encasement of salivary ductules may be evident with an invasive neoplasm. Intrinsic salivary gland tumors may show retention of contrast media in postevacuation films, whereas extrinsic tumors near salivary glands allow complete emptying of the ductal system following gland stimulation.

Much study recently has been devoted to the application of scintigraphy to tumor diagnosis. Initial results seem to indicate that the adenolymphoma (Wharton's tumor) tends to manifest as a scintiphoto "hot spot" in that it accumulates the isotope to a greater degree than normal glandular tissue.[51] Evidence has shown that pleomorphic adenomas tend to present as scintiphoto "cold areas" indicating a glandular filling defect. Some authors recommend that scintiphotography be included as part of a routine workup of a patient with a suspect salivary gland tumor. It should be remembered, however, that this technique of tumor diagnosis must be considered experimental.

Salivary Gland Swelling—Differential Diagnosis

When a patient has an apparent enlargement of one or more salivary glands, certain aspects of a differential diagnosis must be considered. The following paragraphs discuss conditions that may mimic enlargement of the salivary glands. These conditions must be considered along with disease states such as sialadenitis, sialolithiasis, sialadenosis, neoplasms, and the like, that are discussed elsewhere.

Lymphadenopathy

Lymph nodes lie in close association with salivary gland tissue in several areas; enlargement of these nodes can be confused with salivary gland swellings.

The outer surface of the parotid gland is intimately associated with lymph nodes in the preauricular and lower pole areas of the gland. Inflamed preauricular nodes can be differentiated from partial parotid infection because the parotid's upper pole usually does not become infected by itself; examination should be made for sources of infection on the face or temple. The cause of lymphadenopathy of the lower pole nodes may be less obvious; these nodes drain the tonsillar regions. It should be remembered that an obstruction in the intraglandular portion of Stensen's duct may cause swelling of the lower pole only; plain radiology or sialography may be useful in this instance.[18]

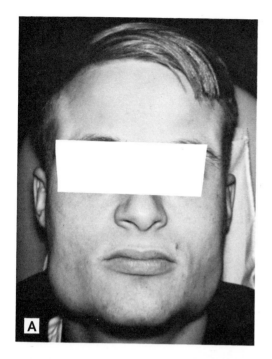

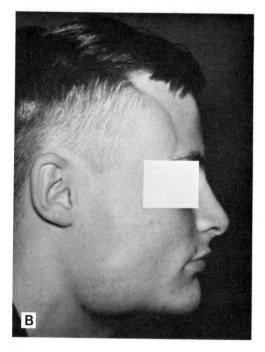

Fig. 22-49. Bilateral masseteric hypertrophy. (A) Frontal view (compare with Fig. 22-4). (B) Lateral view. Note enlargement of masseter and temporalis muscles. Radiographically, the patient's mandibular angle was enlarged.

Lymph nodes are also found along the lower border of the mandible on the superficial portion of the submandibular gland. Lymphadenopathy of these nodes must be distinguished from submandibular gland involvement. These lymph nodes are usually more inferior and further from the midline than the submandibular gland. These respective locations can usually be distinguished with bimanual palpation.

Cellulitis

Sublingual cellulitis of dental origin may be confused with an infection of the submandibular gland. This cellulitis may show swollen sublingual plica and a prominent submandibular duct papilla. If the salivary gland is involved, purulent material can be milked from the duct. If the salivary flow is clear, the possiblitiy of a periodontal abscess or radicular infection of a mandibular tooth should be investigated.[18]

Anatomic Abnormalities

Unilateral or bilateral masseteric hypertrophy may be confused with parotid gland enlargement. This condition is not uncommon; it may be an inherited condition (Fig. 22-49). Palpation reveals a soft mass with no distinct border that parallels the course and extent of the masseter muscle. This mass increases in size and hardens greatly with occlusion. This condition usually exhibits characteristic changes on the radiographs: the area of the mandibular masseteric attachment is enlarged.

Rarely, an apparent parotid mass between the mastoid process and the angle of the mandible may be caused by prominent transverse process of the atlas. Radiographs are useful in establishing this diagnosis.[52]

Complications of Salivary Gland or Associated Surgery

As has been previously noted, surgical excision is the treatment of choice for many salivary gland neoplasms and obstructions. This section will deal with the most common complications of these procedures as well as those arising from surgical procedures in close proximity to salivary structures.

Ductal Stricture

Salivary duct stricture may occur following a surgical biopsy or other surgical procedure near Wharton's or Stensen's duct or their orifices. Strictures also occur following transverse incisions through a ductal wall. Clinical symptoms caused by salivary duct strictures have been discussed in the section on obstructive salivary gland problems.

Frequently, a mild stricture from wound scarring or inflammation may be treated with the administration of a sialagogue. Strictures close to the duct opening may be treated by papillectomy. Strictures located along the ductal course often may be successfully treated by a surgical repositioning of the ductal orifice. In this procedure, the duct is isolated, sectioned proximal to the stricture, and the distal end of the proximal section repositioned to a new, surgically created opening. Ductal strictures close to the gland require removal of the gland. Strictures of the

parotid duct can usually be treated by mechanical dilatation of the duct at several-day intervals over a two-week period. This procedure, however, may afford only temporary remission.

Fistulas

A salivary fistula is an abnormal pathway through which saliva exits to the skin or mucosal surface. Fistulas may be congenital in origin, may result from ulceration caused by ductal calculi, or from surgery on the gland or duct proper.

External fistulas are draining tracts on the skin surface; they are obviously troublesome to the patient. Swelling may accompany the condition. Internal fistulas, since they discharge the saliva into the oral cavity, usually present no symptoms; treatment, therefore, is rarely necessary.

Treatment of salivary fistulas is usually with surgical repair, ductal ligation (with subsequent glandular atrophy), or glandular excision.

Frey's Syndrome (Gustatory Sweating)

An uncommon complication of parotid surgery is gustatory sweating. This syndrome consists of mild to profuse perspiration over cutaneous distribution of the auriculotemporal nerve (regions of the forehead and cheek) following a stimulus to salivary secretion. This condition usually appears within the first year following surgery and may last for an indefinite period.

This condition occurs because of healing between secretory branches of the auriculotemporal nerve proximal to the distal transected fibers controlling sweating and vasodilator pathways.[3]

This condition is curable by division of the intracranial portion of the glossopharyngeal nerve. The condition rarely warrants this procedure; the condition is explained to the patient and is usually left untreated.

Facial Nerve Paresis

Not uncommonly following a major surgical procedure on the parotid gland, temporary or permanent paresis of the facial nerve occurs.[3] This temporary paresis is probably due to a decrease in the conductivity of the nerve secondary to repeated stimulation during the surgery and to postoperative edema. Permanent facial nerve paralysis produces serious results; treatment is necessary and complex.

Allied Conditions

In addition to the specific disease entities affecting the salivary glands proper such as sialolithiasis and neoplasms, there exist certain other conditions that affect the salivary glands as well as other organ systems. Some of these have been discussed earlier (see sialadenosis). This section will discuss Sjögren's syndrome, sarcoidosis, and Mikulicz's disease.

Sjögren's Syndrome (Gougerot-Sjögren Syndrome)

In 1933, Sjögren described a symptom complex of keratoconjunctivitis sicca, pharyngolaryngitis sicca, rhinitis sicca, polyarthritis, enlargement of the parotid glands, and xerostomia. This disease consists of chronic inflammation of the lacrimal and salivary glands leading to dryness of the eye (keratoconjunctivitis sicca), dryness of the mouth (xerostomia), and in some patients, lacrimal and/or salivary gland enlargement. In approximately 50 to 60 per cent of patients, these symptoms are associated with a connective tissue disorder: usually rheumatic arthritis, polymyositis, polyarteritis nodosa, progressive systemic sclerosis (scleroderma), and systemic lupus erythematosus. The term "sicca syndrome" or "sicca complex" is employed when there is no associated connective tissue disorder.

Some investigative work has indicated that there may be a genetic predisposition to this disease; the majority of the cases, however, seem isolated.

Features. This disease is usually seen in women 50 or more years of age. It frequently appears as an insidious development of the sicca complex in a patient with a prior history of rheumatic arthritis. Patients thus affected may complain of a dryness and a burning sensation of the eyes; xerostomia; and nasal, pharyngeal, vaginal, and vulvar dryness. Salivary gland enlargement is clinically variable; usually the parotid is involved bilaterally. This involvement, however, may only be clinically apparent in 15 per cent of the cases.[3] Xerostomia may have the clinical features common to this disorder, as have been discussed previously (Fig. 22-50).

Microscopically, this disease is characterized by a focal lymphocytic sialadenitis of the salivary glands in approximately 70 per cent of the patients.[3] Initially there is infiltration of lymphocytes and plasma cells about the interlobular and centroacinar ducts. Finally, the lymphoreticular tissue overgrows the parenchyma, so that only ducts or their remnants may be found.[10] Microscopic changes may be evident in all the salivary tissue (both major and minor glands); the clinical significance of this will be discussed later.

In addition to the inflammatory infiltrate in the salivary tissue, a type of epi-

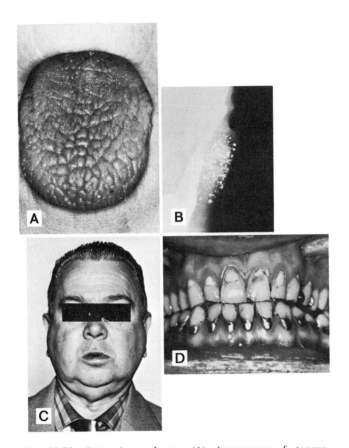

Fig. 22-50. Sjögren's syndrome. (A) Appearance of tongue. (B) Sialogram. (C) Salivary gland enlargement. (D) Evidence of cervical caries due to xerostomia. (Bertram, U.: Xerostomia. Clinical aspects, pathology and pathogenesis. Acta Odontol. Scand. (Suppl. 49), 25:1–126, 1967)

thelial proliferation may be present. This proliferation may be that of the myoepithelial cells only, or it may consist of both cell layers of the terminal salivary duct.[10]

Sjögren's syndrome usually manifests a remarkable prevalence of abnormal immunologic features; the disease ranks second only to systemic lupus erythematosus in the number of serum autoantibodies. Rheumatoid factor is present in 52 to 100 per cent of patients with Sjögren's syndrome, even in the absence of rheumatoid arthritis.[3] Antinuclear antibodies are found in approximately 66 per cent of the patients.[3] Earlier work seemed to indicate the presence of salivary duct antibody in Sjögren's syndrome.[28] This antibody is now considered to be a reflection of rheumatoid arthritis alone, rather than a manifestation of Sjögren's syndrome per se.[12]

Diagnostic Aids. A clinical examination and patient history must be accomplished to rule out other causes of salivary gland enlargement or xerostomia.

Sialography may be of use in the diagnosis of Sjögren's syndrome; the hydrostatic technique is recommended.[3] Varying degrees of sialectasis ("bunch of grapes" appearance) are consistent findings.

Scintigraphy appears to have value in the assessment of salivary gland involvement in Sjögren's syndrome. The uptake of the radioactive compound ^{99m}Tc pertechnetate has been shown to be reduced in patients with Sjögren's syndrome. This method of examination may represent a safe, objective means of evaluating salivary gland involvement in this disease.

Minor salivary gland biopsy has recently also shown much promise in the diagnosis of Sjögren's syndrome. Focal lymphocytic sialadenitis has been demonstrated in approximately 70 per cent of patients with Sjögren's syndrome. The changes manifest in the major salivary gland tissue are reflected in the minor salivary glands. Minor gland biopsy technique affords, therefore, a safe, accessible method of determining salivary gland involvement (Fig. 22-51). This minor salivary gland tissue may be taken from anywhere within the oral cavity; the inner aspect of the lower lip and the palate are the common sites.

Treatment. Sjögren's syndrome has shown remarkable resistance to successful treatment. A broad, symptomatic treatment is usually employed. This treatment is aimed at the multisystem symptoms of the disease.

Oral treatment consists of measures to keep the oral mucous membranes moist. The use of sialagogues such as sour, sug-

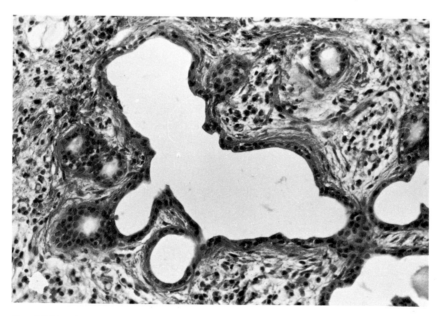

Fig. 22-51. Photomicrograph of minor salivary glands of lip of patient with Sjögren's syndrome. Ductal dilatation with minute sacculations is apparent in addition to chronic inflammation of stromal areas. (Courtesy of Dr. D. E. Waite)

arless candy work well. Patients should be encouraged to increase their fluid intake with frequent sips of water.

Because the patient with Sjögren's syndrome is especially susceptible to infections such as candidosis, frequent monitoring of the patient and prompt adequate treatment of these infections are necessary.

The patient should be instructed and followed in methods of proper oral hygiene. Drugs that tend to cause xerostomia should be avoided.

Some clinical evidence has been presented which indicates that removal of the affected salivary glands of patients with Sjögren's syndrome results in a general improvement in the patients.[53] It is thought that this glandular excision results in the improvement of the immunologic status of the patient. This treatment, however, must be considered experimental.

Complications. Clinical and pathologic evidence seems to indicate that a patient with this disease may have a tendency to develop extrasalivary lymphoid abnormalities, including lymphoreticular malignancies such as malignant lymphomas.[10] Persons with Sjögren's syndrome, therefore, should be followed with suitable blood studies to detect early change from the benign course.

Sarcoidosis

Sarcoidosis is a generalized disease first described by Hutchinson in 1875. The condition was originally known as "Mortimer's malady" after the name of Hutchinson's patient. Sarcoidosis is a systemic granulomatous disease of undetermined origin. Lesions of sarcoidosis may involve any body site; the salivary glands are involved in 3 to 10 per cent of the cases.[54]

Features. Most patients are young or middle-aged adults; no sex difference has been observed. The most common manifestation of this disease is the cutaneous lesion. These lesions are multiple, raised red patches that occur in groups and enlarge slowly. Ulceration or crusting of these cutaneous lesions is uncommon.

Salivary gland involvement, when present, manifests as hard, painless, slow enlargement of usually the parotid glands. Involvement of other salivary tissue usually follows. Xerostomia may be present.

An acute manifestation of systemic sarcoidosis that affects the parotid glands and the uveal tracts of the eyes (uveoparotitis) is termed Heerfordt's syndrome. This manifestation occurs in only 2 to 3 per cent of all patients with sarcoidosis.

The characteristic feature of this disease is the formation of noncaseating granulomas. These granulomas are composed of epithelioid cells, macrophages, multinucleated giant cells, and occasional eosinophils. No acid-fast organisms can be demonstrated; this being one of the few distinguishing features allowing differentiation from the granuloma of tuberculosis.

Diagnostic Aids. The diagnosis of sarcoid sialadenitis is based on the history, the presence of salivary gland symptoms such as asialia and enlargement, and positive results from other systemic tests.

Sialography may show slight changes only, since there are no gross changes in glandular ducts or parenchyma.[14]

Examination of minor salivary gland biopsy specimens has recently been shown to be of some value in the diagnosis of sarcoidosis.[54] As in the case with Sjögren's syndrome, these minor salivary glands lend themselves to safe, uncomplicated diagnostic biopsy procedures.

Treatment. Specific treatment for sarcoidosis is unknown; cortisone therapy has been useful in the treatment of Heerfordt's syndrome.

Mikulicz's Disease (Lymphoepithelial Lesion)

In 1888, von Mikulicz described a case of asymptomatic symmetrical enlargement of the salivary and lacrimal glands. Since that time, much confusion has existed concerning the true nature of this condition. There is increasing evidence that this disease is closely related to Sjögren's syndrome and that both are autoimmune diseases.[31]

Features. This disease manifests as a unilateral or bilateral enlargement of the parotid or submandibular glands. This glandular enlargement is diffuse and poorly outlined. Pain and xerostomia are occasionally present.

This disease is characterized by lymphocytic infiltration of the salivary gland tissue. The acini are destroyed; islands of epithelial cells remain. This remaining epithelium may exhibit ductal formation or may form solid nests of poorly defined cells.

Treatment and Complications. Both surgical excision and radiation treatments have been used with success in the treatment of this condition. Since this condition usually follows a benign course, conservative treatment is probably the treatment of choice.

Recently, reports of malignant behavior with the formation of lymphomas and carcinomas within a benign lymphoepithelial lesion have been published.[3,55] This would indicate that patients with this condition be reviewed on a regular basis and that irradiation as a treatment modality is contraindicated.

References

1. Schneyer, L. H., and Levin, L. K.: Rate of secretion by exogenously stimulated salivary gland pairs in man. J. Appl. Physiol., 7:609–613, 1955.
2. Batsakis, J. G.: Neoplasms of the minor and lesser major salivary glands. Surg. Gynecol. Obstet., 135:289–298, 1972.
3. Mason, D. K., and Chisholm, D. M.: *Salivary Glands in Health and Disease.* Philadelphia, W. B. Saunders Co., 1975.
4. Waite, D. E.: Secretory sialography of the salivary glands. Oral Surg., 27:635–641, 1969.
5. Yune, H. Y., and Klatte, E. C.: Current status of sialography. Am. J. Roentgenol. Radium Ther. Nucl. Med., 115:420–428, 1972.
6. Blair, G. S.: Hydrostatic sialography. Oral Surg., 36:116–130, 1973.
7. Pappas, G. C., and Wallace, W. R.: Panoramic sialography. Dent. Radiogr. and Photogr., 43:27–33, 1970.
8. Eneroth, C. M., Franzen, S., and Zajicek, J.: Cytologic Diagnosis on Aspirate from 1000 Salivary Gland Tumors. Acta Otolaryngol. (Suppl.), 224:168–172, 1967.
9. Spiro, R. H., Huvos, A. G., and Strong, E. W.: Cancer of the parotid gland. Am. J. Surg., 130:452–459, 1975.
10. Rauch, S., Gorlin, R. J., and Seifert, G.: Diseases of the salivary glands. In *Thoma's Oral Pathology*, 6th ed., Vol. 2. R. J. Gorlin and H. M. Goldman (Eds.). St. Louis, C. V. Mosby Co., 1970.
11. Huebuer, G. R.: A Study of Submandibular and Parotid Gland Sialography and Histopathology. M.S.D. Thesis, University of Minnesota, 1971.

12. Chisholm, D. M., and Mason, D. K.: Salivary gland disease. Br. Med. Bull., 31:156–158, 1975.

13. Prowler, J. R., Bjork, H., and Armstrong, G. F.: Major gland sialectasis. J. Oral Surg., 23:421–430, 1965.

14. Diamant, H.: The investigation and management of non-neoplastic diseases affecting the salivary glands. J. Laryngol. Otol., 88:705–716, 1974.

15. Robbins, S. L.: Pathologic Basis of Disease. Philadelphia, W. B. Saunders Co., 1974.

16. Kashima, H. K., Kirkham, W. R., and Andrews J. R.: Postirradiation sialadenitis. Am. J. Roentgenol. Radium Ther. Nucl. Med., 94:271–291, 1965.

17. Gilchrist, R. K., and McAndrew, J. R.: Surgical parotitis. Arch. Surg., 76:863–867, 1958.

18. Seward, G. R.: Anatomic surgery for salivary calculi, Part I. Oral Surg., 25:150–157, 1968.

19. Seward, G. R.: Anatomic surgery for salivary calculi, Part V. Oral Surg., 25:810–816, 1968.

20. Seward, G. R., Anatomic surgery for salivary calculi, Part VI. Oral Surg., 26:1–7, 1968.

21. Seward, G. R.: Anatomic surgery for salivary calculi, Part III. Oral Surg., 25:525–531, 1968.

22. Seward, G. R.: Anatomic surgery for salivary calculi, Part II. Oral Surg., 25:287–293, 1968.

23. Moose, S. M.: Transoral surgical removal of a sialolith in the submandibular gland. Int. J. Oral Surg., 3:318–320, 1974.

24. Waterhouse, J. P., Chisholm, D. M., Winter, R. B., Patel, M., and Yale, R. S.: Replacement of functional parenchymal cells by fat and connective tissue in human submandibular salivary glands: An age related change. J. Oral Pathol., 2:16–27, 1973.

25. Miller, A. S., and Winnick, M.: Salivary gland inclusion in the anterior mandible. Oral Surg., 31:790–797, 1971.

26. Stafne, E. C.: Bone cavities situated near the angle of the mandible. J. Am. Dent. Assoc., 29:1969–1972, 1942.

27. Tolman, D. E., and Stafne, E. C.: Developmental bone defects of the mandible. Oral Surg., 24:488–490, 1967.

28. Bertram, U.: Xerostomia. Acta Odontol. Scand. (Suppl. 49): 25:11–126, 1967.

29. Laskin, D. M.: Treatment of xerostomia and xerophthalmia in Sjögren's syndrome. J.A.M.A. 235:1157, 1976.

30. Krolls, S. O., and Boyers, R. C.: Mixed tumors of salivary glands. Cancer, 30:276–281, 1972.

31. Shafer, W. G., Hine, M. K., and Levy, B. M.: A Textbook of Oral Pathology, 3rd ed. Philadelphia, W. B. Saunders Co., 1974.

32. Patey, D. H., and Thackray, A. C.: The treatment of parotid tumors in the light of a pathological study of parotidectomy material. Br. J. Surg., 45:477–487, 1958.

33. Chandhry, A. P., Vickers, R. A., and Gorlin, R. J.: Intra-oral minor salivary gland tumors. Oral Surg., 14:1194–1226, 1961.

34. Baden, E., Pierce, M., Selman, A. J., Roberts, T. W., and Doyle, J. L.: Intra-oral papillary cystadenoma lymphomatosum. J. Oral Surg., 34:533–541, 1976.

35. Abrams, A. M., Melrose, R. J., and Howell, F. V.: Necrotizing sialometaplasia. Cancer, 32:130–135, 1973.

36. Dunlap, C. L., and Barker, B. F.: Necrotizing sialometaplasia. Oral Surg., 37:722–727, 1974.

37. Argnelles, M. T., Viloria, J. B., Talens, M. C., and McCrory, T. P.: Necrotizing sialometaplasia. Oral Surg., 42:86–90, 1976.

38. Eversole, L. R.: Mucoepidermoid carcinoma. J. Oral Surg., 28:490–494, 1970.

39. Eversole, L. R., Rovin, S., and Sabes, W. R.: Mucoepidermoid carcinoma of minor salivary glands; report of 17 cases with follow-up. J. Oral Surg., 30:107–112, 1972.

40. Tarpley, T. M, and Giansanti, J. S.: Aden-

oid cystic carcinoma. Oral Surg., 41:484–497, 1976.

41. Spiro, R. H., Huvos, A. G., and Strong, E. W.: Adenoid cystic carcinoma of salivary origin. Am. J. Surg., 128:512–520, 1974.

42. Eby, L. S., Johnson, D. S., and Baker, H. W.: Adenoid cystic carcinoma of the head and neck. Cancer, 29:1160–1168, 1972.

43. Berdal, P., de Besche, A., and Mylins, E.: Cylindroma of salivary glands. Acta Otolaryngol, (Suppl.), 263:170–173, 1970.

44. Couley, J., and Dingham, D. L.: Adenoid cystic carcinoma in the head and neck. Arch. Otolaryngol., 100:81–90, 1974.

45. Eneroth, C. M.: Incidence and prognosis of salivary gland tumors at different sites. Acta Otolaryngol Suppl. 263:174–178, 1970.

46. Eneroth, C. M.: Salivary gland tumors in the parotid gland, submandibular gland, and the palate region. Cancer, 27:1415–1418, 1971.

47. Krolls, S. O., Trodahl, J. N., and Boyers, R. C.: Salivary gland lesions in children. Cancer, 30:459–469, 1972.

48. O'Riordan, B.: Phleboliths and salivary calculi. Br. J. Oral Surg., 12:119–131, 1974.

49. Hébert, G., Ouimet-Oliva, D., and Ladouceur, J.: Vascular tumors of the salivary glands in children. Am. J. Roentgenol., 123:815–819, 1975.

50. Couley, J., Myers, E., and Cole, R.: Analysis of 115 patients with tumors of the submandibular gland. Ann. Otol. Rhinol. Laryngol., 81:323–330, 1972.

51. Kraaijenhagen, H. A., Heydendal, G. A. K., and Van Der Ent, G. M.: Salivary gland scintiphotography. Int. J. Oral Surg., 3:326–329, 1974.

52. Einstein, R. A., and Katz, A. D.: Parotid area swelling caused by a prominent transverse process of atlas. Arch. Otolaryngol., 101:558–559, 1975.

53. Berényi, B.: Oral surgical approach to the treatment of Sjögren's syndrome. Int. J. Oral Surg., 3:309–313, 1974.

54. Hughes, G. R. V., and Gross, N. J.: Diagnosis of sarcoidosis by labial gland biopsy. Br. Med. J., 3:215, 1972.

55. Batsakis, J. G., Bernacki, E. G., Rice, D. H., and Stebler, M. E.: Malignancy and the benign lymphoepithelial lesion. Laryngoscope, 85:389–399, 1975.

23 The Temporomandibular Joint

DANIEL E. WAITE

The diagnosis and management of temporomandibular joint disorders are primarily the responsibility of the dentist. For many years the temporomandibular joint has been considered a "no man's land" because different clinical disciplines failed to fully understand and appreciate this complex area. Much remains to be learned; however, great strides have been made in recent years. Not only have anatomic and organic problems been solved by surgical techniques and treatment methods, but the complex area of referred pain mechanisms and the central pain phenomenon is better understood. The role of emotion in producing headache, backache, migraine, and other psychosomatic illnesses (which the pain dysfunction syndrome of the temporomandibular joint may well be) points to the breadth of knowledge necessary to adequately understand the total problem of a patient with temporomandibular joint complaints. This also implies the necessity of cooperation among the many dental and medical disciplines that may be involved in the final analysis and management of the myriad disease processes that the dentist is called upon to treat.

This chapter is intended to serve as a cursory review, and it is hoped that the dental student will utilize the references and current literature for additional knowledge in this dynamic and interesting field.

Anatomy and Physiology

Action

The temporomandibular joint is an intricate biomechanical structure whose movements are complicated by an equally complex system of coordinated masticatory muscles and the presence of teeth in the opposing jaws. The interdigitation of the teeth obviously affects the relation of the jaws in occlusion; however, the muscles of mastication also influence the position of the joint and may dictate jaw position during pain or spasm.

Anatomy

The anatomy of the temporomandibular joint is unique compared to other stress-bearing joints. The condylar head is convex anteroposteriorly and elongated mediolaterally, although variations in the shape of the condyle are frequent. A concavity of the temporal bone, the glenoid fossa, is the seat of the condylar head.

DISC AND LIGAMENTS. In contrast to fibrous and cartilaginous joints, this artic-

422

ulation does not have opposing cartilaginous elements, but has a fibrocartilaginous covering with a dividing articular disc called the meniscus. The disc essentially separates the joint proper into two cavities lined with a synovial membrane and containing synovial fluid.

The articular disc is thin in the central portion and quite thick at the posterior border prominence. The anterior portion of the disc is attached to the fibrous capsular ligament, which blends into the more broadly shaped and reinforcing temporomandibular ligament.

Other ligaments are the stylomandibular and sphenomandibular ligaments. Their function has never been clearly demonstrated, but it appears likely that they serve as limiting ligaments (i.e., suspensory in nature), and are not responsible for any guiding movement of the mandible (Fig. 23-1).

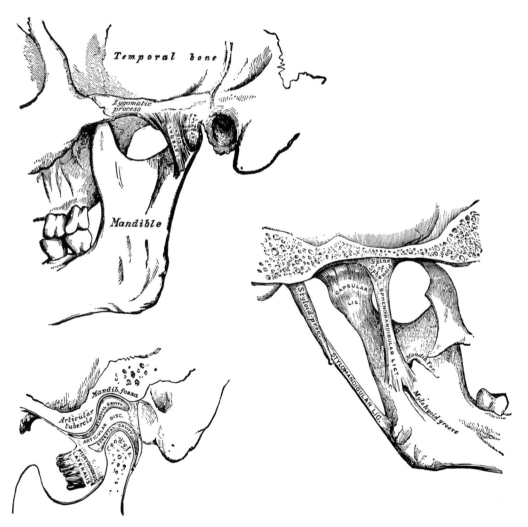

Fig. 23-1. Ligaments of the temporomandibular joint. (Goss, C. M. (Ed.): *Gray's Anatomy of the Human Body*, 28th Am. ed. Philadelphia, Lea & Febiger, 1973)

Growth

The growth of the mandible largely depends upon the growth potential of the condylar head. There seems to be no question that damage to the condyle during early life affects mandibular growth (Fig. 23-2). Surgical intervention or removal of the condyle stunts the growth in height of the ramus and affects other facial changes. The mandible is a membranous bone and the connective tissue of the mandibular condyle serves as the impetus for mandibular growth.[1] As the body of the mandible develops and grows downward as well as forward, adequate space between the jaw bones is provided for the growth of alveolar bone that ultimately will support the dentition. It must also be remembered that a contributing factor to overall growth and development is physiologic function; therefore, the soft tissue environment, osteogenesis, and especially muscle development become important. An intrinsic (genetic) or extrinsic (environmental) defect in any part of a functional matrix may cause secondary defects in related skeletal and dental structures. In cases of partial and total anodontia, congenital or postsurgical, the growth of the alveolar process in children and the maintenance of this bone in adults are dependent on the teeth.

Other growth centers are the coronoid process related to the temporal muscle, the mandibular angle related to the masseter externally and to the medial pterygoid internally, and the alveolar process related to teeth[2,37] (Fig. 23-3).

Muscles

The associated musculature can be discussed as it relates to opening and closing the jaws, which are complex movements. A single hinge action exists, but only as a

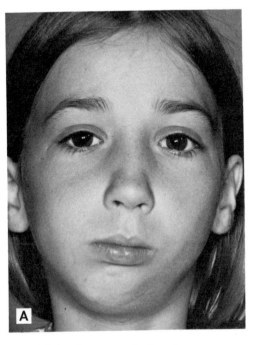
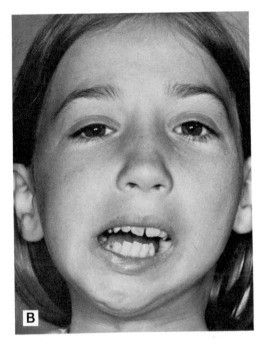

Fig. 23-2. See facing page for legend.

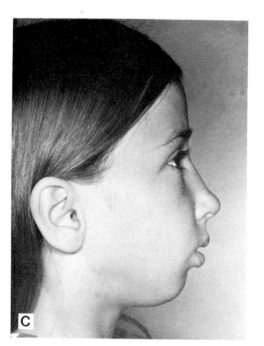

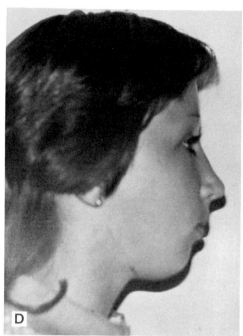

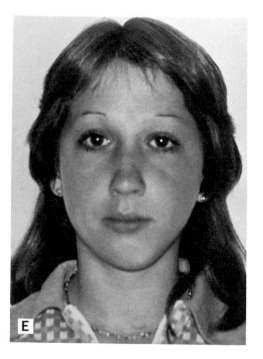

Fig. 23-2. (A and B) Patient, age seven years, at five years of age had a fracture of the condyle causing ankylosis. Note the asymmetry and lack of antero-posterior growth. (C) At seven years of age, arthroplasty with insertion of Silastic was performed. (D and E) At sixteen years of age, the patient has good function. Note the improved developmental growth and symmetry.

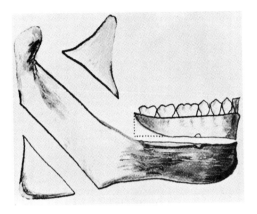

Fig. 23-3. Growth centers of the mandible. (Freese, A. S., and Scheman, P.: *Management of Temporomandibular Joint Problems.* St. Louis, C. V. Mosby, 1962)

passive motion; a gliding-sliding action provides downward and anterior movement. A combination of both actions is necessary for retrusive, protrusive, and lateral excursive movements.

The muscles of mastication that are normally credited for primary mandibular movements are the temporalis, masseter, and pterygoid muscles (Figs. 23-4 and 23-5). Although they are primarily referred to as elevators and depressors, these muscles are also intricately involved with lateral, protrusive, and retrusive movements. The suprahyoid muscles also contribute to jaw movements: the anterior belly of the digastric muscle is specifically involved in opening the mouth. In fractures of the neck of the condyle, it is the limiting lateral aspect of the capsular ligament and the strong pull of the lateral pterygoid muscle that prevent lateral displacement of the condylar head and pull it medially.

Dentition

The teeth and their occlusal relationship are important to temporomandibular joint harmony. However, it must be emphasized that joint position is largely dictated by the muscles. Following muscular relaxation, slow closure of the jaws to the point of occlusal interdigitation will demonstrate the muscular effect on closure. When the inclined surfaces of the teeth begin to contact, it is entirely possible for the jaw position to be different from that intended by muscular harmony. A normal occlusal relation is of prime importance for physiologic muscle function. Bell proposes that normal occlusal relation or

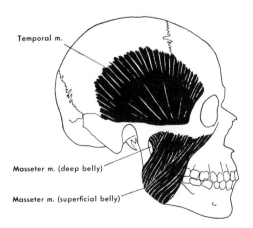

Fig. 23-4. Muscles of mastication. (Kawamura, Y Mandibular movement. *In* Swartz, L., and Chayes, C. M.: *Facial Pain and Mandibular Dysfunction.* Philadelphia, W. B. Saunders, 1968)

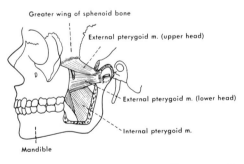

Fig. 23-5. Muscles of mastication. (Kawamura, Y.: Mandibular movement. *In* Schwartz, L., and Chayes, C. M.: *Facial Pain and Mandibular Dysfunction.* Philadelphia, W. B. Saunders, 1968)

harmony depends upon the following four conditions:[3]

1. The presence of interocclusal clearance when the muscles relax.
2. Terminal closure such that the clenched occlusal position does not require shifting from the initial position of primary contact.
3. Return from protrusion and lateral excursion with freedom from cuspal interference.
4. Proper muscle coordination.

Many opinions have been published on the role of occlusion in temporomandibular joint pain.[4-6] Although there is no question that occlusal relation is important as an etiologic factor in pain of the jaws, headache, and facial pain, its true role is confusing. It is probably best understood when we recognize that the dynamics of occlusion are not limited to specific tooth contact only. A broader concept would be that, as teeth contact, deep and superficial neural stimuli are involved, as are various muscular mecha-

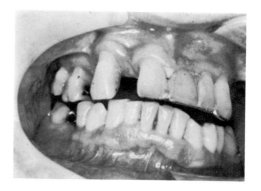

Fig. 23-7. Acute malocclusion with deviation, premature contacts, and pain.

nisms. The problem of acute and chronic malocclusion has been referred to as an important consideration.[3] Chronic malocclusion usually occurs unconsciously and is long-standing in nature. It predisposes to masticatory symptoms, which are usually precipitated by a period of bruxism or tension.

In contrast to this, acute malocclusion results from masticatory dysfunction such as myospasm. Therefore, it is important to be sure of the cause before undertaking occlusal equilibration. In this case, occlusal grinding would tend to relieve the symptoms but do nothing for the etiologic myospasm, at the same time costing the patient the loss of sound tooth structure. (Figs. 23-6 and 23-7).

The Examination

Examination of the temporomandibular joint, as in any other examination, requires a complete history and a review of pertinent local and systemic factors. This cannot and should not be done in the dental chair. The overlying potential problems of this disorder are such that a

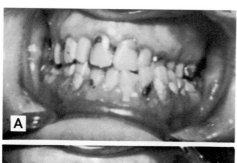

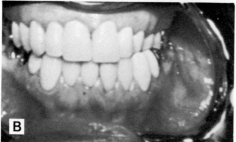

Fig. 23-6. (A) Long-standing chronic malocclusion. (B) Dental reconstruction with disappearance of joint pain.

total and complete history can best be elicited in a quiet and comfortable environment, such as a private office, with the patient seated in a relaxed and comfortable position. While the patient must be permitted to give his own historical data, specific questions by the doctor will lead him through the areas that will reveal pertinent information. Questions relating to the chief complaint, the severity of symptoms, and the type of pain and its location should be discussed. Some assessment of the patient's threshold of pain and his general attitude, types of stress, emotion, and personality factors should be observed. The use of any drugs is significant, since certain tranquilizing medications can produce muscle-related jaw dysfunction. The duration of the pain and its stimulus, and whether or not the patient can do anything to relieve it, may be significant.

Systematic diseases, such as parkinsonism, the arthritides, or any resultant dystonia of the jaw need careful evaluation. Obesity, hypertension, migraine, ulcerative colitis, or gastritis, as they relate to emotional stress, are also important. In many instances, patients will resent giving this information; if so, they should not be pushed to reveal these problems, although the fact that they are hostile may be significant. The examiner should note other dentists or physicians whom the patient has consulted, since information from them may prove helpful. (See Chapter 3 for additional information on conducting the patient interview.)

The initial clinical evaluation might begin with observing coordinated muscular movements of jaw positions. Abnormal deviation from any of the normal accepted patterns should be recorded. Evaluation of the nerve supply to the general area of the temporomandibular joint is also significant. The fifth, seventh, and ninth cranial nerves should be evaluated from both the sensory and motor standpoints. Check for evidence of numbness or hyperesthetic areas. The use of a sharp needle and the brushing effect of cotton give a good variation in stimuli. Any abnormality in these areas suggests the desirability of further neurologic evaluation.

If jaw opening is limited, use calipers to record the degree of opening with or without pain. Asymmetry of the face and especially of the mandible should be noted if present, including the condylar heads upon opening. Examination of the joint includes auscultation and palpation. Even though crepitus may be heard without a stethoscope, it is best to employ one. Differentiation between crepitus and clicking is important, since a joint may function normally but click repeatedly. This is not likely if actual crepitation exists. The temporomandibular joint is best palpated by placing the forefingers in the external auditory canal bilaterally and asking the patient to open and close his mouth. Exerting similar pressure on both joints, the painful joint will become immediately evident. When the palpating finger is placed laterally over the joint surface, the extent of luxation and gross mandibular movement can be noted (Fig. 23-8).

The musculature relating to the joint must also be examined for normal function and the elicitation of painful areas. Each muscle of mastication can be palpated, and while the patient clenches his teeth, the muscles will assume relaxed and rigid positions helpful in the examination. Masseter muscle hypertrophy may be noted in some individuals but is not necessarily related to temporomandibular joint dysfunction[7] (Fig. 23-9). However, the asymmetry is important to differentiate the condition from true mandibular asymmetry.

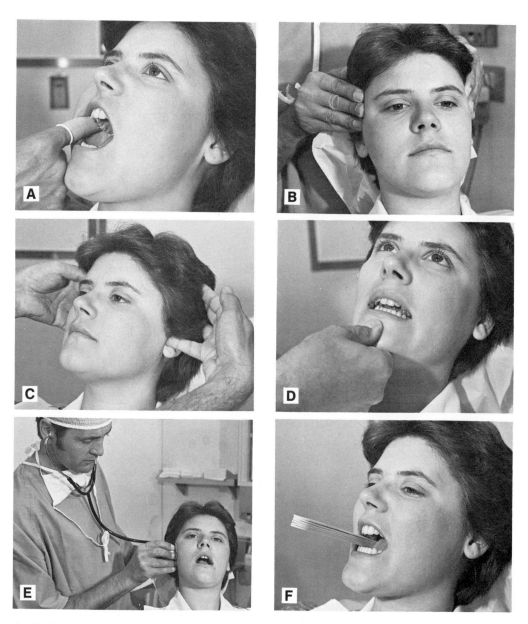

Fig. 23-8. (A) Palpation for intraoral muscular tenderness in the painful temporomandibular joint. (B) Palpation of the temporalis muscles. (C) The palpating finger is placed within the ear canal to determine crepitus or pain as the patient opens and closes the jaws. (D) Temporomandibular joint complaints are evaluated in relation to the most retruded position of the mandible. (E) The stethoscope is used to hear any snapping or cracking of the joint in coordination with exact movements of the mandible. (F) Biting force is evaluated bilaterally to determine muscular weakness or tenderness.

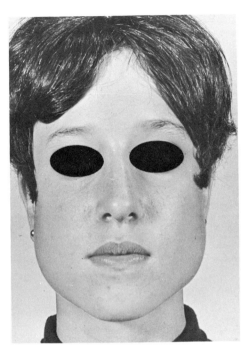

Fig. 23-9. Masseter muscle hypertrophy. (Courtesy Dr. R. Gorlin)

Dental Examination

The first portion of the dental examination is the same as that for any dental evaluation. It is important to establish a routine pattern. One should start with the soft tissue in the pharynx and work forward to the lips, then examine the teeth. The usual evaluation for caries, calculus, periodontal disease, malposition, and missing teeth should be made. Excessive wear and any suggestion of bruxism and occlusal interference must be recorded. The use of articulating paper, tape, and wax may be helpful, or models may be mounted to give additional information.

Roentgenology

Roentgenographic examination is a necessary adjunct to the evaluation even though the report will often be negative. The complex anatomy and superimposed osseous structures in this area make radiographic interpretation difficult. In order to circumvent the anatomic problems of viewing this area, several radiologic techniques and views are available. The dental x-ray machine can be used for some views, but other projections may require different equipment.

The most common radiograph taken at the hospital by a radiologist will be the transcranial oblique view (Fig. 23-10). A transorbital projection gives excellent information on the head of the condyle and the neck (Fig. 23-11).

The panoramic projection as regularly taken provides a good opportunity to observe both joints (Fig. 23-12); however, an additional adjustment with this technique gives even better information (Fig. 23-13). The Towne's projection is another standard view best taken on conventional hospital equipment; it is ideal for the demonstration of condylar fracture (Fig. 23-14). Laminography, a special technique that projects a particular structure in focus while all surrounding structures are out of focus, may be employed. Several projections are usually made, permitting evaluation of the joint from lateral to medial aspects (Fig. 23-15). Cinefluorography, stereoroentgenography, and cephalometry are yet additional methods.

As with the interpretation of all radiographs, the clinician must look for the normal, so that any deviation from the normal will be immediately evident. In general, joint structure and form and a normal range of movement should be observed. A specific series of projections described by Bell involves making two x-ray exposures: (1) while the patient is clenching the teeth, and (2) while the teeth are

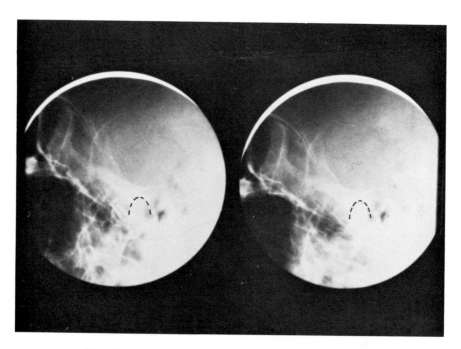

Fig. 23-10. Transcranial view of the temporomandibular joint.

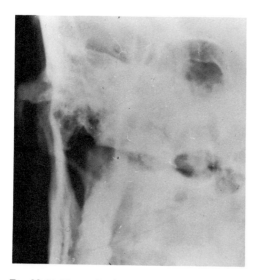

Fig. 23-11. Transorbital view of the temporomandibular joint.

in light occlusal contact. In interpreting the film, the normal joint will reveal no change in the intra-articular space (Fig. 23-16).

The information gained from the roentgenograms will be in accord with the knowledge of the individual interpreting the films. In general, restriction of condylar movement or hypermobility is not difficult to detect, and one may need a laminogram to verify these findings. A finding worthy of note is diffuse enlargement of the condylar head, which may be related to asymmetry of the mandible (i.e., unilateral condylar hyperplasia) (Figs. 23-17 and 23-18). A consultation with a radiologist may be indicated for appropriate interpretation of this area.

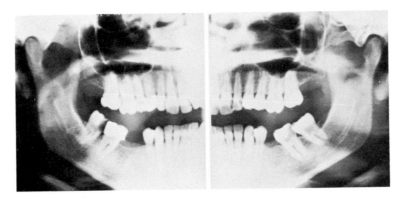

Fig. 23-12. Panoramic view of the mandible, including the temporomandibular joint.

Temporomandibular Joint Disorders

Any attempt to classify these disorders will be incomplete and will not adequately bring to light all of the ramifications of the many individual problems. However, the following categories will direct the student to major areas of concern in which he can expand his reading for further information. Broadly categorized, they are:

1. Dislocation
2. Trauma
3. Pain dysfunction syndrome
4. Arthritides
5. Hypomobility
6. Neurologic disorders
7. Growth deformities (see also Chapter 24.)
8. Neoplasms

A recent study has shown that the pain dysfunction syndrome associated with a masticatory muscle disorder as the initiating symptom is first in the order of incidence.[8]

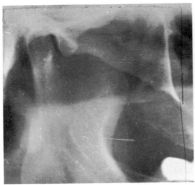
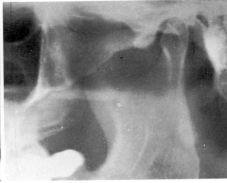

Fig. 23-13. Specific view of the temporomandibular joint taken with Panorex.

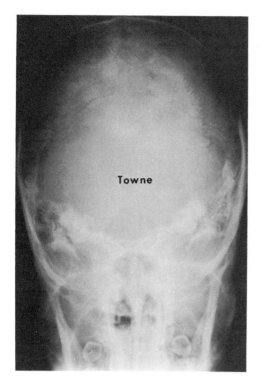

Towne

Fig. 23-14. Towne's projection for the temporomandibular joint.

Dislocation

Dislocation of the temporomandibular joint is usually acute, although chronic and recurrent problems are ever present. Mild injury is the most frequent cause, although sudden stretching, yawning, or wide opening can produce dislocation. A typical facial appearance ensues, and the patient is often frightened when he discovers he cannot close his mouth (Fig. 23-19). Pain may or may not be a significant factor.

Usually, reduction of the dislocation is simply accomplished (Fig. 23-20). When difficulty in reduction is encountered manually, additional procedures, such as infiltration of the joint with a local anesthetic or sedation, may be helpful. General anesthesia may also be required.

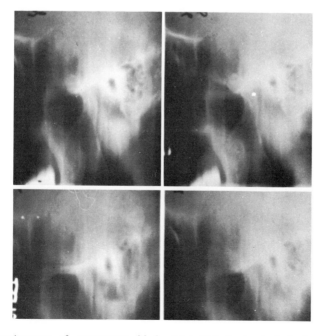

Fig. 23-15. Laminogram of temporomandibular joint. Note foreign body in the upper right cut.

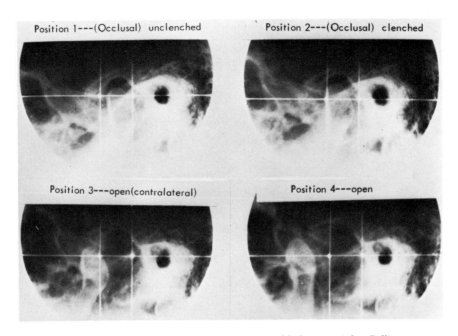

Position 1---(Occlusal) unclenched   Position 2---(Occlusal) clenched

Position 3---open(contralateral)   Position 4---open

Fig. 23-16. Transcranial view of temporomandibular joint (after Bell).

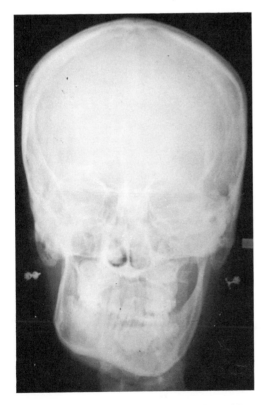

Fig. 23-17. Unilateral condylar hyperplasia. Note enlarged condyle and asymmetry.

The control of chronic dislocation can cause considerable concern for both the patient and the clinician. Chronic recurrent dislocation requires serious habit training to control the opening movements. Surgical procedures have been described for the chronically dislocating joint (Fig. 23-21), but they are rarely indicated.[9,10] If nocturnal dislocation occurs, an elastic head bandage may be of value and is easily constructed (Fig. 23-22). The injection of a sclerosing solution has also been advocated; this solution should not be placed within the joint capsule, but limited to the surrounding tissues with the intent of stimulating fibrosis and limiting movement. In some instances, the dislocation may be a voluntary attention-getting mechanism and may indicate emotional or psychologic problems.

Dislocation of the disc may occur unrelated to dislocation of the condylar head. It may occur in either the anterior or posterior position. If anterior, the pain occurs upon opening, if posterior, upon closing. Treatment is directed at obtaining total

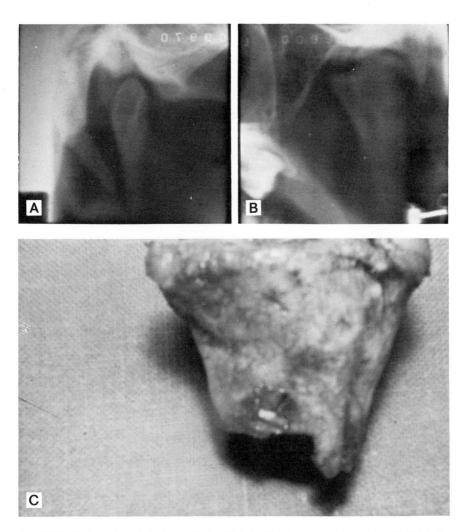

Fig. 23-18. Unilateral condylar hyperplasia. (A) Left side shows normal condyle. (B) Right side shows hyperplasia of condyle. (C) Gross specimen of hyperplastic head of condyle.

relaxation of the joint and manually repositioning the disc, followed by temporarily restricting jaw movement.

Trauma

Trauma to the joint constitutes a wide range of injuries, and may indicate condylar fracture or a mild inflammatory disorder such as discitis. Fractures of the condyle are relatively common because the condylar neck is anatomically one of the weakest points in the mandible. A blow received in the symphysis region causes bowing of the condyle, and possible fracture. The immediate complaint of the

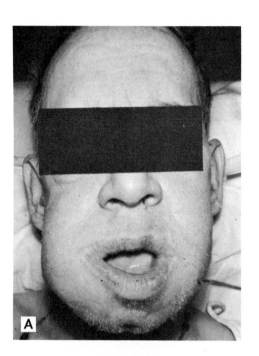

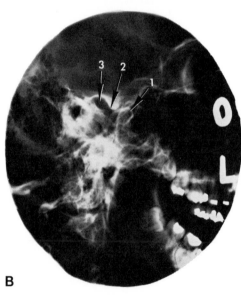

B

Fig. 23-19. Dislocation of temporomandibular joint. (A) Clinical appearance. (B) Radiograph of dislocated condylar head (1), articular eminence (2), and glenoid fossa (3).

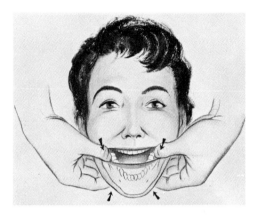

Fig. 23-20. Reduction of dislocation. (Schwartz, L. (Ed.): *Disorders of the Temporomandibular Joint.* Philadelphia, W. B. Saunders, 1959)

patient following condylar fracture is a "changed bite" or deviation of the mandible upon opening or closing. An open bite in the anterior region may also be evident. An adequate history, clinical examination, and appropriate radiographs will usually verify the fracture. The most helpful films for suspected condylar fracture are lateral views of the joint and the Towne's projection.

Conservative treatment is the primary goal in the management of fractures of the condyle. It usually involves re-establishment of occlusion, the application of arch bars, and intermaxillary fixation. Brief immobilization (two weeks or less) is generally sufficient, followed by jaw exercises which include opening and lateral excursive movements. Complicating factors in the treatment of temporomandibular joint fractures are the degree of proximal fragment displacement, the level at which the fracture occurs, additional fractures of the mandibular body or symphysis, and whether the patient is edentulous. Bleed-

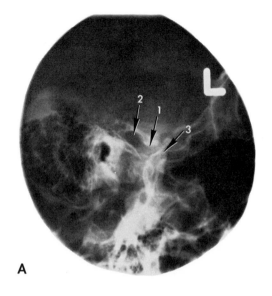

A

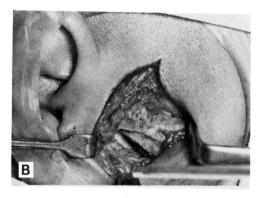

B

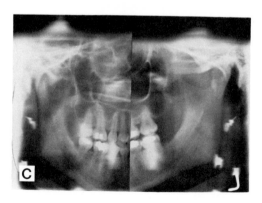

C

Fig. 23-21. Eminectomy for chronic dislocation on left side. (A) Radiograph showing articular eminence (1), glenoid fossa (2), and condyle (3). (B) Preauricular approach for eminectomy. (C) Radiograph of left side after surgical removal of eminence. Compare to radiograph on right showing steep eminence on right side.

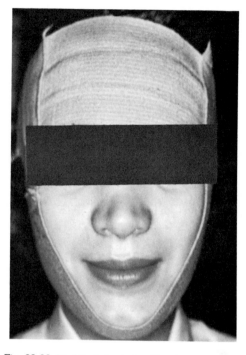

Fig. 23-22. Modified elastic head bandage to prevent chronic dislocation.

ing into the joint space and the tendency to develop ankylosis of the joint occur in condylar fractures in pediatric patients and in adults in particular when the head of the condyle is involved. When high fractures occur and the complicating effects of hematoma develop, earlier mobilization and functioning according to a guided exercise program are indicated.

The main concern for a child with injuries to the temporomandibular joint involves impaired growth and development of the injured side. The altered growth is not due to the reduced or altered function but is a direct result of injury to the growth zone of the condyle, and the risk of such lesions is probably increased by further operative intervention[11] (Fig. 23-23).

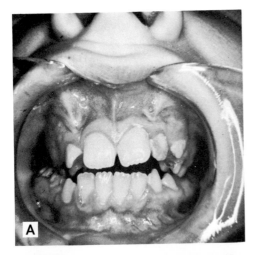

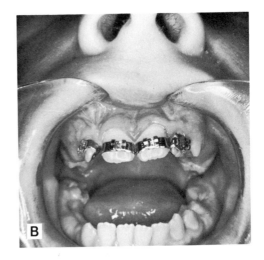

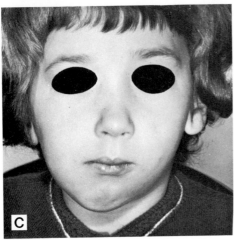

Fig. 23-23. (A) Ankylosis resulting from fracture of temporomandibular joint. (B) Opening after arthroplasty. (C) Clinical view of patient with ankylosed mandible.

Pain Dysfunction Syndrome

It was not until the 1920s that much attention was paid to the dental factors involved in pain of the temporomandibular joint. About this time, publications appeared relating malocclusion and loss of teeth to deafness and auriculotemporal pain.[12,13] Goodfriend, a dentist, reported in 1936 on the relationship of a closed vertical dimension to hearing loss and temporomandibular joint pain.[14,15] Costen wrote extensively on Goodfriend's theories and enlarged them, and this condition eventually became known as Costen's syndrome.[16]

Although the original symptom complex of the syndrome has been disproved, at least as the anatomic and physiologic basis for the syndrome, this theory did serve to focus the problem on the dentition, and hence the interest in and continued treatment of temporomandibular joint problems by the dental profession. Even though the dental occlusion is a potential contributing factor to the pain dysfunction syndrome, it is generally not the total cause. If one accepts the fact that muscle action is indeed a key to normal occlusal relation, then gross malocclusion may occur as a result of muscle action.

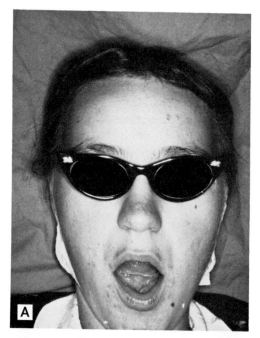

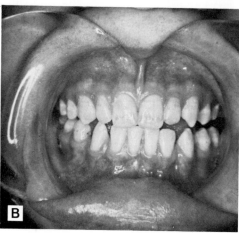

Fig. 23-24. Patient demonstrates the typical deviation and premature contact on closing the jaws with pain of the temporomandibular joint.

Conversely, then, myospasm and pain may also occur as a result of malocclusion (Fig. 23-24).

It is now well accepted that pain in the temporomandibular joint must be evaluated in relation to neuromuscular physiology and the potentiality of referred pain and the phenomenon of central pain.[17] Many people, notably the late Laszlo Schwartz, have devoted much time to the understanding of pain and the temporomandibular area. Refer to Schwartz's monumental text on the temporomandibular joint for details.[18] It was he who coined the term "pain dysfunction syndrome." The basic work of Wolff and associates[19] and of Janet Travell[20] should not be overlooked. In 1952, Travell presented a concept of myofascial pain trigger mechanisms and referred pain that has altered the therapeutic regimes employed for pain in the temporomandibular joint. The investigations of Travell indicated that muscles are the source of pain; she referred to them as myalgias.[21,22] There are many examples of similar disorders, such as tennis elbow, sciatica, tense neck pain, and others. Her concept of pain reference is in relation to myofascial trigger zones that may exist in muscle areas completely free of disease. In such instances, local anesthetic blocking of the trigger area may relieve the painful symptoms some distance away.

Muscle fatigue is the most frequent cause of myospasm. From a dental standpoint, this fatigue can result from bruxism and clenching habits, thus illustrating a probable relationship of the pain dysfunction syndrome to psychosomatic disease. Personality characteristics of patients with these problems support this relationship. Lupton found that 70 per cent of his patients with pain of the temporomandibular joint area were similar in personality to those with conditions such as obesity, ulcers, migraine headache, and hypertension.[23] The majority of these people were women with overly neurotic personalities.

In evaluating 100 patients with atypical face pain, Rushton found that 53 per cent had psychiatric illness, 33 per cent had identifiable organic disease, and 14 per cent had neither psychiatric nor organic illness.[24] Pilling reported on 562 psychiatric patients, of whom 32 per cent gave pain as the primary symptom; the most frequent location of the pain was in the head and neck.[25] Smith and associates reported that, of 32 patients with a diagnosis of atypical facial pain ultimately referred for psychiatric evaluation, 2 patients lacked evidence of psychopathologic conditions and 9 had questionable organic disease.[26] Post-treatment records of these 9 patients indicated that they had undergone a collective total of 22 unsuccessful surgical procedures. All patients had abnormal scores of the Minnesota Multiphasic Personality Inventory.

The most important consideration to recognize is that temporomandibular joint disorders may well derive from a highly complex symptomatology that may or may not be related to specific physical findings. In the general management of pain in the oral cavity and its environment, one must also consider emotional tension, oral consciousness, and personality.

The pain dysfunction syndrome, then, is facial pain with jaw dysfunction. The pain comprises a unilateral, constant jaw ache that extends to earache and headache. The dysfunction comprises restricted jaw movement, poorly coordi-nated movement with clicking of the joint, and a probable dysharmony of occlusion. It is interesting to note that this syndrome occurs four times as often in women as in men. The face and mouth have a very personal significance throughout life, and many psychologic factors are involved in this problem, as Moulton has described.[27-29] The whole concept of the body image becomes involved. Emotional tension, hysterical mechanisms, resentment, and the role of pain as a justification or excuse to gain attention are ramifications of this problem. Asking the right questions, being clear in describing findings, and ruling out organic disease are extremely important in these cases. There should be a special effort to seek consultation opinion when any of the aforementioned problems are noted.

The Arthritides

Temporomandibular joint arthritis may be discussed according to the following types: infectious, rheumatoid, degenerative, and traumatic. The degenerative and traumatic types are the two most common forms of arthritis that the dentist will encounter (Fig. 23-25). Although the temporomandibular joint may be the last joint to be involved in cases of rheumatoid arthritis, the condition is more prevalent than once thought. Russel and Bayles[30] and more recently Hatch[31] have reported that involvement of the temporomandibular joint in patients with rheumatoid arthritis is as high as 50 per cent.

Rheumatoid arthritis is an inflammation that progresses from a synovitis to a characteristically painful and increasingly immobilizing deformity of the joint.

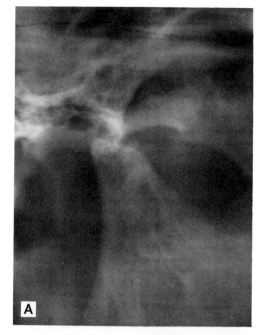

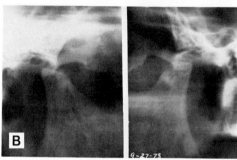

Fig. 23-25. Radiographic evidence of degenerative joint disease associated with long-standing temporomandibular joint pain.

In the young individual, severe facial deformity may develop (Still's disease). Radiographic studies may show degenerative changes in the joint surface (Fig. 23-26). At the least, restricted motion is evident. Treatment in the early stages is directed to the general aspects of the disease—systemic salicylates, cortisone, and occasionally, local intra-articular injection of hydrocortisone may relieve acute pain and allow continued function. Diet, local heat, and exercise are additional important factors in the regime of treatment. In severe cases, surgical intervention may be indi-

cated, and the technique of high condylectomy is advocated.[32]

Traumatic arthritis is preceded by a history of trauma and may range in degree from a painful joint to severely restricted movement and positive radiographic findings (Fig. 23-27).

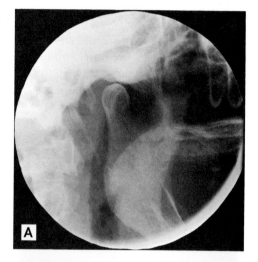

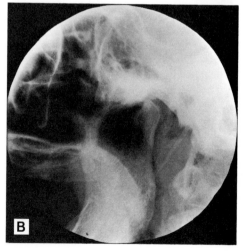

Fig. 23-26. (A and B) Degenerative arthritis. Note areas of demineralization and facet on head of condyle.

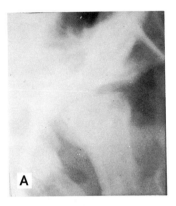

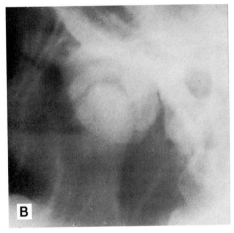

Fig. 23-27. (A and B) Traumatic arthritis in 14-year-old boy; injury seven years previous.

Hypomobility

Hypomobility due to ankylosis may vary from minor degrees of limited function to complete inability to open the jaws. If not treated, the patient will be unable to eat normally, cannot masticate, oral hygiene will deteriorate, and speech will become difficult. If the ankylosis occurred early in life, deformity of the mandible, referred to as micrognathia, may occur. The ankylosis may be fibrous or bony in nature.

The cause of ankylosis, although occa-sionally congenital, inflammatory, or ar-thritic, is usually traumatic. It may be unilateral or bilateral. If unilateral, the jaw will deviate toward the affected side upon attempted opening. Placing the fin-gers into the external auditory canals will reveal whether any motion is evident. Roentgenographic studies aid in deter-mining the extent of the ankylosis, which may range from condylar ankylosis only to ankylosis that involves the coronoid proc-ess with complete obliteration of the sig-moid notch. There may even be extreme fusion with the zygomatic arch, the tem-poral bone, and the base of the skull.

Surgical intervention is the treatment of choice for ankylosis. Several techniques are available, and the surgical approaches are shown in Figures 23-28 and 23-29. In some instances, no interposing substance

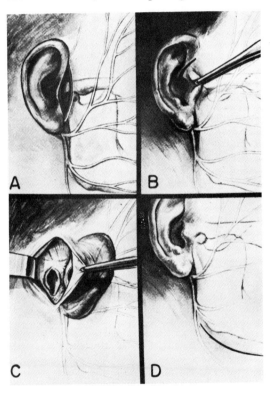

Fig. 23-28. Surgical approaches to the temporoman-dibular joint. (A) Preauricular. (B) Endaural. (C) Postauricular. (D) Submandibular. (Sarnat, B. G.: *The Temporomandibular Joint.* Springfield, Ill., Charles C Thomas, 1964)

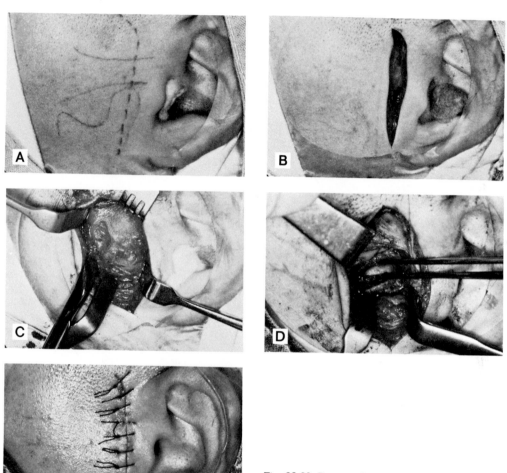

Fig. 23-29. Preauricular approach for a high condylotomy. (A) Outline of planed incision. Note: zygomatic arch and condylar head outlined. (B) Incision. (C) Soft tissue. (D) Exposure of condylar head. (E) Skin closure with 5-0 black silk sutures.

is placed following arthroplasty, whereas others utilize Vitallium chrome cobalt castings[33] or an alloplast such as Silastic; others use fascia or cartilage (Fig. 23-30).

Neurologic Disorders

Many neurologic and related muscular disorders may affect mandibular movement, such as Parkinson's disease, chorea, and dystonia. Muscle disorders in this category include myasthenia gravis, muscular dystrophy, and cerebral palsy. Drug-induced dyskinesia is of particular interest, since many patients taking tranquilizing medication may produce symptoms similar to the neurologic disorders (Fig. 23-31).

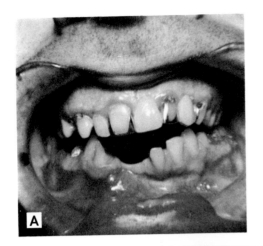

Fig. 23-30. Bilateral ankylosis. (A) Patient was unable to open the mouth for 15 years. Note the loss of teeth in anterior to aid in eating. (B) Radiographs showing ankylosis (above) and result of arthroplasty with chrome cobalt castings (below). (C) Clinical photograph of arthroplasty. (D) Clinical result with prosthesis in place.

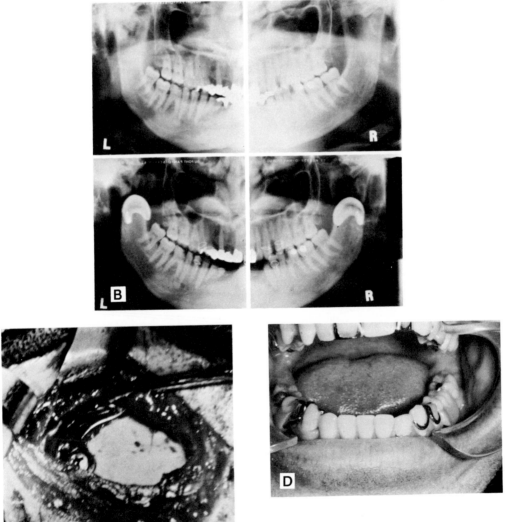

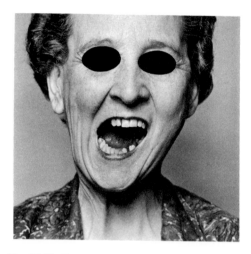

Fig. 23-31. Dystonia. (Courtesy of Dr. J. Gibilisco)

Growth Deformities

The growth potential of the condyloid process as well as other areas in the mandible has been mentioned. Growth deformities are frequently not traceable to the actual causes; nevertheless, injury is undoubtedly high on the probable incidence of origin. Some disorders are congenital. Since many problems become manifest during the developmental period, differentiating the true cause is often difficult.

The deformity of the jaw must be determined not only according to the severity and duration of the injury, but also the time of occurrence in the developmental period. The effect will be greater if the injury occurs during the greatest growth period. Sarnat has suggested that unilateral disorders of the condyle are generally due to local factors, whereas bilateral disturbances of the condyle are often a result of some systemic condition.[34] Bilateral growth deformities are perhaps seen in prognathism and micrognathism. An ex-ample of unilateral developmental problems would be unilateral hyperplasia of the mandibular condyle. Growth deformities are discussed in Chapter 24.

Neoplasms

Intracranial tumors may produce problems relating to jaw dysfunction if associated nerves are involved, as with pituitary adenoma and cerebellopontine angle tumors. Squamous cell carcinoma of the pharynx and posterior one third of the tongue can simulate the pain dysfunction syndrome. During the early stages of the tumor growth, referred pain of the local area is important, and specific involvement of the fifth and seventh cranial nerves may complicate the establishment of the diagnosis (Fig. 23-32).

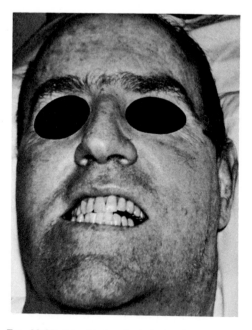

Fig. 23-32. Mandibular deviation and joint pain; etiology was a nasopharyngeal tumor.

Specific tumors of the temporomandibular joint may also arise, of which chondroma and osteoma constitute the majority. There are also reports, though more rare, of fibrous dysplasia, myxoma,[35] and several malignant tumors.[36]

The Therapeutic Program

In general, conservatism is the treatment of choice for many of the disorders discussed in this chapter. Tumors, infections, and fractures are not the major temporomandibular joint problems most commonly seen; when they do appear, they require special handling. When conservative methods do not provide relief for a patient, a high condylotomy may be performed (Fig. 23-33). The general principles of management should be directed toward establishing the diagnosis and correcting the cause. This will necessitate a knowledge of the foregoing material and an attempt to classify the type of disorder. As previously stated, if occlusal disharmony is present, one should first look for muscle pain and/or spasm that has altered the occlusal relation. If selective grinding is attempted, it must be done with care and knowledge of the full complexities of equilibration. Further treatment may include replacement of teeth by bridges or partials, or opening or closing the bite. In cases of a locked occlusion, an extraction may well be indicated or the use of bite splints (Fig. 23-34).

Careful consideration should be given to emotional stress, personality, and anxiety. Habits such as bruxism, clenching, or other abuse to the dentition may need attention. The proper handling of many of these problems will depend upon the doc-

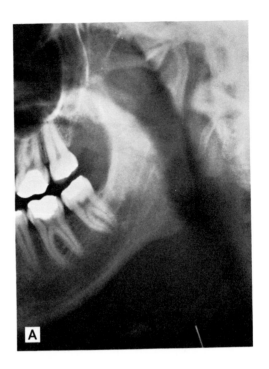

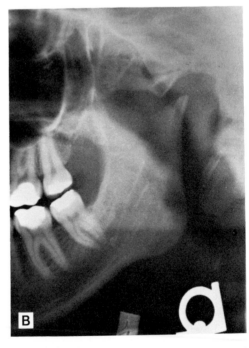

Fig. 23-33. High condylotomy. (A) Note abnormal condylar head and neck. (B) One-year postsurgical radiograph of condylar head which functions well. Patient had no pain.

tor's skill in establishing confidence and rapport with the patient. Medical consultation may become important, and careful, knowledgeable selection of referrals is paramount. The appropriate medical and dental specialties will often become involved in handling these complicating problems.

Since the pain dysfunction syndrome and degenerative joint disease occur most frequently, their differential diagnosis is significant. The pain dysfunction syndrome appears in patients of a wide variety of ages, there is often the possibility of psychogenic factors, and the syndrome will present negative radiographic findings. Degenerative joint disease, on the other hand, should have positive x-ray findings, occurs in older patients, and may reveal a history of additional arthritis. The occlusal dysharmony that may result is due to capsular swelling, and the presence of intracapsular fluid will often cause pain and probable jaw deviation. These same symptoms, of course, may occur from the pain dysfunction syndrome initated by myospasm. In neither instance will occlusal grinding provide anything more than temporary relief.

The following five therapeutic principles have been suggested by Bell with special reference to the pain dysfunction syndrome.

1. Temporary disengagement of the occlusion.
2. Voluntary restriction of use within painful limits.
3. Controlled physiotherapy.
4. Interruption of cycling myospasm by analgesic blocking.
5. Muscle relaxant therapy.

The disengagement of the occlusion is particularly important in cases of acute malocclusion. This can be done through careful discussion of the problem and getting the patient's cooperation in restricting movement of the joint and/or with the use of splints. The avoidance of abrasive foods, heavy chewing, and wide opening will tend to minimize the discomfort and limit the stimulation of already painful muscles. While all of these techniques are methods of physiotherapy, the use of refrigeration, especially in the form of ethyl chloride spray, has been well described. Local anesthetic injections are an additional method of interrupting a cycling myospasm. The painful area is located and the anesthetic infiltrated into the

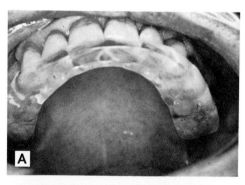

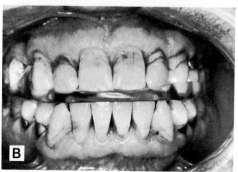

Fig. 23-34. (A and B) Splints.

muscle. Medication encompassing the tranquilizers, skeletal muscle relaxants, and sedatives all have their place in the therapeutic regime. Side effects, however, must be carefully considered, especially in the ambulatory patient.

References

1. Sarnat, B. G.: The Temporomandibular Joint, 2nd ed. Springfield, Ill., Charles C Thomas, 1964.
2. Washburn, S. L.: Growth and Development of Dental and Skeletal Tissue— Clinical and Biological Aspects. Report of 17th Ross Pediatric Research Conference. Boston, Mass., March 28–30, 1955.
3. Bell, W. E.: Temporomandibular Joint Disease. Dallas, The Egan Co., 1960.
4. Ramfjord, S. P., Kerr, D. A., and Ash, M. M.: World Workshop in Periodontics. University of Michigan, 1966.
5. Krogh-Paulsen, W. G., and Olsson, A.: Occlusal disharmonies and dysfunction of stomatognathic system. Dent. Clin. North Am., pp. 627–635, Nov., 1966.
6. Freese, A., and Scheman, P.: Management of Temporomandibular Joint Problems. St. Louis, C. V. Mosby Co., 1962.
7. Barton, R. T.: Benign masseteric hypertrophy. J.A.M.A., 164:1646, 1957.
8. Bell, W. E.: Personal communication, 1970.
9. Merrill, R. G.: Habitual subluxation and recurrent dislocation in a patient with Parkinson's disease. J. Oral Surg., 26:473–477, 1968.
10. Myrhaug, H.: A new method of operation for habitual dislocation of the mandible. Acta Odontol. Scand., 9:247, 1954.
11. Husted, E.: Surgical management of temporomandibular joint disorder. Dent. Clin. North Am., pp. 601–607, Nov., 1966.
12. Monson, G. S.: Occlusion supplied to crown and bridgework. J. Natl. Dent. Assoc., 7:399, 1920.
13. Wright, W. H.: Deafness as influenced by malposition of the jaw. J. Natl. Dent. Assoc., 7:979–992, 1920.
14. Goodfriend, D. J.: Dyarthrosis and subarthrosis of the mandibular articulation. Dent. Cosmos, 74:523–535, 1932.
15. Goodfriend, D. J.: The role of dental factors in the cause and treatment of ear symptoms and disease. Dent. Cosmos, 78:1292, 1936.
16. Costen, J. B.: Neuralgia and ear symptoms associated with disturbed temporomandibular joint. J.A.M.A. 107:252–264, 1936.
17. Alling, C. C., III: Facial Pain, 2nd ed. Philadelphia, Lea & Febiger, 1977.
18. Schwartz, L.: Disorders of the Temporomandibular Joint. Philadelphia, W. B. Saunders Co., 1959.
19. Wolff, H. G., and Hardy, J. D.: The nature of pain. Physiol. Rev., 27:167–199, 1947.
20. Travell, J., and Rinzler, S.: The myofascial genesis of pain. Postgrad. Med., 11:425, 1952.
21. Travell, J.: Referred pain from skeletal muscles; the pectoralis major syndrome of breast pain and soreness and the sternocleidomastoid syndrome of headache and dizziness. N.Y. J. Med., 55:331–339, 1955.
22. Travell, J.: Temporomandibular joint dysfunction. J. Prosthet. Dent., 10:745–763, 1960.
23. Lupton, D. E.: A preliminary investigation of the personality of female temporomandibular joint dysfunction patients. Psychother. Psychosom., 14:199, 1966.
24. Rushton, M. A.: Some aspects of anteroposterior growth of the mandible. Dent. Rec., 68:80–87, 1948.
25. Pilling, L. F., et al.: Psychologic characteristics of psychiatric patients having pain as a presenting symptom. Can. Med. Assoc. J., 97:387–394, 1967.
26. Smith, D. P., et al.: A psychiatric study of atypical face pain. (Unpublished data.)
27. Moulton, R. E.: Oral and dental manifestations of anxiety. Psychiatry, 18:261, 1955.
28. Smith, D. P., et al.: Psychiatric consideration in maxillofacial pain. J. Am. Dent. Assoc., 51:408–414, 1955.
29. Smith, D. P., et al.: Emotional factors in

non-organic temporomandibular joint pain. Dent. Clin. North Am., pp. 609–620, Nov., 1966.

30. Russel, L. A., and Bayles, T. B.: The temporomandibular joint in rheumatoid arthritis. J. Amer. Dent. Assoc., 28:535–539, 1941.

31. Hatch, G.: The Temporomandibular Joint in Patients with Rheumatoid Arthritis. Mayo Clinic Thesis, 1967.

32. Henry, F. A., and Baldridge, O. L.: Condylectomy for the persistently painful temporomandibular joint. J. Oral Surg., 15:24–31, 1957.

33. Husted, E., and Hjorting-Hansen, E. (eds.): International Association of Oral Surgeons Second Congress. Oral Surgery Transactions. pp. 265–267. Los Angeles, Scandinavian University Books, 1967.

34. Sarnat, B. J.: Developmental facial abnormalities. In Facial Pain and Mandibular Dysfunction. L. Schwartz and C. Chayes (Eds.). Philadelphia, W. B. Saunders Co., 1968.

35. Thoma, K., and Goldman, H. M.: Oral Pathology, 5th ed., pp. 866–871. St. Louis, C. V. Mosby Co., 1960.

36. Thoma, K.: Tumors of the condyle and temporomandibular joint. Oral Surg., 7:1091–1107, 1954.

37. Moss, M. L.: The Functional Matrix. Vistas in Orthodontics, pp. 85–98. Philadelphia, Lea & Febiger, 1962.

24 Developmental Jaw Deformities

EMIL W. STEINHAUSER
DANIEL E. WAITE

Normal Facial Configuration and Cephalometric Measurements

IDEAL STANDARDS AND RACIAL PECULIARITIES. Beauty and harmony of the face have great significance for mankind. In the oldest scriptures we find facial characteristics described in such terms as "noble," "beautiful," or "courageous." Even today, the appearance of an individual certainly has great importance in any professional or social position. Therefore, the perpetual desire of man to be more beautiful and more perfect is understandable; understandable too, is man's feeling that his face, the focal point of his communication with the rest of the world, should assume great importance in his striving for perfection.

The fine arts have always engaged in trying to find certain ideals of beauty for representing human faces. One of the many artists who committed himself to certain ideal measurements of the face was Leonardo da Vinci, who recorded the different proportions of the face with mathematical accuracy. Many others followed his example, and naturally their conceptions of an ideal face differed a great deal. This became evident in a synopsis by Schwarz, a Viennese orthodontist who, on the basis of famous sculptures, determined three principal facial configurations.[1] His classification into a straight forward face, a straight backward face, and an intermediate face constituted an early analysis system. Racial peculiarities were not considered, however, and negroid and mongoloid people have a quite different concept of the ideal face. Even in the white race there exists a great variety of facial configurations—just consider the relatively oblong facial forms of Scandinavian people and the more or less round facial appearance of southern Europeans.

REGULAR CEPHALOMETRIC LINES AND ANGLES. As stated by E. H. Angle in 1908, the position of the jaws is the most important factor in defining the character of a face.[2] The appearance of the tissue contours largely depends upon the structure of the skeleton and the dentition. The analysis of the profile, the facial skeleton, and the dental structure enables us to determine the relationship of these three components by measurements. To evaluate the relationship of the different parts of the face and the jaws, we use cephalometry, which provides a relative method for measuring. Most of these measurements are expressed by angles, which are more reliable than lines, especially when comparing one person to another. Average values have been established by serial examinations; these subdivide again into age, sex, and racial groups.

The lateral x-ray view of the head, taken from a standard distance with a precisely fixed position of the head, is largely recognized to be the most exact method of measurement. With relatively soft rays, the picture obtained in this manner reproduces the soft tissue contours as well as the skeletal configuration (Fig. 24-1). After the appropriate landmarks are connected by straight lines, the angles necessary for the analysis can be measured.

The oldest and best known measurement line is that from the tragus of the ear to the infraorbital rim, which in anthropology is known as the "Frankfort horizontal plane." However, since this plane cannot always be determined exactly, the line from the middle of the sella turcica to the root of the nose, which is generally termed the "cranial base plane" and marked with the letters SN, is used more often. The root of the nose is the starting point for further lines, which are drawn to the apical base of the front teeth in the maxilla (creating the angle SNA) and the

analogous position of the mandible (creating the angle SNB). Thereby the anteroposterior position of the maxilla and the mandible can be related to the cranial base plane. The difference between these two angles gives the anteroposterior relationship between the maxilla and the mandible (angle ANB). Abnormalities in skeletal profile can thus be diagnosed if these angles are measured. Besides the analysis of the relationship of maxilla and mandible, the dental analysis is diagnostically important. Treatment planning, of course, is based upon the exact diagnosis which this analysis provides. For this purpose a line is drawn through the long axis of the maxillary incisors intersecting the cranial base plane SN. The angle thereby created may be decisive as to whether surgical or only orthodontic treatment is indicated. In the mandible, the line drawn through the long axis of the lower incisors intersects the mandibular plane, which is determined by the line connecting the point gonion (GO) and the point gnathion (GN) (Fig. 24-2). For the total corrective possibilities of the treatment and diagnosis, the evaluation of soft tissue and vertical proportionality must be recognized, as well as dental and skeletal measurement.

The simplest and most important angle in soft tissue analysis is the facial contour angle suggested by Burstone—glabella-subnasale-pogonion (the average measurement of $-11° \pm 4°$) (Fig. 24-3).

As a rule, the total facial height between the eye and soft tissue menton can be divided into fifths. The upper facial height (eye-subnasale) is two fifths, and lower facial height (subnasale-menton) is three fifths.[60]

These measurements permit a compari-

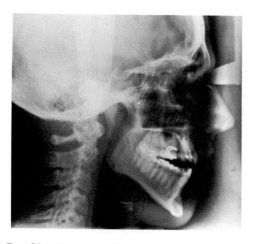

Fig. 24-1. Regular cephalometric x-ray view. The relatively soft x rays make it possible for the soft tissue contours to be visible.

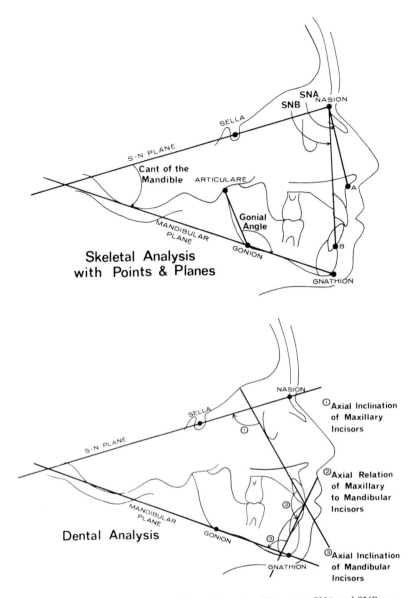

Fig. 24-2. Cephalometric x-ray studies with tracing. The points SNA and SNB are connected by lines. Also, the inclination of the upper teeth to the cranial base plane SN and of the lower teeth to the mandibular plane GO-GN can be measured.

son of the anteroposterior relationship of the jaws to the cranial base and of the teeth to the jaws. The values obtained are compared to normal values for the corresponding population. In some cases, further measurement points may be necessary. The determination of the angle of the jaw, a prominent chin, and the config-

uration of the nose and lips is also important. The facial height, measured in vertical distances, should be considered as well.

It is recommended that the student refer to an orthodontics textbook for further details of cephalometric analysis. The analysis of developmental deformities

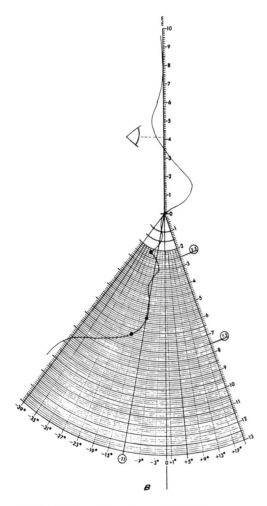

Fig. 24-3. Diagnostic contour protractor.

without proper interpretation of the cephalometric x-ray view is usually insufficient and often followed by inappropriate treatment and poor surgical results.

Etiology of Growth Disturbances

GENETIC OR CONGENITAL DEFORMITIES. Whether a developmental deformity in the maxillofacial region is hereditary or

congenital cannot be determined exactly. In cleft palate or Pierre Robin syndrome, the congenital character of the deformity is already evident at birth, and other jaw deformities may appear during the period of growth. If no other cause such as trauma, general or constitutional affection, disturbances of nutrition, or bad habits can be registered, a hereditary cause must be considered.

In general, it is usually seldom possible to prove inheritance in jaw deformities. Exceptions are cleft lip and palate, of which 20 to 25 percent have been proved to be inherited. Occasionally, an inheritance of true mandibular prognathism during several generations has been observed. The so called "Hapsburg jaw" is a classic example, and was a typical characteristic of the imperial Hapsburg family that reigned over Austria and Central Europe for centuries. The prominent lower jaw of numerous male members of this imperial family can still be observed in several well-preserved portraits. Furthermore, a family history is present in certain syndromes connected with jaw deformities. Examples are craniofacial dysostosis, also known as Crouzon's disease, mandibulofacial dysostosis, and progressive hemifacial atrophy. These aspects of disease are discussed in detail with the different deformities of the maxilla and mandible.

ACQUIRED DEFORMITIES. Disturbances occurring during the period of growth of an individual may lead to serious deformities and malformations of the facial skeleton and the covering soft tissues. Since all of the soft tissues functionally relate to a given skeletal element, the defect or alteration of the soft tissues will be significant in any given anomaly. The causes of disturbances are classified into two basic groups, inflammation and trauma.

Inflammations may lead to deformities if they involve regions of growth. The area with the greatest growth potential in the mandible is the condyle itself; the other growth areas in the jaw angle and in the alveolar process are less significant. When damage occurs in an important growth center, a greater deformity naturally results. Maxillary hypoplasia probably occurs less frequently because the maxilla does not have an essential growth center as does the mandible. An exception is the cleft palate case.

The main cause of inflammation is infection. Otitis media often appears in childhood, and because of the immediate vicinity of the temporomandibular joint, may sometimes cause a purulent arthritis. As a consequence, fibrous or eventually bony ankylosis may appear and partially or totally destroy the main growth areas. Hematogeneous osteomyelitis may also damage the growth area in childhood. Other inflammatory diseases affect the joint, although less frequently.

The second large group of acquired disturbances of the facial growth results from trauma (Fig. 24-4). The fracture of one or both temporomandibular joints in a growing person may result in uni- or bilateral growth restraint, which is the main cause of malformation in this group. Although extracapsular fracture of the temporomandibular joint is not as significant to growth, fracture of the condylar head seriously endangers the growth area that is located there. In spite of appropriate treatment, serious articular transformation and ankylosis may appear. As a consequence, there may be a total cessation in

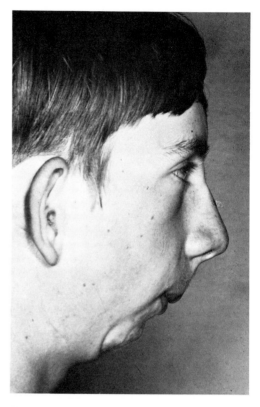

Fig. 24-4. Growth deformity from childhood injury to mandibular condyle.

the growth of the jaw on the affected side of the mandible.

Functional activity is essential for growth. If the mandible is limited in its movements by unilateral ankylosis, it will practically grow no further in spite of viable cartilage cells in the growth area of the nonaffected side. Therefore, in a unilateral ankylosis that occurs in childhood, the intact side of the mandible scarcely continues growing. The result is retrognathia with microgenia and only very little of the asymmetry seen in unilateral condylar hypertrophy (Fig. 24-5).

Fractures of the mandible that do not involve the joint, as well as fractures in the maxilla, have little influence on growth if treated appropriately. However, surgical procedures involving detachment of the periosteum and exposure of large bone areas should be avoided if possible in a growing patient. Typical examples of growth disturbances provoked by operative trauma are the deformed and underdeveloped maxillas seen in cleft palate patients (Fig. 24-6). These disturbances can be attributed to the surgical closure of the clefts in early childhood, since patients with an unoperated cleft show normal growth of the maxilla. More protective operative techniques, as well as pre- and postoperative orthodontic treatment, have resulted in remarkable improvements.

In addition to inflammation and

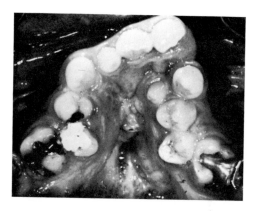

Fig. 24-6. Acquired maxillary deformity. Heavily compressed and malformed maxillary arch in an adult patient with unilateral cleft palate.

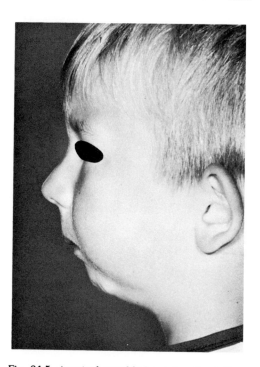

Fig. 24-5. Acquired mandibular deformity. Inflammation in early childhood caused a unilateral ankylosis of the temporomandibular joint. A remarkable retrognathia of the mandible is already present at the age of six.

trauma, there are other rare causes of acquired deformities. These are certain tumors and systemic diseases of childhood, such as juvenile fibrous dysplasia, causing jaw deformities (Fig. 24-7). Acromegaly may also lead to a spectacular longitudinal growth of the mandible.

Therapeutic Principles for Functional and Cosmetic Rehabilitation

TIMING AND PLANNING OF CORRECTION. An important principle in the treatment of developmental deformities is to delay the operative correction until the period of growth has been completed. This means that a girl should be at least 15 and a boy 16 years old before a correction should be carried out. However, these age limits should not be considered inflexible, because racial and individual physical growth factors determine whether the period of growth is completed sooner or later.

There are several logical reasons for not

planning an operation before completion of growth. The surgical procedure might disturb the growth of bone areas, and the operative result may become unsatisfactory owing to further growth. An additional surgical operation can be avoided with more patience on the part of the doctor and the patient. There are certain exceptions to these principles, and we, as well as others, have sometimes operated on patients of an earlier age. This is indicated if the unfavorable appearance of a patient causes serious complexes or other psychic upsets and disturbances. In such cases, it should always be pointed out to the parents and to the patient that another operation might be necessary after growth has been completed. In hemifacial microsomia (mandible), there are sound advantages for early surgical intervention: improvement of symmetry, reduction of maxillary deficiency, establishment of normal occlusal table, and early expansion of the skeletal structure and maintenance of the soft tissue covering and muscle development. However, in mandibular prognathism it is preferable to wait until growth has been completed in order to avoid relapses. Operation may be considered earlier in a retrognathic mandible.

Obviously, the treatment plan greatly influences the final result. Therefore it should be projected with great precision, considering all operative possibilities as

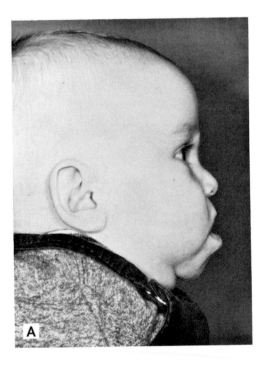

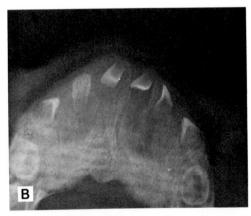

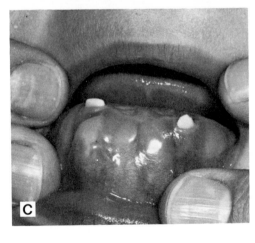

Fig. 24-7. Juvenile fibrous dysplasia causing both intraoral and facial deformity in three-month-old patient. (A) Profile. (B) Radiograph. (C) Clinical appearance of mouth.

well as complications. For the planning of treatment we consider it important to have the following records prepared:

1. Case history with special consideration of hereditary occurrence.
2. Precise extraoral and intraoral examination.
3. Cephalometric x-ray views with analysis.
4. Study models with mounting and sectioning (two sets).
5. Photographs, frontal and lateral views.
6. Periapical x-ray films and tooth vitality tests.
7. Special x-ray pictures like laminograms, anteroposterior skull view, lateral mandibular view, and so forth.

As an example of the planning for the correction of a jaw deformity, the management of a case of maxillary retrusion is demonstrated.

1. In a 42-year-old healthy man, the medical history was unremarkable. His family history revealed no jaw deformities other than his own, which had been present since his early childhood in the form of a prominent lower jaw. Two premolars in the maxilla had probably been extracted many years ago. A general dentist called the patient's attention to the possibility of an operative correction and referred the patient to us.
2. The extraoral examination showed a hypoplasia of the entire maxilla as well as a pseudoprognathism of the mandible (Fig. 24-8A). The oral examination showed a 7-mm. reverse overjet of the incisors. In relation to the mandible, the maxilla was relatively broad (Fig. 24-8B).

3. The cephalometric x-ray view showed clearly the discrepancy between maxilla and mandible. There was an abnormal SNA angle and the relationship of the ANB was negative. The dental analysis demonstrated a normal position of the lower front teeth, the upper incisors being retruded. The chin prominence in relationship to nasion (SNB) was in a good position (Fig. 24-8C).
4. The study models demonstrated the malrelation of the teeth. The sectioning of the mounted models showed that a good intermaxillary relationship could be obtained when advancing the maxilla anteriorly for 9 mm. (Fig. 24-8D). Also, a sagittal splitting of the maxilla was necessary in order to adjust the broad maxilla to the mandibular arch. For this, a narrowing of 8 mm. in the posterior part of the maxilla was necessary.
5. The enlarged frontal and lateral photographs of the face were studied and cut. On the photographs, the maxilla was brought forward in an attempt to get a better shape of the face. The result obtained by this method was not instructive because the actual postoperative shape of the nose could not be estimated.
6. The periapical x-ray films in the maxilla showed neither an inflammatory process in the root region nor impacted teeth. The vitality of all teeth in the maxilla was positive.
7. An additional Waters' sinus x-ray projection was obtained, which revealed clear sinus bilaterally.

After the evaluation of all these preliminary measures, the diagnosis of maxillary retrusion was confirmed.

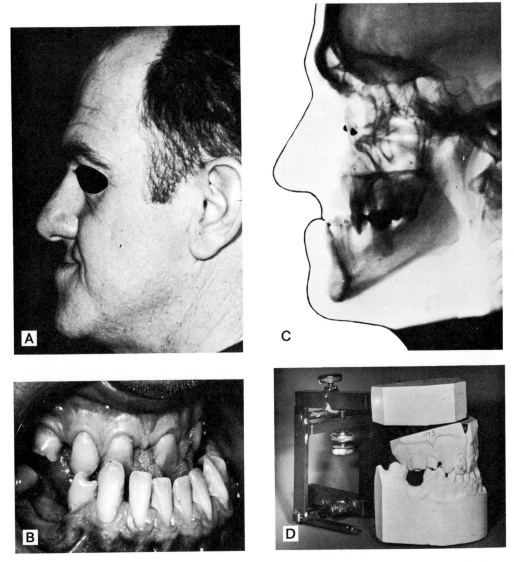

Fig. 24-8. Treatment planning in a case of maxillary deficiency. (A) Profile preoperatively. (B) Occlusion preoperatively. (C) Cephalometric x-ray view clearly showing the maxillary retrusion. (D) Model operation that indicates a forward movement of the maxilla of 9 mm. and a drop-down in the posterior area. (E) Profile postoperatively. (F) Occlusion postoperatively.

Now the therapy was obvious: it should consist of a maxillary advancement with simultaneous sagittal splitting and narrowing of the maxilla. The final result confirmed the correctness of the procedure in this case (Fig. 24-8E and F).

PRE- AND POSTOPERATIVE TREATMENT. Preoperative orthodontic treatment is necessary in a great number of cases. This is especially true if in spite of sectioning the model, no satisfactory occlusion can be obtained. If there are only small disorders in occlusion, selective grinding of single

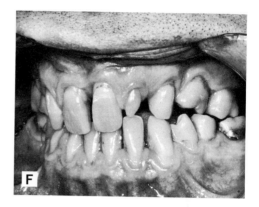

Fig. 24-8. Continued

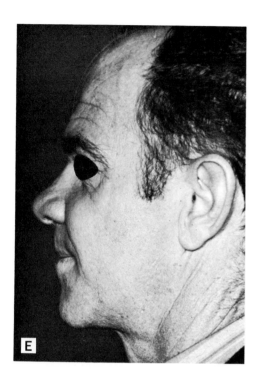

protuberances or tooth pairs might be sufficient. After each grinding, impressions should be retaken. The model operation should also be repeated in some cases in order to have a reliable guide during the actual operation.

If the disturbance of occlusion is serious enough to prevent a good result, the assistance of an orthodontist is indispensable. He can position the teeth in the alveolar arch so that, after surgical repositioning of the jaw, the teeth fit together in harmony. A typical example would be the correction of true mandibular prognathism. In these cases, the lower front teeth are often in a retruded position, so that just obtaining an overbite of the incisors often leaves the patient with

insufficient skeletal correction. The lower face will still be prominent and the chin protruded in spite of the seemingly good dental relationship. In such cases, the lower front teeth should first be erected with the aid of orthodontics. This will result in a greater surgical retrusion to obtain a good dental relationship so that the push-back of the mandible will, in correcting this position of the teeth, also correct the proportions of the face.

The correction of the prognathic open bite is a further example. If the osteotomy is made in the ascending ramus, the strong masticatory muscles will be overstretched by the necessary rotation of the body of the mandible. Naturally, these muscles have a tendency to retract, and a relapse of the open bite might result. In such a case the orthodontist will make an interdental splint, also called a wafer, in order to produce an open bite in the molar region (Fig. 24-9). Thus the expected relapse will be counteracted. We call this a "controlled or regulated relapse" and expect the occlusion in the molar region to

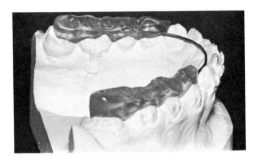

Fig. 24-9. Interdental splint. The splint, which opens the occlusion in the posterior area, is used to find the right occlusal relationship as well as to avoid relapses.

re-establish itself spontaneously when the wafer has been removed after bony healing is complete.

Another important preoperative measure is the splinting of the partially or completely edentulous jaw. First determine whether intermaxillary fixation is necessary. One can use different types of splints for intermaxillary fixation, such as arch bars, cap splints, acrylic splints, or continous loop wiring. According to his training and laboratory facilities, the surgeon selects the type of splint. The only important consideration is to obtain a reliable intermaxillary fixation.

For an operative movement of single parts of the alveolar process (e.g., in correcting maxillary protrusion, mandibular alveolar protrusion or retrusion, or many kinds of open bite deformities), we use a splint technique that does not require intermaxillary fixation, which is naturally more convenient for the patient. The principle of the splinting is to fix the moved parts to the stable parts of the operated jaw. For this we use a strong arch bar that is tied to the teeth with the aid of orthodontic bands (Fig. 24-10).

After the operation, the patient receives special care. Begin careful mouth hygiene from the first postoperative day. This is not always easy because of the impediment of the splints. The toothbrush is the best aid, and the patient, as well as the nurses, has to be instructed exactly in its use. The splint is being controlled and eventually reinforced, and the patient and his relatives are given special advice regarding nourishment. Because differences arise from case to case, no exact statement can be made concerning the time for opening the intermaxillary fixation. Normally we maintain it for six weeks, but intersegmental fixation in one jaw is usually retained for one or two weeks longer.

The postoperative phase also includes the removal of the splints, the making of the necessary models for demonstration and study purposes, postoperative photographs, x-ray and cephalometric views.

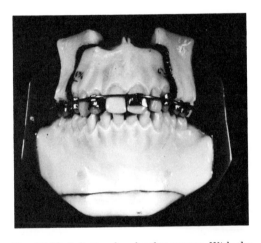

Fig. 24-10. Splinting for alveolar surgery. With the aid of orthodontic bands, brackets, tubes, and round wire, the moved premaxilla is fixed to the stable posterior maxilla. No intermaxillary fixation is necessary. (Courtesy of Dr. Obwegeser, University of Zurich, Switzerland)

The latter are especially important in order to reveal relapes at an early time. Besides the examination of the sensory and motor nerves in the operative field, a vitality test of the teeth is important. Follow-up studies have shown that, even with an osteotomy of the alveolar process, regeneration of the sensory nerves to the teeth occurs after an average of six to nine months in the maxilla and nine to twelve months in the mandible. According to our experience, the most reliable test method is the application of CO_2 snow.[3]

In many cases, the cooperation of the orthodontist is also necessary postoperatively to move teeth and tooth groups that are still not in an ideal position. More important, in some cases, is the preparation of a retention appliance that helps to stabilize the occlusion and keep the operatively moved jaw segments in their position.

Mandibular Deformities

Prognathism (Prognathia Inferior)

Protrusion of the lower part of the face may have different causes. The total lower jaw, including the alveolar process and the chin prominence, may be overdeveloped in comparison to the facial profile, but a prominence of only the alveolar process or the chin may also cause a remarkable disturbance in the harmony of the face. Therefore it is of great importance to have an exact analysis of the facial skeleton as well as a dental occlusal analysis before an operative correction is performed. The best aid for this analysis is the cephalometric x-ray view, which shows the deviation from normal most clearly (Fig. 24-11).

TRUE MANDIBULAR PROGNATHISM. The most common and therefore clinically most important disturbance of the facial proportions is true mandibular prognathism. The cause of this overdevelopment is, as in many jaw deformities, unknown.

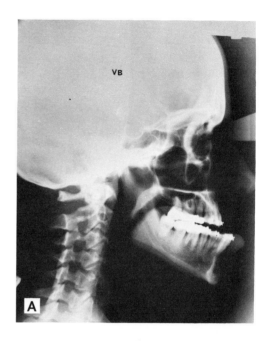

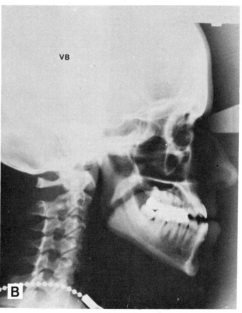

Fig. 24-11. Severe mandibular prognathism. (A) Preoperative cephalometric x-ray film. (B) Postoperative cephalometric x-ray film.

The only exceptions are the cases with familial occurrences in which a hereditary component must be assumed. One per cent of the Caucasian population demonstrates prognathism and the statistic is up to 10 per cent in first-degree relatives. Rare adenomas of the eosinophilic cells of the anterior part of the hypophysis result in a similar condition of the mandible and is systemically acromegaly. The clinical symptoms of true mandibular prognathism are impressive. The lower face and chin prominence are enlarged, and there is usually a negative overjet varying from 0 mm. (edge to edge) to 30 mm. In addition to their anterior crossbite relation to the upper incisors, the lower incisors are often inclined lingually, as reflected by the angle of the axis of the lower anterior teeth to the mandibular plane. Furthermore, the contour of the mandibular angle may be flat and elongated. The most significant change in the cephalometric x-ray view is found in the angle SNB, which is larger than normal, whereas SNA remains within normal limits. The gonial angle may also be abnormal.

The therapy of mandibular prognathism has been discussed in many textbooks and publications. Up to now, the opinions regarding the "ideal method" are divided and many variations of the operative technique have been reported. Principally, a distinction is made between procedures in the ascending ramus and in the body of the mandible. It is impossible to describe all methods practiced, and only the most common techniques will be explained (Fig. 24-12).

Osteotomy in the Condylar Neck. This method for the correction of mandibular prognathism is one of the oldest, having

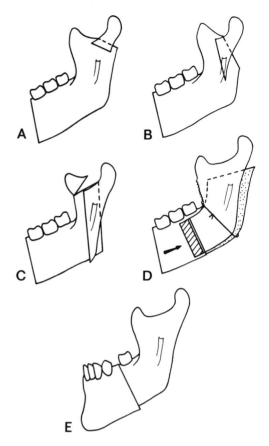

Fig. 24-12. Common techniques for the correction of mandibular prognathism. (A) Osteotomy in the condylar neck. (B) Subcondylar oblique osteotomy. (C) Vertical osteotomy of the ramus. (D) Sagittal splitting of the ramus. (E) Ostectomy of the body.

first been reported in 1898 by Jaboulay and Berard.[4] Later, Dufourmentel,[5] Kostecka,[6] and Lindemann[7] preferred this procedure and reported good results. Although the sectioning of the condylar neck originally was performed blindly with the Gigli saw, Lindemann altered this technique by using an extraoral approach through a broader incision. In this way, the view of the operative field became more favorable and the danger of damaging the facial nerve, the main risk in this operation, was considerably diminished if not completely eliminated. Another change of technique was reported by Moose, who chose an intraoral approach.[8]

Because of the poor view in the operative field, osteotomy in the condylar neck had only a few adherents. Besides causing possible damage to the nerves, the small contact surface of the bone is another disadvantage of this method, because bony union is achieved slowly. Also, numerous local autonomic disturbances such as gustatory hyperhydrosis have been observed. The advantage of this method is the short operating time and the small skin incision. However, the disadvantages are so significant that few surgeons apply the osteotomy in the condylar neck.

Subcondylar Oblique Osteotomy. In this method, the line of the osteotomy is begun midway between the coronoid process and the condylar neck and proceeds diagonally downward to the posterior margin of the mandible. The principal difference in this technique, first described by Robinson[9] and Hinds,[10] is the use of the submandibular approach. Access to the mandibular notch and condylar neck is quite good, and the osteotomy of the thin bone in this area can be readily performed with bur and chisel or with a nasal saw. After the osteotomy, the proximal fragment with the condylar head is moved laterally, providing a reasonable overlapping of the bony fragments. The musculus pterygoideus lateralis pulls the small fragment medially, ensuring bony contact. Therefore direct bone wiring is not necessary. The advantage of this method is the relatively short operating time, owing to the simple technical procedure. Furthermore, there is minimal danger of damaging the main branch of the facial nerve. However, as in any submandibular approach, there is the possibility of involvement of the mandibular branch of this nerve. Other disadvan-

tages are the small contact surface of the bone, which requires an immobilization time of six to eight weeks, and the possibility of visible scars resulting from the extraoral approach, which may be unpleasant to some patients, and especially to those who have a tendency for keloid formation (Fig. 24-13).

Because of the relative ease of this approach, it is frequently used for the correction of mandibular prognathism. According to the reports of Caldwell, the subcondylar oblique osteotomy should be limited to cases of mild or moderate mandibular prognathism.[11]

Vertical Osteotomy in the Ramus. In this method, which was published by Caldwell and Lettermann in 1954,[12] the osteotomy line proceeds vertically, from the lower aspect of the mandibular notch to the lower border of the mandible in the angle area. The mandibular foramen remains in the anterior side of the osteotomy line, and the small proximal fragment together with the condyle is moved laterally. When

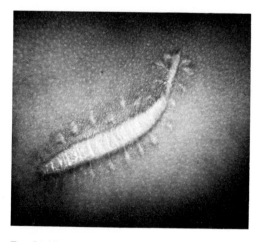

Fig. 24-13. Keloid formation.

the main fragment with the mandibular body is pushed posteriorly, correction of the chin prominence and the position of the lower teeth, and improvement of the mandibular angle are all achieved. This is quite desirable in many cases of true mandibular prognathism (Fig. 24-14).

In their original paper, Caldwell and Lettermann recommended the decortication of the overlapping cortical surfaces. In a later publication, however, the decortication of the buccal side of the main fragment was regarded as sufficient. The bony union is thereby favored and the

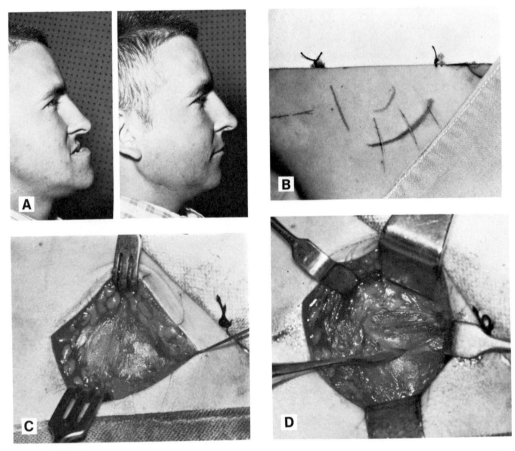

Fig. 24-14. Mandibular prognathism. (A) Preoperative and postoperative photographs. (B) Draping and skin marked with ink to outline the planned incision for a vertical osteotomy. Note the earlobe as a landmark at the apex of the drapes. (C) The first incision is through the skin and subcutaneous tissues, exposing the platysma muscle. (D) The platysma muscle is transected and dissection is continued to the masseter muscle. (E) The planned osseous surgery is to include the coronoidectomy and the vertical ramus section. (F) The rotating surgical handpiece is used to make the bony cut from the mandibular notch to the angle of the mandible. (G) The proximal segment is permitted to overlap the distal segment. (H) The deep tissues are closed as are the skin margins. Note that the cross-hatch marks are reapproximated to verify original skin position.

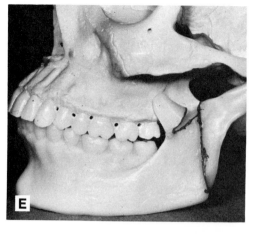

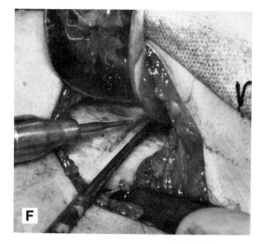

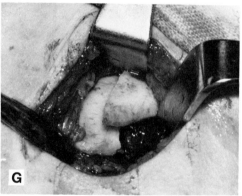

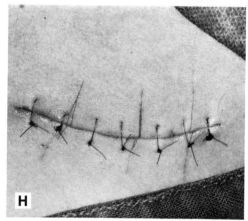

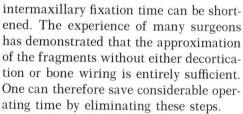

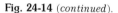

Fig. 24-14 (*continued*).

intermaxillary fixation time can be shortened. The experience of many surgeons has demonstrated that the approximation of the fragments without either decortication or bone wiring is entirely sufficient. One can therefore save considerable operating time by eliminating these steps.

According to Caldwell and Lettermann, if the mandible is set back 10 mm. or more, sectioning of the coronoid process should be performed.[12] This is based on the fact that the inelasticity of the temporalis muscle fibers hinders a push-back of the large mandibular fragment and may contribute to relapse or cause an anterior open bite postoperatively. Sectioning of the coronoid process is not a difficult procedure and it can be carried out by the same submandibular approach.

The advantages of this method, which is used by many surgeons, are evident. The mandible can be pushed back to the extreme extent of 30 mm., the cosmetic result is good, especially in the region of the jaw angle, and the bony union is reliable. Furthermore, damage to the inferior alveolar nerve can be avoided. The minimal disadvantage of the extraoral approach is that of involvement with the mandibular ramus branch of the facial nerve, and the possibility of unfavorable scarring.

Sagittal Splitting of the Ramus. This method was published by Obwegeser in 1952 and is preferred by many surgeons because of its essential advantages.[13] The principle of this operative technique is the sagittal splitting of the ramus by an intra-oral approach. The broad bone contact surfaces thereby produced are greatly advantageous for establishing bony union. After exposing the horizontal ramus by a mucosal incision, the masseter-pterygoideus sling is bluntly detached from the angle area. The periosteum is carefully detached from the lingual side between the mandibular notch and the mandibular foramen. The exposed cortical surface is cut with a long Lindemann bur, protecting the lingual soft tissues with a special retractor. The lingual cut should extend just distal to the mandibular foramen. A natural split will usually occur, leaving

the heavy thick angle of the mandible and the medial pterygoid muscle as part of the condylar segment. This permits movement of the mandible in either the anterior or posterior direction with minimal influence by the medial pterygoid muscle, thus minimizing relapse or open bite. According to the proposal of Dal Pont, the cut through the buccal cortical plate is preferably performed in the region of the second molar.[14] After the connection of both cortical cuts, the sagittal splitting is performed with osteotomes. Normally the mandibular nerve together with the big fragment is now on the medial side, and the condyle with the small fragment remains laterally (Fig. 24-15). The mobile main fragment of the lower jaw can now be moved posteriorly for the correction of a mandibular prognathism, or anteriorly

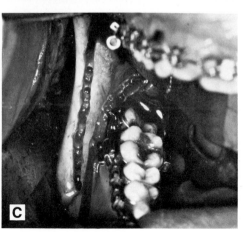

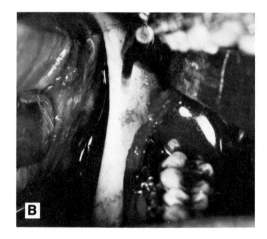

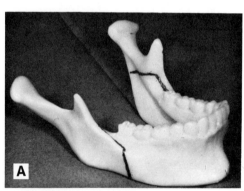

Fig. 24-15. Sagittal split osteotomy. (A) Bony incision (cut) outlined on model. (B) After reflection of the mucosa overlying the ramus, the first bony cut is made. (C) The bony cut is continued along the ascending ramus. (D) A vertical cut is made from the inferior border of the mandible between the first and second molars. (E) The split is completed with chisels. (F) If an impacted third molar is present, it can be removed through the split ramal segments. (G) After the jaw is repositioned, a direct bone wire can be placed to immobilize the segments in the new position. (H) Model indicates the overlap as the anterior segment is repositioned, as in procedure for prognathism. (I) The normal anatomy of the osseous and soft tissue structures is an important consideration in the sagittal split operation on the ramus.

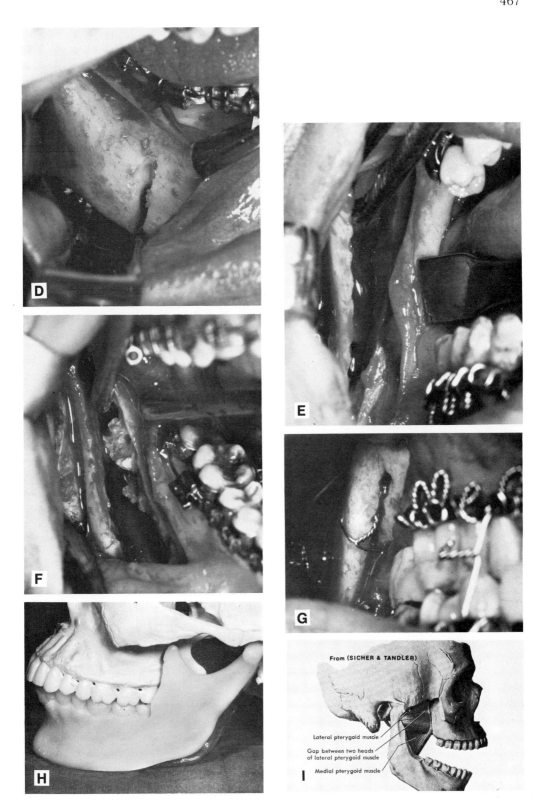

Fig. 24-15 (continued).

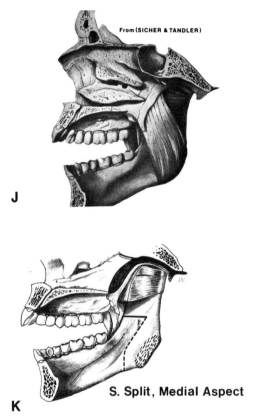

J

K

S. Split, Medial Aspect

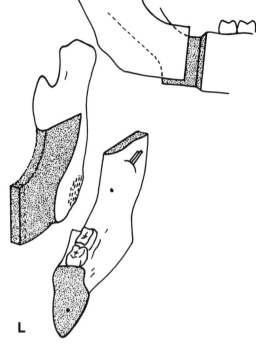

L

Fig. 24-15 (*continued*). (J) In jaw advancement procedures, the medial pterygoid muscle can contribute to relapse unless it is left undisturbed as in K and L.

in cases of mandibular retrusion. The correction of certain open bite cases is also possible with the same technique. As in the other methods described for the correction of mandibular prognathism, the occlusion is stablized by an intermaxillary fixation. The splints used for this purpose vary, according to dentition and laboratory facilities, from arch bars, continuous loop wires, cap splints, and acrylic splints to denture splints for edentulous patients. Of course, orthodontic appliances may be used. Obwegeser recommends additional stabilization of the fragments with circummandibular wires,[13] whereas other authors report no disadvantages when omitting this wiring. After four to six weeks the rigid intermaxillary fixation may be opened, but in some cases it is advisable to have elastic bands for one to two weeks longer.

The advantages of this method are the use of the intraoral approach whereby visible scars can be avoided (Fig. 24-16), the certain preservation of the facial nerves, and the broad bone contact surfaces which accelerate a bony union. This method also has some disadvantages, specifically considerable postoperative swelling and the high possibility of injury to the mandibular nerve during the splitting. We know from experience that this nerve has good regenerative ability; however, in different follow-up studies, a small percentage of permanent hypesthesia disturbances has been reported.[15,16]

Ostectomy of the Body of the Mandible. In this procedure, contrary to the formerly described method, a measured section of the horizontal ramus of the mandible is excised. Blair described this technique for the first time in 1907,[17] and it was later published in a modified manner by other authors. Finally, in 1944 and 1948, Dingman proposed the ostectomy of the mandible in two steps.[18] The main reasons for proceeding in two stages were to avoid

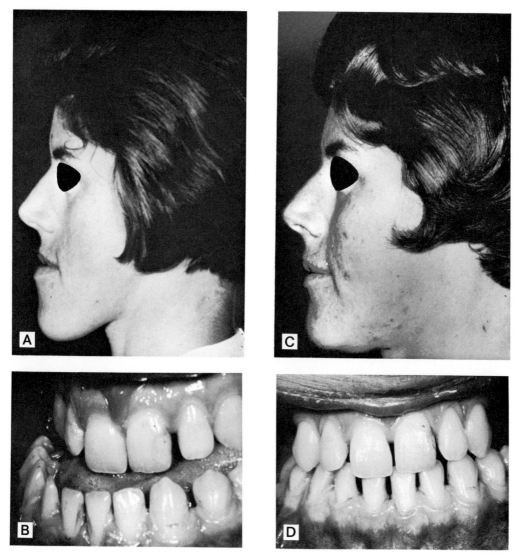

Fig. 24-16. Case of mandibular prognathism corrected by sagittal splitting. (A and B) Profile and occlusion preoperatively. (C and D) Profile and occlusion postoperatively.

infection in the region of the fracture line and to better preserve the mandibular nerve (Fig. 24-17).

In the first stage, which is done intraorally, the extraction of a tooth, usually a molar, or the sectioning of a corresponding piece of bone in cases of partial dentition, is carried out. The mucosa is sutured afterwards. About three weeks later, the second stage is performed by an extraoral approach. The lower border of the mandible is exposed and an exactly measured bone section is removed. The contents of the mandibular canal can thereby be well preserved. After the adaption of the fragments and placement of intermaxillary

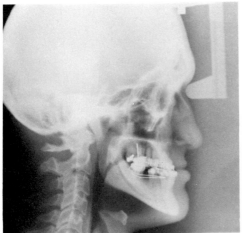
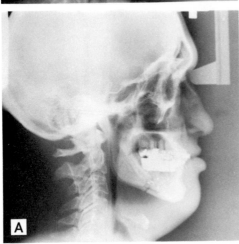
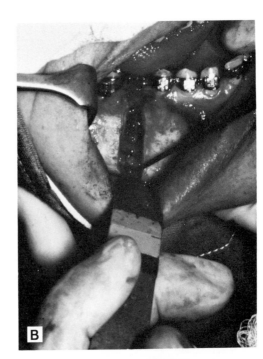
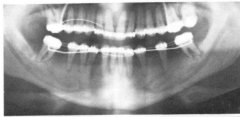
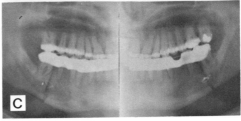

Fig. 24-17. The body osteotomy is also used for the correction of jaw deformity. (A) Preoperative and postoperative radiographs with splint still in place. (B) In the intraoral operative approach, a section of the mandibular body is removed, preserving the neurovascular bundle. (C) Preoperative and postoperative panoramic radiographs.

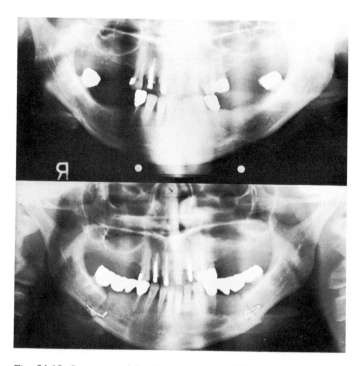

Fig. 24-18. Ostectomy of the body of the mandible, radiographic view. The upper film shows the preoperative situation. The picture below shows the fixation two months after surgery with lower border wiring and stabilization of the upper border by means of fixed bridgework.

fixation, bone wiring is applied at the lower border. The stabilization of the upper border is done by adequate splinting (Fig. 24-18). This two-stage procedure was later also described by Dingman as a one-stage operation, but he still recommended an oral and extraoral approach.[19] Again, other authors perform the total procedure in one step by the oral route only, and report good results.[20] However, antibiotic protection is especially emphasized.

The advantages of this operative technique are that the correction of an extremely long and extended horizontal ramus can be performed in an ideal manner, and that the vascular-nerve bundle can be protected. The procedure is clearly indicated in some open bite cases and to avoid any change in musculature. The disadvantages, on the other hand, are so considerable that this formerly popular method has few adherents today. The difficulties begin when measuring the piece of bone to be resected. Most important is the delayed bony union mentioned in different reports. The straight bone surfaces in the fracture line have only small bone contact surfaces, and this must be considered a reason for the delayed bony union. Therefore, the intermaxillary fixation has to be maintained longer—

most authors recommend 8 to 10 weeks. In spite of increased fixation time, a pseudarthrosis may result, especially in older patients. Another disadvantage is that the flat jaw angle in a true mandibular prognathism is not improved by this method, as it is in the operations performed in the ascending ramus. Also, compression of the soft tissues occurs more often, which results in additional wrinkling of the skin. Therefore, some authors recommend a face-lifting in older patients following the procedure.[21,22]

In order to avoid a delayed bony consolidation, different "step form" resections have been described.[23,24,25] These techniques are principally also ostectomies in the horizontal ramus.

PSEUDOPROGNATHISM. "Pseudoprognathism" means a seeming protrusion of the normal mandible in relation to a deficient maxilla. Again, the cephalometric x-ray study is of great importance for the diagnosis. While the angle SNB is within normal limits, contrary to the case in true mandibular prognathism, the angle SNA is decreased. This indicates that the deformity lies within the maxilla, and is not due to an overgrowth of the mandible.

The causes for pseudoprognathism may be hereditary, congenital, or acquired as a result of different diseases or trauma. They are discussed together with the therapeutic possibilities on page 490 under "Maxillary Retrusion." Surgeons often prefer to perform the correction for pseudoprognathism in the mandible because the procedures in the maxilla are more complicated, although maxillary procedures achieve a much better result. Occasionally a combined procedure is recommended in which, after the mandible has been pushed back, the contours of the

middle face (i.e., of the maxilla) are improved by prosthetic measures or by onlays of bone or cartilage.[26]

MANDIBULAR ALVEOLAR PROTRUSION. The correction of an alveolar protrusion in the mandible was probably the first surgical treatment performed in order to correct a developmental deformity. Hullihen described a case in 1849 in which a patient who was burned in early childhood had a downward and forward growth of the alveolar process caused by scar traction.[27] Although the body of the mandible together with the chin prominence was normally developed, the lower lip was strongly vaulted by the protrusion of the alveolar process. Hullihen planned and performed an operation on the patient with logical consistency by bilaterally sectioning a wedge from the alveolar process and pushing it back, thereby overcoming the protrusion. Today, most cases of mandibular alveolar protrusion are treated orthodontically by extracting a bicuspid bilaterally and moving the lower anterior teeth back slowly. Occasionally in adults a surgical correction is indicated which is performed orally. In this operation, after removal of a tooth and corresponding bone section, a subapical osteotomy is carried out (Fig. 24-19). The fragment, pedicled only on the lingual soft tissues, is moved posteriorly. Intersegmental fixation is sufficient for splinting and intermaxillary fixation is not necessary. With a correct diagnosis, for which cephalometric x-ray studies are important, this relatively small surgical procedure often has a surprising functional and aesthetic effect (Fig. 24-20).

MACROGENIA. Even with normal occlusion, the patient may have a prognathic appearance if the chin is too strongly developed. The chin prominence may be not only protruded, but also too high or too broad. An operative reduction of the bony chin is involved in all these cases. The dimension of the reduction can be determined exactly with the aid of preoperative

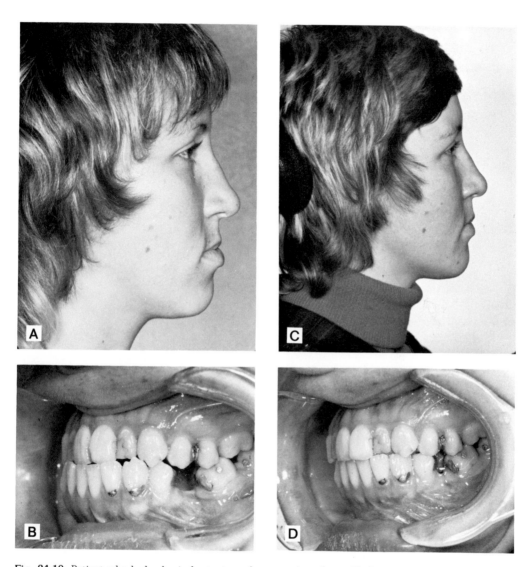

Fig. 24-19. Patient who had subapical osteotomy for correction of mandibular protrusion. (A) Preoperative profile. (B) Preoperative occlusion. (C) Postoperative profile. (D) Postoperative occlusion.

cephalometric x-ray views and templates. The exposure of the chin prominence is easily accomplished with the so-called degloving procedure in which, from an incision in the vestibulum, the total soft tissues are pushed over the bony chin.

Then, using a saw and burs, the chin prominence can be formed correspondingly (Fig. 24-21). Although most authors reduce just the chin, Koele recommends an osteotomy whereby a wedge is removed from the middle of the chin.[28] The chin

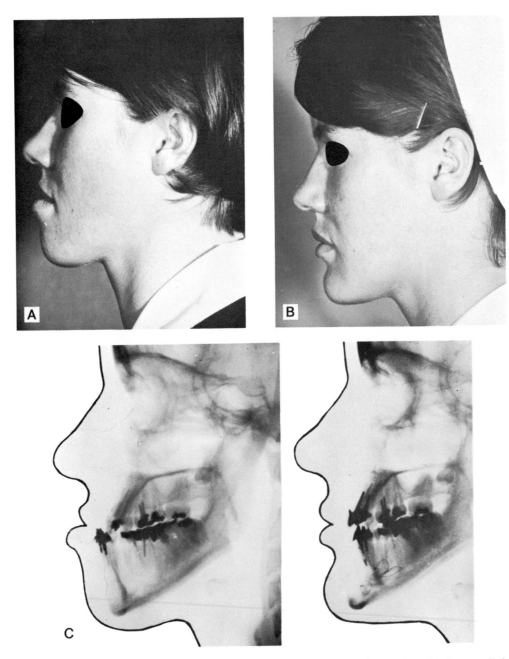

Fig. 24-20. Mandibular alveolar protrusion. (A) Preoperative view. The profile is unfavorable because of the protruding lower lip. (B) Facial configuration postoperatively. (C) In the cephalometric x-ray studies, the set-back of the lower alveolar process and the change in the profile are evident.

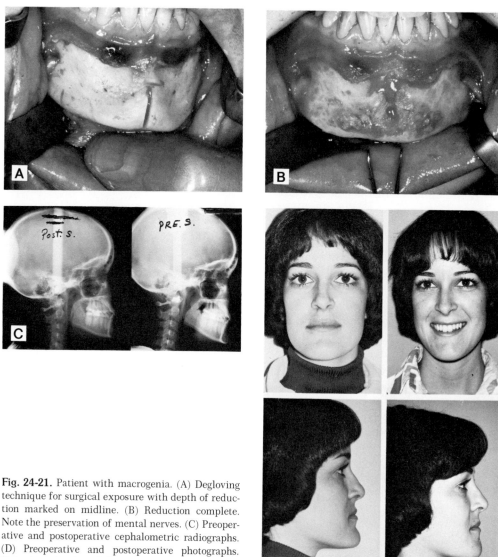

Fig. 24-21. Patient with macrogenia. (A) Degloving technique for surgical exposure with depth of reduction marked on midline. (B) Reduction complete. Note the preservation of mental nerves. (C) Preoperative and postoperative cephalometric radiographs. (D) Preoperative and postoperative photographs. Note the reduction of the square jaw and improved feminine profile.

border then is flipped upward and fixed, and the original form of the chin can be maintained. Occasionally, after a mandibular prognathism operation, it may be necessary to perform a corresponding correction of the chin area. This can be done simultaneously, but it is more favorable to do this in a second procedure since the extent of the correction can be judged better.

Retrognathism

Underdevelopment of the mandible was formerly thought to always be related to ankylosis of the temporomandibular joint. The first operative procedures for the lengthening of the mandible were described for the correction of the so-called bird-face deformity, which is a typical consequence of ankylosis during the pe-

riod of growth. Today we know that retrognathism does not result only from ankylosis but may have different causes,
such as congenital hypoplasia, disturbances in the branchial arch development,
or rheumatoid arthritis in children,
known as Still's disease (Fig. 24-22). According to the extent of the underdevelopment of the mandible, we distinguish between total mandibular retrusion, alveolar
mandibular retrusion and retrogenia, or
microgenia.

MANDIBULAR RETRUSION. In these cases,
which also are called distal bites, there is
a malocclusion because the teeth and the
alveolar process are dislocated distally
(Class II according to Angle[2]). Therefore,
the deformity may be combined with retroposition of the chin. Frequently an additional alveolar protrusion of the maxilla
and a deep overbite exist. The main cause
for mandibular retrusion is usually related to a growth disturbance, unless it is
one of the congenital forms, which is discussed in the next section. The growth
disturbance may result from ankylosis in
one or both mandibular joints, most commonly resulting from trauma and infection. These cause a partial or total destruction of the growth center of the
condylar process, leading to a partial or
total cessation of growth. The extent of
the disturbance depends upon the age of
the patient at the time of the inflammation or trauma. Other causes for retrognathia of the mandible are not well
known, apart from certain bad habits such
as thumb-sucking. Occasionally, hereditary factors have been observed, although
these occur even more seldom than in
mandibular prognathism.

The treatment of mandibular retrusion,

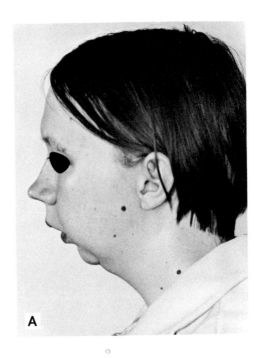

A

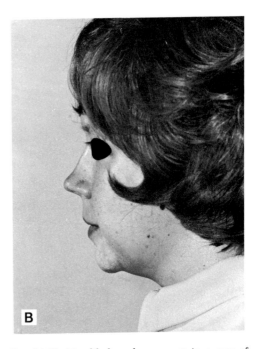

B

Fig. 24-22. Mandibular advancement in a case of
underdevelopment of the mandible. (A) Rheumatoid
arthritis (Still's disease) caused a severe mandibular
retrusion with microgenia. (B) Situation after mandibular advancement by the sagittal splitting method
and simultaneous chin enlargement.

similar to that of mandibular prognathism, is characterized by many operative techniques (Fig. 24-23). It is generally acknowledged that the advancement of the mandible is more difficult than the push-back procedures. Many authors recommend bone grafting in order to bridge the defect resulting from the advancement procedure. The presence of this defect is the reason why different osteotomies in "step" form have been specified. We mention here only the techniques according to Eiselsberg[29] and Dingman,[19] Pichler,[23] Kazanjian,[30] Converse,[24] and Limberg,[31]

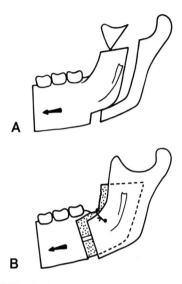

Fig. 24-24. Methods of mandibular advancement. (A) With the vertical L-osteotomy, bone contact is maintained only at the lower border. (B) The advancement by sagittal splitting shows the broad area of bony contact.

which are all carried out in the horizontal ramus. The L-form osteotomies performed in the ascending ramus are more common, and we also refer the student to the publications of Wassmund,[32] Schuchhardt,[33] Robinson,[34] and Thoma,[20] who mostly recommend a bone grafting procedure. The frequently used L-form osteotomy in the ascending ramus will be reported separately, as will the methods of sagittal splitting, which we think is excellent (Fig. 24-24).

Vertical L-osteotomy. This method was reported by Caldwell, Hayward, and Lister and is principally a modification of the formerly described vertical osteotomy for correction of mandibular prognathism.[35] By the same approach and after the resec-

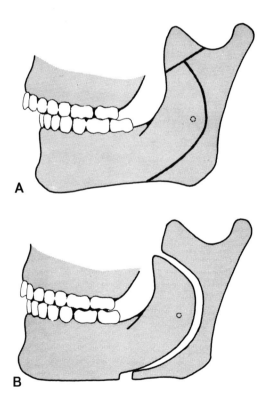

Fig. 24-23. (A) Outline of bony cut for C osteotomy with coronoidectomy. (B) C osteotomy advancement of mandible without coronoidectomy (different case).

tion of the coronoid process, the vertical osteotomy is not carried through to the lower border of the mandible, but instead proceeds in a L-form anteriorly. In this manner, when advancing the mandible, the bony contact is maintained between the fragments and bone grafting is often not necessary. After the intermaxillary fixation, wiring of the fragment is recommended in order to get additional stabilization.

Sagittal Splitting. Even more ideal than the L-form osteotomy seems to be the mandibular advancement with the intraoral sagittal splitting procedure described earlier (see p. 465) (Fig. 24-25). Even after extensive advancement, there are still broad bone contact surfaces and bone grafting is not necessary. The additional stabilization with bone wiring is easy to carry out and follow-up studies reveal only a slight tendency for relapse.[36] Both methods have a certain relapse tendency, which Caldwell tries to avoid by sectioning the musculus temporalis and Obwegeser by cutting the m. pterygoideus internus at its insertion on the mandible. We recommend a small overcorrection during surgery, which can be done using the previously mentioned occlusal splint. Furthermore, a frequent cause of relapse is the pulling of the condylar head from the fossa during the procedure. Temporomandibular joint x-ray films are strongly recommended in the operating room or immediately postoperatively.

CONGENITAL MANDIBULAR HYPOPLASIA. In these congenital malformations, of which only the most important ones shall be discussed, it is a question of deformities with various typical symptoms being generally designated as syndromes. One of the symptoms in these deformities is hypoplasia of the mandible.

Pierre Robin Syndrome. This deformity, described by Robin in 1923, has three typical symptoms: micrognathia, glossoptosis and cleft palate.[37] The small and retroposed mandible together with the posteriorly positioned tongue often causes serious respiratory difficulties that may appear immediately after birth. If all symptoms are present, as well as a cleft of the hard or soft palate, the tongue will block the nasal airways. If pharyngeal obstruction occurs owing to the position of the tongue, and there is an additional sternal retraction, immediate surgical aid is necessary in order to prevent the infant from suffocating.

Different methods have been described to move the tongue anteriorly with respect to the mandible. Probably the most common method is that published by Douglas, who, after excising a mucosal area under the tongue and the vestibular side of the lower lip, connected the two wound surfaces to fix the tongue to the lip.[38] This fixation is maintained until respiration and nourishment have been secured. Another technique has been described by Eschler, who detached the masseter-pterygoideus sling from the lower border and placed it posteriorly around the ascending ramus.[39]

If the child survives the first postnatal stage, the main difficulties have been overcome. Under the influence of function the mandible starts growing and, by the time the second dentition begins erupting, the length of the lower jaw is usually normal so that no further corrections have to be done. A corresponding orthodontic treatment, in order to stimulate the

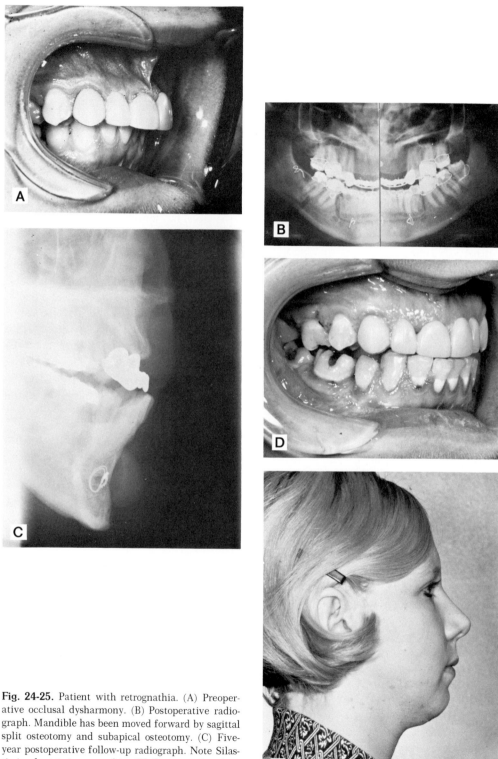

Fig. 24-25. Patient with retrognathia. (A) Preoperative occlusal dysharmony. (B) Postoperative radiograph. Mandible has been moved forward by sagittal split osteotomy and subapical osteotomy. (C) Five-year postoperative follow-up radiograph. Note Silastic implant to increase chin. (D) Postoperative clinical appearance of occlusion. (E) Postoperative profile.

growth of the mandible, is favorable. Naturally, the closure of the cleft palate has to be performed before speech and masticatory function will be normalized.

Agenesis of the Condyle. Agenesis of a condyle can be combined with a deficiency of all or part of the ascending ramus. In addition, the external or internal ear, the temporal bone, the zygoma, and the total soft tissue covering in this area may be involved. This disease is designated as first branchial arch syndrome, or otomandibular dysostosis; it is caused by a faulty cellular differentiation of the derivatives of the first and/or second branchial arches. The absence of the condylar growth center results in an asymmetry of the mandible and a generalized retroposition of the total lower face.

In this deformity, severe occlusal disturbances are present, and the therapeutic measures are protracted and difficult. During the period of growth orthodontic treatment is preferred, although some authors recommend early bone grafting.[40] After completion of growth, one of the procedures for lengthening of the mandible may be used, possibly in combination with a genioplasty. In addition, a reconstruction of the affected mandibular area with auto- or homoplastic cartilage grafts may be necessary.

Mandibulofacial Dysostosis. Mandibulofacial dysostosis, also called Treacher-Collins syndrome, differs from the previously described disease in several respects. The syndrome appears to be familial, inherited as an autosomal dominant trait; furthermore, the deformity is bilateral. Besides the microgenia, as seen in the typical bird-face, this syndrome demon-

strates hypoplasia of the malar bones, colobomas of the lower eyelids, fish-like mouth, and antimongoloid obliquity of the eyes. Similar to conditions associated with agenesis of the condyle, ear deformities and deafness are present, and severe occlusal disturbances have been observed (Fig. 24-26). According to the severity of the deformities, the therapy is complicated. The correction of the coloboma and the securing of hearing aids are usually the first measures. After completion of growth, the operative correction of the occlusion by lengthening the mandible and using transplants for the correction of the zygomatic bones may be considered. However, a satisfactory cosmetic result can hardly be obtained.

MANDIBULAR ALVEOLAR RETRUSION. Sometimes the mandibular retrusion is due only to the position of the alveolar process while the chin region is normally developed. The occlusion is Class II and there are considerable masticatory difficulties. These patients are also bothered by the retracted lower lip and the pronounced sublabial fold.

The correction of mandibular alveolar retrusion is best performed surgically ac-

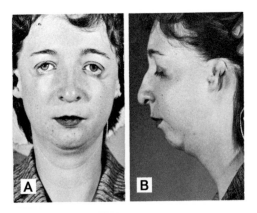

Fig. 24-26. Mandibulofacial dysostosis. (A) Note antimongoloid obliquity of eyes, colobomas of lower lids, and underdevelopment of malar bones. (B) Significant are the microgenia and the deformed ears. (Gorlin, R. J., and Pindborg. J. J.: *Syndromes of the Head and Neck.* New York, McGraw-Hill, 1964)

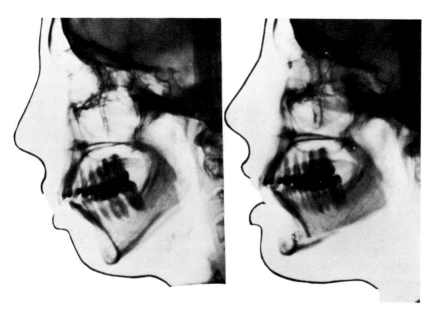

Fig. 24-27. Obwegeser's technique for chin enlargement. The pre- and postoperative cephalometric x-ray studies show the improvement of the profile by sliding genioplasty.

cording to the method recommended by Hofer.[41] In this method, a subapical osteotomy is carried out, similar to the one described for the correction of mandibular alveolar protrusion. In order to pull the alveolar segment forward, which is detached from the mandibular base, the mucosa must also be released on the lingual side. The defects created in the bicuspid area are either filled with homoplastic bone or, if possible, with bone from the vicinity. The stabilization of the alveolar segment is guaranteed by bone wires and an intersegmental splint.

MICRO- OR RETROGENIA. Underdevelopment of the chin can exist alone or in combination with a retroposition of the whole mandible. In the first case the correction is purely an aesthetic problem, since occlusion and masticatory function are normal. In discussing the operative

correction of deficient chins, we must principally distinguish between the use of autogenous bone and the use of other materials for the improvement of the chin. In the procedures utilizing transplants from the vicinity, the lower border of the chin is cut and moved anteriorly, as reported and accomplished by Hofer[42] extraorally and by Obwegeser[13] and Converse[43] intraorally. The bone cut is thereby adapted to the necessary forward movement (Fig. 24-27). In the other methods, distant transplants are used, whereby different materials like autoplastic bone and cartilage transplants or homoplastic materials are preferred, according to the particular experience of the surgeon. Several authors use alloplastic transplants exclusively, such as Silastic, and report good results.[44] The advantage of these materials is that they are not subject to resorption, although there is the danger of incompatibility and rejection. Autoplastic materials show some resorption, as a matter of fact, but undergo a harmonic union with the host site.

Laterognathism

Laterognathism is essentially an asymmetry of the lower third of the face. In severe cases the middle third of the face may also be involved. The causes are mostly due to an irregular growth of the lower jaw, but fractures, tumors, or bone diseases may also be etiologic factors. Other frequent causes for asymmetry are soft tissue disturbances such as hypertrophy or atrophy of single parts of the tissue, as occurs in masseter hypertrophy.

UNILATERAL MANDIBULAR HYPOPLASIA. The causes of unilateral hypoplasia of the mandible are various. Congenital disturbances may exist, such as the previously described agenesis or otomandibular dysostosis, but acquired factors such as osteomyelitis, fractures or tumors of the growth center may lead to a unilateral growth retardation. Ankylosis of the temporomandibular joint, if unilateral, may produce asymmetry. The appearance of patients with unilateral mandibular hypoplasia is typical, the underdeveloped and retropositioned chin being most conspicuous. With the underdevelopment of one side, a deviation of the mandible toward the affected side results. This is contrary to unilateral hyperplasia, in which the deviation occurs away from the affected side.

There are also disturbances in occlusion that appear as a unilateral or even bilateral crossbite. Occasionally, deformities of the maxilla such as protrusion may accompany this condition. This might be explained by secondary functional influences. The therapy of mandibular unilateral hypoplasia is complicated and requires a treatment plan different from the one for normal mandibular corrections. Usually, the horizontal ramus of the affected side is lengthened by bone implantation. In some cases, unilateral sagittal

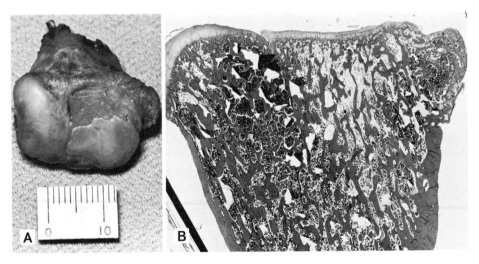

Fig. 24-28. Condylar hyperplasia in an 18-year-old patient from whom the condyle was removed. (A) Condyle specimen from a top aspect. (B) Low-power photomicrograph of enlarged slightly irregular mandibular condyle. Note irregularity of cartilage covering, but properly organized bone.

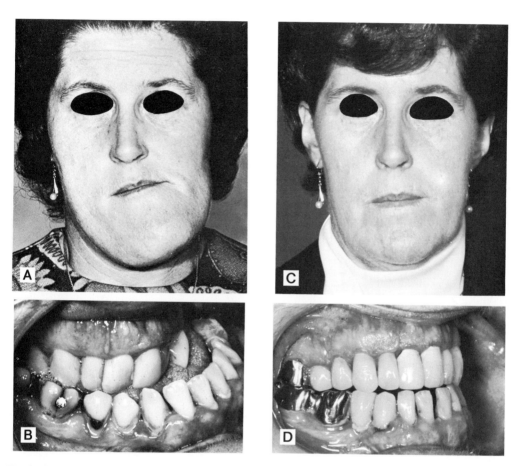

Fig. 24-29. Laterognathism and facial asymmetry caused by condylar hyperplasia. (A) Preoperative facial view of a 35-year-old patient with condylar hyperplasia on the right side. Remarkable are the deviation of the chin to the left and the downward bowing of the mandible on the right side. (B) Severe malocclusion with contact only in the molar area. (C) Aesthetic and functional correction. In a one-stage procedure, bilateral sagittal splitting, V-shaped ostectomy on the right side, and chin-shaping were performed. The hyperplastic condyle was not removed in this case, because there was no growth within the last ten years. (D) Final occlusion after dental restoration.

splitting is sufficient. In other cases, the shape of the chin must be corrected in a further operation, which may be performed by shifting the chin border. In combined occlusal disturbances in the maxilla and mandible, additional orthodontic treatment is indispensable.

UNILATERAL MANDIBULAR HYPERPLASIA.

The cause of this disease is not clear. In most cases excessive growth of the condyle suddenly appears around the ages between 15 and 20 years. It is interesting to note that the histologic examination of the enlarged condyle does not show any pathologic cells or bone substance (Fig. 24-28). Such authors as Gottlieb,[45] Rushton,[46] and others call this a true or progressive hyperplasia. In certain cases a lengthening of the condylar neck can also be noticed, either in combination with or without enlargement of the condyle. With the progressive growth of one condylar head or neck, a deviation of the mandible toward the healthy side results, so that the chin may be extremely protruded and asymmetric. A marked downward bowing of the inferior border of the mandible on the affected side is typically present. An open bite develops on the affected side, whereas a crossbite often develops on the other side (Fig. 24-29). Different possibilities exist for the correction of this deformity, which is functionally but above all aesthetically unfavorable (Fig. 24-30). If the condyle is still in the period of growth, most surgeons recommend extirpation of the hyperplastic condylar head. Usually this operation is not sufficient and additional osteotomies on the healthy side or in the chin region have to be performed. Ostectomies of the enlarged horizontal

ramus as well as shaping of the inferior border are occasionally necessary. In most cases a satisfactory symmetry of the lower face and a stable occlusion can be obtained only after two or three operative procedures. Extirpation of the condyle is not always necessary, especially when no further growth has been observed.

Maxillary Deformities

Maxillary Protrusion (Prognathia Superior)

In protrusion of the maxilla, one must distinguish between enlargement of the total maxilla and enlargement of the alveolar process. Occasionally, the protrusion is produced by the position of the upper front teeth, in which case they frequently show a diastema.

MAXILLARY MACROGNATHIA. The enlargement of the total maxilla is not common but has also been observed in connection with a generalized bone disease. Paget's

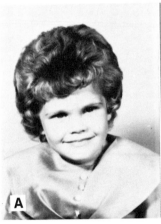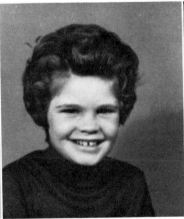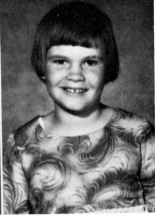

Fig. 24-30. Unilateral condylar hyperplasia. (A) Deformity was evident at an early age. (B and C) Preoperative and postoperative photographs.

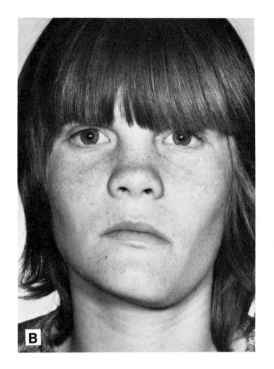

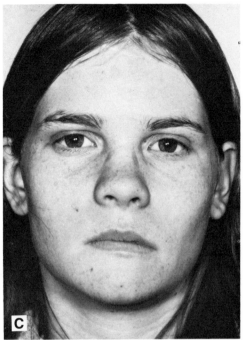

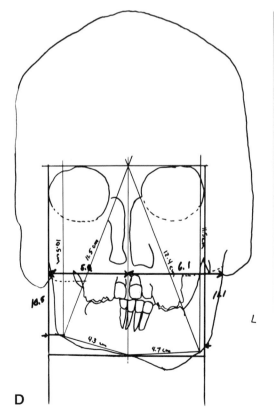

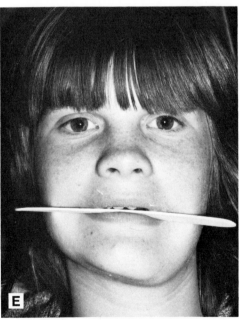

Fig. 24-30 (*continued*). (D and E) Presurgical work-up to note the area of the deformity.

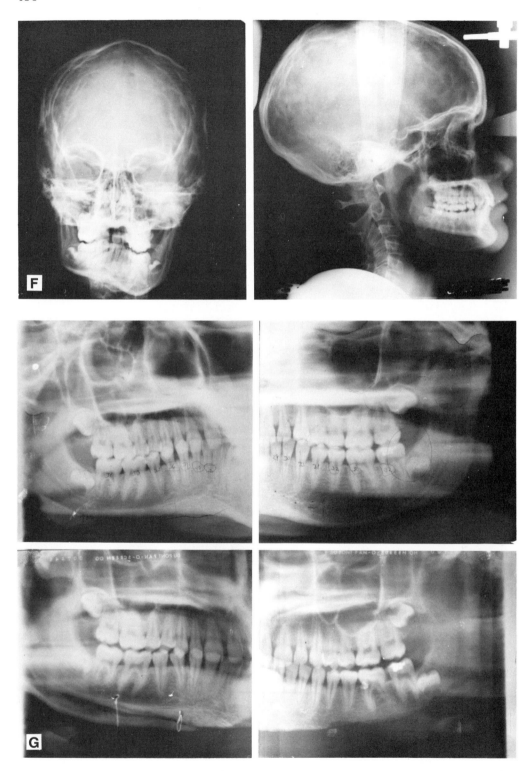

Fig. 24-30 (*continued*). (F) Preoperative posteroanterior and cephalometric radiographs. (G) Preoperative and postoperative panoramic radiographs showing inferior mandibular ridge trim and onlay graft.

disease may be localized in the maxilla, leading to a lengthening and broadening of the jaw base as well as to a broadening of the tooth arch. Leontiasis ossea causes similar deformities.

The therapy of deformities caused by such diseases is symptomatic and restricted mostly to masking procedures whereby the excessive bone is removed. As relapses tend to occur, these procedures have to be repeated in order to re-establish aesthetic and functional qualities.

MAXILLARY ALVEOLAR PROTRUSION. The protrusion of the alveolar process in the maxilla is unfavorable cosmetically and functionally, especially if combined with a deep bite and retroposition of the mandible. Frequently these patients also have a short upper lip, and lip closure is impeded or quite impossible (Fig. 24-31).

For the correction of this deformity, extraction of the teeth and leveling of the alveolar process had been recommended, because an operative set-back of the maxilla was regarded too risky. Cohn-Stock in 1921 was probably the first to set back the anterior part of the upper jaw.[47] This procedure was later modified by Wassmund,[32] and it is still performed in almost the same manner today. Usually, a bicuspid is extracted bilaterally in these procedures. The anterior segment is detached from the maxillary base by sectioning the bone lateral to the nasal aperture; following this, it is detached from the palate and from the nasal septum as well. After removal of the necessary quantity of bone, the fragment can be set back and also be brought higher up. The latter step is necessary to shorten the teeth in relation to the lip line. Splinting is done with the aid of prepared acrylic or cap splints. Frequently, however, orthodontic bands in

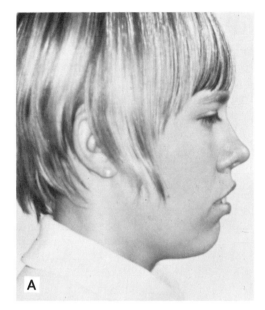

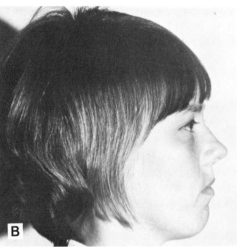

Fig. 24-31. (A) Preoperative profile of maxillary protrusion. (B) Postoperative profile. Note lip posture.

connection with an arch bar are used. With this splinting technique, intermaxillary fixation is not necessary. Variations of this technique have been made by (1) Wunderer, who no longer tunnels the palatal mucosa, and keeps the anterior segment pedicled to the buccal soft tissue only[48] (Fig. 24-32), and (2) Heiss, who recommends an additional split in the midline to create two completely separate fragments in order to better form the tooth arch.[49]

As already mentioned, maxillary alveolar protrusion is often combined with deformities of the mandible. In order to correct these and to re-establish the harmony of the facial profile, the same operative methods described for the retrognathism of the mandible may be used. According to the results of the profile analysis and the case model studies, an advancement of the whole mandible, the lower alveolar process, or the chin area alone may be performed.

If a deep bite is combined with protrusion of the maxilla, the lower front incisors often touch the palatal mucosa, which may produce periodontal diseases of the anterior teeth. In such cases, besides the set-back of the upper anterior segment, lowering of the anterior alveolar process in the mandible is also indicated (Fig. 24-33).

BIALVEOLAR PROTRUSION. This deformity shows a protrusion of the upper and lower alveolar processes and the profile is very unfavorable; in many cases lip closure is also impossible. The often used term "bimaxillary protrusion" is not quite correct in this case, as it mostly implies a protrusion of the alveolar process and not an enlargement of the jaw base. True bimaxillary protrusion is mainly a racial peculiarity characteristic of Negroes.

The correction may be done by orthodontic means, extracting either incisors or bicuspids. In older patients a surgical set-back of the upper and lower alveolar proc-

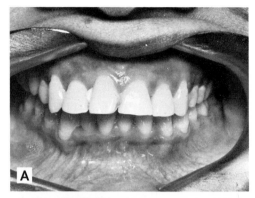

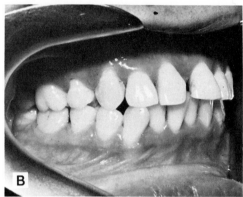

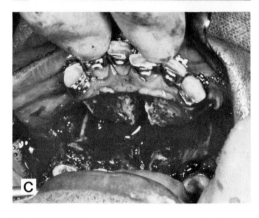

Fig. 24-32. (A) Preoperative appearance of occlusion. (B) Clinical photograph of occlusion following the surgical technique of Wunderer for maxillary protrusion. (C) Note palatal flap and direct access for the bone cut and midline split.

ess is indicated, which can be carried out in a one-stage procedure. In order to gain the necessary space, a bicuspid has to be extracted bilaterally in both jaws. The operation and splinting technique are the

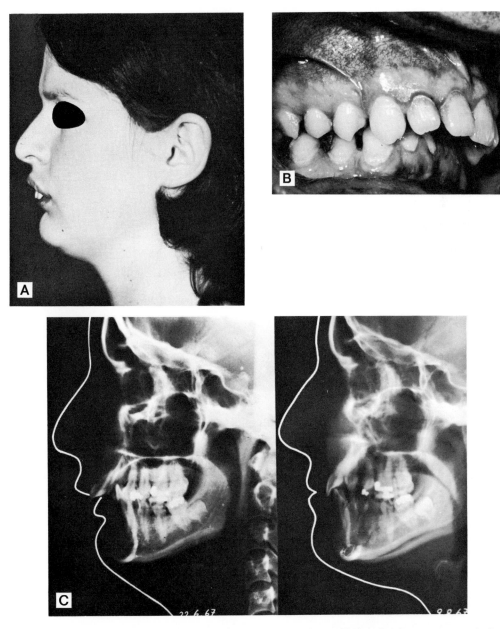

Fig. 24-33. Case of combined maxillary alveolar protrusion and mandibular alveolar retrusion with deep overbite. (A) Profile preoperatively. (B) Occlusion preoperatively; note the deep overbite as well as the Class II occlusal relationship. (C) The cephalometric x-ray studies show the change in profile and occlusion achieved by setting back and raising the anterior maxillary segment; simultaneously, the lower anterior alveolar process was advanced and lowered.

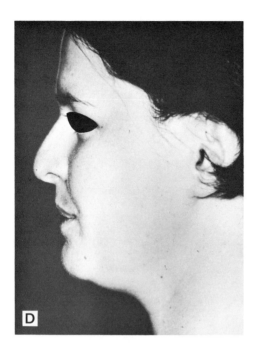

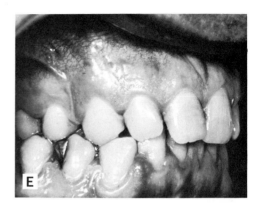

Fig. 24-33 (*continued*). (D) Profile postoperatively. (E) Occlusion postoperatively.

same as those described for mandibular alveolar and maxillary protrusion (Fig. 24-34).

Maxillary Retrusion

The cause for a retroposition of the maxilla is rarely congenital underdevelopment. In most cases, it results from acquired growth disturbances in the maxilla or postoperative sequelae following fractures, tumors, or other bone diseases. In all cases, however, the retroposition of the middle face, nasal base, and upper lip is characteristic. A mentioned in the discussion on "pseudoprognathism," an important sign for diagnosis is the angle SNA, which is smaller than normal, whereas SNB measurements are normal in cephalometric x-ray views. Also, racial peculiarities should be considered, since a

flattening of the middle face is especially typical of Asiatic races.

CONGENITAL UNDERDEVELOPMENT OF THE MAXILLA. Craniofacial dysostosis, also known as Crouzon's syndrome,[50] is characterized by hypoplasia of the maxilla, exophthalmos, hypertelorism, and craniosynostic malformations (Fig. 24-35). Because the growth of the mandible is normal, the term "pseudoprognathism" may be applied. Considerable functional disturbances are produced by the repositioned and mostly V-shaped form of the maxilla.

Previously, orthodontic therapy was considered the only possible means of obtaining a "certain" improvement of occlusion. Today, different authors recommend total maxillotomy with advancement of the maxilla. Tessier[51] and Obwegeser[52] correct, in some cases, the

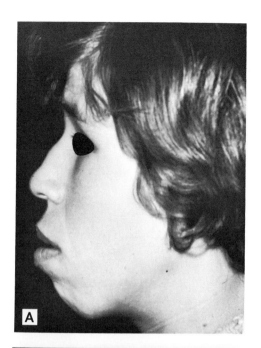

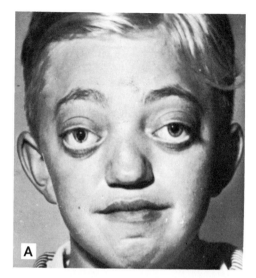

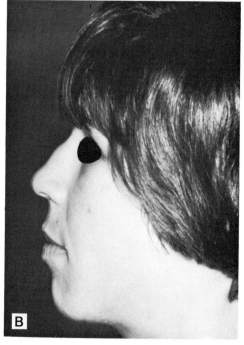

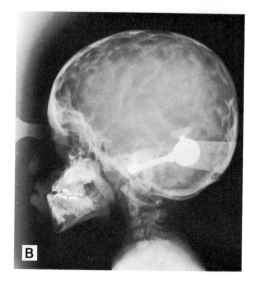

Fig. 24-34. Bimaxillary alveolar protrusion. (A) Profile preoperatively. (B) Postoperative view after setting back the anterior alveolar process in maxilla and mandible.

Fig. 24-35. Crouzon's disease in a six-year-old boy. (A) The main symptoms of Crouzon's disease, i.e., exophthalmos, hypertelorism, and hypoplasia of the maxilla, are all present in this case. (Gorlin, R. J., and Pindborg, J. J.: Syndromes of the Head and Neck. New York, McGraw-Hill, 1964) (B) The lateral head plate shows a remarkable retroposition of the maxilla (pseudoprognathism) even at this early age. Note the change in the bone structure of the skull (digital impressions).

hypertelorism as well as the retroposition of the middle face by extended osteotomies that basically correspond with the fracture lines of a Le Fort III. After the advancement of the middle face, the exophthalmos disappears. The aesthetic results are really remarkable.

ACQUIRED MAXILLARY RETRUSION. The majority of patients with maxillary underdevelopment are those with cleft lip and palate deformities. Until now it has not been completely clear whether the deformity of the maxilla is primarily connected with the cleft formation, or whether the diminished growth may be attributed to operative trauma during the closure of the palate. We are of the opinion that it is an acquired deformity rather than a congenital one. Support for this traumatic genesis has been documented by Monasterio, who found that unoperated cleft patients of Indian tribes in Mexico had a normal or in some cases enlarged growth of the maxilla.[53] Animal experiments further demonstrated that operative trauma to the palate at an early age causes growth disturbances. In the opinion of different authors, it is best to postpone the operation until two and one-half to three years or even longer.

In patients with bilateral cleft lip and palate, the hypoplasia and retroposition of the maxilla can take dramatic aspects. Deformations are also frequent in unilateral clefts. The best way to avoid these deformities is to provide early orthodontic treatment. At a later age, the surgical advancement of the maxilla, sometimes together with the broadening of the maxilla, is indicated.

Another form of a maxillary retroposition, which is not rare, occurs with dislocation and subsequent healing of mal-united maxillary fractures. The maxilla is often dropped in the posterior part, so that there is an open bite in the front. In such cases, the therapy of choice is surgical repositioning of the maxilla. As already mentioned, many cases of maxillary retrusion have been corrected by a set-back of the mandible, since the advancement of the maxilla is relatively complicated; also, one assumes a great relapse tendency. Gillies[21] and Axhausen[54] were probably the first to perform a total osteotomy in the maxilla. Later, Converse and Shapiro changed this technique by advancing, not the total maxilla, but only the alveolar process.[24] According to Obwegeser, the total high osteotomy of the maxilla is preferred, since this improves not only the occlusion and the form of the lips, but also the position of the nose and cheeks.[52] Stabilization of the osteotomized maxilla should be done by bone transplants, which are placed between tuberosity and pterygoid plate and along the osteotomy lines (Fig. 24-36). The results obtained in this manner are reliable, as follow-up studies have shown. If there are no occlusal disturbances, onlays of bank bone or cartilage onto the canine fossa may bring good cosmetic results (Fig. 24-37).

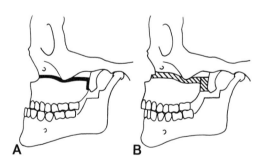

A   B

Fig. 24-36. Technique of total maxillary advancement. (A) The osteotomy line shown on the drawing corresponds with a high fracture line in a Le Fort I type fracture. (B) After the advancement of the maxilla, the gap between the tuberosity and the pterygoid plate is filled with a block of cancellous bone. Also bone grafts, which are marked by diagonal strokes, are inserted along the fracture line.

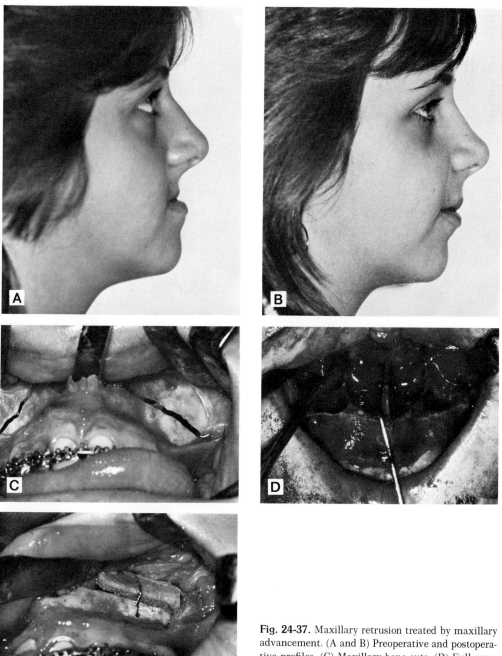

Fig. 24-37. Maxillary retrusion treated by maxillary advancement. (A and B) Preoperative and postoperative profiles. (C) Maxillary bone cuts. (D) Full maxilla in the down-fractured position. (E) Advancement of the maxilla with bilateral bone grafts.

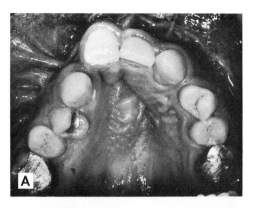

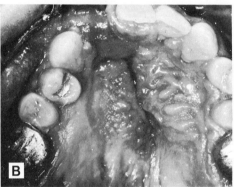

Maxillary Asymmetry

Apart from malformations in cleft palate patients, asymmetry of the maxilla is rare. Here again, conditions after improper treatment of fractures or unilateral bone growth, as seen in bone tumors, are the primary causes. The occlusal disturbances in agenesis of the condyle or otomandibular dysostosis are remarkable. In these cases the upper teeth on the affected side are lower and the occlusal plane is oblique instead of horizontal; the midline is also usually displaced. In patients with a unilateral cleft of the palate, the so-called small segment frequently occurs in a palatal collapsed position. The resulting crossbite is functionally unfavorable and complicates the desirable dental reconstruction of the cleft area with fixed bridgework (Fig. 24-38A). From an aesthetic and functional point of view, a surgical correction is desirable. This is performed as follows: the palatal positioned fragment is cut and swiveled laterally. The center of rotation is the tuberosity area, which usually is in a normal position. If the cleft in the alveolar process is reopened or enlarged during this procedure, it should be closed in a further operation by implanting bone in the defect. In this manner, a symmetric and regular alveolar arch may well be reconstructed (Fig. 24-38B).

Fig. 24-38. Maxillary asymmetry caused by collapse of the "small segment" in a patient with unilateral cleft. (A) Occlusal disturbance due to crossbite on the cleft side. Also note the unfavorable situation for bridgework. (B) Situation after outward rotation of the "small segment." Thus the crossbite is corrected and the space between cuspid and medial incisor now allows for a regular bridge construction.

Open Bite Deformities

The open bite is a deformity of the jaws in which one or both tooth lines do not reach the occlusal plan. The open bite may occur largely in the anterior alveolar segments of the jaws or it may occur as a result of a skeletal deformity. The ramus may be short, causing anterior rotation, or the maxilla may be long in the posterior, creating the anterior rotation of the mandible which results in the open bite. Treatment is directed to the origin of the deformity.

Origin in the Mandible

Some typical disturbances in the mandibular skeleton causing open bite can be observed. The ascending ramus may be shortened, the horizontal ramus bent downward, and the mandibular plane angle as well as the gonial angle enlarged. In some cases, a curve in the mandibular body anterior to the insertion of the masseter-pterygoideus sling can be recognized. The open bite may be present only in the front or it may extend to the last molars. In regard to the profile, the lower third of the face is enlarged, frequently also in an anterior position.

Numerous methods have been described for the operative correction of the open bite conditioned by the mandible. As in the treatment of mandibular prognathism, a distinction is made between the procedures performed in the ascending ramus and those performed in the body. In the ascending ramus, arched or oblique bone cuts are made in order to obtain better rotation possibilities.[20,31,32,55] All authors refer, however, to the high relapse tendency. Attempts to avoid relapse have included longer intermaxillary fixation and the use of a chin cup.

An overcorrection by opening the bite in the molar region with the aid of occlusal splints is recommended. In operations in the jaw body, V-shaped bone cuts are recommended so that the anterior fragment can be rotated upward more easily. Here

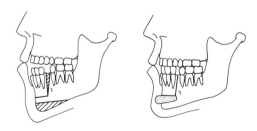

Fig. 24-39. Correction of open bite in the mandible. With a subapical osteotomy the alveolar process is moved upward and the open bite is closed. The lower border of the chin prominence is wedged into the created defect in the mandible. Thus the chin height and the chin contour can be corrected at the same time.

the original method of Koele, in which a subapical osteotomy is used to lift only the alveolar process, should be mentioned.[56] In cases of an overly high chin prominence, the chin can be simultaneously reduced and the bone removed used as a wedge for stabilizing the alveolar segment (Fig. 24-39). Although all operations performed in the ascending ramus and in the jaw body have a high relapse tendency, the prognosis for the subapical osteotomy seems to be much better.

Origin in the Maxilla

In the maxilla, the open bite can be caused by an infraocclusion of the maxillary anterior teeth, but in most cases there is a relative overgrowth of the maxillary posterior alveolar process. The vertical dimensions of the face are enlarged as compared to normal facial measurements, and the aesthetic and functional disturbances are considerable. If the disturbance is anterior, it can be corrected by a bilateral osteotomy and lowering of the premaxilla. However, this method can be applied only in a few cases, since the upper lip is usually too short and the lip closure would be impeded, resulting in a considerable aesthetic disadvantage. For these reasons, an upward movement of the posterior part of the maxilla, as proposed by Schuchhardt,[57] is more often indicated. In this method, which can be carried out in one or two stages, a corresponding quantity of bone is removed from the buccal wall of the maxilla. The anterior open bite can then be closed by positioning the teeth higher in the posterior region (Fig. 24-40). Follow-up examinations have shown that this theoretically ideal method is also affected by relapses.

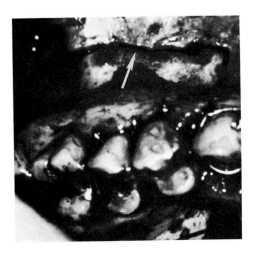

Fig. 24-40. Posterior maxillary osteotomy for closure of open bite (operation view). Following the horizontal osteotomy line (arrow), a corresponding amount of bone is removed. After a bone cut is made on the palate, this segment of the alveolar process can be pushed upwards.

Origin in Both Jaws

The origin of an open bite can be related to deformity of both jaws, with a downward bowing of the mandibular body as well as a raising of the upper front teeth (Fig. 24-41). Occasionally, the open bite is also combined with mandibular prognathism. Correction must be performed in both jaws. This may require operative procedures in the ramus and the mandibular body, as well as in the anterior or posterior part of the maxilla (Fig. 24-42). It is preferable to do these corrections in one stage, as the proper occlusion can then be determined with more certainty.

Complex Developmental Deformities

From the foregoing discussion it is obvious that complicated procedures are often necessary to obtain a functional and aesthetic result. This is not only true for open bite, but concerns all complex deformities of the maxillofacial skeleton. In some cases it is impossible to obtain the desired result in one operation. Therefore, it is important to proceed according to a precisely fixed plan arrived at preoperatively. Often it is advantageous to reestablish a normal occlusion first, since this will serve as a basis for further corrections. Then plan the next step. It should be a principle to perform corrections on the bone first, and later, if necessary, on the soft tissues. In order to treat a complex case or a relatively simple one, a knowledge of all the operative possibilities at one's disposal is necessary. Naturally, each surgeon will prefer the operative methods in which he is most experienced. However, he should never try to solve all problems with only a few methods. A good surgeon will recognize, admit, and observe his own limitations. Cooperation with the orthodontist, who can provide valuable pre- and postoperative help, is emphasized again.

References

1. Schwarz, A. M.: Die Roentgenostatik, Wien, Urban and Schwarzenberg, 1958.
2. Angle, E. H.: Okklusionsanomalien der Zaehne. Berlin, H. Meusser, 1913.
3. Obwegeser, H., and Steinhauser, E.: Ein neues Geraet zur Vitalitaetspruefung der Zaehne. Schweiz. Mschr. Zahnheilk., 73:1001, 1963.
4. Jaboulay, M., and Berard, I.: Traitement chirurgical du prognathisme inferieur. Presse Med., 6:173, 1898.
5. Dufourmentel, L.: Le traitement chirurgical du prognathisme. Presse Med., 29:235, 1921.
6. Kostecka, F.: Die chirurgische Therapie

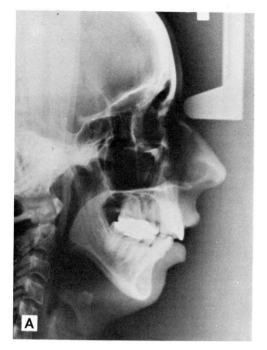

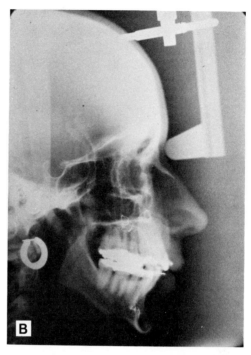

J.B. ♀	PRE TX	POST TX
AGE	34-0	34-6
ANB	10°	7°
MPA	52°	42°
FCA	-33°	-23°
OJ	3.5 mm	2.0 mm
OB	0.5 mm	2.0 mm

MAX IMP	
ANT	11 mm
POST	9 mm
A-P	+2 mm
GENIOPLASTY	
A-P	+9 mm
MP	35°

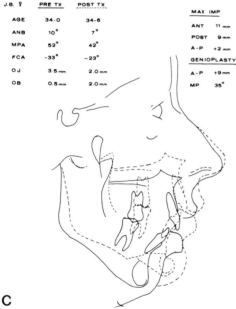

C

J.B. ♀	GENIOPLASTY
A-P	+9 mm
MP	35°
34-0	———
34-2	—·—·—
34-6	-------

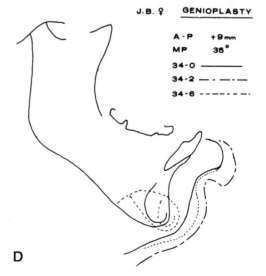

D

Fig. 24-41. (A) Cephalometric radiograph of a patient with open bite, elongation of anterior maxilla, and downward rotation of mandible. (B) Cephalometric radiograph following reduction of maxillary excess by a maxillary down fracture and genioplasty. (C) Superimposed cephalographs. —— Preoperative cephalographic analysis. – – – Postoperative cephalographic analysis. (D) Superimposed tracings to show change with genioplasty.

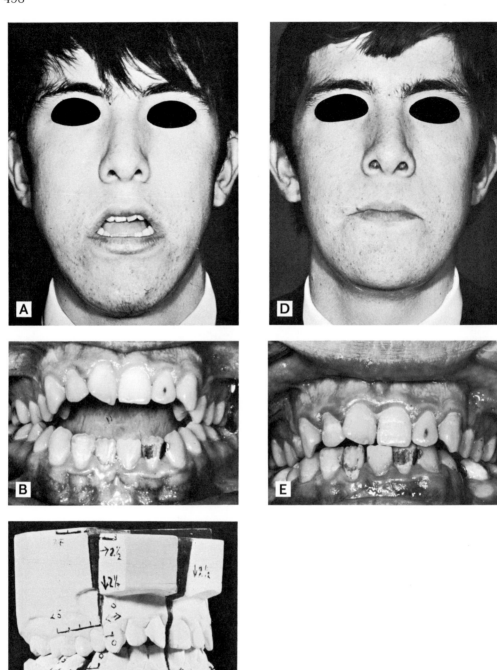

Fig. 24-42. Open bite deformity with its origin in both jaws. (A) Preoperative view; lip closure is impossible. (B) Severe open bite with raising of the upper front teeth and downward bowing of the lower front teeth. (C) Model operation showing the planned procedure. The arrows and numbers indicate direction and distance of the movement of the bone segments. (D) Postoperative view; spontaneous lip closure is now possible. (E) Occlusion postoperatively.

der Progenie. Zahnärztl. Rdsch., *40:*669, 1931.

7. Lindemann, A.: Leitfaden der Chirurgie und Orthopaedie des Mundes u. der Kiefer. Leipzig, J. A. Barth, 1938–1954.

8. Moose, S. M.: Surgical correction of mandibular prognathism by intraoral subcondylar osteotomy. Oral Surg., 22:197, 1964.

9. Robinson, M.: Prognathism corrected by open vertical subcondylotomy. J. Oral Surg., *16:*215, 1958.

10. Hinds, E. C.: Correction of prognathism by subcondylar osteotomy. J. Oral Surg., *16:*209, 1958.

11. Caldwell, J. B.: Textbook of Oral Surgery, 3rd ed., pp. 453–465. St. Louis, C. V. Mosby Co., 1968.

12. Caldwell, J. B., and Lettermann, G. S.: Vertical osteotomy in the mandibular rami for correction of prognathism. J. Oral Surg., *12:*185, 1954.

13. Obwegeser, H.: The surgical correction of mandibular prognathism and retrognathia with consideration of genioplasty. Part I. Surgical procedures to correct mandibular prognathism and reshaping of the chin. Oral Surg., *10:*677, 1957.

14. Dal Pont, G.: Retromolar osteotomy for the correction of prognathism. J. Oral Surg., *19:*42, 1961.

15. Egyedi, P.: Medical Dissertation. University of Zurïch, 1964.

16. Koele, H.: Ergebnisse, Erfahrungen und Probleme zur operativen Behandlung der Progenie. Deutsch. Zahn Mund Kiefer-heilk., *40:*177, 1963.

17. Blair, V. P.: Operations on jaw bones and face. Study of etiology and pathological anatomy of developmental malrelations of maxilla and mandible to each other and to facial outline and to operative treatment. Surg. Gynecol. Obstet., *4:*67, 1907.

18. Dingman, R. O.: Surgical correction of mandibular prognathism, an improved method. Am. J. Orthod. (Oral Surg. Section), *30:*683, 1944.

19. Dingman, R. O.: Surgical correction of developmental deformities of the mandible. Plast. Reconstr. Surg., 3:124, 1948.

20. Thoma, K. H.: Oral Surgery, 4th ed., p. 1135. St. Louis, C. V. Mosby Co., 1963.

21. Gillies, H.: Fractures of the facial skeleton. Edinburgh, Rowe and Killey, 1955.

22. Kufner, J.: Personal communication, 1968.

23. Pichler, H.: Ueber Progenieoperationen. Klin. Wschr. (Wien.), *41:*1333, 1928.

24. Converse, J. M.: and Shapiro, H. H.: Treatment of developmental malformations of the jaws. Plast. Reconstr. Surg., *10:*473, 1952.

25. Toman, J.: Prispevek chirurgicke terapii progenie. Inlayova ostektomie tela dolni celisti. Czas. Stomatol., 316, 1958.

26. Koele, H., Reichenbach, E., and Brueckel, H.: Chirurgische Kieferortho-paedie, p. 114. Leipzig, J. A. Barth, 1965.

27. Hullihen, S. R.: Case of elongation of the under jaw and distortion of the face and neck, caused by burn, successfully treated. Am. J. Dent. Sci., 9:157, 1849.

28. Koele, H.: Korrekturen am Kinn und Kieferwinkel. Fortschritte der Kiefer-u. Gesichtschirurgie. Bd. VII. Stuttgart, G. Thieme, 1961.

29. Eiselsberg, A.: Ueber schiefen Biss infolge Arthritis eines Unterkieferkoepfchens. Arch. klin. Chir. (Berlin), 79:587, 1906.

30. Kazanjian, V. H.: Surgical correction of deformities of the jaws and its relation to orthodontia. Int. J. Orthod., 22:259, 1936.

31. Limberg, A.: Treatment of open bite by means of plastic oblique osteotomy of the ascending rami of the mandible. Dent. Cosmos, 67:1191, 1925.

32. Wassmund, M.: Lehrbuch der praktischen Chirurgie des Mundes und der Kiefer, Bd. I. Leipzig, J. A. Barth, 1935.

33. Schuchhardt, K.: Erfahrungen bei der Be-handlung der Microgenie. Langenbeck Arch, klin. Chir., *289:*651, 1958.

34. Robinson, M.: Open vertical osteotomies

of the rami for correction of mandibular deformities. Am. J. Orthod., 46:425, 1960.

35. Caldwell, J. B., Hayward, J. R., and Lister, R. L.: Correction of mandibular retrognathia by vertical L-osteotomy: A new technique. J. Oral Surg., 26:259, 1968.

36. Perko, M.: Retrognathia. Transactions II Congress of the Internat. Assoc. Oral Surg. Copenhagen, Munksgaard, 1967, p. 76.

37. Robin, P.: La chute de la base de la langue consideree comme une nouvelle cause de gene dans la respiration naso-pharyngienne. Bull. Acad. Med. (Paris), 89:37, 1923.

38. Douglas, B.: Treatment of micrognathia associated with obstruction by plastic procedures. Plast. Reconstr. Surg., 1:300, 1946.

39. Eschler, F.: Personal communication, 1968.

40. Hovell, J. H.: The surgical treatment of some of the less common abnormalities of the facial skeleton. Dent. Pract., 10:170, 1960.

41. Hofer, O.: Die operative Behandlung der alveolaeren Retraktion des Unterkiefers und ihre Anwendungsmoeglichkeit fuer Prognathie und Mikrogenie, Deutsch. Zahn Mund Kieferheilk., 9:122, 1942.

42. Hofer, O.: Die osteoplastische Verlaengerung des Unterkiefers nach von Eiselsberg bei Mikrogenie. Deutsch. Zahn Mund Kieferheilk., 27:81, 1957.

43. Converse, J. M.: Micrognathia, Br. J. Plast. Surg., 16:197, 1963.

44. Walker, R.: Textbook of Oral Surgery, p. 343. Boston, Little, Brown and Co., 1968.

45. Gottlieb, O.: Hyperplasia of the mandibular condyle. J. Oral Surg., 9:118, 1963.

46. Rushton, M. A.: Unilateral hyperplasia of the mandibular condyle. Proc. R. Soc. Med. (London), 39:431, 1945.

47. Cohn-Stock, G.: Die chirurgische Immediatregulierung der Kiefer, speziell die chirurgische Behandlung der Prognathie. Vjschr. Zahnheilk. (Berlin), 37:320, 1921.

48. Wunderer, S.: Die Prognathieoperation mittels frontal gestieltem Maxillafragment. Öst. Z. Stomat., 59:98, 1962.

49. Heiss, J.: Ueber die chirurgische Unterstuetzung der Dehnung im komprimierten Oberkiefer. Dtsch. Zahnärztebl., 8:56, 1963.

50. Crouzon, O.: Dysostose Cranio-faciale Heriditarie. Bull. Mem. Soc. Med. (Paris), 33:545, 1912.

51. Tessier, P.: Transactions of IV International Congress of Plastic Surg. Amsterdam, Excerpta Medica Co., 1968.

52. Obwegeser, H.: Surgical corrections of small or retrodisplaced maxillae. Plast. Reconstr. Surg., 43:351, 1969.

53. Monasterio, F.: Personal communication, 1964.

54. Axhausen, G.: Zur Behandlung veralterter disloziert geheilter Oberkieferbrueche. Dtsch. Zahn Mund Kieferheilk., 1:334, 1934.

55. Shira, R. B.: Surgical correction of open bite deformities by oblique sliding osteotomy, J. Oral Surg., 19:275, 1961.

56. Koele, H.: Fromen des offenen Bisses und ihre chirurgische Behandlung. Dtsch. Stomat., 9:753, 1959.

57. Schuchhardt, K.: Experiences with the surgical treatment of some deformities of the jaws: prognathia, micrognathia and open bite. Transactions of II International Congress of Plastic Surg. Edinburgh and London, E. and S. Livingstone, 1960.

58. Converse, J. M. and Cocaro, P. J.: Diagnosis and treatment of maxillomandibular dysplasia. Am. J. Orthod., 68:625, 1975.

59. Moss, M. L.: The Functional Matrix. Vistas in Orthodontics, pp. 85–98. Philadelphia, Lea & Febiger, 1962.

60. Worms, F. W., Isaacson, R. J. and Speidel, T. M.: Surgical orthodontic treatment planning: Profile analysis and mandibular surgery. Angle Orthod., 46:1–25, 1976.

61. Waite, D. E., and Worms, F.: Orthodontic and surgical evaluation and treatment of maxillo-mandibular deformities. In Current Advances in Oral Surgery, 5th ed. W. B. Irby (Ed.). St. Louis, C. V. Mosby Co., 1974.

25 Cleft Lip and Cleft Palate

EMIL W. STEINHAUSER

Cleft lip and cleft palate are congenital deformities which, because of their frequency and localization in the maxillofacial region, are of great significance for the dentist, especially the pedodontist, orthodontist, oral surgeon, and prosthodontist, who inevitably play essential roles in the oral rehabilitation of the patient. Other specialists taking part in the treatment of cleft lip and cleft palate patients are plastic surgeons, pediatric surgeons, and otolaryngologists, as well as speech therapists, psychotherapists, and social workers. In most instances these specialists work as a team, since it has been demonstrated that better results can be obtained by coordinating the skill and experience of different specialists. Cleft palate teams are located all over the United States; in 1968, 244 teams were registered by the American Cleft Palate Association. The concept and value of a cleft palate team have been increasingly recognized and other countries are beginning to organize similar arrangements for treatment.

Etiology

For a long time, a genetic basis was regarded the most important factor in the formation of a cleft lip and palate. Further studies have demonstrated, however, that true inheritance can be observed in only 20 to 25 per cent of cleft lip or cleft palate patients.[1] Although the type of genetic tendency cannot be determined with certainty, it can be said to be multigenic, so that a single mendelian dominant or recessive inheritance cannot be established.[2,3] Furthermore, in identical twins a cleft was present in both infants only 44 per cent of the time, which shows the significance of exogenic influences.[4] Some of the most important exogenic factors responsible for the cleft lip and cleft palate formation in utero include (1) attacks of infectious viral diseases, such as rubella, measles, or mumps during the mother's first trimester of pregnancy; (2) x-rays; (3) oxygen deficiency; (4) dietary disturbances; (5) certain drugs and medicaments; and (6) increased maternal age. That exogenic factors can prevent the fusion of lip and palate parts also has been demonstrated in animal research. The administration of different medicaments, especially cortisone,[5] and starvation and even noise have produced clefts in experimental animals.[6]

In summary, it can be said that a complex concatenation of genetic as well as exogenic factors are responsible for the origin of cleft lip and palate. Human geneticists suppose that a multifactorial sys-

501

tem is frequently present in cleft lip and palate patients.[4,7] Although the number of clefts that can be attributed to heredity can be rather accurately estimated at 25 per cent, the exogenic and environmental factors are, in many cases, still unknown. Therefore, the possibility of taking precautionary measures during pregnancy in order to prevent cleft lip and cleft palate formation is limited.

Embryology

The manifestation of cleft lip and palate occurs during the first weeks of embryonic life. Disturbances in the formation of the primitive nose and palate causing clefting are embryologically separated and appear at different times. This explains why isolated deformities of only the lip or only the palate can develop. A combination of failures in normal embryonic development may lead to a complete cleft formation of the upper lip, the alveolar ridge and of the hard and soft palate (Fig. 25-1).

Disturbances during the development of the nose between the thirty-sixth and forty-second day of pregnancy result in a cleft lip deformity. Normally, the epithelia of the medial and lateral nasal processes, which are separated from each other by shallow grooves, fuse and a broad epithelial wall develops which closes the nose from dorsal to ventral to form the normal orifice of the nose. This epithelial wall is then penetrated by proliferating mesoderm. This is a basic requirement for the normal development of the lip as well as the nostril.

The factors responsible for a cleft formation of the lip are not quite clear. However, Toendury, who examined embryos at this critical stage of development, states that there are two possible ways for the cleft formation to occur:[8] (1) The medial and lateral nasal processes fail to fuse together. In this instance, the epithelial wall does not develop at all, resulting in a complete cleft of the lip and the alveolar bone. Also, the processes may fuse only partially, resulting in an incomplete cleft that appears as a notch in the lip. (2) The epithelial wall does develop, but is not penetrated by mesoderm. This results in instability, since mesoderm must always separate two layers of epithelium if they are to remain as a permanent structure.

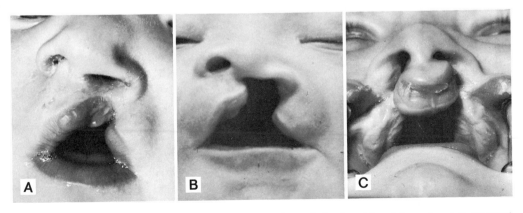

Fig. 25-1. Different types of cleft lip. (A) Incomplete cleft lip with developed but deformed nostril. (B) Total and exceptionally wide unilateral cleft lip. (C) Bilateral cleft lip; there is also a bilateral cleft of the palate.

The buccopharyngeal membrane is an example of two layers of epithelium *not* normally invaded by mesoderm; it, of course, breaks down during normal embryonic development. The same type of breakdown can occur in this epithelial wall, resulting in formation of an incomplete or complete cleft in those areas where no mesoderm invades the wall.

The mechanism for the formation of a cleft of the palate appears to be less complicated. During approximately the sixth to eighth weeks of embryonic life, the mouth and nose form a joint cavity in which the large, developing tongue is situated. The palatal shelves then expand medially and the tongue descends (Fig. 25-2). Now the septum also descends from the roof of the nose and, at the beginning of the third fetal month the palatal shelves and the septum of the nose fuse in the midline.[9] This fusion occurs from anterior to posterior, which accounts for the fact that clefts may form solely in the soft palate, but are never isolated only in the hard palate. In contrast to the cleft of the lip, which may be uni- or bilateral, the

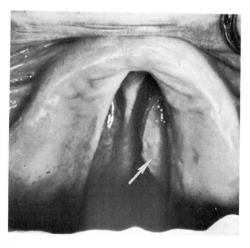

Fig. 25-3. Isolated cleft of the hard and soft palate. Lateral to the vomer, the inferior conchae are visible (arrow).

isolated cleft palate is always located in the midline (Fig. 25-3). In a complete cleft of the lip and palate, however, the cleft of the anterior palate and alveolar ridge may be uni- or bilateral (Fig. 25-4).

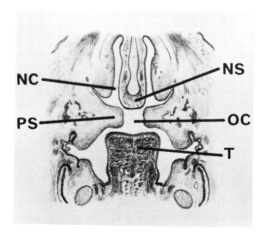

Fig. 25-2. Transverse section of the developing palate, situation in the seventh to eighth prenatal week. NC, nasal cavity; PS, palatal shelves; NS, nasal septum; OC, oral cavity; T, tongue. (Redrawn from Avery, J. K. *In* Bunting R. W.: *Oral Hygiene*, 3rd ed. Philadelphia. Lea & Febiger, 1957)

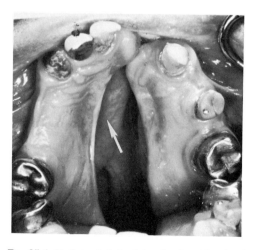

Fig. 25-4. Unilateral cleft of the alveolar ridge, hard and soft palate in an adult patient. The vomer represents one border of the cleft (arrow).

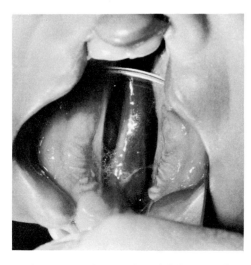

Fig. 25-5. Bilateral incomplete cleft lip in combination with a bilateral total cleft of the hard and soft palate (mirror view). This is an example of the different occurrence of cleft lip and palate deformities.

Incidence and Classification of Cleft Deformities

In general, the frequency of cleft lip and palate deformities in newborns is estimated to be 1:1000. However, interesting racial differences can be observed. Although an average of one cleft occurs in 800 to 900 live births in the total population of the United States a separate evaluation of Negro children reveals a rate of clefting of only 1:2000. In the Oriental and Indian races, however, clefts are more frequent and registrations show almost 3:1000 children born with a cleft formation.[10]

The types of cleft appear with different frequency, and often are unequally distributed with regard to sex. The incidence of clefts is greater in males than in females by a ratio of 3:2. However, isolated clefts of the palate occur more frequently in females in a ratio of 3:2. In bilateral total clefts, the incidence in the male sex is higher, about 2:1.[11]

The unilateral cleft lip deformity is observed three times more frequently than the bilateral cleft lip; also, the left side is more often involved than the right side. In the entire cleft morphology, total unilateral cleft of the lip and palate appears most frequently. Generally speaking, clefts seem to occur more often today than in the past, which probably can be explained by better chances for marriage of cleft palate patients owing to improved treatment results, as well as by a reduced infant mortality rate.

The classification of the cleft lip and palate deformities is complicated by the fact that all types of clefts, total or subtotal, as well as unilateral or bilateral, may occur and may be combined in different ways (Fig. 25-5). Of all the numerous and often complicated classification systems, only that of the American Cleft Palate Association is shown here. This classification principally divides the clefts into two groups:

1. *Prepalate*   2. *Palate*
   (a) Lip   (a) Hard palate
   (b) Alveolar   (b) Soft palate
       process

With this basic classification, however, it is also necessary to determine the following for each case: (1) the location, extent, and width of the cleft, and (2) any other specific modification of the deformity.

Timing for Operative Closure

Except for the cleft deformity, the newborn infant is usually normal and healthy and its birth weight does not differ from the average child. However, there is some indication that these children might have associated deformities, such as heart defects, and finger and toe abnormalities, more often than normal infants.[11] Difficulties in nourishment can be anticipated and overcome by exact instruction of the mother or, in some cases, by the use of a feeding aid in the form of an obturator splint (this could be considered the first orthodontic measure).

For psychologic reasons, it is important to assure parents that their child's intelligence will not be affected because of the cleft. Investigations and follow-up studies have indicated that performance intelligence quotients were the same in groups of children with cleft deformities when compared to their siblings.[13,14] The parents' frequent desire to have the lip closure performed as soon as possible after birth is understandable, since they do not want their child to be seen in public before the lip is closed. For these reasons over half of the surgeons perform the lip closure shortly after birth. Other surgeons, however, wait until an age of three to six months, whenever the child has reached a body weight of 10 pounds. Since the operation is not an emergency but an elective procedure, the age of the child makes no primary difference. Once the proper body weight has been attained, other criteria are that the infant is healthy and has a satisfactory blood hemoglobin count of at least 10 gm. If a two-stage closure is preferred in a bilateral cleft lip, the closure of the second cleft side is performed about six to eight weeks later.

The timing of the closure of the palate is a controversial subject, especially since it is known that early surgical intervention may affect the growth of the maxilla unfavorably. The opinions of surgeons differ widely. Palatal closure has been performed at ages ranging from six months to twelve years. According to an inquiry published by Lewin in 1964, 80 per cent of surgeons in the United States performed the closure of the palate between the first and second years of age; 12 per cent, between the second and fourth years; and 8 per cent, either earlier or later.[15]

Today there is a general tendency to perform the closure of the palate at a later time; for example, individual surgeons in Europe go so far as to wait until school entrance or even until ten to twelve years of age.[16] However, closure of the soft palate is performed in these patients at an age of one to one and one-half years in order not to disturb the speech development. Only a few surgeons share this rather extreme point of view; however, the idea of postponing the closure of the palate until the complete eruption of the first dentition is becoming increasingly accepted. The main reason for the preference of this timing is to diminish the danger of producing an iatrogenic maxillary deformity. Early orthodontic treatment is also easier, since retention and expansion splints can be better stabilized on the fully developed deciduous dentition.

It is not easy to make a statement regarding the perfect timing for closure of the palate since there are still too many unknown factors influencing speech development and maxillary growth. Only an exact evaluation of a great number of follow-up investigations may give the right answer.

Cheilorrhaphy

The goals of cheilorrhaphy are the reestablishment of the continuity of the musculus orbicularis oris, and thereby the function of the upper lip, as well as the aesthetic rehabilitation of the patient. Many techniques for lip closure have been described and different methods are being practiced.

Basically, the operative technique can be divided into two types: those employing linear and those employing angular incision lines (Fig. 25-6). The first method, which has been used frequently in the past, may yield good primary results, but often a shortening of the upper lip on the cleft side is later observed, necessitating a second corrective operation.[17,18] It is possible to avoid this shortening of the lip with the angular incision line by breaking the scar line with quadrangular flaps[19] or triangular flaps.[20-22] With these methods, the deviated ala of the nose is simultaneously rotated medially and the anterior part of the nasal floor is closed. With the angular incision lines commonly used today, the rehabilitation of the length and form of the lip and Cupid's bow is possible at the same time as the improvement of the oral vestibule in this area (Fig. 25-7).

Much more difficult, however, is the

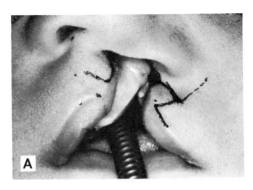

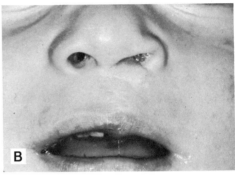

Fig. 25-7. Cleft lip repair according to Tennyson's technique. (A) The incision lines outlined. (B) One year after the lip closure. Note the equal length of both sides of the upper lip. (Courtesy of Dr. M. Perko, Zurich, Switzerland)

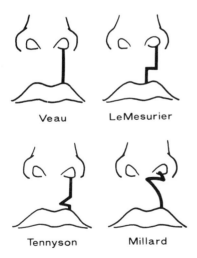

Veau   LeMesurier

Tennyson   Millard

Fig. 25-6. Suture lines resulting from different techniques in cleft lip repair.

closure of the lip in a complete bilateral cleft. If the premaxilla is too protruded it should never be resected because severe maxillary deformities may result. It is preferable to move the protruding premaxilla posteriorly by preoperative orthodontic means, which makes the lip closure much easier. Lip closure may be performed first on one side and six to eight weeks later on the opposite side, or both sides may be closed simultaneously, depending upon the width of the cleft and the position of the premaxilla. If the angular incision line technique is chosen, it is suggested that the lip closure be performed in a two-stage operation in order to avoid disturbing the blood supply of the premaxillary tissue. The scars following repair of a bilateral cleft are sometimes aesthetically unfavorable, and combined with the shortening of the middle part of the upper lip, often make further corrective procedures necessary.

The so-called primary osteoplasty should also be mentioned. In this procedure, lip closure is performed simultaneously with closure of the bony cleft in the alveolar process, using an autogenous bone transplant. This method, which formerly had many adherents, has been abandoned more and more since it demonstrates no advantages; in fact, growth disturbances of the maxilla have been observed.[23] The bone transplant, which is not growing, has the effect of a clamp, and consequently the growth of the maxillary arch is inhibited. In addition, the removal of the bone graft, usually a rib, is associated with more complications in the small child.

Palatorrhaphy

Closure of the palate is of greater interest for the dentist than closure of the lip, since occlusal disturbances with all their possible effects on the dentition may result if the closure of the hard palate is not performed appropriately. In closure of the palate the functional result is the primary concern, aesthetic aspects being less important. A result that allows normal speech is most essential; closure of the oral cavity from the nose is important for masticatory and hygienic reasons as well. The aims of palatal closure then are to obtain a long and mobile soft palate capable of producing normal speech, and a complete closure from the nose. In order to fulfill these requirements, several operative techniques have been developed. The one basic principle employed in all these methods is that a double layer clo-

sure between the oral cavity and the nose must be achieved. Only the double layer closure guarantees complete habilitation of palatal function. Generally, closure is achieved first by mobilizing the nasal mucosa from the lateral wall of the nose and the pharynx and sometimes also from the nasal septum by means of vomer flaps. Following this, the oral mucosa also is mobilized and closed, and thus the whole defect is covered by a double layer of mucosal tissue. Some surgeons perform an additional suture of the muscles in the region of the soft palate, which is practically equivalent to a triple layer closure.

Of all the different methods used for the closure of cleft palates, the principles of only two techniques shall be discussed. These are the bridge flap technique of Von Langenbeck[24] (Fig. 25-8) and the arterial

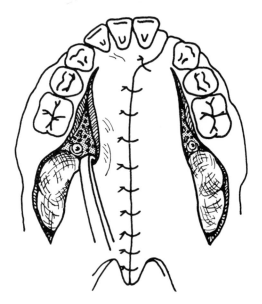

Fig. 25-8. Von Langenbeck's technique for the closure of the cleft palate. The palatal flaps remain attached in the anterior part: the palatine vessels are ligated.

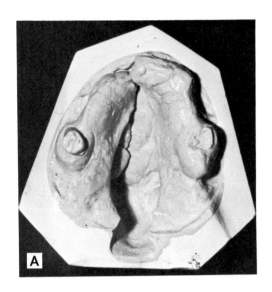

flap or pedicled flap technique according to Veau[17] (Fig. 25-9). The advantage of the first technique is that closure can be achieved without tension. It does, however, require the ligation of the main palatal vessels, and nutrition and growth disturbances of the maxilla may occur as a consequence of the affected blood supply. In the method according to Veau, the artery can be preserved, but tension results at the border of the soft palate, which may cause residual openings in this area. With an exact and careful technique, however, both methods may obtain the same result: the accurate closure of the nasal floor and a sufficient length and mobility of the soft palate (Fig. 25-10).

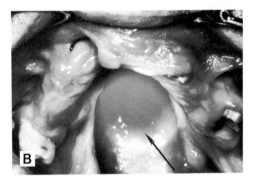

In so-called incomplete clefts of the palate, only a part of the hard or soft palate is separated. Closure is absolutely necessary in such instances, especially for the development of proper speech. The principle of

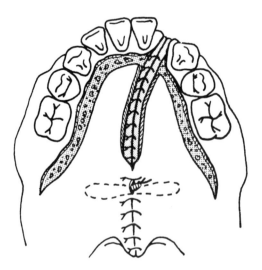

Fig. 25-9. Closure of the cleft palate according to Veau. The nasal floor has been closed, and the palatal flaps are widely detached from the hard palate; however, the palatine vessels remain intact.

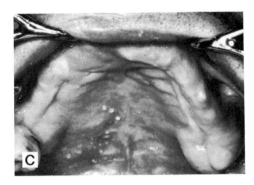

Fig. 25-10. Closure of a wide palatal cleft in an adult patient. (A) Stone model showing the wide cleft of the hard and soft palate. (B) Direct view of residual cleft in the alveolar ridge and extremely wide cleft of the palate. The posterior wall of the pharynx is indicated by the arrow. (C) The principles of Veau's technique have been applied in the closure of the palate.

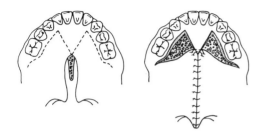

Fig. 25-11. Principle of lengthening the palate by Wardill's push-back operation. The tissue over the denuded bone area regenerates rapidly.

the double layer closure is the same as in total clefts. However, the lengthening of the soft palate should be stressed; this can be achieved by different techniques. Of these so-called push-back procedures, we especially refer to Wardill's method, in which the palate is lengthened by a relatively simple technique[25] (Fig. 25-11). Velopharyngeal closure—of great importance for normal speech—is greatly improved.

The submucosal or occult cleft palate may lead to speech defects as severe as with a complete cleft. The cleft is not obvious because the mucosa is intact on the nasal and oral side (Fig. 25-12). The

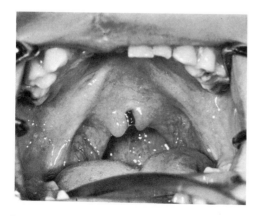

Fig. 25-12. Bifid uvula in a submucous cleft.

muscles of the soft palate, however, are underdeveloped and not united. Because there is no lifting action of the soft palate, the velopharyngeal closure mechanism is insufficient. Important diagnostic signs of a submucosal cleft are a bifid uvula, a notch at the posterior border of the hard palate, and a pale line in the middle of the soft palate which indicates the nonunion of the muscle bundles.[26] The operative procedure consists of uniting the muscle bundles after opening the soft palate in the midline; of course, the nasal and oral mucosae must also be closed in two layers as in other cleft palate deformities.

Secondary Surgical and Rehabilitation Measures

By secondary surgical procedures in cleft palate patients we mean operations not directly related to the primary closure. The timing for these operations is different and the procedures are performed according to growth, deficiencies in function, and aesthetic desires of the patients. For the complete rehabilitation of a patient, several measures are usually necessary, and only the main ones are discussed.

Secondary Closure of Alveolar Cleft Defects

The management of residual congenital osseous clefts of alveolar bone has long been a problem for the clinician who is faced with the restoration of function and aesthetics in this area. In addition to the osseous defects, the residual oral/nasal soft tissue cleft or clefts permit direct communication between the vestibule of the oral cavity and the nasal cavity.

Some of the primary problems that occur here are (1) malocclusion of the teeth in the alveolar segments related to the cleft, (2) eruption of teeth into the cleft space leading to the early loss of teeth, (3) the escape of oral secretions including food into the nose during mastication, (4) the continual drainage of nasal secretions into the oral cavity, and (5) although there is some loss of oral seal and air escape, there seems to be only minimal effect on pronunciation and resonance. This is in contrast to the escape of air through posterior palatal fistulas, which can greatly affect speech. Additional complications resulting from lack of grafting to this void are further collapse of the maxillary segments contributing to additional malocclusion and adding difficulty to the potential prosthodontics.

Alveolar bone grafting of this defect is considered the treatment of choice, although some differences of opinion exist in regard to timing of the graft (Fig. 25-13A and B).

Primary bone grafting is done at the time of the primary lip repair, usually within the first few weeks of the patient's life. Those favoring early bone grafting advocate the advantage of minimizing the original deformity (1) by early prevention of the collapse of the maxillary segments, (2) by providing early continuity to the alveolar arch, (3) by the provision of a

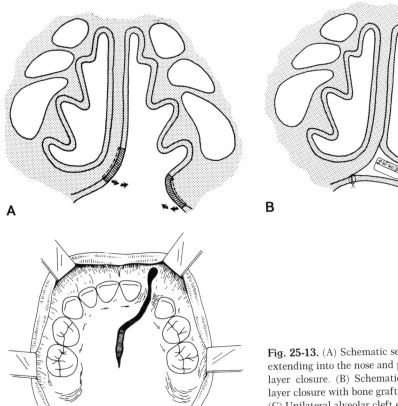

Fig. 25-13. (A) Schematic section to show oral cleft extending into the nose and planned flaps for double layer closure. (B) Schematic illustration of double layer closure with bone graft between the two layers. (C) Unilateral alveolar cleft extending into the labial vestibule with oral-nasal fistula.

A

B

C

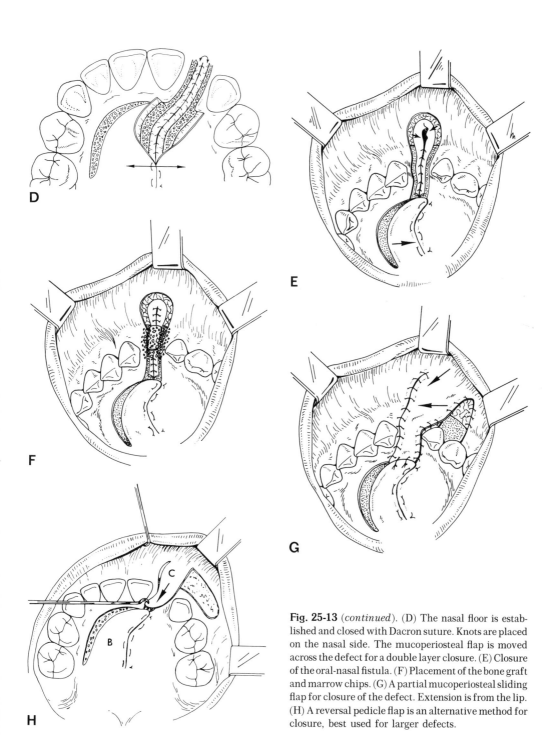

Fig. 25-13 (*continued*). (D) The nasal floor is established and closed with Dacron suture. Knots are placed on the nasal side. The mucoperiosteal flap is moved across the defect for a double layer closure. (E) Closure of the oral-nasal fistula. (F) Placement of the bone graft and marrow chips. (G) A partial mucoperiosteal sliding flap for closure of the defect. Extension is from the lip. (H) A reversal pedicle flap is an alternative method for closure, best used for larger defects.

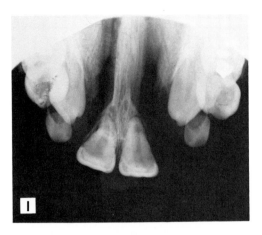

Fig. 25-13 (*continued*). (I) Bilateral cleft with alveolar bone defects. The cuspid teeth have not erupted. (J) Grafts are complete and cuspid teeth are erupting through the graft. (K) Occlusal radiograph to show good continuity of the alveolar arch. Cuspid teeth are nearing normal position and ready for final orthodontic management. (L) Clinical photograph showing good soft tissue closure. When orthodontic treatment is completed, patient will be ready for final fixed bridge.

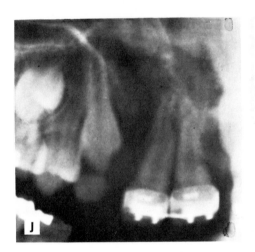

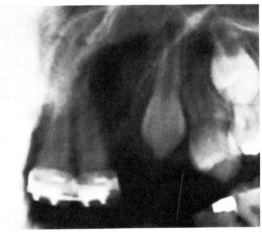

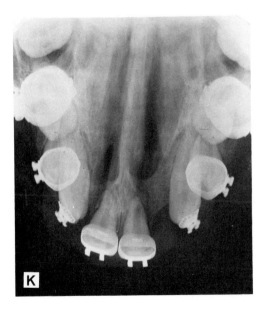

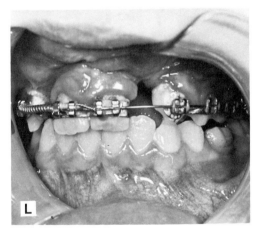

bony bed for deciduous teeth to erupt into, and (4) maxillary growth continues as a unit to minimize the overall deformity. In contrast to this, secondary bone grafting is done after the major maxillary growth is complete, near the ages of seven or eight years. Surgery done at this time will permit final orthodontic management of tooth alignment with key permanent teeth in position, that is, the maxillary centrals and the first molars. A bone graft placed in the defect during this period of growth will provide bony continuity of the arch and bony alveolus for the permanent cuspids to erupt into. There seems to be less of a problem with occlusion when surgery is delayed until this time than when the osseous surgery and grafting are done at the time of primary lip closure.

A surgical technique for secondary bone graft repair will be described (Fig. 25-13). Usually autogenous bone grafting is best, with the particulate bone graft obtained from the iliac crest. The surgical site in the region of the cleft or clefts is prepared. A mucoperiosteal incision is made on the palatal side next to the maxillary teeth. This incision is carried forward to isolate the cleft and the mucoperiosteal flap is reflected. Mucosa is then elevated toward the cleft to become the nasal floor when joined by the opposite side and sutured into position (Fig. 25-13D). The oral/nasal fistula is closed by splitting the mucosa and inverting it upon itself to complete the nasal floor (Fig. 25-13E). At this point, bone on the sides of the cleft should be exposed. The cortical medullary bone is then fashioned to fill the defect (Figs. 25-13F and 25-14). Additional cancellous chips are packed around the graft. When this is accomplished, a labial mucoperiosteal sliding flap (Fig. 25-13G) or a pedicle

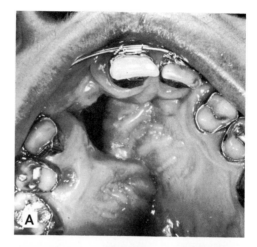

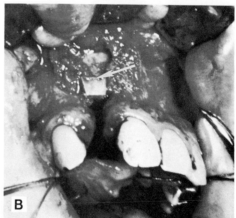

Fig. 25-14. Closure of oronasal fistula with simultaneous bone grafting procedure. (A) Oronasal fistula in the anterior portion of the hard palate. (B) An autogenous graft of iliac crest bone has been wedged into the defect of the alveolar process (arrow).

flap is created from the buccal vestibule in such a manner that it will cover the bone (Fig. 25-13H). The flap is sutured to the palatal mucosa and the site of the donor flap is undermined and closed (Fig. 25-13H). A splint is then placed over the palatal surface for about 10 days. (This section, courtesy of Dr. D. E. Waite)

Occlusal Corrections

Generally, the operative trauma of the cleft closure and the tension and fibrosis caused by an inadequate amount or inferior quality of the tissue with which to close the defect are assumed to cause growth disturbances of the maxilla. These may manifest themselves as (1) asymmetry of the maxilla (see Fig. 24-38), (2) a retrusion of the maxilla (Fig. 25-15), or (3) a remarkable collapse of all maxillary segments, as may be seen in bilateral clefts. In order to correct occlusal disturbances, surgical procedures such as the lateral movement of the small segment of the cleft maxilla only, or the advancement of both segments of the maxilla should be considered. The advancement may be carried out in one stage when a good occlusion can be achieved in this manner. Reopening the cleft and moving both maxillary parts anterolaterally is often necessary when the segments have collapsed. In this case, the segment on the cleft side is usually in a more unfavorable position. When anterolateral repositioning is done, the cleft in the alveolar and palatal region becomes broader and a larger oronasal fistula may result. The closure of the oronasal opening is then performed in a second operation with simultaneous bone grafting,[28] as described in the section on secondary closure of alveolar cleft defects.

The correction of occlusal disturbances resulting from bilateral clefts is more difficult. In addition to the two lateral segments, the premaxilla may be in an unfavorable position. In such a case the lateral segments should be adjusted first. The osteotomy and repositioning of the premaxilla may be performed in a second stage; a bone graft may be done simultaneously for stabilization purposes. Naturally, the closure of residual openings to the nose can be achieved at the same time.[27] With these techniques, it is possible to obtain a functional rehabilitation even in the most severe occlusal deformities of the maxilla. Of course, the change in the profile of the patient can be dramatic. The so-called pseudoprognathism owing to the underdeveloped maxilla can be corrected in the most physiologic way by these maxillary surgical procedures. Only a few cases might require additional surgical intervention in the mandible. These would be (1) true mandibular prognathism in combination with a cleft, (2) a protruding lower alveolar process, and finally (3) enlarged chin areas. Correction measures of these deformities have been previously described in Chapter 24.

Pharyngeal Flap Procedures

Velopharyngeal insufficiency is frequently caused by shortness and inflexibility of the soft palate. In most cases, this is a consequence of an inadequate operative closure, which may necessitate further operative procedures. Scar tissues resulting from closure can impair the mobility of the soft palate remarkably. Also, paralysis of the velum, which may occur, for example, following diphtheria in childhood or atrophy of the palatal muscles, as in a submucosal cleft, may cause "nasality" in speech. The evaluation of the speech by speech therapists is important in deciding whether a pharyngeal flap procedure is indicated.

Several surgical methods are available for connecting the soft palate to the posterior wall of the pharynx in order to reduce

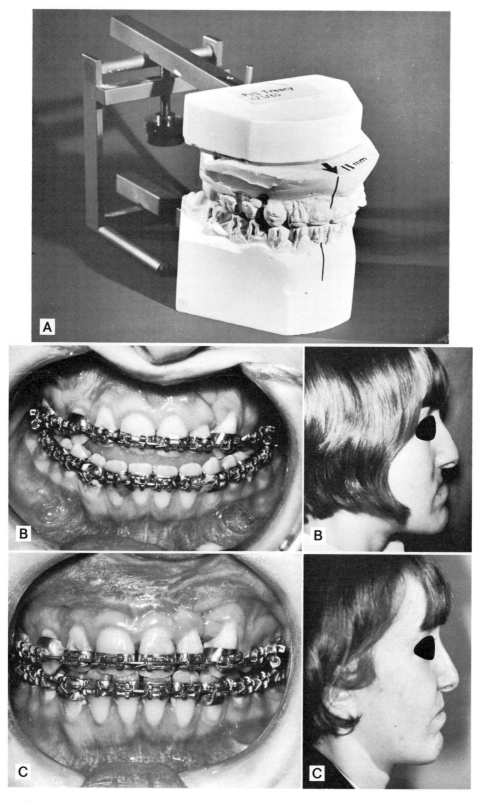

Fig. 25-15. Surgical correction of maxillary retrusion in combination with open bite in a patient with unilateral cleft lip and palate. (A) On the models the maxillary advancement is indicated. (B) Profile and occlusion preoperatively. (C) Profile and occlusion postoperatively, after advancement of the maxilla and closure of the open bite.

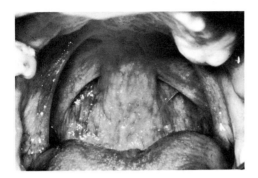

Fig. 25-16. Pharyngeal flap with inferiorly attached base.

the air stream into the nasopharynx (Fig. 25-16). Pedicled flaps from the soft tissues of the posterior wall of the pharynx can be formed, with their bases attached superiorly or inferiorly. Usually, the superiorly based flap is preferred. In addition to the soft palate, the muscles of the lateral pharyngeal wall and of Passavant's bar are important parts of the palatopharyngeal sphincter mechanism. In cleft palate patients, these muscle groups are usually well developed to compensate for the palatal deficiency.

Pharyngeal flap procedures are not difficult to perform, but results are not always satisfactory. In spite of speech therapy—which is indicated after pharyngeal flap procedures—the phonetic result may still be poor, especially when the operation is carried out in older patients. This is one more reason why the primary closure of the palate should be done by an experienced surgeon, since damage to the tissues in this area can be irreparable.

Nose and Lip Correction

The primary closure of a cleft lip is usually sufficient from the standpoint of function. However, quite often aesthetic deficiencies still exist which may become more apparent in time. Therefore, secondary corrections of the nose and lip are frequently necessary. Severe deformities are better corrected before the patient enters school in order to avoid psychologic and emotional problems. The final corrections should not be performed before the completion of facial growth, which usually occurs between 15 to 17 years of age. In these procedures there is one basic principle to consider: the correction of the bone, such as maxillary advancement, bone grafts, or premaxillary repositioning, should always be carried out before the final correction of the soft tissues. Otherwise the corrective bone surgery may influence the shape of the lip and the nose. Since there is such a variation in techniques and surgical opinions regarding reoperation for soft tissues correction, we shall not make specific statements here.

Orthodontic Therapy

Orthodontic treatment of cleft palate patients may begin prior to lip closure. The most common preoperative orthodontic measures include (1) the utilization of an obturator for eating purposes, and (2) the approximation of the segments of the cleft. The latter can be helpful in simplifying the operative closure of the lip, especially in total bilateral clefts (Fig. 25-17). McNeil was the first to prove the advantage of preoperative orthodontics;[29] other orthodontists have since reported similar results.[30,31]

After the closure of the hard palate, orthodontic measures are often indicated again in order to avoid a collapse of the maxillary segments. For this reason several surgeons postpone the closure of the palate until the eruption of the deciduous dentition has been completed, because the fully developed teeth provide better retention for a palatal splint. It may be several years before orthodontic therapy is insti-

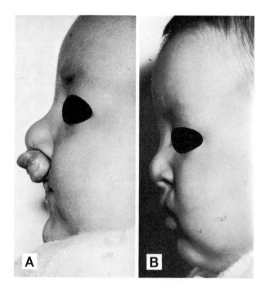

Fig. 25-17. Preoperative orthodontic treatment for repositioning of the premaxilla. (A) Protruding premaxilla in a bilateral cleft before treatment. (B) Improved position of the premaxilla following preoperative orthodontic therapy. Now the lip closure is much easier to perform. (Courtesy of Dr. M. Hotz, Zurich, Switzerland)

tuted again. All kinds of anomalies of the position of the upper teeth are possible, but often the teeth adjacent to the cleft area are in malocclusion. The lateral incisors are often deformed, or even absent, and eruption of the cuspids delayed. Straightening the upper alveolar arch and aligning the teeth are helpful in achieving occlusal harmony, and may also create better tooth relationship when an operative procedure for the correction of the occlusal disturbances is indicated. Thus preoperative and eventually postoperative orthodontic therapy is a distinct advantage in the overall treatment of cleft palate patients.

Prosthetic Therapy

The cooperation of the prosthodontist is important for the rehabilitation of speech and masticatory function. In an insufficient velopharyngeal mechanism, a speech aid appliance in form of a speech bulb can be fixed to the prosthesis or to the teeth. In this manner the velopharyngeal isthmus can be narrowed, and the muscle action of the lateral pharyngeal wall is augmented by the stimulation resulting from a speech bulb. Therefore, the speech bulb is regarded as a preoperative measure to promote the success of a pharyngeal flap operation. If the flap procedure is not performed for some reason, the speech bulb can be left in place as a permanent speech aid[32] (Fig. 25-18). Naturally, spe-

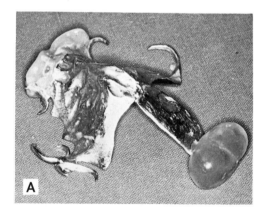

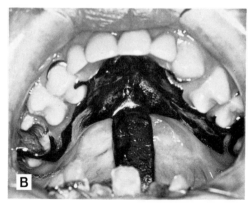

Fig. 25-18. (A) An acrylic speech bulb is connected to the arm of a stainless steel prosthesis. (B) The prosthesis that replaces the anterior teeth is connected with the speech bulb appliance which is in place.

cial care must be taken to preserve the teeth, which are important for the retention of the prosthetic appliance. Palatal fistulas can be closed with an obturator when surgical closure is not preferred.

On the other hand, surgical procedures can be of great value for the work of the prosthodontist. The bony reconstruction of the alveolar process by secondary osteoplasty and the stabilization of the premaxilla with bone grafting are of great advantage in preparing the area for the construction of fixed bridgework. The anterior part of an edentulous, atrophic alveolar ridge reconstruction by bone transplants will create a better base for a prosthesis. This is especially helpful in case of partial or total loss of the premaxilla. Finally, the retention for a total prosthesis, which eventually may have to include a speech bulb, can be improved by preprosthetic surgical methods. This can be achieved by sulcus extensions with skin or mucosal grafts (Fig. 25-19). The cooperation of prosthodontist and surgeon affords a typical example of the value and the necessity of a team approach in the complicated treatment of cleft palate patients.

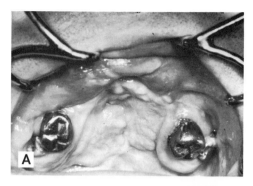

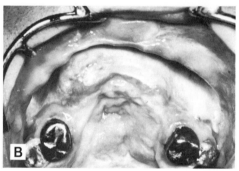

Fig. 25-19. Value of preprosthetic surgery in cleft lip and palate patients. (A) Poor situation for a denture due to the unfavorable labial sulcus resulting from closure of the cleft. (B) Improvement of the vestibular area following split-thickness skin graft procedure.

References

1. Gabka, J.: Allgemeine Missbildungsaetiologie unter besonderer Beruecksichtigung der Lippen-Kiefer-Gaumenspalten. Dtsch. Zahn-Mund-, u. Kieferheilk., 20:9–10, 1953.
2. Grob, M.: Lehrbuch der Kinderchirurgie. Stuttgart, G. Thieme, 1957.
3. Woolf, C. M.: et al.: Cleft lip and heredity. Plast. Reconstr. Surg., 34:11, 1964.
4. Joergensen, G.: Zur Aetiologie der Lippen-, Kiefer- und Gaumenspalten. Med. heute, 18:293, 1964.
5. Fraser, F., Walker, B., and Trasler, G.: Experimental production of congenital cleft palate: Genetic and environmental factors. Pediatrics. 19:782, 1957.
6. Peters, S., and Strassburg, M.: Erzeugung von Gaumenspalten durch Laerm und Hunger. Dtsch. Zahnärztl. Z., 23:843, 1968.
7. Schulze, C.: Anomalien, Missbildungen und Krankheiten der Zaehne, des Mundes und der Kiefer. Handbuch Humangenetik II. Stuttgart, G. Thieme, 1964.
8. Toendury, G.: On the mechanism of cleft formation. In Congenital Anomalies of the Face and Associated Structure, p. 85. S. Pruzansky (Ed.) Springfield, Ill., Charles C Thomas, 1961.
9. Bunting, R.: Oral Hygiene. Philadelphia, Lea & Febiger, 1957.

10. Gorlin, R., and Goldman, H.: Thoma's Oral Pathology, 6th ed., vol. 1. St. Louis, C. V. Mosby Co., 1970.

11. Fogh-Anderson, P.: Inheritance of Hare-lips and Cleft Palate. Kopenhagen, Nyt Nordisk Forlag, Arnol Busck, 1942.

12. Harkins, C., et al.: A classification of cleft lip and cleft palate. Plast. Reconstr. Surg. 29:31, 1962.

13. Goodstein, L.: Intellectual impairment in children with cleft palates. J. Speech Res., 4:287, 1961.

14. Ruess, A.: A comparative study of cleft palate children and their siblings. J. Clin. Psychol., 21:354, 1965.

15. Lewin, M.: Management of cleft lip and palate in the United States and Canada. Plast. Reconstr. Surg., 33:383, 1964.

16. Schweckendiek, H.: Ergebnisse bei Lippen, Kiefer-, Gaumenspaltoperationen mit der primaeren Veloplastik. Fortschr. Kiefer- u. Gesichtschir., 4:167, 1958.

17. Veau, V.: La Division Palatine. Paris, Masson et Cie, 1931.

18. Rose, W. In Textbook of Oral Surgery, 3rd ed., G. O. Kruger (Ed.). St. Louis, C. V. Mosby Co., 1968.

19. LeMesurier, A.: A method of cutting and suturing the lip in the treatment of complete unilateral clefts. Plast. Reconstr. Surg., 4:1, 1949.

20. Tennyson, C.: The repair of the unilateral cleft lip by the stencil method. Plast. Reconstr. Surg. 9:115, 1952.

21. Randall, P.: A triangular flap operation for the primary repair of unilateral clefts of the lip. Plast. Reconstr. Surg., 23:331, 1959.

22. Millard, D.: Complete unilateral clefts of the lip. Plast. Reconstr. Surg., 25:595, 1960.

23. Rehrmann, A., Koberg W., and Koch, H.: Long-term postoperative results of primary and secondary bone grafting in complete clefts of lip and palate. Cleft Palate J., 7:206, 1970.

24. Von Langenbeck, B.: Die Uranoplastik-mittels Abloesung des Muco-periostalen Gaumenueberzuges. Arch. klin. Chir., 2:205, 1862.

25. Wardill, W.: The technique of operation for cleft palate. Br. J. Surg., 25:117, 1937.

26. Hayward, J.: Cleft lip and cleft palate. In Textbook of Oral Surgery, 3rd ed. G. O. Kruger (Ed.). St. Louis, C. V. Mosby, 1968.

27. Perko, M.: Surgical correction of the position of the pre-maxilla in secondary deformities of cleft lip and palate. IVth Internat. Congress Plastic Surg., p. 410. Amsterdam, Excerpta Medica Foundation, 1969.

28. Obwegeser, H.: Surgery as an adjunct to orthodontics in normal and cleft palate patients. Europ. Orthodont. Soc. Rep. Congr., 42:343, 1966.

29. McNeil, C.: Oral and Facial Deformity. London, Pittman & Sons, 1949.

30. Notz, M. A., and Gounski, W.: Comprehensive care of cleft lip and palate children at Zürich University: A preliminary report. Am. J. Orthod., 70:481, 1976.

31. Pruzansky, S.: Pre-surgical orthopedics and bone grafting for infants with cleft lip and palate. Cleft Palate J., 1:164, 1964.

32. Millard, R. T.: Training for optimal use of the prosthetic speech appliance. Cleft lip and palate. pp. 861–867, Boston, Little Brown and Co., 1971.

33. Epstein, L. I., Davis, B. W., and Thompson, L.: Delayed bone grafting in cleft palate patients. Plast. Reconstr. Surg., 46:363–367, 1970.

34. Boyne, P. J., and Sands, N. R.: Secondary bone grafting of residual alveolar and palatal defects. J. Oral Surg., 30:87–92, 1972.

35. Robertson N. R. E., and Jolleys, A.: Effects of early bone grafting in complete clefts of lip and palate. Plast. Reconstr. Surg., 42:414–421, 1968.

36. Robinson, F., and Wood, B.: Primary bone grafting in the treatment of cleft lip and

palate with special reference to alveolar collapse. Br. J. Plast. Surg., 22:336–342, 1969.

37. Georgiade, N. C., Pickrell, K. L., and Quinn, G. W.: Varying concepts in bone grafting of alveolar palatal defects. Cleft Palate J., 1:43–51, 1964.

38. Stenstrom, S. J., and Thilander, B. L.: Bone grafting in secondary cases of cleft lip and palate. Plast. Reconstr. Surg., 32:353–360, 1963.

39. Broude, D. J., and Waite, D. E.: Secondary closure of alveolar defects. J. Oral Surg., 37:829–840, 1974.

40. Georgiade, N. G.: Anterior palatal-alveolar closure by means of interplated flaps. Plast. Reconstr. Surg., 39:162–167, 1967.

41. Koberg, W. R.: Present view on bone grafting in cleft palate (a review of the literature). J. Maxillofac. Surg., 1:185–193, 1973.

Surgery has been made safe for the patient: we must now make the patient safe for surgery.   MOYNIHAN

26 General Supportive Therapy

NORMAN O. HOLTE

General supportive therapy encompasses a wider circumspection of the dental patient than the terms "preoperative" and "postoperative" care imply. The teeth and indeed the oral cavity are no longer regarded an isolated area of interest to the dentist, but rather an integral part of the physiology and personality of a human being. The specialist in the care of the teeth and mouth, therefore, must relate his professional judgment and skills to all functions of the human body, namely, the digestive, circulatory, respiratory, muscular, nervous, and excretory systems. In the presence of disease, the patient may require a temporary functional readjustment for his comfort and well-being. In a broad sense, this defines general supportive therapy, which is provided by the dentist through the use of drugs, physical agents, and psychologic principles.

The best support that any doctor can provide his patient is to establish confidence and a professional relationship that is above reproach. This kind of attitude on the part of the dentist arises out of happiness and satifaction with one's work and is involved in the magic of giving nothing less than one's best. To do this, one must have a good background in dental education and be willing to represent the profession well. This can only be done if one

strives for continuing education by participating in postgraduate courses, keeping up on professional reading, and maintaining a continual dialogue with dental colleagues. This is more easily accomplished in group practice than in solo practice. We should be grateful for our education, respect our educators, and appreciate the legacy of our past and present dental pioneers.

A dental office should be clean, bright, and cheery. All office personnel should be courteous, pleasant, and fully supportive of the professional staff. The office should be well organized and reflect the fact that the entire purpose of the office is to serve the patient. Each member within the office should be positive in his approach, knowledgeable, and personable, yet professional. At all times, office personnel should maintain an outward calm even though activities of the day may not always be harmonious. It should be obvious to the patient that the dentist enjoys what he is doing, and if one consistently operates within his limits of experience and preparation, the transferral of confidence to the patient will become obvious.

It is important to establish the habit of having the patient's record before you at each appointment. The presence of a record permits you to review quickly the past visits by the patient and, of course, to make

521

additional notes relative to the present visit. A quick reference to the record may bring to mind a conversational point permitting a more relaxed interview. Equally and perhaps even more important is to have the patient's name in front of you: no word is more pleasant to the ears than one's own name. To call a patient by his or her first name and relate a personal incident relative to the last visit or the intervening period provides an additional means to promote a confident relationship.

In order to deliver adequate treatment for the variety of problems that patients will bring to the dentist, one must, of course, be able to make an accurate diagnosis. The foregoing chapters, if carefully interpreted, plus experience and continued preparation will provide the dentist with these skills.

Nutrition

The general nutrition of the surgical patient is most important. The specific dietary requirements are obviously significant for healing tissue. However, the adequate ingestion of a good diet is impaired in any surgical patient and particularly one undergoing surgery of the oral cavity. Most important is adequate fluid intake. The patient can tolerate the deferment of solid food intake for a few days, but he cannot do without sufficient fluids. These fluids should be qualitatively nutritional and quantitatively adequate. Two or three quarts (2000 to 3000 ml.) per day are ample for the average adult, although it may be necessary to urge an increased fluid intake for the postsurgical patient. This may be done by providing palatable fluids according to his tastes. Soup broth, tea, and a variety of nutritional protein supple-

ments are helpful. When a patient cannot swallow or refuses to take adequate oral fluids, the intravenous route must be considered.

Drug Therapy

Sedatives and Tranquilizers

Adequate rest both pre- and postoperatively for minor surgical procedures is much more important than patients often recognize. Unfortunately, dental patients view their surgical procedures as far less important than they really are.

In dental therapeutics, sedatives and tranquilizers are used extensively to control nervousness, allay apprehension, and induce sleep. The pharmacologic agents that evoke these responses are many in number, produce a degree of hypnosis that is desirable and necessary in dental practice, and yet possess varied and sometimes formidable effects on the central nervous system.

The central nervous system depressant drugs may be classified into two broad categories on the basis of their beneficial therapeutic effects as follows: (1) Drugs that depress the central nervous system (CNS). These include sedatives, hypnotics, some narcotic drugs such as the barbiturates, alcohols, chloral derivatives, and miscellaneous CNS depressants. (2) Drugs that selectively modify CNS function. In this category are the non-narcotic analgesics, antipyretics, narcotic analgesics, anticonvulsants, central skeletal muscle relaxants, the major and minor tranquilizers, and miscellaneous psychotherapeutic agents.

Much of a patient's discomfort can be managed by the correct use of sedatives and other medications and by careful preparation of the patient for dental procedures. It may be advisable to give a patient a sedative the night prior to surgery. Many patients have sufficient anxiety that they will not sleep well and therefore come to the office tired, tense, and incapable of relaxing or remaining calm during the dental procedures. A variety of sedatives and hypnotics are available for pre- and postoperative management (Table 26-1, p. 530 to 537).

Analgesics

It is unfortunate that pain has been almost synonymous with dentistry from time immemorial. Dental discomfort has been the object of humorous etchings, jokes, and cartoons throughout the ancient and modern history of the profession. That dentists have made many significant contributions to the knowledge and control of pain is clearly stamped in the history of medicine. For example, the introduction of general anesthesia by Wells and Morton, both dentists, left an impact of such magnitude that their ingenuity is credited with making the remarkable advancements in modern surgery possible.

Despite all of the contributions and scientific advancements in neurophysiology, neuroanatomy, and neuropharmacology, attempts to define pain quantitatively have been discouraging indeed. However, many drugs have been introduced for modifying or blocking the reception, transmission, or perception of painful stimuli. Local anesthetics interfere with conduction of nerve impulses. Analgesic drugs alter pain perception, interpretation, and reaction by the central nervous system. Many diverse systemic analgesic agents are available and used extensively in the control of dental pain (Table 26-2), p. 538 to 547). These may be classified, for convenience, as opiates (narcotics derived from opium), opioids (synthetic narcotics), and non-narcotic agents.

The narcotic analgesics possess two pharmacologic actions that distinguish them from other pain-relieving drugs. First, these agents are capable of relieving severe, intractable pain, and second, they possess an addicting liability that imposes a limit on the duration and frequency of their use. The manufacture and distribution of opiates and opioids are strictly controlled by federal legislation. A drug enforcement agency (DEA) number (formerly called a BNDD number) is available to licensed practitioners of medicine, dentistry, and veterinary medicine at an annual fee of five dollars. If a practice is conducted at more than one location, a separate permit number is required for each address. Anyone prescribing or in possession of narcotics without a DEA permit is in violation of the law and subject to severe penalties. The non-narcotic analgesics are effective in varying degrees in obtunding mild to moderately severe pain without posing the danger of habituation. The sale and distribution of these agents are restricted to prescription by licensed practitioners in the healing arts.

Antibiotics

In the prevention and control of infection, a variety of choices among antibiotics must be available to the clinician (Table 26-3, p. 548 to 554). New antibiotics are being offered to the profession constantly. The proper use of antibacterial agents is essential to the elimination of dental infection and the prevention of secondary systemic complications. Penicillin, or one of its analogues, remains the drug of choice for most infections of dental origin; however, its many limitations often make the selection of another antibiotic necessary or clinically desirable.

In order to ensure the selection of the most effective antibiotic, sensitivity tests should be performed whenever infecting organisms can be obtained for bacteriologic culture. The "agar-plate" testing method determines only the resistance or sensitivity of microorganisms to a specific drug. More precise data are obtained by the "tube-dilution" method, which determines the concentration required to destroy or control the growth of organisms, i.e., the number of micrograms of the antibiotic per milliliter of fluid (culture media or circulating plasma). Laboratory results are usually not available for 18 to 24 hours. Since it is usually necessary to begin antibiotic therapy without delay, selection of the antibacterial agent, therefore, is based on the dentist's tentative diagnosis, experience, and clinical judgment.

In addition to choosing the effective antibiotic, the dentist must carefully consider the indications, contraindications, complications, side effects, adverse reactions, and adequate dosage. These considerations are extremely important and must not be overlooked in clinical practice. Detailed information is available from voluminous scientific articles. Each medication should be chosen wisely and appropriate prescriptions written. The specific drugs should be selected according to the individual patient's need.

Antihistamines

The antihistamines are useful in dentistry to prevent or reverse the symptoms produced by the release of histamine in the body. These drugs can reduce or decrease the intensity of allergic and anaphylactic manifestations, such as capillary permeability, edema, itching (e.g., that produced by local anesthetics), and symptoms of vasodilation (Table 26-4, p. 555 and 556).

Prescription Writing

A variety of unusual reactions may be encountered in the use of medications, including those resulting from individual idiosyncrasies and overdosage. The taking of a medical history is of paramount importance in revealing previous untoward reactions to drugs. The Physician's Desk Reference (PDR) is an excellent index to prescription drugs, commercial pharmaceutical specialties, biologicals, and general information relating to contraindications, precautions, warnings, adverse reactions, and dosage forms.

Statutory and federal laws permit a licensed dentist the privilege of prescribing drugs in practicing his profession. He must prescribe whatever he believes is the most effective and safest drug for the treatment of dental disease in retoring the patient to health. He must consider the possible interactions that might occur when he adds a drug to other medications that the patient is receiving at that time. He must know and understand the mechanisms of drug action and interaction to ensure that his prescription will provide the most desirable therapeutic effect. Therefore, the dentist must review, from time to time, the basic principles of pharmacology, absorption, distribution, bioavailability, biotransformation, toxicity, and other factors that modify drug dosages.

Prescription writing is an art dating back to the ancient history of medicine. It has been called "the most significant communication of the human race."[1] Within the past 30 years, the pendulum has swung from writing secret multi-ingredient prescriptions to those that contain only one or two specific drugs. The principles and practices of writing a prescription have become increasingly important today with the release of new and potentially hazardous drugs. A dentist who is afforded the legal right and privilege to write prescriptions must likewise assume certain responsibilities pertaining thereto.

By definition, a prescription is a legal document that the pharmacist must keep on file for future reference. Errors or omissions must be avoided in order to preclude ethical or legal action against the prescriber and the pharmacist. Good prescription practice calls for a few simple rules:

1. It must be legible, written in ink, printed, or typewritten.
2. It must include the patient's name and address and the date of issue.
3. The name of the drug and the amounts should be stated clearly and accurately.
4. The instructions to the pharmacist should specifically indicate the amount and type of preparation to be dispensed.
5. The directions to the patient should be concise, specific, complete, and accurate. Avoid instructions such as "as directed" or "as often as necessary."
6. Limitations for refill should be included.
7. The name of the drug may be printed on the label if the prescriber considers it desirable.
8. The DEA number must appear on the prescription when certain habit-forming drugs are dispensed.
9. The prescription must be signed by the doctor.

The prescriptions illustrated in Figure 26-1 are acceptable examples for form and completeness. The official names or formulas might well be written in the body of the prescription; however, commonly used medications of these types are prepared and distributed under the trade names of specific pharmaceutical manufacturers rather than by the pharmacist himself. Despite our intentions to avoid commercialism in a professional practice, trade names inevitably find their way into prescription writing. Most commercial preparations undergo strict quality and quantity control in manufacture and packaging that meets the requirements established by the federal Food and Drug Administration. If a practitioner prefers the product of a specific manufacturer, he may write the proprietary or trade name; otherwise, the official names are usually used in prescriptions. Pharmacists, like physicians and dentists, are ethically bound to provide the patient with the best professional service they have to offer.

Prescribing for a patient involves several techniques, many of which are under legal control and jurisdiction. Verbal orders may constitute a prescritpion, but this method is subject to error and hazards that must be avoided. Office dispensing of drugs is a hazardous practice and, for most drugs, is usually prohibited by law. An order written in a hospital chart is a prescription. Most prescriptions, however, are written orders to a pharmacist to provide specific medications for a specific person under professional care.

The mere writing of a prescription is important to the patient-doctor relationship when the patient observes the confidence, attention to detail, and the personal nature of the treatment recommended for his ailment. A few hints may be helpful in writing a prescription:[2,3]

1. It should be written in the presence of the patient.
2. It should be written without interruption.
3. It should be written with confidence and concentration on the task.
4. Erasing or crossing out errors should be avoided.
5. Discarding a prescription in the presence of a patient leaves a poor impression.

6. Before signing a prescription, proofread and verify the accuracy of its content, dosage, and directions to the patient.
7. Inform the patient regarding the nature of the drug, his disease, and the treatment regimen.
8. If the drug is expensive, the patient should be so informed.
9. Allow the patient to select his own pharmacist.

The practice of writing prescriptions for one's self or for one's family is medically unsound, unethical, and sometimes in

---

JOHN J. DOE, D.D.S.

503 PHYSICIAN'S AND DENTIST'S BLDG.

Off: 332–3958   Center City, State   Res: 866–5117

For: Mrs. Jane Roe   Date: Aug. 31, 1971

Address: 123 Main Street, Center City   State: State

Rx: Phenoxymethyl Penicillin   250 mg.
Dispense such tablets #24
Sig: One (1) q6h

Label X

DEA No. ___—___

REFILL: 0-①-2-3-4-_____

John J. Doe, D.D.S.

John J. Doe, D.D.S.

JOHN J. DOE, D.D.S.

503 PHYSICIAN'S AND DENTIST'S BLDG.

Off: 332–3958   Center City, State   Res: 866–5117

For: Mrs. Jane Roe   Date: Aug. 31, 1971

Address: 123 Main Street, Center City   State: State

Rx: A.S.A. Compound c̄ Codeine   30 mg.
Dispense such capsules #12
Sig: One (1) q4h if needed for pain

Label X

DEA No. AH 0000000

REFILL: 0-①-2-3-4-_____

John J. Doe, D.D.S.

John J. Doe, D.D.S.

Fig. 26-1. Sample prescription forms.

violation of the law. This point is well depicted in the old proverb: "The doctor who prescribes for himself, has a fool for a patient, and a fool for a doctor."

Physical Therapy

In addition to the use of medication, appropriate physical therapy and the utilization of heat and cold have a place in good postoperative management of surgical problems. Gentle massage of a postsurgical swelling and stretching of the jaws when muscular trismus occurs may be helpful. In general, cold would be beneficial in the form of an ice compress immediately following surgical trauma; this seems to help limit or control excessive edema. However, after the first 24 hours, cold has little value and the use of heat is then indicated.

It is generally thought that moist heat is more effective than dry heat, however, both will be comforting to the patient, have some minimal effect in dilating blood vessels, and generally aid in circulating the blood. Physical exercise of the injured part and the application of heat do much to return the circulation within the surgical site to normal.

Oral Surgery as an Art *

If a practitioner has the right instruments and knows his oral surgical skills, yet cannot use them effectively on patients, his knowledge and training will be of no use to him. As the dentist applies his knowledge to care for the needs of his patients he is performing an art, and this skill or aptitude should be recognized for

* Adapted from Clark, H. B., Jr.: *Practical Oral Surgery*, 3rd ed. Philadelphia, Lea & Febiger, 1965.

what it is. Science is the knowledge of facts, particularly those relating to natural phenomena of the physical world. Art is the application of that knowledge to man's use. In the finer sense, the art of practice denotes the finesse, smoothness, timing, rhythm, insight, and understanding with which professional care is rendered.

As in all forms of well-executed art, oral surgical care should be not a disjointed sequence of mechanical steps, but a well-integrated, smooth flowing series of actions that are adjusted to the patient's needs.

To illustrate the necessity for integration of surgical technique, judgment, and sympathetic concern for the patient, the recommended method of testing for anesthesia is described.

1. Approximately two minutes after the local anesthetic has been injected, the operator says with a slow distinct voice, "We are going to start now, very carefully and slowly at first. If at any time you would like me to stop, just raise your hand and I will do so. Do you understand me?" (Note that there has been no mention of the words pain, hurt, pressure, or too much pain. This would plant the thought in the patient's mind that the dentist thinks there may be pain—a terrifying prospect! The operator should radiate confidence in his anesthetic solution and the method in which it was injected. The affirmative approach is important.)

2. When the patient indicates that he understands, the operator initates his operation in either one of two ways:
   a. He places the forceps beaks lightly on the tooth and gradually applies pressure, watching the patient's

hands out of the corner of his eye. If there is no signal to stop, he gradually increases the amount of force until it is evident that he is past the point where pain would have been felt if anesthesia were inadequate.
b. Every patient who sits in a dental chair to have a tooth removed is frightened or apprehensive to some degree. Both mental and physical suffering combine to make many dental procedures unpleasant for the patient. The operator must care for both by his anesthetic agents, his attitude, and his spoken words.

3. The strength of the force is increased to the required amount necessary to extract the tooth. This is done with slow, resolute, purposeful movements.
4. If at any time the patient raises his hand the operator must remove fingers and forceps from the mouth and gently inquire if anything is wrong. Depending upon the reply, he will allow further time for deepening of the anesthesia or, if some complaint other than pain was reported, he will care for the patient's need in the correct manner.
5. If the patient does not interrupt the operation and the tooth is extracted promptly, it is laid on the table and the dentist observes whether it is intact. Upon confirming the fact to himself, he says in a calm, pleasant voice something to this effect, "The tooth is out now and you were an excellent patient." Both the mental and physical aspects of the apprehension have been satisfied, and when the realization comes over the patient that the ordeal is over, his mental attitude is frequently favorable.

Sometimes patients cry out or squirm about but fail to raise the hand. Under such circumstances, it is well to pause and repeat the instructions, adding that crying out does not help, but will simply disturb patients in the waiting room. If this behavior continues, and the patient does not listen or cooperate, the operation should be discontinued until rational conversation can be resumed. If in spite of a highly agitated state the patient gives no report of actual pain, heavy sedation or general anesthesia is indicated. If the patient states upon calming down that there was true pain, there should be no feeling of ill will if the first stimulating surgical movements were made gradually. In some instances patients will raise the hand just to see if the dentist means what he says (!), then urge him to continue.

The Care of Children

Some of the greatest pleasures in the dentist's life come from the care of little children because of their freshness, frankness, and ready appreciation of true sincerity. Although they are not receptive to complicated explanations, children react well to honesty and badly to deceit.

The general practitioner is more fortunate than the specialist in that the former has the opportunity to get to know the child patient through a series of appointments for routine dental care. When the need for oral surgery arises, he already has the child's confidence. On the other hand, the specialist must establish communication with the young patient at the first and crucial visit. When the subject is suffering from severe pain owing to acute infection, the psychologic problems are often complex.

Children react well to all drugs and anesthetics that are suitable for adults, providing the correct dosage is used, but their high metabolic rate often makes the estimation of the correct dosage somewhat difficult. Owing to the high activity of their vital processes they often make remarkably prompt recoveries from serious illnesses. Further, since their mental processes are simpler, they tend to forget unpleasant experiences more quickly than adults.

It must be remembered that no operation should be performed upon a child without the consent of the parent or guardian, preferably written.

General Considerations

Although the surgical appointment is most significant and frequently the appointment for which the patient is most concerned, emphasis should also be directed to the postoperative appointment. It has been often said that once the patient is anesthetized and the surgical procedure is underway, he feels no pain and is really unaware of the details of the procedure. If the postoperative course has been stormy and the patient has had unanticipated pain, a poor night's sleep, and severe trismus, extreme skill, kindness, tenderness, and empathy will be necessary to manage the postoperative course. It is here that the skill of the clinician perhaps will be most completely evident. While caring for patients with oral surgical problems, the dentist will find that it takes considerable self-restraint to remain calm and pleasant in the presence of patients whose disposition is not of the best owing to the condition of stress. Yet it is imperative that he do so, for the patient subconsciously wants the dentist to be strong and confident and wishes to become dependent on him.

Practitioners of dentistry who are naturally of the extrovert type have no difficulty establishing and maintaining contact with the patient from the moment of first encounter; their problem is curbing discussions somewhat so that too much is not said, so that work gets done. On the other hand, the introvert type of dentist will realize, after some reflection, that he must make some willful effort to affect a role which is midway between modesty and self-confidence if he is to achieve a satisfactory level of rapport with his clientele. It is comforting to recall the words of the great psychologist William James on this point. He has well described the way in which one who is depressed or apathetic can forcibly alter his mood to a more desirable state by concentrating on the things that will bring about an improved state of mind. Assuming an erect posture, forcing up the corners of the mouth, and otherwise employing psychomotor activity consistent with a cheerful outlook *will actually bring about the desired mental state.* By the same token, as every child knows, sadness can be brought on by frowning, and forcing the tears to come. We feel the way our body acts.

Although not strictly a component of personality, the status of personal cleanliness and grooming is so closely related that it must be given some mention. Whiskers, dirty fingernails, unkempt hair, neglected clothing—all serve as distractors to the patient, and reduce the effectiveness of otherwise effective professional care. The same is true of the office furnishings and equipment. All these things help to prepare the patient for the pending surgical ordeal with a calm mental attitude that is conducive to a feeling of confidence.

Table 26-1. Sedatives and Tranquilizers

OFFICIAL AND COMMERCIAL NAME	PREPARATIONS AVAILABLE	ADMINISTRATION	USUAL DOSAGES	IMPORTANT PHARMACOLOGIC CONSIDERATIONS
Pentobarbital Na Nembutal® Na (Abbott)	*Tablets:* Gradumet® (long-release) 100 mg. *Capsules:* 30 mg., 50 mg., 100 mg. *Elixir:* 20 mg./5 ml. tsp. *Suppositories:* 30 mg., 60 mg., 120 mg., 200 mg. *Ampules:* 50 mg. per ml.	Oral Oral Oral Rectal I.M., I.V.	*Adults:* 30 mg. to 200 mg. q6h to q8h *Children:* 8 mg. to 60 mg. q6h to q8h	*Indications:* 1. Insomnia, simple anxiety. *Contraindications:* 1. Refer to phenobarbital. *Precautions:* 1. Short duration of effect. 2. Drowsiness, impairment of judgment. 3. May be habit-forming. *Possible Adverse Effects:* 1. Refer to phenobarbital.
Phenobarbital Luminal® (Winthrop)	*Tablets:* 16 mg., 32 mg., 100 mg. *Elixir:* 20 mg./5 ml. tsp. *Ampules:* 100 mg., 300 mg.	Oral Oral S.C., I.M., I.V.	*Adults:* 30 mg. to 100 mg. q8h to q12h *Children:* 16 mg. to 100 mg. q12h or hs	*Indications:* 1. Insomnia, simple anxiety, apprehension. 2. Convulsions. *Contraindications:* 1. History of previous reactions. 2. Liver and kidney disease. 3. Blood dyscrasias (e.g., agranulocytosis). 4. Pulmonary insufficiency. *Precautions:* 1. Drowsiness, impaired judgment. 2. Diminished response to CO_2. 3. Produces induction of liver enzymes.

Drug	Preparations	Route	Dose	Indications / Contraindications / Precautions / Adverse Effects
				4. Alteration of drug responses (e.g., anticoagulants, diphenyl-hydantoin).
				5. May be habit-forming.
				Possible Adverse Effects:
				1. Depression of respiration.
				2. Hypotension or circulatory collapse.
				3. Decreased motility of G.I. tract.
				4. Hypothermia, decreased B.M.R.
				5. Delirium and confusion (large doses).
				6. Respiratory and cardiac failure.
Amobarbital Na Amytal® Na (Lilly)	*Tablets:* 15 mg., 30 mg., 50 mg., 100 mg.	Oral	*Adults:* 65 mg. to 200 mg. hs	*Indications:* 1. Insomnia, simple anxiety.
	Capsules: 65 mg., 200 mg.	Oral	*Children:* 30 mg. to 100 mg. hs	*Contraindications:* 1. Refer to phenobarbital.
	Elixir: 22 mg./5 ml. tsp. 44 mg./5 ml. tsp.	Oral		*Precautions:* 1. Intermediate duration of effect.
	Suppositories: 200 mg.	Rectal		2. Drowsiness, impairment of judgment.
	Ampules: 65 mg., 125 mg., 250 mg., 500 mg.	I.M., I.V.	*Adults:* 65 mg. to 500 mg. I.M. or I.V.	3. May be habit-forming.
			Children: 30 mg. to 200 mg. I.M. or I.V.	*Possible Adverse Effects:* 1. Refer to phenobarbital.

531

Table 26-1. (*Continued*)

OFFICIAL AND COMMERCIAL NAME	PREPARATIONS AVAILABLE	ADMINISTRATION	USUAL DOSAGES	IMPORTANT PHARMACOLOGIC CONSIDERATIONS
Secobarbital Na Seconal® Na (Lilly)	*Tablets (Enteric Coated):* 100 mg. *Capsules:* 30 mg., 50 mg., 100 mg. *Elixir:* 22 mg./5 ml. tsp. *Suppositories:* 30 mg., 60 mg., 120 mg., 200 mg. *Ampules:* 50 mg. per ml. *Disposable Syringes:* 50 mg. per ml.	Oral Oral Oral Rectal I.M., I.V. I.M., I.V.	*Adults:* 30 mg. to 200 mg. q6h to q8h *Children:* 8 mg. to 60 mg. q6h to q12h	*Indications:* 1. Insomnia, simple anxiety. *Contraindications:* 1. Refer to phenobarbital. *Precautions:* 1. Short duration of effect. 2. Drowsiness, impairment of judgment. 3. May be habit-forming. *Possible Adverse Effects:* 1. Refer to phenobarbital.
Chloral hydrate Noctec® (Squibb) Kessodrate® (McKesson) Somnos® (Merck, Sharp & Dohme)	*Capsules:* 250 mg., 500 mg., 1000 mg. *Syrup:* 500 mg./5 ml. tsp.	Oral	*Adults:* 250 mg. to 500 mg. hs or preop.	*Indications.* 1. Insomnia. *Contraindications:* 1. Severe liver or kidney impairment. 2. Previous hypersensitivities. 3. Severe heart disease (large doses). *Precautions:* 1. Avoid simultaneous use with alcohol. 2. Metabolism of anticoagulants increases. *Possible Adverse Effects:* 1. Drowsiness and sound sleep may be produced.

532

Drug	Dosage Forms	Route	Dose	Clinical Information
Ethinamate Valmid® (Lilly)	*Tablets:* 500 mg.	Oral	*Adults:* 500 mg. to 1000 mg.	2. Only slight depression of respiration. 3. Gastric irritation. *Indications:* 1. Insomnia, mild apprehension. *Contraindications:* 1. Hypersensitive reactions previously. 2. Pregnancy. *Precautions:* 1. Avoid with use of alcohol. 2. Impaired judgment. 3. Use lower doses in elderly patients. 4. Not recommended for small children. *Possible Adverse Effects:* 1. Idiosyncrasy (rare). 2. Thrombocytopenia (rare). 3. Mild gastrointestinal symptoms.
Prochlorperazine Compazine® (Smith Kline & French)	*Tablets:* 5 mg., 10 mg., 25 mg. *Capsules (Sustained Release):* 10 mg., 15 mg., 30 mg., 75 mg. *Suppositories:* 2½* mg., 5 mg., 25 mg. *Syrup:* 5 mg./5 ml. tsp.	Oral / Oral / Rectal / Oral	*Adults:* 5 mg. to 10 mg. q6h to q8h Sustained release capsules: 10 mg. to 15 mg. q12h *Children:* 2½ mg. to 5 mg. q8h to q12h	*Indications:* 1. Anxiety, agitation, confusion. 2. Nausea and vomiting. *Contraindications:* 1. Depressed states due to drugs. 2. Bone marrow depression. 3. Pediatric diseases.

* In this case, write 2½ instead of 2.5 to preclude error through confusion with 25 mg. dose.

Table 26-1. (*Continued*)

OFFICIAL AND COMMERCIAL NAME	PREPARATIONS AVAILABLE	ADMINISTRATION	USUAL DOSAGES	IMPORTANT PHARMACOLOGIC CONSIDERATIONS
Prochlorperazine (*continued*)	*Concentrate:* 10 mg. per ml. *Vials:* 5 mg. per ml.	Oral I.M., I.V.		*Precautions:* 1. Blood dyscrasias, jaundice. 2. Impaired mental and physical abilities. 3. Potentiates other drugs. *Possible Adverse Effects:* 1. Drowsiness, dizziness, hypotension. 2. May produce leukopenia, jaundice. 3. May produce restlessness, insomnia. 4. Occasional dystonias, neurologic signs.
Perphenazine Trilafon® (Schering)	*Tablets:* 2 mg., 4 mg., 8 mg., 16 mg. *Sustained Release:* 8 mg. *Syrup:* 2 mg./5 mg. tsp. *Concentrate:* 16 mg./5 ml. tsp. *Injection:* 5 mg. per ml.	Oral Oral Oral I.M., I.V.	*Adults:* 2 mg. to 16 mg. q8h to q12h Sustained release tablets: 8 mg. q12h to q24h *Children:* 1 mg. to 2 mg. q8h	*Indications:* 1. Psychomotor overactivity, anxiety. 2. Protracted hiccoughs. 3. Nausea and vomiting. *Contraindications:* 1. CNS depression from drugs. 2. Presence of bone marrow depression. *Precautions:* 1. May mask other diagnostic symptoms. 2. May potentiate other drug activity.

Trimethobenzamide HCl
Tigan® (Roche)

Capsules:
  100 mg., 250 mg.
Suppositories:
  200 mg.
Vials:
  100 mg. per ml.

Oral

Rectal

I.M.

Adults:
  250 mg. q6h to q8h
Children:
  100 mg. to 200 mg.
  q6h to q8h

Indications:
1. Vomiting (prophylaxis and treatment).
2. Motion sickness.

Contraindications:
1. Hypersensitivity or intolerance.
2. Injectable not used in children.
3. Suppositories not used in premature or newborn infants.

Precautions:
1. Drowsiness and incoordination possible.
2. Avoid barbiturates and atropine drugs.

Possible Adverse Effects:
1. May obscure diagnostic signs.
2. Hypersensitive reactions.
3. Hypotension (occasionally).
4. Blurring of vision, drowsiness.
5. Jaundice, blood dyscrasias (rare).

Possible Adverse Effects:
1. Blurred, double vision.
2. Possible autonomic side effects.
3. Dizziness, dryness of mouth.
4. Anorexia, constipation (uncommon).
5. Insomnia, motor restlessness.
6. Dystonia in children.
7. Allergic reactions, laryngeal edema.

Table 26-1. (Continued)

OFFICIAL AND COMMERCIAL NAME	PREPARATIONS AVAILABLE	ADMINISTRATION	USUAL DOSAGES	IMPORTANT PHARMACOLOGIC CONSIDERATIONS
Meprobamate Equanil® (Wyeth) Kesso-Bamate® (McKesson) Miltown® (Wallace)	*Tablets:* 200 mg., 400 mg. *Capsules (Sustained Release):* 200 mg., 400 mg. *Oral Suspension:* 200 mg./5 ml. tsp.	Oral Oral Oral	*Adults:* 400 mg. q4h to q8h Sustained release capsules: 400 mg. q12h *Children:* 100 mg. to 200 mg. q8h to q12h	*Indications:* 1. Anxiety, tension, muscle spasm. 2. Neuromuscular disorders. 3. Insomnia due to muscular spasm. *Contraindications:* 1. Hypersensitivity and intolerance. *Precautions:* 1. Drowsiness, ataxia, impaired judgment. 2. Careful supervision during treatment. 3. May potentiate other drugs. 4. Seizures on discontinuing drug (rare). *Possible Adverse Effects:* 1. Allergic reactions (rare). 2. Ecchymosis and petechiae (occasionally). 3. Fainting, hypotension, fever (rare). 4. Blood dyscrasias, visual disturbances.
Diazepam Valium® (Roche)	*Tablets:* 2 mg., 5 mg., 10 mg. *Vials:* 5 mg.	Oral I.M. or I.V.	*Adults:* 5 mg. to 10 mg. q4h to q8h	*Indications:* 1. Anxiety, tension and stress reactions. 2. Reflex skeletal muscle spasm.

Contraindications:

1. Hypersensitivity and intolerance.
2. Glaucoma.

Precautions:

1. Potentiation of drugs (e.g., barbiturates, narcotics, antidepressants).
2. Caution in renal and hepatic disease.
3. Laryngeal spasm and cough increased.
4. Avoid use with barbiturates, alcohol.
5. Avoid use in children under age 12.

Possible Adverse Effects:

1. Hypotension, muscle weakness.
2. Drowsiness, ataxia, muscle fatigue.
3. Nausea, changes in salivation, hiccoughs.
4. Jaundice, urinary retention (rare).
5. Vertigo, blurred vision, syncope.
6. Muscle spasm, insomnia.

Table 26-2. Analgesic Agents

OFFICIAL AND COMMERCIAL NAME	PREPARATIONS AVAILABLE	ADMINISTRATION	USUAL DOSAGES	IMPORTANT PHARMACOLOGIC CONSIDERATIONS
Opiates (derived from opium)				
Morphine	*Tablets:* 5, 8, 10, 15, and 30 mg. *Hypodermic Tablets:* 5, 8, 10, and 30 mg. *Ampules:* 10 mg., 15 mg., 30 mg./ml.	Oral S.C., I.M., I.V.	*Adults:* 8 mg. to 20 mg.	*Indications:* 1. Moderately severe to severe pain. *Contraindications:* 1. Increased intracranial pressure (e.g., head injury). 2. Emphysema, asthma, etc. 3. Biliary and renal colic. 4. Simultaneous use of barbiturates and tranquilizers. *Precautions:* 1. Hypotension. 2. Narcotic addiction. *Possible Adverse Effects:* 1. Carbon dioxide retention. 2. Respiratory depression. 3. Constriction of sphincter muscles. 4. Depression of cough reflex.
Methylmorphine (Codeine)	*Tablets:* 8 mg., 15 mg., 30 mg., 60 mg. *Hypodermic Tablets:* 8 mg., 15 mg., 30 mg., 60 mg.	Oral S.C., I.M. (not I.V.)	*Adults:* 15 mg. to 60 mg.	*Indications:* 1. Moderately severe pain. *Contraindications:* 1. Respiratory diseases. 2. Hypersensitivity to codeine. 3. Not administered intravenously.

Drug	Preparation	Route	Dosage	Precautions / Indications
Codeine in Combination				
	Ampules: 30 mg./ml., 60 mg./ml.	S.C., I.M. (not I.V.)		*Precautions:* 1. May support addiction. 2. Psychologic dependence. 3. May produce nausea. 4. May produce constipation. 5. May depress cough center. *Possible Adverse Effects:* 1. Large doses in children may produce convulsions. 2. Gastrointestinal effects similar to morphine.
Ascodeen-30® (Burroughs Wellcome) A.S.A.® and Codeine Compound (Lilly)	*Tablets:* Codeine 30 mg. Aspirin 325 mg. *Capsules:* Codeine 8, 15, 30, or 60 mg. Aspirin 227 mg. Phenacetin 160 mg. Caffeine 32 mg.	Oral Oral	*Adults:* 1 tablet q4h to q6h *Adults:* 1 tablet q4h to q6h	*Indications:* 1. Moderately severe pain. *Contraindications:* 1. Respiratory diseases. 2. Allergy to ingredients. *Precautions:* 1. Cough suppression. 2. May be habit-forming. *Possible Adverse Effects:* 1. Gastrointestinal complications.
Empirin® Compound with Codeine Phosphate (Burroughs Wellcome)	*Tablets:* Codeine 8, 15, 30, or 60 mg. Aspirin 220 mg. Phenacetin 150 mg. Caffeine 30 mg.	Oral	*Adults:* 1 tablet q4h to q6h	*Indications:* 1. Moderately severe pain.
Phenaphen® with Codeine (Robins)	*Tablets or Capsules:* Codeine 15, 30, or 60 mg. Phenobarbital 15 mg. Hyoscyamine 0.03 mg. Aspirin 150 mg.	Oral	*Adults:* 1 cap. or tab. q4h to q6h	*Indications:* 1. Moderately severe pain. *Contraindications:* 1. Allergy to ingredients. 2. Glaucoma (hyoscyamus).

Table 26-2. (Continued)

OFFICIAL AND COMMERCIAL NAME	PREPARATIONS AVAILABLE	ADMINISTRATION	USUAL DOSAGES	IMPORTANT PHARMACOLOGIC CONSIDERATIONS
Phenaphen® with Codeine (continued)				*Precautions:* 1. Sedation (phenobarbital). 2. Drug interaction (phenobarbital). *Possible Adverse Effects:* 1. Increase in intraocular pressure. 2. Gastrointestinal effects (codeine). 3. Impaired judgment, drowsiness.
Tylenol® with Codeine (McNeil)	*Tablets:* Codeine 8, 15, 30, or 60 mg. Acetaminophen 300 mg.	Oral	*Adults:* 1 tablet q4h to q6h	*Indications:* 1. Moderately severe pain. 2. Fever. *Contraindications:* 1. Presence of kidney disease. 2. Children under 3 years. *Precautions:* 1. Treatment should not exceed 10 days. *Possible Adverse Effects:* 1. Methemoglobinemia (prolonged use). 2. Nausea, vomiting, anorexia. 3. Possible nephrotoxicity. 4. Gastrointestinal effects (codeine).
Percodan® (Endo)	*Tablets:* Oxycodone HCl 4.5 mg. Oxycodone terephthalate 0.38 mg. Homatropine 0.38 mg. Aspirin 224 mg. Phenacetin 160 mg. Caffeine 32 mg.	Oral	*Adults:* 1 tablet q6h	*Indications:* 1. Moderately severe to severe pain. *Contraindications:* 1. Allergy to ingredients. 2. Glaucoma (homatropine). *Precautions:* 1. Addiction (oxycodone).

540

				Possible Adverse Effects: 1. Increase in intraocular pressure. 2. Gastrointestinal effects. 3. Impaired judgment, drowsiness.
Opioids (synthetic narcotics)				

Meperidine
Demerol® (Winthrop)
	Tablets:
	  50 mg., 100 mg.
	Elixir:
	  50 mg./5 ml. tsp.
	Ampules:
	  50 mg./ml.
	  75 mg./ml.
	  100 mg./ml.
	Disposable Syringes:
	  50 mg./ml.
	  75 mg./ml.
	  100 mg./ml.
		Oral
		Oral
		S.C., I.M., I.V.
		S.C., I.M., I.V.
			Adults:
			50 mg. to 100 mg.
			q4h to q6h
				Indications:
				1. Moderately severe to severe pain.
				Contraindications:
				1. Allergy.
				2. With barbiturates, antidepressants.
				Precautions:
				1. Respiratory impairment.
				2. Addiction possible.
				Possible Adverse Effects:
				1. Respiratory depression.
				2. Sedation.
				3. Postural hypotension.
				4. Convulsions.

Methadone HCl
Dolophine® HCl
(Lilly)
	Tablets:
	  5 mg., 10 mg.
	Syrup:
	  10 mg./30 ml.
	Ampules:
	  10 mg./ml.
		Oral
		Oral
		S.C., I.M., I.V.
			Adults:
			2.5 mg. to 10 mg.
			q3h to q4h
				Indications:
				1. Moderately severe to severe pain.
				Contraindications:
				1. Same as morphine.
				2. Bradycardia.
				Precautions:
				1. Addicting liability is great.
				2. Decreased pulmonary ventilation.

Table 26-2. (*Continued*)

OFFICIAL AND COMMERCIAL NAME	PREPARATIONS AVAILABLE	ADMINISTRATION	USUAL DOSAGES	IMPORTANT PHARMACOLOGIC CONSIDERATIONS
Methadone HCl (*continued*)				*Possible Adverse Effects:* 1. Prolonged analgesic effect. 2. Sedation and respiratory depression. 3. Smooth muscle effects similar to morphine. 4. Postural hypotension.
Levorphanol Levo-Dromoran® (Roche)	*Tablets:* 2 mg. *Ampules:* 2 mg./ml.	Oral S.C., I.M., I.V.	*Adults:* 2 mg. to 3 mg. q6h to q8h	*Indications:* 1. Severe pain. *Contraindications:* 1. Same as morphine. *Precautions:* 1. More potent than morphine. 2. Addicting liability is great. 3. Decreased pulmonary ventilation. *Possible Adverse Effects:* 1. Sedation and respiratory depression. 2. Smooth muscle effects increased. 3. Potent antitussive.
Non-narcotic Agents Acetylsalicylic Acid (Aspirin) A.S.A.® Enseals® (Lilly) Ecotrine® (enteric coated) (Smith Kline & French)	*Tablets:* 300 mg., 325 mg., 650 mg.	Oral	*Adults:* 1 or 2 tablets q3h to q6h	*Indications:* 1. Mild to moderate pain. 2. Analgesic, antipyretic, anti-rheumatic. *Contraindications:* 1. Gastrointestinal irritation, ulcers. 2. Blood coagulation disorders.

Precautions:
1. Tolerated poorly by young children.
2. Gastric irritation.

Possible Adverse Effects:
1. Gastrointestinal bleeding.
2. Acid-base balance changes.
3. Tinnitus, blurring of vision, dizziness.

Drug	Composition	Route	Dosage	
Aspirin in Combination Empirin® Compound (Burroughs Wellcome)	Tablets: Aspirin 310 mg. Phenacetin 150 mg. Caffeine 30 mg.	Oral	Adults: 1 or 2 tablets q4h to q6h	Indications: 1. Mild to moderately severe pain. 2. Fever. Contraindications: 1. Gastrointestinal irritation, ulcer. 2. Blood coagulation disorders. Precautions: 1. Gastric irritation. 2. Tolerated poorly by young children. Possible Adverse Effects: 1. Nausea, vomiting, anorexia. 2. Gastrointestinal bleeding. 3. Tinnitus, visual disturbances. 4. Dizziness.
Equagesic® (Wyeth)	Tablets: Ethoheptazine 75 mg. Meprobamate 150 mg. Aspirin 250 mg.	Oral	Adults: 1 tablet q4h to q6h	Indications: 1. Analgesic, antianxiety. 2. Tension and skeletal muscle spasm.

Table 26-2. (*Continued*)

OFFICIAL AND COMMERCIAL NAME	PREPARATIONS AVAILABLE	ADMINISTRATION	USUAL DOSAGES	IMPORTANT PHARMACOLOGIC CONSIDERATIONS
Equagesic® (*continued*)				*Contraindications:* 1. Allergy and intolerance to ingredient. 2. Avoid in pregnancy and lactation. 3. Avoid in children 12 years and younger. *Precautions:* 1. Avoid prolonged and excessive doses. 2. Potentiation of drugs and alcohol. 3. Possible habituation. *Possible Adverse Effects:* 1. Seizures with abrupt withdrawal. 2. Reaction time and judgment impaired. 3. Blood dyscrasias (rare).
Propoxyphene Darvon® (Lilly)	*Capsules:* 32 mg., 65 mg.	Oral	*Adults:* 1 capsule q4h to q6h	*Indications:* 1. Moderately severe pain. *Contraindications:* 1. Allergy or intolerance to ingredients. 2. Orphenadrine-containing compounds.
Darvon® with A.S.A.® (Lilly)	*Capsules:* Propoxyphene 60 mg. Aspirin 325 mg.	Oral	*Adults:* 1 capsule q4h to q6h	*Precautions:* 1. Reaction time and judgment impaired. 2. Avoid using for young children.

Drug	Preparation	Route	Dosage	Indications / Contraindications / Precautions / Possible Adverse Effects
Darvon® Compound-65 (Lilly)	*Capsules:* Propoxyphene 65 mg. Aspirin 227 mg. Phenacetin 162 mg. Caffein 32.4 mg.	Oral	*Adults:* 1 capsule q4h to q6h	*Possible Adverse Effects:* 1. Dizziness, excitement, insomnia. 2. Sedation or euphoria (rare). 3. Gastrointestinal disturbances. 4. Skin rashes. 5. Convulsions (with overdose).
Ethohepatzine Zactirin® Compound (Wyeth)	*Tablets:* Ethoheptazine 100 mg. Aspirin 227 mg. Phenacetin 162 mg. Caffeine 32.4 mg.	Oral	*Adults:* 1 tablet q4h to q6h	*Indications:* 1. Moderately severe pain. *Contraindications:* 1. Hypersensitivity or intolerance. 2. Gastric irritation or bleeding. *Precautions:* 1. Dizziness and light-headedness. 2. Drowsiness and impaired judgment. *Possible Adverse Effects:* 1. Gastrointestinal disturbances. 2. CNS stimulation (rare).
Acetaminophen Tylenol® (McNeil)	*Tablets:* 325 mg. *Elixir:* 120 mg./5 ml. tsp.	Oral Oral	*Adults:* 1 or 2 tablets q6h *Children:* ½ to 2 tsp. q6h	*Indications:* 1. Analgesic and antipyretic. *Contraindications:* 1. Hypersensitivity or intolerance. *Precautions:* 1. Presence of kidney disease. 2. Children under 3 years. *Possible Adverse Effects:* 1. Nausea, vomiting, anorexia. 2. Possible nephrotoxicity. 3. Methemoglobinemia on prolonged use.

Table 26-2. (Continued)

OFFICIAL AND COMMERCIAL NAME	PREPARATIONS AVAILABLE	ADMINISTRATION	USUAL DOSAGES	IMPORTANT PHARMACOLOGIC CONSIDERATIONS
Mefenamic Acid Ponstel® (Parke-Davis)	*Capsules:* 250 mg.	Oral	*Adults:* 2 capsules for first dose—then 1 capsule q6h	*Indications:* 1. Analgesic, anti-inflammatory. *Contraindications:* 1. Intestinal ulceration, kidney disease. 2. Women of childbearing age. 3. Not used in children under 14 years. 4. Intolerance or allergy. *Precautions:* 1. Asthma. 2. Allergy or hypersensitivity. *Possible Adverse Effects:* 1. Drowsiness, dizziness, nervousness 2. Gastrointestinal disturbances.
Pentazocine Talwin® (Winthrop)	*Tablets:* 50 mg. *Parenteral Solution:* 30 mg. per ml.	Oral S.C., I.M., I.V.	*Adults:* 30 mg. to 60 mg. q4h	*Indications:* 1. Moderately severe to severe pain. *Contraindications:* 1. Head injury (increased pressure). 2. Pathologic brain conditions. 3. Pregnancy. *Precautions:* 1. May support drug addiction. 2. Avoid in children under 12 years. 3. Respiratory depression (any cause).

4. Liver and kidney disease.

Possible Adverse Effects:

1. Hallucinations, disorientation (rare).
2. Dizziness, sedation, uncoordination.
3. Narcotic antagonism in addicts.
4. Gastrointestinal effects.
5. Hypotension, tachycardia.

Table 26-3. Antibiotics

OFFICIAL AND COMMERCIAL NAME	PREPARATIONS AVAILABLE	ADMINISTRATION	USUAL DOSAGES	IMPORTANT PHARMACOLOGIC CONSIDERATIONS
Potassium Penicillin G Hyasorb® (Key) Kesso-Pen® (McKesson) Pentids® (Squibb) Pfizerpen® (Pfizer) Sugracillin™ (Upjohn) Penicillin G Potassium for injection (Many suppliers)	*Tablets:* 200,000 U., 250,000 U., 400,000 U., 800,000 U. *Capsules:* 400,000 U., 800,000 U. *Syrup:* 125,000 U./5 ml. tsp. 200,000 U./5 ml. tsp. 250,000 U./5 ml. tsp. 400,000 U./5 ml. tsp. *Vials (Sterile Powder):* 400,000 U., 800,000 U., 1,000,000 U., 5,000,000 U., 10,000,000 U., 20,000,000 U.	Oral Oral Oral I.M., I.V., I.V. drip	*Adults:* 1 or 2 capsules or tablets q3h to q8h 1 or 2 tsp. q3h to q8h Parenteral dosage and frequency of administration determined by severity of disease.	*Indications:* 1. Gram-positive organisms (strep., staph.). 2. Oral and parenteral use. *Contraindications:* 1. Previous reaction to penicillin. *Precautions:* 1. Oral dosages—avoid mealtime. 2. Water solutions deteriorate rapidly. *Possible Adverse Effects:* 1. Anaphylactoid reactions (rare). 2. Overgrowth of some organisms. 3. Allergic reactions. 4. Anemia, leukopenia, thrombocytopenia.
Benzathine Penicillin G Bicillin® (Wyeth) Permapen® (Pfizer) Benzathine Penicillin G with Procaine Penicillin G Bicillin® C-R (Wyeth)	*Disposable Syringes:* 300,000 U. per ml. 600,000 U. per ml. *Disposable Syringes:* 300,000 U. per ml. (150,000 U. of each), 600,000 U. per ml. (300,000 U. of each)	Deep I.M. injection only	*Adults:* 1 or 2 ml. I.M. every 5 to 7 days.	*Indications:* 1. Gram-positive organisms (strep., staph.). 2. Deep I.M. use only. *Contraindications:* 1. Previous reaction to penicillin. *Precautions:* 1. Avoid accidental I.V. injection. 2. Not for oral administration.

548

Drug	Form & Strength	Route	Adults	Notes
Procaine Penicillin G Crysticillin® 300 A.S. Crysticillin® 600 A.S. (Squibb) Duracillin® A.S. (Lilly) Pentids®-P 300 A.S. Pentids®-P 600 A.S. (Squibb) Wycillin® (Wyeth)	*Vials:* 300,000 U. per ml., 600,000 U. per ml.	Deep I.M. injection only	*Adults:* 1 or 2 ml. q24h	*Possible Adverse Effects:* 1. Anaphylactoid reactions (rare). 2. Overgrowth of some organisms. 3. Allergic reactions. 4. Anemia, leukopenia, thrombocytopenia. *Indications:* 1. Gram-positive organisms (strep., staph.). 2. Deep I.M. use only. *Contraindications:* 1. Previous reaction to penicillin. 2. Not for oral administration. *Precautions:* 1. Avoid accidental I.V. injection. 2. Use deep I.M. injection (e.g., buttock).
Phenoxymethyl Penicillin (Penicillin V) Compocillin® (Abbott) Ledercillin® (Lederle) Pen-Vee® (Wyeth) V-Cillin® (Lilly)	*Tablets:* 125 mg., 250 mg., 500 mg. *Chewable Tablets:* 125 mg., 250 mg.	Oral Oral	*Adults:* 1 or 2 tablets q4h to q8h 1 or 2 wafers q4h to q8h	*Possible Adverse Effects:* 1. Anaphylactoid reactions (rare). 2. Overgrowth of some organisms. 3. Allergic reactions. *Indications:* 1. Gram-positive organisms (strep., staph.). 2. Oral use only. *Contraindications:* 1. Previous reaction to penicillin. *Precautions:* 1. Not for parenteral use.

Table 26-3. (Continued)

OFFICIAL AND COMMERCIAL NAME	PREPARATIONS AVAILABLE	ADMINISTRATION	USUAL DOSAGES	IMPORTANT PHARMACOLOGIC CONSIDERATIONS
Phenoxymethyl Penicillin (Penicillin V) (continued) V-Cillin®, Pediatric (Lilly)	*Oral Solutions:* 125 mg./5 ml. tsp. 250 mg./5 ml. tsp. *Oral Suspensions:* 180 mg./5 ml. tsp. *Pediatric Drops:* 125 mg./2.5 ml. dropper	Oral Oral Oral	*Adults:* 1 or 2 tsp. q4h to q8h 2.5 ml. to 5.0 ml. q4h to q8h	*Possible Adverse Effects:* 1. Anaphylactoid reactions (rare). 2. Overgrowth of some organisms. 3. Allergic reactions. 4. Anemia, leukopenia, thrombocytopenia.
Ampicillin Alpen® (Lederle) Amcill® (Parke-Davis) Omnipen® (Wyeth) Penbritin® (Ayerst) Polycillin® (Bristol) Principen® (Squibb) Totacillin® (Beecham)	*Capsules:* 250 mg., 500 mg. *Chewable Tablets:* 125 mg. *Oral Suspension:* 125 mg./5 ml. tsp. 250 mg./5 ml. tsp. *Pediatric Drops:* 100 mg. per ml. *Vials (parenteral use):* 125 mg., 250 mg., 500 mg., 1000 mg., 2000 mg.	Oral Oral Oral Oral I.M., I.V.	*Adults:* 250 mg. to 500 mg. q6h *Children:* 6.25 mg. to 12.5 mg. per kg. body weight q6h *Adults:* 250 mg. to 500 mg. I.M. or I.V. q6h *Children:* 12.5 mg. to 25 mg. per kg. body weight I.M. or I.V. q6h	*Indications:* 1. Broad spectrum (gram pos. and neg.). 2. Oral and parenteral use. *Contraindications:* 1. Previous reactions to penicillins. 2. Penicillinase-producing organisms. *Precautions:* 1. Not used in pregnancy. 2. Reserve the parenteral form for severe infections in patients unable to take the oral forms. *Possible Adverse Effects:* 1. Anaphylactoid reactions (rare).

Drug	Dosage Forms	Route	Dosage	Indications / Contraindications / Precautions / Adverse Effects
Methicillin Na Staphcillin® (Bristol)	Vials: 1 gm., 4 gm., 6 gm.	I.M., I.V.	Adults: 1 gm. q4h to q6h I.M. or I.V. Children: 25 mg. per kg. body weight q4h to q8h I.M. or I.V.	2. Overgrowth of some organisms. 3. Allergic reactions. 4. Anemia, leukopenia, thrombocytopenia. Indications: 1. Resistant staph. infection only. 2. Penicillinase-resistant organisms. Contraindications: 1. Previous reaction to penicillin. Precautions: 1. I.M. or I.V. use only. Possible Adverse Effects: 1. Allergic reactions. 2. Overgrowth of some organisms.
Tetracycline Achromycin® (Lederle) Kesso-Tetra® (McKesson) Panmycin® (Upjohn) Steclin® (Squibb) Tetracyn® (Roerig) Tetrachel® (Rachelle)	Capsules: 50 mg., 100 mg., 125 mg., 250 mg., 500 mg. Tablets: 100 mg., 250 mg. Syrup: 125 mg./5 ml. tsp. Oral Suspension: 250 mg./5 ml. tsp. Pediatric Drops: 100 mg. per ml. Vials (intramuscular use): 100 mg., 200 mg., 250 mg.	Oral Oral Oral Oral Oral I.M.	Adults: 250 mg. to 500 mg. q6h to q12h Children: 5 mg to 10 mg. per kg. body weight q6h to q12h Adults: 150 mg. to 250 mg., I.M. q12	Indications: 1. Broad spectrum (gram pos. and neg.). 2. Oral and parenteral use. Contraindications: 1. Previous reaction to tetracyclines. 2. Some resistant strains (strep., staph.). 3. Renal impairment. Precautions: 1. Forms calcium complex in teeth and bones. 2. Avoid dosage with milk, food. 3. Pain with I.M. injection.

Table 26-3. (*Continued*)

OFFICIAL AND COMMERCIAL NAME	PREPARATIONS AVAILABLE	ADMINISTRATION	USUAL DOSAGES	IMPORTANT PHARMACOLOGIC CONSIDERATIONS
Tetracycline (*continued*)	*Vials* (*intravenous use*): 100 mg., 250 mg., 500 mg.	I.V. only	*Children:* 2.5 mg. to 5 mg. per kg. body weight q12h *Adults:* 150 mg. to 500 mg. q12h I.V. Drip *Children:* 2.5 mg. to 5 mg. per kg. body weight q12h I.V. Drip	*Possible Adverse Effects:* 1. Liver toxicity. 2. Photosensitivity to sunlight (skin). 3. Overgrowth of some organisms. 4. Allergic reactions. 5. Gastrointestinal disturbances. 6. Anemia, leukopenia.
Lincomycin Lincocin® (Upjohn)	*Capsules:* 250 mg., 500 mg. *Solution* (*parenteral use*): 50 mg. per ml.	Oral I.M., I.V.	*Adults:* 500 mg. q6h to q8h *Children:* 10 mg. to 15 mg. per kg. body weight q6h to q8h *Adults:* 600 mg. q8h to q12h I.M. or I.V. *Children:* 2 mg. to 5 mg. per kg. body weight q8h to q12h I.M. or I.V.	*Indications:* 1. Gram-positive organisms (strep., staph.). 2. Oral and parenteral use. *Contraindications:* 1. Previous reaction to lincomycin. *Precautions:* 1. Use in pregnancy not established. 2. Use in liver disease not established. 3. Impaired renal function: decrease dose. 4. Cross resistance with clindamycin.

| | | Capsules:
75 mg., 150 mg.
Syrup:
50 mg. per ml. | | Adults:
150 mg. to 450 mg.
q6h
Children:
2 mg. to 5 mg. per
kg. body weight q6h | Oral
Oral | *Possible Adverse Effects:*
1. Hypersensitive reactions (rare).
2. Gastrointestinal disturbances.
3. Overgrowth of some organisms.
4. Anemia, leukopenia (rare). |

Clindamycin
Cleocin® (Upjohn)

Indications:
1. Anaerobic organisms.
2. Oral administration only.

Contraindications:
1. Previous reaction to clindamycin.

Precautions:
1. Cross resistance with lincomycin.
2. Possible antagonism with erythomycin.
3. Use in pregnancy not established.
4. Impaired renal function: decrease dose.

Possible Adverse Effects:
1. Hypersensitive reactions (rare).
2. Gastrointestinal disturbances.
3. Overgrowth of some organisms.
4. Anemia, leukopenia (rare).

Table 26-3. (*Continued*)

OFFICIAL AND COMMERCIAL NAME	PREPARATIONS AVAILABLE	ADMINISTRATION	USUAL DOSAGES	IMPORTANT PHARMACOLOGIC CONSIDERATIONS
Erythromycin E-Mycin (Upjohn) Erythrocin® (Abbott) Ilosone® (Lilly) Ilotycin® (Lilly) Ilotycin® Gluceptate, I.V. (Lilly) Pediamycin™ (Ross)	*Capsules:* 125 mg., 250 mg. *Tablets:* 100 mg., 125 mg., 250 mg. *Chewable Tablets:* 125 mg. *Drops:* 100 mg. per ml. *Oral Liquid:* 125 mg./5 ml. tsp. 250 mg./5 ml. tsp. *Oral Suspension:* 125 mg./5 ml. tsp. 200 mg./5 ml. tsp. *Suppositories:* 125 mg.	Oral Oral Oral Oral Oral Oral Oral	*Adults:* 250 mg. to 500 mg. q6h *Children:* 10 mg. to 15 mg. per kg. body weight q6h	*Indications:* 1. Gram-positive organisms (strep., staph.). 2. Oral and parenteral use. *Contraindications:* 1. Previous reaction to erythromycin. *Precautions:* 1. Water solutions deteriorate rapidly. 2. Pain with I.M. injection. 3. Venous irritation with I.V. injection. *Possible Adverse Effects:* 1. Allergic reactions. 2. Gastrointestinal disturbances. 3. Overgrowth of some organisms.
	Vials (intramuscular use): 200 mg., 500 mg.	I.M. only	*Adults:* 100 mg. to 250 mg. I.M. q4h to q6h *Children:* 1 mg. to 2 mg. I.M. per kg. body weight q4h to q6h	*Caution:* 1. Use I.V. route for short periods of time until patient can take drug orally. 2. Make *initial* solution with sterile water from glass-sealed ampules *only* to ensure complete solution and preclude gel formation. Further dilution with saline or glucose solution may be made according to directions.
	Ampules (intravenous use): 250 mg., 500 mg., 1000 mg.	I.V.	*Adults:* 250 mg. to 500 mg. I.V. q6h	

554

Table 26-4. Antihistamines

OFFICIAL AND COMMERCIAL NAME	PREPARATIONS AVAILABLE	ADMINISTRATION	USUAL DOSAGES	IMPORTANT PHARMACOLOGIC CONSIDERATIONS
Diphenhydramine Benadryl® (Parke-Davis)	*Capsules:* 25 mg., 50 mg. *Ampules:* 10 mg. per ml., 50 mg. per ml.	Oral I.M., I.V.	*Adults:* 10 mg. to 50 mg. q6h to q8h *Children:* 12.5 mg. to 25 mg. q6h to q12h	*Indications:* 1. Histamine reactions, allergic reactions. 2. Nausea and vomiting, motion sickness. 3. Insomnia. *Contraindications:* 1. Asthma, glaucoma. 2. Bladder neck obstruction, prostatitis. 3. Peptic ulcer, pyloric obstruction.
Tripelennamine Pyribenzamine® (Ciba)	*Tablets:* 25 mg., 50 mg. *Tablets (long acting):* 50 mg., 100 mg. *Elixir:* 25 mg./5 ml. tsp.	Oral Oral Oral	*Adults:* 50 mg. to 100 mg. q4h Long acting tablets: 100 mg. q12h *Children:* 25 mg. to 50 mg. q6h to q8h	*Precautions:* 1. Possesses an atropine-like activity. 2. Addictive effects with CNS depressants. 3. Blurring of vision, diplopia. *Possible Adverse Effects:* 1. Convulsions, confusion, restlessness. 2. Impaired judgment and motor skills. 3. Dryness of mouth, nose, throat. 4. Vertigo, hypotension, insomnia. 5. Drug rash, urticaria, photosensitivity. 6. Hemolytic anemia.

Table 26-4. (*Continued*)

OFFICIAL AND COMMERCIAL NAME	PREPARATIONS AVAILABLE	ADMINISTRATION	USUAL DOSAGES	IMPORTANT PHARMACOLOGIC CONSIDERATIONS
Chlorpheniramine Chlor-Trimeton® (Schering) Teldrin® (Smith, Kline & French)	*Tablets:* 4 mg.	Oral	*Adults:* 8 mg. to 12 mg. q6h to q12h Repeat action tablets: 8 mg. to 12 mg. q12h to q24h	*Indications:* 1. Histamine reactions, allergic reaction. 2. Bronchial cough.
	Tablets (repeat action): 8 mg., 12 mg.	Oral		*Contraindications:* 1. Hypersensitivity and intolerance.
	Syrup: 2 mg./15 ml. tsp.	Oral	*Children:* 2 mg. to 4 mg. q6h to q8h	*Precautions:* 1. Moderate drowsiness (infrequent). 2. Dryness of mouth, nausea, anorexia. 3. Diplopia.
	Ampules: 100 mg. per ml. (S.C., I.M.) 10 mg. per ml. (I.V.)	S.C., I.M., I.V.	*Adults:* 10 mg. I.V. q6h to q12h; 100 mg. I.M. q24h *Children:* 5 mg. I.V. q6h to q12h; 5 mg. to 10 mg. I.M. q24h	*Possible Adverse Effects:* 1. Impaired judgment and motor skills. 2. Dizziness, weakness, restlessness. 3. Dysuria, polyuria. 4. Hypotension (transient).
Dimenhydrinate Dramamine® (Searle)	*Tablets:* 50 mg. *Oral Solution:* 15 mg./5 ml. tsp.	Oral Oral	*Adults:* 50 mg. q4h *Children:* 12.5 mg. to 50 mg. q8h to q12h	*Indications:* 1. Vertigo, motion sickness, nausea. *Contraindications:* 1. With certain antibiotics.
	Suppositories: 100 mg.	Rectal		*Precautions:* 1. Drowsiness. 2. Inject slowly.
	Ampules: 50 mg. per ml. (I.M.) 10 mg. per ml. (I.V.)	I.M. I.V.	*Adults:* 50 mg. I.M. or I.V. q4h *Children:* 12.5 mg. to 25.0 mg. q8h to q12h	*Possible Adverse Effects:* 1. Vertigo with antibiotic therapy. 2. Drowsiness, motor skills impaired.

References

1. Malloy, D. J.: Personal communication, 1971.
2. Swinyard, E. A.: Principles of Prescription Order Writing. In The Pharmacological Basis of Therapeutics, 4th ed., pp. 1701–1719. L. Goodman and A. Gilman (Eds.), Macmillan, New York, 1970.
3. Friend, D. G.: Principles and practices of prescription writing. J. Clin. Pharmacol. Ther., 6:411–416, 1965.

Additional References

Clark, H. B., Jr.: Practical Oral Surgery, 3rd ed. Philadelphia, Lea & Febiger, 1965.

Jones, R. G.: Antibiotics of the penicillin and cephalosporin family. Am. Sci., 58:404–411, 1970.
Myers, F. H., Jawetz, E., and Goldfien, A.: Review of Medical Pharmacology and Therapeutics, 2nd ed. Los Altos, Calif., Lange Medical Publishers, 1970.
Physician's Desk Reference, 24th and 25th eds. Oradell, N.J., Litton Publications, 1970, 1971.
Weinstein, L.: Antibiotics. In The Pharmacological Basis of Therapeutics. 4th ed., pp. 1277–1278. L. Goodman and A. Gilman (Eds.). New York, Macmillan, 1970.

27 Tracheostomy

CEDRIC A. QUICK

Tracheostomy means the provision of an alternative airway by opening the anterior tracheal wall. The ancient Greeks, about 200 B.C., gave sporadic descriptions of operations that involved opening the trachea. Until the nineteenth century the operation was performed for acute glottic obstructions caused by foreign bodies and suppuration of the throat. During the nineteenth century the place of tracheostomy in the management of diphtheria was recognized, and the majority of tracheostomies performed at that time were for this disease. During the polio epidemic in the United States in the 1950s many lives were saved by the timely performance of this operation. Tracheostomy is now performed for many diverse indications and its application has extended far beyond the realm for which it was originally described. Consequently, its role in general medical care has grown in importance. Dentists may not find it unusual to be confronted with a patient possessing a tracheostomy, or more important, be confronted with the necessity of performing the lifesaving procedure of tracheostomy.

From time to time, fortunately not too often, a tooth or a dental appliance may become dislodged and pass from the oral cavity into the pharynx. From the phar-

ynx the object may pass rapidly into the larynx and bronchus during an inspiratory gasp of the patient (Fig. 27-1A) or to the esophagus when the patient swallows or gags (Fig. 27-1B). At this point the object, now termed foreign body, is beyond retrieval by use of the fingers, or the kind of forceps readily available to the dentist. Most of the aspirated objects are small and pass directly into a bronchus where they are not an immediate threat to life and there is sufficient time to transfer the patient to a medical facility for removal by bronchoscopy. Similarly swallowed foreign bodies are not dire emergencies but should be referred without delay for removal by esophagoscopy. However, if the object should become wedged in the larynx or trachea, an emergency situation exists which may result in complete airway obstruction and fatal asphyxiation.

It is incumbent upon those who work in the proximity of "the airway" to be familiar with the applied anatomy and physiology of the upper airway, and the methods of relieving an obstructed airway including the operation of tracheostomy. Indeed, all who deal with patients of all varieties should know the fundamentals of these procedures.

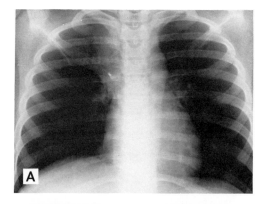

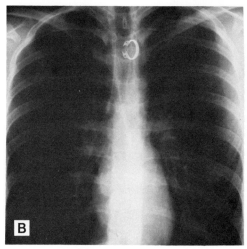

Fig. 27-1. (A) Fragment of tooth with amalgam filling in right upper lobe bronchus. (B) Rubber dam clamp in esophagus.

Applied Anatomy and Physiology

The trachea is a relatively rigid tube lying in the midline of the neck and upper mediastinum. It extends from the lower border of the larynx to its division into the main bronchi at the lower border of the manubrium. In the living erect individual, the trachea may descend a full 2 inches below this level during full inspiration. Its main relations throughout its length are to the esophagus posteriorly and to the main vessels of the neck on either side (Fig. 27-2). In the neck these vessels are enclosed in the carotid sheath. The lobes of the thyroid gland lie along-side the trachea, extending from the larynx down to the sixth tracheal ring, with the thyroid isthmus crossing the trachea approximately between the second and fourth rings. These structures are covered by the pretracheal layer of fascia. As it enters the thorax, the trachea lies close to the undersurface of the manubrium, and just below this level the trachea with the pretracheal fascia is crossed by the innominate vein, which runs horizontally. The recurrent laryngeal nerves lie in the groove between the esophagus and the trachea.

The trachea consists of a musculofibrous tube made rigid by incomplete rings of cartilage. These are incomplete posteriorly. Between each ring and bridging the defect posteriorly is the trachealis muscle, composed of nonstriped muscle fibers. The trachea is lined with pseudostratified ciliated columnar epithelium. Numerous mucus- and serum-secreting glands fill the subepithelial layers (the corium).

Inspired air, having passed through the nose, is approximately 75 per cent saturated and warmed to 36° C. or 96.8° F. Most of the particulate matter has also been removed. The final adjustment to internal body temperature and humidity is accomplished by the trachea. It is estimated that every 24 hours about 0.5 liter of body water is lost to the atmosphere from the lungs. Moving over the surface of the trachea in an upward direction is a layer of mucus—the so-called mucous blanket. This removes any other particulate matter, such as dust and bacteria, that have not been removed by the nose. An accumulation of this mucus stimulates the cough reflex. The mechanism of the cough reflex is that pressure in the chest is

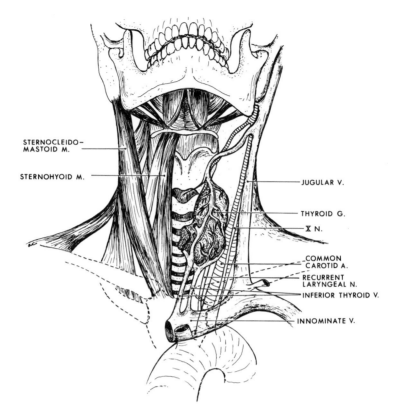

STERNOCLEIDO-
MASTOID M.

STERNOHYOID M.

JUGULAR V.

THYROID G.

X N.

COMMON
CAROTID A.

RECURRENT
LARYNGEAL N.

INFERIOR THYROID V.

INNOMINATE V.

Fig. 27-2. Dissection of the neck. Superficial (patient's right), and deep (patient's left).

raised and a considerable force is exerted on the closed glottis. With simultaneous action the glottis opens and the chest wall muscles and diaphragm contract even harder, forcing the air out of the trachea in an explosive blast. An opening into the anterior wall of the trachea would render the "glottic stop" ineffective.

If the nose and pharynx are bypassed, as in tracheostomy, the task of humidification and warming would rest solely with the trachea, which cannot suddenly cope with this task.

Indications for Tracheostomy

About 40 per cent of all tracheostomies are performed for head injuries or other central nervous system problems; about 10 per cent, for acute laryngeal obstructions of all causes; 10 per cent, in the treatment of chest injuries or lung diseases; and slightly over 30 per cent, to facilitate removal of obstructing secretions. A discussion of all conditions that may be helped by tracheostomy would be too lengthy for this text, but some of the possibilities are outlined below:

1. Central nervous system.
   a. Severe head injury.
   b. Coma.
   c. Cervical cord injury.
   d. Nerve disorders such as poliomyelitis.
2. Chest wall and associated muscles of respiration.
   a. Trauma, "stove-in" chest, or "flail chest."
   b. Prolonged curarization (flaxedilization), as in the treatment of tetanus.
   c. Major chest or cardiac surgery.

3. Airway patency (may involve extrinsic pressure, lesions of the wall, or intrinsic obstruction).

   a. The mouth and pharynx.

      (1) *Trauma*. Severe lacerations of the tongue and palate with swelling; facial fracture involving maxilla or mandible; as a prophylactic procedure prior to extensive surgery in these areas.

      (2) *Infection*. Tooth abscess with cervical cellulitis (Ludwig's angina); severe tonsillitis; quinsy.

      (3) *Edema*. Insect sting of tongue; allergic stomatitis from any cause; pemphigoid.

   b. Larynx and upper trachea.

      (1) *Trauma*. Direct blow to the throat, as occurs in karate, or more commonly, in road traffic accidents.

      (2) *Infection*. Epiglottitis; laryngitis; croup; laryngitis secondary to upper respiratory infection or lung disease.

      (3) *Edema*. Associated with trauma, infection, neoplasm, or allergic response, as in anaphylaxis.

      (4) *Foreign bodies*. Food particles, objects such as coins or toys, dental plates, tooth fragments, dental swabs or instruments.

      (5) *Neoplasia*. Performed because of airway obstruction or preliminary to surgery.

4. Lung diseases; acute or chronic diseases of the terminal bronchi or lung parenchyma.

Tracheostomy is of value in most cases of respiratory insufficiency. It decreases the dead space about 150 ml. Although this is a negligible amount in individuals with a normal tidal volume, it represents a considerable improvement in patients whose tidal volume is reduced to 300 to 400 ml. Tracheostomy reduces the resistance to airflow, making it easier for a patient to breathe. Finally, it allows removal of secretions without physical distress to the patient. These factors result in a considerable increase in the efficiency of respiration. However, in certain emphysema patients, a sudden reduction in airway resistance may be detrimental. These patients may need the controlled resistance provided by the larynx to force air out of the distended alveoli through the bronchioles, which have a tendency to collapse.

The foregoing discussion illustrates many of the conditions for which tracheostomy has been performed or for which tracheostomy may be considered. However, it must be stressed that many of these conditions can be handled by other means (see below). For all these indications, the great question is whether the tracheostomy should be an emergency or elective procedure. In most cases today it is possible to predict the progress of a patient, and with careful planning, the surgeon will be able to perform an elective tracheostomy before an emergency arises. In some instances, such as acute obstruction due to trauma, the prompt performance of emergency tracheostomy may be lifesaving.

Restoration of Airway

The provision of an adequate airway is the first procedure to be done in all cases of obstructed breathing. This may be accomplished by several methods:

1. Positioning the patient, retracting the tongue, elevating the mandible, and inserting an oral airway.
2. Directly visualizing the larynx with a laryngoscope, which allows the removal of foreign bodies, secretions or aspirants, and permits the insertion of an endotracheal tube or bronchoscope.
3. Catheterizing the trachea with a large bore needle (no. 15 intracath).
4. Heimlich maneuver (see Chapter 7). This valuable procedure has saved many lives when total obstruction of the larynx or trachea occurs by aspirated foreign bodies. It is most useful for soft foreign bodies such as meat, fruit, or vegetables. When the objects are sharp and irregular such as a partial dental plate, the procedure is less successful and may cause trauma to the mucosal lining. This procedure is always worth attempting but should not be relied upon as the only resuscitative measure.
5. Laryngotomy or cricothyroidotomy.
6. Tracheostomy.

The method of choice depends largely upon the facilities available, the condition of the patient, and the knowledge and skill of the attendant. Per oral intubation has the merit of being relatively easy, quick, and bloodless (usually). The disadvantages are that secretions are difficult to remove, the endotracheal tube is difficult to clean, and replacement necessitates further laryngoscopy. Swallowing around the tube is also extremely difficult. Prolonged intubation in a conscious patient results in excessive movement causing mucosal ulceration, which may lead to granulomatous lesions and stenosis of the trachea or vocal cords.

Catheterization of the trachea with a large bore needle is not recommended. The choice between cricothyroidotomy and tracheostomy will be discussed following a description of the techniques involved in the performance of these operations.

Technique of Elective Tracheostomy

The operative technique of elective tracheostomy is described first, and those of emergency procedures subsequently. The patient should be taken into the operating room and placed in the most favorable position, which is supine with the foot of the table lowered to about 30° (Fig. 27-3). This empties the major veins of the neck and lessens the risk of excessive bleeding during the operation. A sandbag is placed underneath the shoulders and lower neck, extending the head as far back as is comfortable. The greatest length of the trachea is then brought into the neck. The chin, trachea, suprasternal notch, and axis of the body must all lie in the same line with no rotation. Throughout the procedure it is *imperative* that dissection be confined to the midline structures.

Anesthesia

General or local anesthesia may be used. Local anesthesia (1 per cent Xylocaine with epinephrine) may be injected immediately after skin preparation, making certain that the needle does not run into the deep tissues to cause hematoma. After the appropriate interval the skin incision can be made and deeper structures can then be anesthetized by direct infiltration as necessary. General anesthesia with endotracheal intubation offers many advantages, but the necessity for the operation often contraindicates its use.

Incision

Before starting, ensure that the chosen tracheostomy tubes are adequate and all

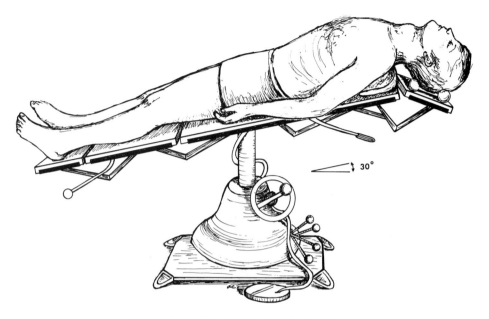

Fig. 27-3. Position of patient for tracheostomy.

components fit and work properly. A horizontal incision is made at the junction of the lower and middle third of the region between the thyroid cartilage (Adam's apple) and the suprasternal notch (Fig. 27-4). It should be about 2 inches in length and extend from the anterior border of one sternomastoid muscle to the other (Fig. 27-5). The incision should be carried through the skin and the platysma.

Subcutaneous Dissection

Reflection of the skin flaps is best accomplished by blunt dissection using a gauze piece over the finger. The deep fascia should then be incised vertically in the midline. Sometimes one or two prominent veins (branches of the superficial jugular) are met and these should be either sealed with cautery or ligated. The strap muscles on either side can then be reflected laterally and retracted by the assistant, which reveals the thyroid isthmus. If this structure is too prominent and prevents sufficient access to the tracheal surface, it should be divided. If there is any doubt, it is better and safer to divide the isthmus definitively between clamps. Transfixion ligatures of strong catgut or silk should be applied to the cut ends of the isthmus and secured firmly.

Exposure of the Trachea

The anterior surface of the trachea should now be cleaned, and the last remnants of the tracheal fascia may be removed by blunt dissection using a gauze piece. Expose only a sufficient length of the trachea to allow an adequate opening

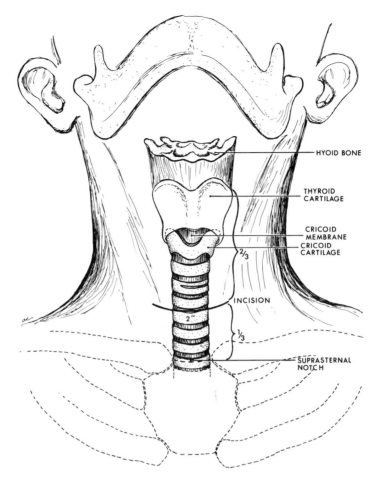

Fig. 27-4. Landmarks of tracheostomy incision.

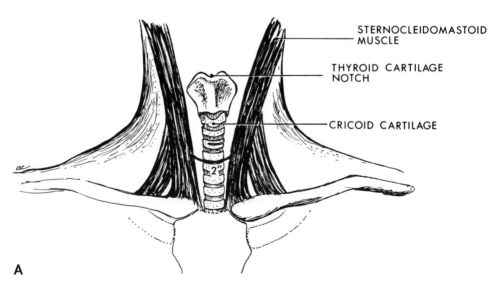

A

Fig. 27-5. Stages in the performance of elective tracheostomy. (A) Skin incision. (B) Incision of pretracheal fascia. (C) Division and ligation of thyroid isthmus. (D and E) Incision of trachea. (F) Insertion of tube.

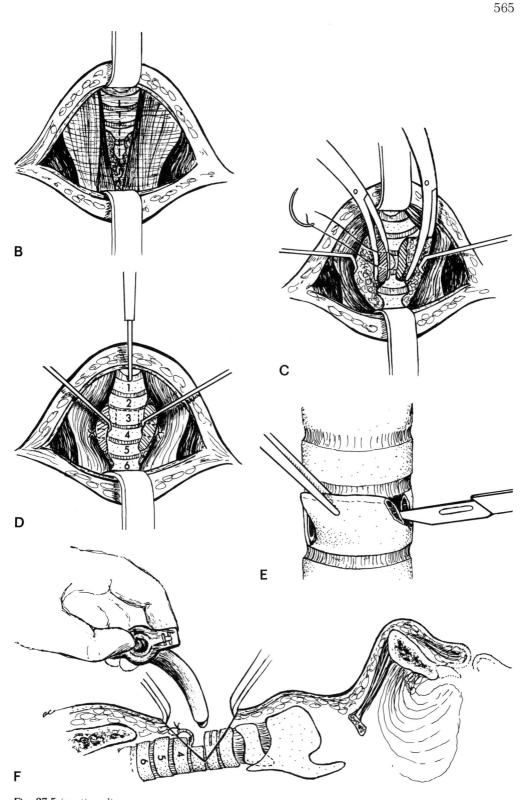

Fig. 27-5 (*continued*).

to be made. No dissection is carried lateral to the trachea, where it might involve the lobes of the thyroid or the great vessels of the neck. Above all, no dissection should be carried down the trachea below the sternal notch, where it might cause damage to the innominate vein or laterally open the dome of the pleura and cause pneumothorax.

Opening of the Trachea (Tracheotomy)

Fortunately the large cricoid cartilage is a prominent landmark and therefore a good reference point. A cricoid hook is placed underneath the cricoid cartilage and held by an assistant. This secures the trachea and prevents excessive movement. Using a clean no. 11 scalpel blade, an incision is made in the trachea, preferably between the second and third rings, and extended down on either side through the third ring. A rectangular flap of trachea based inferiorly is then turned anteriorly, and with two catgut sutures secured to the subcutaneous tissues. It should not be sutured to the skin surface, as this will cause tethering of the scar at a future date. Alternatively, the rectangular flap of trachea can be excised completely. At this stage careful suction of the tracheal lumen is carried out, removing all secretions and blood clots. The tracheal stoma should now be enlarged to accommodate the chosen tracheostomy tube. The operation is now virtually complete. Once the tracheostomy tube is in position, meticulous hemostasis should be performed. Time spent sealing every bleeding point prevents a great deal of the postoperative bleeding that occurs when the neck is flexed and the tissues are no longer under tension. The skin should be loosely closed with

interrupted sutures. It is not necessary to close the layer of subcutaneous tissue with catgut. Should the tracheostomy tube come out in the immediate postoperative period, the anterior tracheal flap facilitates its replacement even by ancillary medical staff. It also prevents the clumsy insertion of a tube alongside the trachea, creating a false passage, bleeding, or pneumothorax. The tracheostomy tube should be held firmly in place by tapes encircling the neck and tied with a knot (Fig. 27-6).

Emergency Situations

Most emergency situations can be dealt with by laryngoscopy and per oral intubation or bronchoscopy. If emergency surgery is necessary, the choice of operation lies between cricothyroidotomy and emergency tracheostomy.

Emergency Tracheostomy

Once the patient has been placed in the most effective position, a vertical midline incision is made in the neck. The incision is carried down to the tracheal surface in one sweep, through the thyroid isthmus if necessary. The trachea is then opened

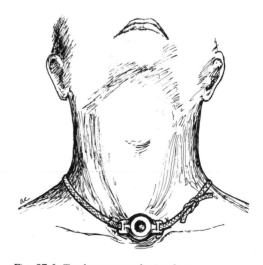

Fig. 27-6. Tracheostomy tube in place.

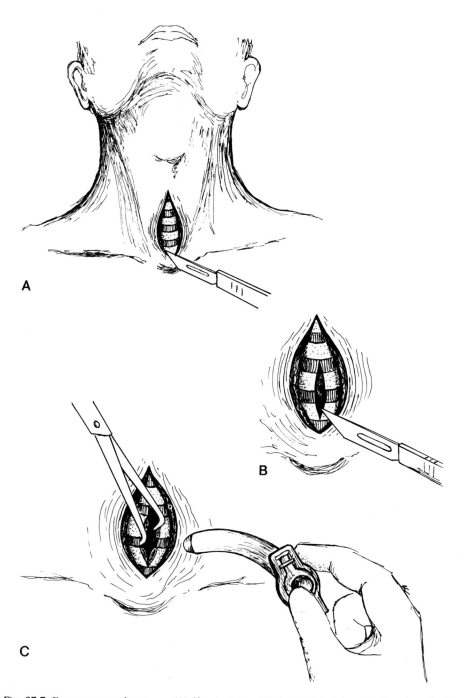

Fig. 27-7. Emergency tracheostomy. (A) Skin incision. (B) Tracheal incision. (C) Insertion of tube.

with a vertical incision extending through two tracheal rings, avoiding the upper two rings. This opening is then spread with dilators and a tracheostomy tube inserted (Fig. 27-7). An airway is now established and the patient is out of danger. Hemostasis can then be secured or the wound can be packed with gauze and the patient transferred to a hospital for formal tracheostomy.

Emergency Laryngotomy or Cricothyroidotomy

With the patient's neck extended, a horizontal incision is made just below the thyroid cartilage. This exposes the cricothyroid membrane, incision into which allows a tube to be inserted just below the level of the vocal cords. Again, once an airway has been established, formal tracheostomy should follow at the earliest possible convenience.

Opinions vary regarding the relative merits of these two procedures. The cricothyroid space is often narrow and insertion of an adequately sized tube cannot be accomplished without damaging the cricoid cartilage or conus elasticus, resulting in voice changes and stenosis. Arteries enter the cricothyroid space in the midline and can be the cause of considerable bleeding. The advantages of cricothyroidotomy are that it needs no specialized equipment and can be performed by nonmedical personnel. Generally, tracheostomy is considered the better and more effective procedure. Whenever emergency surgery is done outside the hospital, once the airway has been established the patient should be transferred to the hospital

where formal elective tracheostomy can be performed. Within a hospital, emergencies can often be adequately dealt with by per oral intubation or insertion of a bronchoscope.

Management of Tracheostomy

As explained in the section on applied physiology, the air entering the trachea through a tracheal stoma is not warmed or saturated with water vapor, and the cough reflex has been rendered ineffective. Therefore, humidification, warming, and removal of secretions by suction must be performed for the patient.

Following the operation, the patient should be placed in a semisupine position with the head supported by pillows. Nursing personnel must be instructed to maintain close observation of the patient. In addition to the routine observation of vital signs, specific instructions must be issued for the observance of the following:

1. Surgical emphysema. A little is normally present, but it should not increase nor extend beyond the soft tissues of the neck.
2. Cyanosis.
3. Blood at the site of incision. There should be no blood loss; the dressing will be soiled, but no increase should occur.
4. Breathing should be quiet and effortless.
5. Humidification. Ideally, the air entering the tracheostomy should be warmed to body temperature and be 100 per cent saturated. This is technically difficult to achieve. Many room humidifiers, such as the Puritan Pot,

are available, but the most effective humidification is achieved by new ultrasonic nebulizers. Humidification in itself helps to liquefy the secretions and make removal easier. Several detergents are available that purport to assist this process. Sometimes the secretions are so tenacious that they cannot be removed adequately by suction and humidification, in which case bronchial washing may be used. About 5 to 10 cc. of warm sterile saline solution can be placed into the trachea and bronchi via the tracheostomy and immediately withdrawn by suction.

6. Removal of secretions. It cannot be stressed enough that sterile precautions should be taken in performing suction toilet of the trachea. A new sterile catheter, preferably disposable, should be used every time, and the attendant should wear gloves. The technique of suction is important. Secretions usually accumulate in the trachea just below the end of the tracheostomy tube. The catheter should be inserted with no suction as far as the trachea. This makes the patient cough which, of course, helps. The suction should be restored and the catheter gradually withdrawn. This procedure should be repeated as often as necessary. Careful listening to the breathing will often suggest the presence of a mucous plug that needs removal. The patient may also go through a series of short, ineffective coughing spells when a mucous plug lingers in the trachea. In some conditions the secretions may accumulate in the lower trachea or main bronchi. These may also be removed by suction. In fact, good bronchial toilet can be performed in this way. Again, the technique is important. The soft sterile catheter is inserted as far as the bronchus, and the negative pressure applied only during its withdrawal.

The care of the tracheostomy has been cogently described as the same care that should be applied to a paraplegic with an indwelling urethral catheter.

Care of the Tracheostomy Wound

A clean, dry dressing is all that is required in the vast majority of patients. Infection of the wound can occur, but it is often preceded by prolonged per oral endotracheal intubation or occurs secondary to a chest infection. The most difficult of the offending organisms are the gram-negative bacilli. Topically applied acetic acid (0.05 per cent) may help rid the organisms from the tracheostomy wound, but systemic therapy may be necessary for the elimination of these organisms from the respiratory tree.

Tracheostomy Tubes

There are many varieties of tracheostomy tubes, but an ideal tube should satisfy the following specifications: It should consist of an outer and an inner cannula so that the inner cannula can be removed and cleaned, leaving the outer cannula in position. The secretions normally accumulate at the end of the tube, and for this reason the inner cannula should be slightly longer than the outer cannula. The walls of the tubes must be thin enough that a maximal lumen is obtained, yet rigid enough that they do not "kink" easily. The tube must not damage the tracheal mucosa. Traumatic abrasions may occur if the tube is too long, too curved, or the angle of the tube to the flange is not correct, and, finally, if the tube is too rigid. Some degree of flexibility and malleability is ideal. The epithelium may also be damaged chemically; rubber tubes are notorious in this respect. Silver tubes are not as active chemically. The most inert tube is the Portex tube; however, a Portex tube does not have an inner cannula.

As yet, no tube satisfies all these criteria, and the tube chosen is often a matter of personal choice influenced by the subsequent job it has to do. Until recently, each metal tracheostomy tube was custom-made so that only one inner cannula would fit each outer cannula. Some manufacturers have now made these components interchangeable, but it would be unwise to assume this. Each component must be checked by the surgeon. An important consideration is whether controlled respiration is to be used, as this necessitates a cuffed tracheostomy tube. There are inherent dangers in the cuffs: they may prolapse, break, or cause great distention of the trachea. The tube most commonly used at the present time is the metallic tube (previously silver but now stainless steel) of the Jackson or Hollinger design. Nylon tubes are also convenient. The tubes must be easy to clean and sterilize. Any tracheostomy tube may be used that satisfies the preceding criteria. However, it must be noted that no tracheostomy tubes on the market today are ideal—all have some defects.

Care of the Tracheostomy Tubes

1. The tube should be cleaned as often as necessary. This varies with each patient.
2. The technique of removal and insertion should be demonstrated to all supervisory staff.

3. The details of sterilization and storage of each variety of tube must be noted.

Complications of Tracheostomy

The mere mention of the word "complication" does the operation of tracheostomy a great disservice. Many reports have been published by many authorities describing the dangers and complications of tracheostomy. The surveys have usually been retrospective and have included the performance of tracheostomy by surgeons at all stages of their training for both emergency and elective procedures and by all varieties of surgeons. Complications encountered by surgeons who are normally accustomed to dealing with the larynx and trachea are almost nonexistent. What remain are the complications owing to the morbidity of the patient's original disease that necessitated the tracheostomy. Therefore, it would seem that the complications and dangers of the tracheostomy procedure itself could be eliminated almost entirely by attention to the technique of the operation and to its subsequent management.

Immediate Complications

HEMORRHAGE. Bleeding usually occurs from the muscle layers or from the thyroid gland. Hemorrhage will be experienced by the clumsy surgeon who strays from the midline and may even come from the great vessels of the neck. Remember that the horizontally placed innominate vein can be encountered in the neck.

PNEUMOTHORAX. Dissection lateral to the trachea and below the suprasternal notch is the greatest cause of rupture of the pleura. Excessive surgical emphysema of the neck may be the first sign of rupture of the dome of the pleura. A little subcutaneous emphysema is inevitable in the operation owing to leakage from the tracheostomy. The extent of this is limited if the wound is closed loosely and the dissection is confined to those procedures necessary to make only a hole in the trachea.

INFECTION. Primary infection at the tracheostomy site is rare. It usually occurs secondary to infection in the trachea and is more frequent when there has been a previous indwelling per oral endotracheal tube.

Late Complications

CHEST INFECTION. This type of infection can sometimes result from (1) inadequate removal of secretion; (2) nonsterile suction toilet technique; (3) failure of adequate humidification. This may be diffuse infection or secondary to atelectasis of one lobe.

TRACHEAL DAMAGE. This may occur as a result of (1) prolonged overinflation of the cuff. There is some doubt about the value of intermittent release of the cuff. Overinflation of the cuff leads to dilatation and subsequent stricture. A fluted cuff may avoid these problems. (2) Cartilage degeneration and stricture may result from erosion by the tip of the tube. (3) The skin may become tethered to the trachea, causing dysphagia and dyspnea.

Conclusion

The provision of an artificial opening in the trachea has some advantages and some disadvantages. The main disadvantages are:

1. The loss of smell.
2. The loss of the glottic stop so that the explosive force of the cough cannot be performed.

3. The loss of the voice, although it can easily be restored by placing a finger over the tracheal opening, allowing the air to pass on either side of the tracheostomy tube.
4. The necessity for humidification and warming of air in the early days of tracheostomy.

The advantages are:

1. Relief of upper airway obstruction.
2. Easy access to the main bronchial tree for removal of secretions.
3. Diminution of the dead space, increasing the efficiency of respiration in those patients who are in respiratory distress.
4. Isolation of the air passage from the alimentary tract.
5. Ease in performing bronchoscopy and induction of general anesthesia.

The operation of tracheostomy may be easy or it may be difficult, depending upon the patient and the facilities available. There should be no fear on the part of any person in surgical training to perform tracheostomy when the situation arises, provided he confines his dissection strictly to midline. For those who need to do formal elective tracheostomy, the attention to surgical detail outlined previously will prevent most of the more frequent complications. The rest of the complications can usually be prevented by insisting upon good management of the patient following the tracheostomy. The time to perform a tracheostomy is when the operation is first thought of. By the time cyanosis or respiratory distress has occurred, the operation has been delayed too long!

Index

Page numbers in *italics* indicate illustrations. Page numbers followed by "t" indicate tables.

573